A MANUAL OF ORTHOPAEDIC TERMINOLOGY

Sixth Edition

A Manual of Orthopaedic Terminology

Sixth Edition

Carolyn Taliaferro Blauvelt
Writer/Editor, Medical-Dental Publications
Member, Midatlantic Chapter
American Medical Writers Association
Bethesda, Maryland

Fred R. T. Nelson, MD, FAAOS
Clinical Instructor
University of California, San Diego
Clinical Assistant Professor
Uniformed Services University of the Health
Sciences
Bethesda, Maryland

Mosby

An Affiliate of Elsevier Science

Mosby

An Affiliate of Elsevier Science

Executive Editor: Robert Hurley
Associate Developmental Editor: Marla Sussman
Project Manager/Project Specialist: David Orzechowski
Manuscript Editor: Lilliane Anstee
Designer: Nancy C. Baker
Manufacturing Manager: William A. Winneberger, Jr.
Cover Design: Hyperdesign, Inc.

Printed in the United States of America

Mosby, Inc.
11830 Westline Industrial Drive
St. Louis, Missouri 63146

Library of Congress Cataloging-in-Publication Data

Blauvelt, Carolyn Taliaferro
    A manual of orthopaedic terminology / Carolyn Taliaferro Blauvelt,
  Fred R. T. Nelson.—6th ed.
      p.   cm.
  Includes bibliographical references and index.
   ISBN 0-8151-2787-1
    1. Orthopedics—Terminology—Handbooks, manuals, etc. I. Nelson,
  Fred R. T., 1941– . II. Title.
    [DNLM: 1. Orthopedics terminology. WE 15 B645m 1998]
  RD723.B53   1998
  616.7′001′4—dc21
  DNLM/DLC   98-10711

FOREWORD

Medical science in general and orthopaedics in particular are advancing so rapidly that each year sees the introduction of new instruments, procedures, techniques, medications, and even new diseases. Each new discovery brings new terminology. Since the fifth edition of this book in 1994, much has been added to orthopaedics; fortunately the authors have been diligent in identifying what is new. For example, the spinal chapter is new, and there is a special emphasis on the myriad of new procedures and advanced use of surgical appliances. The fracture chapter has an extended and consolidated classification system. In the imaging chapter, the usual radiologic views and measurements were supplemented with illustrations to portray the importance of magnetic resonance imaging and other imaging technologies in orthopaedics. The discussion of laboratory evaluations includes newer test markers for bone resorption that are specific in diagnosing patients with metabolic bone disease. A new test for patients with HIV that has recently been implemented to improve diagnosis is included.

The musculoskeletal research section includes the basic language and new terms of biochemistry, biomechanics, immunology, physics, prosthetics, and engineering. The result is that now non-physicians have a handy source that will allow better communication with the clinician and vice versa.

Many acronyms and abbreviations, which can be challenging even to physicians, are included. Some have been replaced by simple descriptive terms. Just as in previous editions, the authors have reviewed these terms for relevance. The authors also requested more than one reviewer for a number of chapters to enhance the expertise from several different geographic areas.

Orthopaedic surgeons and other health care providers and paraprofessionals are concerned with the musculoskeletal system. To have meaningful communication, these individuals with different training and experience must be able to communicate effectively. This valuable book improves communication by providing precise definitions and detailed explanations where necessary. The writing style and print make for easy reading. The secretary typing a report, the nurse executing an order, and a technician performing a procedure will have clear understanding of the instructions given by the physician.

There is an old saying that tends to minimize the value of words: A picture is worth a thousand words. On the other hand, another old story illustrates the value of the ability to understand words! A tourist in a foreign country could not speak the language. Wanting a steak and mushrooms, the tourist went to a restaurant, but unfortunately, waiter and tourist could not speak a common language. The tourist drew a picture of a steer and a mushroom. The waiter brought him an umbrella and a ticket to a bullfight. The value of accurate communication is clear.

Happily, users of this book will acquire a clear understanding of orthopaedic terminology and the tools for accurate communication, thereby fulfilling the editors' goals. The orthopaedic community and all who must communicate about the musculoskeletal system owe authors Carolyn Taliaferro Blauvelt and Fred R. T. Nelson a debt of gratitude for this extremely useful book.

Charles H. Epps, Jr., MD
Special Assistant to the President for Health Affairs, Howard University
Dean Emeritus and Professor Emeritus Orthopaedic Surgery

PREFACE

Since the inception of *A Manual of Orthopaedic Terminology* in 1977, the manual has continued to grow in keeping with the many changes taking place in the orthopaedic specialty. The manual was translated into Japanese in 1986, and again with the fifth edition (1994). As we present this sixth edition, the purpose and objectives remain the same: to describe with brevity and clarity the language of orthopaedics and, hopefully, to contribute to the understanding of this specialty. We have attempted to find a convenient way of sorting, rearranging, and distributing the many terms in their proper category to assist the professional and the layman.

Usually one must refer to many textbooks to obtain specific meanings of the terminology within the specialty. This compendium of terms under one cover will enable the reader to deal with the language of orthopaedics more effectively. The manual was designed to assist office assistants, nurses, medical students, orthopaedic interns and residents, technicians, researchers, librarians, allied health professionals, and others who interface with or are a part of the orthopaedic community.

Unlike a standard dictionary, the chapters are defined according to areas of orthopaedic specialty. A reader interested in a certain radiographic technique, disease process, or surgical procedure refers to that chapter. Each chapter is divided into sections to give greater coherence to related terms. The expanded index lists and cross-references all key words and their appropriate pages. However, with increasing familiarity and knowledge of orthopaedics, the user will recognize the terms and their place in a certain chapter.

Proper names (eponyms) are listed in alphabetic order and grouped together in context within a chapter, which will readily assist those looking for a specific name that is related to a disease process or surgical procedure. Appendix D covers the eponymic ICD codes along with the page references. This important addition will assist those who work in medi-

cal records, billing, and medical insurance to understand the coding system for diseases that go by proper names.

With each new edition, a significant amount of new material surfaces, reflecting many changes. We have updated, expanded, and revised the chapters in which constant revision is necessary to keep with the rapid growth in the field. Although fundamentals do not change, materials, methods, and techniques do.

As we enter the twenty-first century, we will see a tremendous surge in the application of biochemical and biophysical knowledge in clinical orthopaedics, including applications in electrobiology, diagnostic imaging, oncology, and immunology. Changes in pharmacology and nonsurgical modalities will have a wide influence in orthopaedic practice.

Updated material for the sixth edition includes:

- *Fractures.* In addition to the general, classic, and descriptive terminology of fractures and dislocations, the AO and Orthopaedic Trauma Association systems of fracture classifications have been updated, extended, and consolidated, as has the compendium of grading systems. The formats of these classifications were revised to best describe the "original intent" of the system for educational purposes. An extensive reference list is included. Discussion of sports-related terms also has been expanded to reflect the current terminology of this subspecialty.
- *Musculoskeletal Diseases.* As the genetic and biochemical understanding of musculoskeletal diseases has changed, these changes have been made to existing terms. With the benefit of an orthopaedic oncologist, information on musculoskeletal tumor types and treatments has been expanded. Included as well is the World Health Organization (WHO) classification system for tumors.
- *Imaging Techniques.* The field of radiology has

changed dramatically with the use of magnetic resonance imaging, computed tomography scans, and other computed technology with direct effect on orthopaedic evaluations. Many new views and measurements have been added, and sections have been supplemented with illustrations to portray the importance of this technology.

- *Tests, Signs, Maneuvers.* Important to diagnosing joint mechanics, many new terms have been added from different geographic regions to give a wider point of view of these examinations.
- *Laboratory.* In addition to the general blood and serum tests, sections have been added to highlight the serum tests specific to metabolic bone disease, i.e., bone turnover markers, bone formation, and bone resorption.
- *Casts, Splints, Dressings.* The chapter has been reviewed and updated.
- *Prosthetics and Orthotics.* This allied health field specialty uses many abbreviations. Many terms have been defined for the user of this book to better understand the nomenclature.
- *Anatomy and Surgery.* This chapter continues to expand with the addition of many internal fixation devices for fracture repair and many newer types of prosthesis components. A section on the management of tumors has been included.

SUBSPECIALTIES

There are now three subspecialty areas addressed in this manual, where the advantage of having these terms in close proximity improves the use of the manual for readers who will find 95% of the terms they use within a dozen pages.

- *The Spine.* New to this edition is a chapter on the spine. This unique and intricate part of the anatomy is long overdue for a chapter to itself and includes in detail the anatomy, diseases, and surgery of the spine. With the extended use of surgical appliances and a myriad of new procedures, this chapter is a welcomed addition to the manual.

- *The Hand and Wrist.* In this edition, traumatic disorders, nail and skin disorders of the hand and wrist were added to the disease section; to the surgery section, the eponymic arthrodeses of the wrist and procedures for amputation revisions were added to this subspecialty.
- *The Foot and Ankle.* This chapter has been revised, rearranged, and expanded to clarify the many terms in this subspecialty.

Professionals in the field of orthopaedics work closely with members of their allied health specialties in patient care—*occupational therapy* and *physical therapy*. For that reason, terms from those associated areas are included. The current trends and services of the specialties of occupational therapy and physical therapy have been brought up-to-date with revisions in both areas. Many physical therapy modalities and procedures have been added, offering a wider range of management options.

Musculoskeletal Research. This chapter was rewritten in part to reflect the better understanding of biomechanical forces and the body's response to physical maneuvers and to bring the terminology to the edge of the twenty-first century. Research terminology is unique and rapidly expanding and is unlike that which is used in a clinical setting. It includes the language of biochemistry, biomechanics, immunology, physics, engineering, and prosthetics. The introduction to Chapter 13 outlines the various stages of research, from the idea to the written protocol, the research in progress, and the end results and findings. Advances in technology are presented, incorporating clinical and biomedical research. Terms that might overflow into applied orthopaedics are maintained.

Appendices. The appendices were included as supporting information on: A. Orthopaedic Abbreviations, B. Anatomic Positions and Directions, C. Orthopaedic Etymology—The Origin of Orthopaedic Terms (new), and D. ICD Eponymic Codes.

The authors requested more than one reviewer for a number of chapters, and most were new to the process, to add their breadth of experience. We believe that the new reorganization of material will make this manual a more practical office guide and resource for more advanced medical use.

CONTRIBUTORS

No one can write a book on all areas of orthopaedics and keep it current without the help of many competent people. This manual is no exception. We have chosen contributors whose background and experience make them well qualified to assist in updating material for each edition and who work directly or indirectly in this specialty. These people have generously given their time, in view of other professional commitments, to improve the correctness and accuracy of information, provide an update, and give constructive criticism. We can share in the success of this manual with them, and we wish to express our appreciation and thanks to our past contributors, and the following persons and organizations who participated in the revisions of the sixth edition:

Fractures/Dislocations
C. E. Brooks, MD, FRCS(C)
Division of Orthopaedic Surgery
Queen Elizabeth Hospital
Charlottetown, Prince Edward Island
Canada

David Collon, MD
Chairman, Department of Orthopaedics
Henry Ford Hospital
Detroit, Michigan

Sports Medicine
Stephen B. Gunther, MD
Orthopaedic Fellow
Shoulder and Elbow Surgery
Prince of Wales Hospital
Sydney, Australia

MS Diseases—Tumors
Alan D. Aaron, MD
Assistant Professor
Department of Orthopaedic Surgery
Georgetown University Hospital
Washington, D.C.

Imaging Techniques
Kae S. Yingling, MD
Member, Groover, Christie & Merritt Radiology Group
Department of Radiology
Suburban Hospital
Bethesda, Maryland

David Fessell, MD
Department of Radiology
Henry Ford Hospital
Detroit, Michigan

Joseph Craig, MB, ChB
Department of Radiology
Henry Ford Hospital
Detroit, Michigan

Tests, Signs, Maneuvers
Eric L. Radin, MD
Chairman Emeritus
Department of Orthopaedics
Henry Ford Hospital
Detroit, Michigan

Laboratory Evaluations
Jeffrey M. Ogorzalek, MD
Commander, Medical Corps, US Navy
Head, Laboratory Medicine Department
National Naval Medical Center
Bethesda, Maryland

Nayana Parikh, BS
Laboratory Supervisor
Bone and Mineral Research Lab
Henry Ford Hospital
Detroit, Michigan

Casts, Splints, Dressings
Jeff Virgo, OTC, OPA-C, RSA
National Association of Orthopaedic Technologists (NAOT)
NBCOT, Raleigh, North Carolina

Prosthetics and Orthotics
Norman Berger, Prosthetist
Aspen, Colorado

Anatomy and Surgery
Charles H. Epps, Jr., MD
Special Assistant to the President for Health Affairs
Dean, Emeritus
Professor, Emeritus
Orthopaedic Surgery
Howard University
Washington, D.C.

The Spine
Lee H. Riley, III, MD
Assistant Professor of Orthopaedic Surgery
Assistant Professor of Neurosurgery
Johns Hopkins University Hospital
Baltimore, Maryland

The Hand and Wrist
Leo M. Rozmaryn, MD, FAAOS
Attending Hand Surgeon
Shady Grove Adventist Hospital
Rockville, Maryland

The Foot and Ankle
Kent Wu, MD
Foot and Ankle Section
Department of Orthopaedics
Henry Ford Hospital
Detroit, Michigan

Physical Medicine and Rehabilitation
Charles M. Dilla, PT, PA
Physical Therapist
Silver Spring, Maryland

Musculoskeletal Research
James H. Kimura, PhD
Head, Section of Biochemistry
Henry Ford Hospital
Detroit, Michigan

David P. Fyhrie, PhD
Head, Section of Biomechanics
Henry Ford Hospital
Detroit, Michigan

Advisor
John J. Gartland, MD
University Medical Editor
James Edwards Professor Emeritus of Orthopaedic
     Surgery
Jefferson Medical College of the Thomas Jefferson
     University
Philadelphia, Pennsylvania

For contributions to the first five editions, we wish to acknowledge The American Occupational Therapy Association, Rockville, MD, The American Physical Therapy Association, Alexandria, VA, Mark A. Berman, CO; Wilton H. Bunch, MD, PhD; John F. Burkart, MD; Robert W. Chambers, MD; Helen F. Delaney, OT; J. M. Dennis, DPM; Terry Elan, Prosthetist; Jean Flint, Orthotist; Gary E. Friedlaender, MD; Joshua Gerbert, DPM, MS; Stephen F. Gunther, MD, FAAOS; Carole Hays, MA, OTR, FAOTA; Donald L. Hiltz, PT; Donald P. Jenkins, PhD; Emily Jeter, OTR/L; Steve Kramer, CPO; David M. Lichtman, MD, FACS; Frederick G. Lippert, III, MD; Donna M. Mathisen, GPT; W. Patrick Monaghan, PhD; Francesca C. Music, MS, MT; Thomas Neviaser, MD; James M. Salander, MD, FACS; Barton K. Slemmons, MD, FAAOS; Samuel Wiesel, MD; David Q. Wilson, MD, FAAOS; and William D. Wurzel, MHA, MD.

We wish to remember the late Charles V. Heck, MD, the former executive director of the American Academy of Orthopaedic Surgeons, who, through his support and encouragement, gave us the incentive to pursue this awesome task.

The success of the first five editions proved the need for a reference of this kind for this specialty. It is with pleasure that we present this sixth edition with many, many thanks not only to our contributors but also to the editorial staff and those "behind the scenes" at Mosby, Inc., whose continued guidance, support, and publication skills have contributed much to the book's success.

Carolyn Taliaferro Blauvelt
Fred R. T. Nelson

INTRODUCTION TO THE ORTHOPAEDIC SPECIALTY

Or"tho-pae'dic. Orthopaedic means correction or prevention of bony deformities (formerly, especially in children). The word comes from the Greek *orthos,* meaning straight, upright, right, or true—hence, also correct or regular—and from the Greek *pais,* meaning child.

The scope of orthopaedic surgery includes the treatment, management, and rehabilitation of patients with musculoskeletal conditions affecting bones, muscles, joints, tendons, ligaments, cartilage, blood vessels, nerves, and related tissues through surgical, nonsurgical, and other medical measures. The nature of these conditions may involve congenital abnormalities, metabolic disease processes, metastatic (tumor) pathology, or traumatic injuries (fractures), to name a few conditions requiring the expertise of the orthopaedic specialty. When surgery is indicated, postoperative rehabilitation is equally important in the continued care and treatment of musculoskeletal conditions.

The orthopaedic surgeon is a specialist on the musculoskeletal system as applied to adult and childrens' orthopaedics and the management of trauma. In addition, he or she possesses a working knowledge of neurology, cardiopulmonary physiology, and bioengineering in the care of the orthopaedic patient. This expertise has expanded to include computed tomography, magnetic resonance imaging, electrical and magnetic bone stimulation, microsurgery, and knowledge of the advances in internal and external fixation devices. Orthopaedic medicine is continually changing, and the orthopaedic surgeon is challenged with the responsibility of keeping informed of new techniques through continuing education in the field.

The orthopaedic surgeon develops many skills in the practice of this specialty. Nonoperative measures include the artful application of casts for immobilization and management of fractures or scoliosis, to the treatment of diseases and disabilities through conservative management. In the operating room, the orthopaedist is skilled in the repair and reconstruction of major skeletal defects, which include replacing diseased joints with plastic implants, inserting metallic rods and other devices for stability, or performing fusions, revisions, or amputations. Of a more delicate nature, he or she performs surgery that applies arthroscopic and microvascular techniques that encompass skin grafts, finger transplantations, nerve repairs, and similar difficult procedures.

From a team approach, the orthopaedic specialty depends on many other disciplines in the treatment of patients. The immediate team members are the professional nurses who provide and participate in the primary care of patients and who are assisted by the services of the orthopaedic technicians, both in the clinic and hospital setting. The second group of team members includes the allied health professionals, the physiatrist, physical therapist, and occupational therapist. These professionals are directly involved in, and may be consulted for, the development of a treatment plan in a patient's rehabilitation. The next group of team members to provide assistance include the prosthetists (artificial limbs) and orthotists (braces), who measure, fit, design, and fabricate devices for the orthopaedic patient. Indirectly, the manufacturer of orthopaedic appliances plays an important role, as does the researcher who tests the biocompatibility of materials used in the musculoskeletal system.

All of these specialties are an important and integral part of the orthopaedic team, and provide a combination of skills that benefits thousands of patients with musculoskeletal problems. Other disciplines that interface with orthopaedics include bioengineering, electrobiology, transplantation, diagnostic imaging, oncology, biochemistry, and similar areas.

Orthopaedic medicine has become so diverse that there is specialization within the specialty. In addition to general orthopaedics, a physician may specialize in diseases and surgery of the spine, soft tissues, the hand, the foot, major joints, trauma, sports medicine, or the ever-changing area of orthopaedic research.

Many physicians are exposed to orthopaedic surgery during their training years, but only a select group actually pursue this difficult and diverse field to the point of certification.

The qualifications for certification by the American Board of Orthopaedic Surgery (ABOS) are 4 or 5 years of graduate education after medical school, and an additional year of practice in which his or her ethical conduct is monitored. The physician must complete all requirements to become "board certified" and a diplomate of the Board. After completion of the certification requirements, an orthopaedic surgeon becomes eligible for fellowship in the American Academy of Orthopaedic Surgeons (AAOS), the national organization of the specialty. The admission to fellowship in the Academy is based on a 2-year practice period beyond certification and certain other specific requirements. The Academy fellowship at present represents about 81% of the orthopaedic surgeons in the United States.

The national organization of the specialty, the American Academy of Orthopaedic Surgeons, developed the accepted definition of orthopaedics in 1952:

Orthopaedic Surgery is the medical specialty that includes the investigation, preservation, restoration, and development of the form and function of the extremities, spine, and associated structures by medical, surgical, and physical methods.

CONTENTS

Foreword   **v**

Preface   **vii**

Introduction   **xi**

1/CLASSIFICATIONS OF FRACTURES, DISLOCATIONS, AND SPORTS-RELATED INJURIES   *1*

Terminology of Fractures and Dislocations   *2*
Classifications of Fractures   *3*
Classic and Descriptive Names (by Anatomic Location)   *6*
Contributing Factors   *12*
Degree and Nature of Healing   *12*
International Classification System and Trauma Registry System   *13*
Classification Systems by Grades, Types, and Mechanisms   *14*
Dislocations   *31*
Subluxations   *33*
Strains and Sprains   *33*
Sports-Related Injuries   *34*

2/MUSCULOSKELETAL DISEASES AND RELATED TERMS   *39*

Bone Diseases   *40*
Miscellaneous Bone Conditions   *49*
Muscle Diseases   *57*
Cartilage Diseases   *60*
Diseases of (Specific) Soft Tissue   *63*
Ligament, Tendon, Bursa, and Fascia Diseases   *65*
Joint Diseases (Arthro-, Synovio-, Capsulo-, Ankylo-)   *66*
Vascular Diseases and Conditions   *69*
Neurologic Diseases   *75*
Metabolic Diseases   *79*
Diseases and Conditions by Anatomic Area   *82*
Associated Disease Terminology   *88*

3/IMAGING TECHNIQUES   *97*

General Radiologic Terms   *98*

Orthopaedic Radiographic Techniques and Procedures   *99*

Routine Radiographic Views   *100*

Radiographic Angles, Lines, Signs, and Methods   *103*

Invasive and Noninvasive Techniques   *114*

Vascular Diagnostic Studies   *117*

Radiation Therapy   *118*

4/ORTHOPAEDIC TESTS, SIGNS, AND MANEUVERS   *119*

Tests, Signs, and Maneuvers   *120*

Gaits   *139*

Scales and Ratings   *139*

Other Physical Examinations   *140*

5/LABORATORY EVALUATIONS   *141*

Routine Evaluations   *141*

General Blood and Serum Tests   *143*

Serum and Urine Tests for Metabolic Disease   *145*

Bacteriologic Studies   *147*

Other Special Studies   *148*

Blood Bank Procedures and Products   *149*

Laboratory Abbreviations   *151*

Annotation of Units   *153*

6/CASTS, SPLINTS, DRESSINGS, AND TRACTION   *155*

Cast Materials   *156*

Cast Immobilization   *157*

Devices Applied to Casts   *159*

Cast Complications   *160*

Splints and Accessories   *160*

Dressings   *161*

Suspension, Traction, and Frames   *163*

Emergency Stabilization   *166*

7/PROSTHETICS AND ORTHOTICS   *169*

Prostheses   *170*

Orthoses   *177*

Shoe Modifications   *187*

8/ANATOMY AND ORTHOPAEDIC SURGERY   *189*

Osteo- (Bone)   *189*
Arthro- (Joints)   *213*
Other Specific Tissue(s)   *217*
Vascular (Blood Vessels) System   *222*
Specific Anatomy and Surgery by Location   *227*
Arm and Forearm   *233*
Pelvis and Hips   *240*
The Lower Limbs   *247*
Skin Grafts   *258*
Surgical Blocks   *259*
Surgical Approaches   *259*
Replantation Microsurgery   *261*
Treatment of Tumors   *262*
Amputations   *262*
Associated Surgical Terms   *264*

9/THE SPINE   *269*

General Anatomy of the Spine   *269*
Cervical Spine Anatomy   *271*
Thoracic Spine Anatomy   *273*
Lumbar and Lower Spine Anatomy   *273*
Diseases and Structural Anomalies   *274*
Surgery of the Spine   *284*

10/THE HAND AND WRIST   *291*

Anatomy of the Hand and Wrist   *291*
Diseases and Structural Anomalies   *301*
Surgery of the Hand and Wrist   *313*

11/THE FOOT AND ANKLE   *323*

Anatomy   *323*
Diseases and Conditions of the Foot and Ankle   *331*
Surgery   *336*

12/PHYSICAL MEDICINE AND REHABILITATION: PHYSICAL THERAPY AND OCCUPATIONAL THERAPY   *347*

Physical Therapy   *347*
Occupational Therapy   *353*

13/MUSCULOSKELETAL RESEARCH   *357*

General Research Terminology   *358*

Measurements   *360*

Bone Healing and Metabolism   *360*

Electrobiology   *361*

Cartilage and Joints   *362*

Collagen   *364*

Biomechanics   *364*

Biomaterials   *369*

APPENDIX A/ORTHOPAEDIC ABBREVIATIONS   *371*

Diseases, Conditions, and Syndromes   *371*

General Anatomy   *372*

Specific Anatomy   *373*

Surgical Procedures and Related Terms   *375*

Imaging Techniques   *376*

Casts, Splints, Dressings   *376*

Prosthetics and Orthotics   *376*

Physical Medicine and Occupational Therapy (Exercises and Tests)   *377*

Research   *378*

Miscellaneous   *378*

Prescriptions   *380*

APPENDIX B/ANATOMIC POSITIONS AND DIRECTIONS   *381*

Surface Location   *381*

Anatomic Planes   *381*

Specific Locations   *383*

Joint Motions   *383*

Anatomic Associated Terms   *386*

APPENDIX C/ETYMOLOGY OF ORTHOPAEDICS   *390*

APPENDIX D/ICD CODES FOR EPONYMIC MUSCULOSKELETAL DISEASE TERMS   *404*

Bibliography   *410*

Index   *417*

Chapter 1

Classifications of Fractures, Dislocations, and Sports-related Injuries

The musculoskeletal reaction to trauma can result in a variety of bone, muscle, and ligamentous disruptions; sometimes fracture and ligamentous injuries occur concurrently. The general types of musculo skeletal trauma are fractures, dislocations, subluxations, sprains, strains, and diastases.

This chapter defines fractures and dislocations in three sections. The first part contains general terms that are easily understood by the nonspecialist, followed by classic, descriptive, and eponymic terms. The second section is a brief outline of the AO system and Orthopaedic Trauma Association system of fracture classification. The third section is a compendium of grading systems. These three sections are followed by the definitions for dislocations, subluxations, strains, sprains, and sports-related injuries.

Most patients with musculoskeletal injuries present to an emergency room in an acute stage and are treated by the emergency room physician until it is determined that an orthopaedic specialist may be required. Good communication is essential, and it is beneficial to the nonspecialist to understand the language of orthopaedics when relating the assessment of acute injuries. A brief and accurate description is vital to the evaluation and treatment of the injured, and familiarity with the classification systems that follow will help in undertstanding the importance of accurate communication. A system of grades, types, and mechanisms is included to supplement the existing information on musculoskeletal trauma.

Familiarity with the correct terms will enable one to identify a fracture immediately. For example, "open, midshaft, femur, comminuted fracture" is a brief description, but much information is related. To achieve this degree of accuracy, learning the classifications is necessary.

A uniformed descriptive system also allows accurate coding of specific diagnostic entities. The bony detail is described by the following:

1. Open vs. closed
2. Portion of bone involved
3. General appearance
4. Alignment of fragments

Interestingly, fractures have specific terminology that varies from time of occurrence to healing. Fractures may be named for an anatomic location, a person, or a place. They are further defined in terms of how they occurred or reason for the break. As fractures begin to heal, the degree and nature of healing are described.

Contributing factors, such as tumors, infections, and repeated stress, are included in the descriptive terminology. This is important for diagnostic coding. Also clarified is the management of fractures. *Closed* management (closed reduction) means that treatment is in the form of a manipulation, cast, or splint/traction application or some combination of the three. *Open* management (open reduction) requires a surgical incision to approximate the fracture fragments into normal position. Often, some form of internal fixation (**osteosynthesis**) is performed with open management of fractures.

Many new advances have been made in the management of fractures including a recent trend from casting to bracing, or a combination of both. The term **cast brace** has been applied to a form of treatment in which the brace design is incorporated into temporary standard cast materials. This method allows for limited motion in the brace during the early healing stage with "controlled" fracture movement. Its use has shown greater callous weld around the fracture site, improved ligamentous healing, and earlier recovery of joint mobility and muscle control.

Another method of fracture management employs magnetic as well as electrical devices, some with *surface electrodes* externally applied to a fracture site. For certain types of fractures, this method has diminished the need for braces.

The mainstay of traumatic fracture management has involved external fixation devices and frames, also known as "fixateurs" or fixators. External fixation is a diverse system for managing loss of skeletal stability with various components placed in bone. Treatment methods and external skeletal fixation devices are discussed in Chapters 6, 7, and 8.

TERMINOLOGY OF FRACTURES AND DISLOCATIONS

fracture (L., *fractura*):   structural break in the continuity of a bone, epiphyseal plate, or cartilaginous joint surface, usually traumatic with disruption of osseous tissue.

fracture-dislocation: fracture of a bone that is also dislocated from its normal position in a joint.

dislocation (L., *luxatio*):   complete displacement of bone from its normal position at the joint surface, disrupting the articulation of two or three bones at that junction and altering the alignment. This displacement affects the joint capsule and surrounding tissues (muscles, ligaments). Dislocation (**luxation**) may be traumatic (direct blow or injury), congenital (developmental defect), or pathologic (as in muscle imbalance, ligamentous tearing, rheumatoid arthritis, or infection).

subluxation: incomplete or partial dislocation in that one bone forming a joint is displaced only partially from its normal position; also, a chronic tendency of a bone to become partially dislocated, in contrast to an outright dislocation, for example, shoulder, patella, and, in infants, hip.

diastasis: may be one of two types: (1) disjointing of two bones that are parallel to one another, for example, radius and ulna, tibia and fibula complex, or (2) rupture of any "solid" joint, as in a diastasis of the symphysis pubis. Such an injury tends to occur in association with other fractures and is then called "fracture-diastasis." A diastasis in children may refer to separation of the epiphysis from the diaphysis without a fracture of the bone.

sprain–ligament rupture (L., *luxatio imperfecta*):   stretching or tearing of ligaments (fibrous bands that bind bones together at a joint), varying in degrees from being partially torn (stretched) to being completely torn (ruptured), with the continuity of the ligament remaining intact. After a sprain, the fibrous capsule that encloses the joint may become inflamed, swollen, discolored, and extremely painful. Involuntary muscle spasm, and sometimes a fracture, may occur. Rest, elevation, and a restrictive bandage, splint, or cast are methods of treating these injuries until properly healed. When a ligament or tendon has been torn completely, dislocation may also occur. Surgical repair may be required in some cases.

strain: stretching or tearing of a muscle or its tendon (fibrous cord that attaches the muscle to the

CLOSED BREAK   OPEN BREAK

From within   From without

FIG 1–1.
Closed vs. open fracture. (From Schneider FR: *Handbook for the orthopaedic assistant,* ed 2, St Louis, 1976, The CV Mosby Co.)

bone it moves) that may result in bleeding into the damaged muscle area, which causes pain, swelling, stiffness, muscle spasm, and, subsequently, a bruise. A strain is serious because muscle damage (scar tissue) may cause muscle shortening. With rest, strains will subside in 2 to 3 days, but symptoms may persist for months.

CLASSIFICATIONS OF FRACTURES

Open vs. Closed (Fig 1–1)

closed f.:   does not produce an open wound of the skin but does result in loss of continuity of bone subcutaneously. Formerly called simple f.

open f.:   one of the fragments has broken through the skin, and there is loss of continuity of bone internally. Formerly called compound f.

Portion of Bone Involved

To denote the portion of bone involved or the point of reference of a fracture, the distal third may be expressed as D/3 or distal/3, the middle third as M/3 or middle/3, and the proximal third as P/3 or proximal/3. Middle/3 fractures are commonly known as midshaft fractures. (The abbreviations are acceptable for clinical notes but should be spelled out in formal correspondence.) For highly specified anatomic locations, the following terms are commonly used.

apophyseal f.: avulsion of or fracture through an apophysis (bony prominence) where there is strong tendinous attachment.

articular f.: involves a joint surface. Also called joint f. and intraarticular f.

cleavage f.: shelling off of cartilage with avulsion of a small fragment of bone such as the capitellum.

condylar f.: involves any round end of a hinge joint; see sections on femoral and distal humeral fractures.

cortical f.: involves cortex of bone.

diacondylar f.: transcondylar fracture (line across the condyle).

direct f.: results at specific point of injury and is due to the injury itself.

extracapsular f.: occurs near, but outside, the capsule of a joint, especially the hip.

intracapsular f.: occurs within the capsule of a joint.

nonphyseal f.: any childhood fracture that does not involve a growth plate.

periarticular f.: occurs near but not involving a joint.

transcondylar f.: occurs transversely between the condyles of the elbow. This term is also used in fractures of the femur and bones with condyles. Also called **diacondylar f.**

tuft f.: involves the distal phalanx (tuft) of any digit. Also called **bursting f.**

General Appearance (Fig 1–2)

avulsion f.: tearing away of a part; a fragmentation of bone where the pull of a strong ligamentous or tendinous attachment tends to forcibly pull the fragment away from the rest of the bone. The fragment is usually at the articular surface.

bursting f.: multiple fragments, usually at the end of a bone; classically, f. of the first cervical vertebra.

butterfly f.: a bone *fragment* shaped like a butterfly and part of a comminuted f. Usually involves high energy force delivered to the bone.

chip f.: a small fragment, usually at the articular margin of a condyle.

comminuted f.: more than two fragments; lines of fracture may be transverse, oblique, spiral, or T or Y shaped. Also called splintered f. Locations of fractures most likely to be comminuted are:

   supracondylar f. of humerus: immediately above humeral condyle.

   supracondylar f. of femur: immediately above femoral condyle.

   intertrochanteric f. of femur: line of fracture extends between lesser and greater trochanters.

   bimalleolar f.: involves inner or outer maleolus of ankle.

   long bone f.: involves proximal, middle, and/or distal third of shaft.

complete f.: the bone is completely broken through both cortices.

compression f.: crumbling or smashing of cancellous bone by forces acting parallel to the long axis of bone; applied particularly to vertebral body fractures.

depressed f.: used to describe skull or articular surface fractures where the fragment is displaced below the overall level of the skill or articular surface.

displaced f.: fragments are moved away from each other.

double f.: segmental f. of a bone in two places.

epiphyseal f.: involves the cartilaginous growth plate of a bone. Also referred to as **epiphyseal slip f., Salter f.,** and **Salter-Harris f.** (Fig 1–3).

fissure f.: crack in one cortex (surface) only of a long bone.

greenstick f.: in children, incomplete, angulated fracture with a partial break. Also called **incomplete f., interperiosteal f., hickory-stick f.,** and **willow f.**

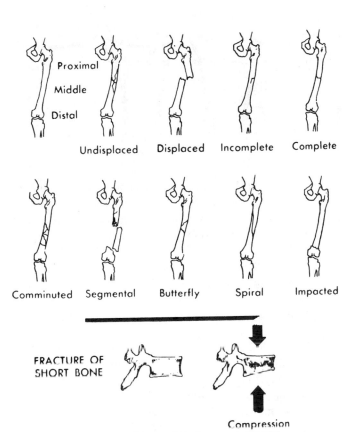

FIG 1–2.
Fracture terminology, general appearance. (From Schneider FR: *Handbook for the orthopaedic assistant,* ed 2, St Louis, 1976, The CV Mosby Co.)

hairline f.:   nondisplaced fracture line (crack) in the cortex of bone.

impacted f.:   fragments are compressed by force of original injury, driving one fragment of bone into adjacent bone.

incomplete f.:   cortices of bone are buckled or cracked but continuity is not destroyed; the cortex is broken on one side and only bent on the other. Microscopically, the fracture is present on bent side, and resorption and callus will occur on this side as well. Types are **greenstick f., torus f.**

infraction f.:   small radiolucent line seen in pathologic fractures, most commonly resulting from metabolic problems.

lead pipe f.:   in children, a forearm fracture in the cortex of long bone shaft where one of the cortices is compressed and bulging at point of impact on one side, with a linear fracture on opposite side.

linear f.:   lengthwise fracture of bone; implies that there is no displacement.

multiple f.:   two or more separate lines of fracture in the same bone.

oblique f.:   slanted fracture of the shaft on long axis of bone.

occult f.:   hidden fracture (undetectable on a radiograph), generally occurring in areas of the ribs, tibia, metatarsals, and navicula.

plastic bowing f.:   curved deformity of a tubular bone without gross fracture.

secondary f.:   pathologic f. of bone weakened by disease.

segmental f.:   several large fractures in the same bone shaft.

FIG 1–3.
Epiphyseal fracture types classified by the Salter method.

I   II   III   IV   V

spiral f.: fracture line is spiral shaped, usually on shaft of long bones. Also called **torsion f.**

stellate f.: numerous fissures radiate from central point of injury.

subperiosteal f.: bone but not its periosteal tube is broken; uncommon, usually the result of a direct blow.

torsion f.: see spiral f.

tortus f.: usually noticed in children; a stable, often incomplete f. in which one distal cortical surface appears to be wrinkled by compression forces, and the opposite cortex may or may not be infracted by tension forces.

transverse f.: line of fracture across the shaft at right angles to the long axis of a bone.

Position and Alignment of Fragments (Fig 1–4)

The position of a fragment refers to any displacement of one bone fragment in reference to the next. Displacement, should it exist, can be in any plane. Alignment refers to rotatory and/or angular deviation of the distal fragment in relation to the proximal fragment. For example:

posterior bow: in a completely displaced midshaft femoral fracture with a 3 cm overriding and 20 degree anterior angulation, the bone ends are not in apposition; there is a 3 cm shortening, and the distal end is angulated in an anterior direction.

bayonet position: the fragments touch and overlap, but there is good alignment. Internal and external rotation can also be stated in degrees.

The descriptive radiographic interpretations of fractures are defined as follows. The *angulation* of the fracture is designated by the direction of the apex of the fracture points. *Fragments* themselves are designated as proximal and distal.

When broken ends of the principal fragments are touching, they are said to be in *apposition.* Accuracy or degree of apposition is defined in percentages, such as 50%, indicating at least one radiographic view.

The *site* may be diaphyseal, metaphyseal, or epiphyseal portions of a specific bone or may be intraarticular. *Extent* may be described as complete, incomplete, cracked, hairline, buckled, or greenstick. The *configuration* may be transverse, oblique, or spiral and is referred to as comminuted when more than two fragments are present. The *fracture fragments* may be undisplaced or displaced.

Thus, a fracture is described radiographically by its site, bone name, extent, configuration, relationship of fragments to each other and to the external environment, and the presence or absence of complications.

CLASSIC AND DESCRIPTIVE NAMES (BY ANATOMIC LOCATION)

Shoulder Fractures (Proximal Humerus and Scapula)

anatomic neck f.: occurs in the area of tendinous attachments, the true neck of humeral metaphysis.

Bankart f.: detachment of a small piece of bone from the anteroinferior rim of the glenoid; seen with anterior shoulder dislocation.

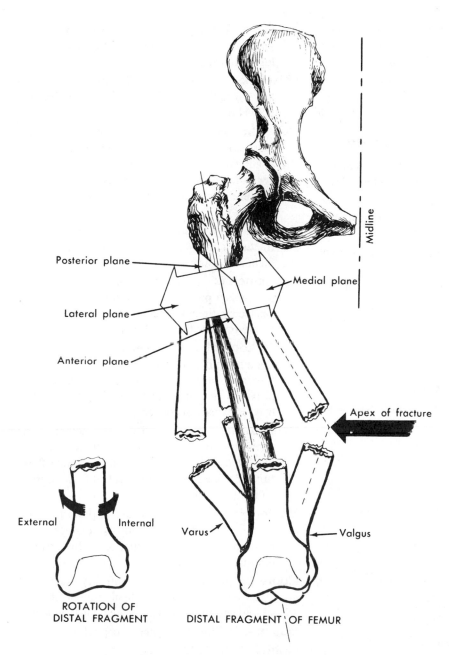

FIG 1–4.
Description of fracture deformity. (From Schneider FR: *Handbook for the orthopaedic assistant,* ed 2, St Louis, 1976, The CV Mosby Co.)

Hill-Sachs (Hermodsson) f.: moderate compression f. of the humeral head usually seen after an anterior dislocation of the shoulder.

surgical neck f.: occurs in area below the anatomic neck of the humerus.

Arm and Elbow Fractures (Distal Humerus)

boxer's elbow: chip f. at the tip of the olecranon caused by a fast extension of the elbow in a missed jab (punch).

condylar f.: occurs at the medial or lateral articular process of the humerus at the elbow.

epicondylar f.: occurs through one of the two epicondyles, medial or lateral.

Holstein-Lewis f.: involves the humerus at the junction of the middle and distal thirds. Associated with radial nerve paralysis because of nerve proximity to posterior septum and bone.

Kocher f.: semilunar chip f. of capitellum with displacement into joint.

Laugier f.: involves the trochlea of the humerus.

Malgaigne f.: extension mechanism supracondylar f. of humerus.

Posada f.: anteriorly angulated fracture of distal humerus associated with posterior dislocation of radius and ulna.

sideswipe f.: comminuted fracture of distal humerus and sometimes radius and ulna caused by direct blow against elbow.

supracondylar f.: occurs through the distal metaphysis of the humerus or femur.

T f.: intercondylar fracture shaped like a T.

Y f.: intercondylar fracture shaped like a Y.

Forearm and Wrist Fractures

Barton f.: a fracture of the dorsal or volar lip of the distal radius, often resulting in subluxation of the radial carpal joint into the fracture site.

chauffeur's f.: oblique fracture of the radial styloid caused by a twisting or snapping-type injury; also called **backfire f., Hutchinson f.,** and **lorry driver's f.**

chisel f.: incomplete, usually involving medial head of radius, with fracture line extending distally about ½ inch.

Colles f.: usually implies a fracture of the distal radius, either articular or nonarticular, with dorsal angulation of the distal fragment producing a silver fork deformity; generally asssociated with a fracture of the ulnar styloid. (Term becoming archaic.)

de Quervain f.: combination of a wrist scaphoid fracture with volar dislocation of scaphoid fragment and lunate.

Dye-punch f.: an intraarticular fracture of the ulnar (volar) portion of the distal radius, usually caused by direct impaction of the lunate onto the lunate fossa of the distal radius.

Essex-Lopresti f.: a comminuted radial head fracture with an injury to the central limb of the forearm; interosseous membrane can cause a proximal migration of the radius if the radial head is excised secondarily.

Galeazzi f.: typically a displaced fracture of the distal third or quarter of the radius with disruption of the distal radioulnar joint; called **fracture of necessity** because surgical fixation is required for reduction.

Monteggia f.: isolated fracture of proximal third of ulna, with posterior or anterior dislocation of radial head allowing angulation and overriding of ulnar fragments.

Moore f.: like a Colles f.; specifically, fracture of distal radius with dorsal displacement of ulnar styloid and impingement on annular ligament.

Mouchet f.: involves humeral capitellum.

nightstick f.: undisplaced fracture of the ulnar shaft caused by a direct blow.

Piedmont f.: oblique f. usually at the proximal portion of distal third of the radius; obliquity runs from proximal ulnar to distal radial aspect, allowing distal fragments to be pulled into the ulna by the pronator quadratus muscle. **Fracture of necessity** requiring operative management.

radial head f.:   involves the most proximal part of the radius, a dish-shaped portion of bone called the radial head.

radial styloid f.:   involves distal radial tip of radius.

reverse Barton f.:   dorsal displacement of carpus on radius, with associated fracture of dorsal articular surface of radius. The mechanism and appearance of this fracture are similar to those of a Colles f.

Skillern f.:   open f. of distal radius associated with greenstick f. of distal ulna.

Smith f. (reverse Colles f.):   fracture of the distal radius in which the distal fragment is displaced volarly. This fracture was defined before the advent of radiography, and, classically, there are three types:
1. Nonarticular
2. Intraarticular (**volar Barton f.**)
3. Oblique nonarticular fracture near the joint line

Hand Fractures

Bennett f.:   fracture of the base of the thumb metacarpal, usually leaving a volar ulnar fragment attached to a retaining ligament.

mallet f.:   avulsion f. of the extensor tendon from the dorsal base of the distal phalanx of any digit that includes insertion of extensor apparatus, thus allowing distal segment to "drop" into flexion. Also called **baseball finger, drop finger, mallet finger deformity.**

Rolando f.:   comminuted fracture of the base of the thumb metacarpal.

unciform f.:   fracture of the "hook of the hamate," usually caused by direct trauma that may or may not be associated with ulnar neuropathy.

Wilson f.:   involves the proximal volar portion of the middle phalanx because of strong attachment of volar plate.

Spine Fractures

Chance f.:   involves vertebra, with horizontal splitting of spinous process and neural arch with disruption through vertebral body; an unstable fracture.

clay shoveler's f.:   involves spinous process(es) C-6, C-7, T-1, T-2, or T-3.

hangman's f.:   posterior element (pedicles) fracture with anterior subluxation of the cervical neck of C-2 on C-3.

Jefferson f.:   bursting f. of the ring of the first cervical vertebra (atlas).

posterior element f.:   broad term used to describe any fracture of the spinous process, lamina, facets, pars interarticularis, or pedicle.

sentinel f.:   a cervical spine fracture characterized by fractures through the lamina on either side of the spinous process.

spondyloptosis: dislocation of one vertebra from another without any bone fracture.

teardrop f.:   exists in two forms: (1) an isolated anteroinferior fracture of the cervical spine (unstable) or (2) a three-part, two-plane fracture of an anteroinferior corner of the vertebral body (the teardrop), a sagittal vertebral body, and the posterior neural arch.

vertebra plana f.:   wafer-thin compression f. of a vertebral body resulting from an intrinsic pathologic condition of the bone.

wedge f.:   anterior compression f. of any vertebra; most common in the dorsal thoracic spine.

Pelvis, Hip, and Proximal Femur Fractures

basal neck f.:   involves base of femoral neck at junction of trochanteric region.

bucket-handle f.:   vertical shear fracture of anterior pubis and opposite ilium.

central f.:   acetabular fracture, centrally displaced through inner wall of pelvis.

dashboard f.:   posterior lip of acetabulum chips when femoral head is driven against it; often caused by a sudden jolt when knee hits dashboard.

dome f.: acetabular fracture involving weight-bearing surface of the acetabulum. This term can also be applied to a fracture of the superior surface of the talus.

Duverney f.: involves ilium just below the anterosuperior spine.

extracapsular f.: occurs outside of joint capsule of humerus or femur.

femoral neck f.: transcervical fracture through midportion of femoral neck.

intertrochanteric f.: occurs along a line joining the greater and lesser trochanters.

Malgaigne f.: occurs through wing of the ilium or sacrum with associated fractures through the ipsilateral pubic rami, allowing upward displacement of hemipelvis. Often associated with internal injuries.

pertrochanteric f.: involves proximal femur where the fracture line passes through both the lesser and greater trochanters.

ring f.: involves at least two parts of pelvic circumference.

shaft f.: occurs between subtrochanteric and supracondylar area.

sprinter's f.: involves anterosuperior or anteroinferior spine of ilium, with a fragment of bone being pulled forcibly by sudden muscular pull.

straddle f.: double f. or dislocation of the pubis usually caused by a straddling mechanism, for example, falling onto a rail with the point of contact between the legs.

subcapital f.: femoral fracture at head-neck junction.

subtrochanteric f.: transverse f. of femur just below lesser trochanter.

Walther f.: transverse ischioacetabular f. where the fracture line passes from ischial spine to acetabular cavity to ischiopubic junction.

Distal Femur, Knee, Tibia, and Fibula Fractures

bumper f.: involves the tibia or femur and is caused by a direct blow in area of the tibial tuberosity; commonly caused by a car bumper accident; may be bilateral.

Hoffa f.: coronal fracture of medial femoral condyle.

patellar f.: involves kneecap.

pillion f.: T-shaped fracture of distal femur with displacement of the condyles posteriorly to femoral shaft, caused by severe blow to knee.

Segond f.: small avulsion f. of superolateral tibia caused by tension on the lateral capsule or ligament. Usually associated with other ligamentous injuries leading to anterolateral knee instability.

sleeve f.: involves a small chip of bone from the superior or inferior portion of the patella associated with loss of integrity of quadriceps extensor mechanism.

Stieda f.: avulsion f. of origin of medial collateral ligament on medial femoral condyle.

supracondylar f.: involves the distal shaft of bone above condyles of femur or humerus.

tibial plateau f.: involves proximal tibial articular surface.

toddler f.: nondisplaced fracture of the tibia seen in toddlers beginning to walk.

wagon wheel f.: involves distal femoral epiphysis in children. Also called **cartwheel f.**

Y and T f.: combined supracondylar and intercondylar f. of the distal femur.

Ankle and Foot Fractures

ankle mortise diastasis: separation of tibia and fibula at ankle; often associated with a fracture or dislocation.

aviator's astragalus: denotes a wide variety of talar fractures caused by sudden impaction of foot into ankle; may be associated with other fractures about the foot and ankle.

boot-top f.:   involves transverse, distal third of tibia, occurring at boot top. Also called **skier's injury.**

Bosworth f.:   fracture-dislocation of the ankle, with oblique fracture of the distal fibula and displacement of the proximal fibular fragment out of fibular groove to a place posterior and medial to the posterolateral ridge of the tibia.

bunkbed f.:   intraarticular f. of the base of the first metatarsal in children.

Cedell f.:   fracture of the posterior process of the talus.

Chaput f.:   involves the anterior tubercle of distal tibia because of strong attachment of anterior tibiofibular ligament.

Conrad-Bugg trapping: incarceration of soft tissue, usually the posterior tibial tendon, between fragments of an ankle fracture. This produces an injury that must be reduced by open methods.

Cotton f.:   partial forward dislocation of the tibia to produce a fracture of the posterior inferior margin of the tibia, sometimes called the **posterior malleolus.** This is most commonly associated with a fibular fracture.

Descot f.:   involves the posterior lip of tibia.

dome f.:   involves the superior articular surface of talus or the weight-bearing portion of the acetabulum.

Dupuytren f.:   spiral f. of the distal end of fibula; associated with ankle diastasis.

Gosselin f.:   V-shaped fracture of the distal tibia into the tibiotalar joint.

Henderson f.:   trimalleolar fracture of the ankle.

Jones f.:   fracture of the base of the fifth metatarsal such that the fracture line extends from the lateral cortex in the direction of the proximal portion of the articulation of the fourth and fifth metatarsals. This term has been misapplied to

fractures in the midcortical area of bone and those at its extremely proximal apophyseal portion.

Kohler f.:   involves the navicular and is associated with avascular necrosis; seen in children.

Lisfranc f.:   usually a fracture-dislocation, with displacement of the proximal metatarsals.

Maisonneuve f.:   spiral f. of proximal end of fibula, near the neck, associated with a tear of the anterior tibiofibular ligament and the potential for ankle diastasis.

march f.:   stress f. of metatarsal caused by excessive marching. Also called **fatigue f.**

midnight f.:   open, oblique fracture of proximal phalanx of little toe.

Montercaux f.:   involves fibular neck and is associated with diastasis of ankle mortise.

paratrooper f.:   involves posterior articular margin of tibia and/or malleolus.

Pott f.:   spiral oblique f. of distal fibula with associated rupture of the deltoid ligament; avulsion of the medial malleolus and lateral displacement of foot on tibia.

plafond f.:   any fracture that involves the surface of the tibia that comes in contact with the dome of the talus.

Shepherd f.:   involves posterior talus with sheared off piece of bone and, in some instances, a separate piece of bone (os trigonum).

Tillaux Kleiger f.:   involves distal lateral tibia, vertically extending into the joint; sometimes associated with diastasis and other fractures about the ankle.

tongue f.:   involves the posterosuperior portion of calcaneus.

triplane f.:   involves the ankle in three planes: coronally through the posterior tibial metaphysis, transversely through the growth plate, and sagittally through the distal tibial epiphysis.

Volkmann f.:   involves a triangular portion of the posterior lateral tibia into the joint, leaving a triangular bone fragment sometimes called **Volk-mann's triangle.**

Wagstaffe f. (Le Fort f.):   separation of a distal anterior fragment of the fibula, that is, the portion of attachment of the anterior tibiofibular ligament.

CONTRIBUTING FACTORS

Aside from a single obvious traumatic event, there are other factors contributing to fractures.

dyscrasic f.:   results from weakening of bone by a disease process.

endocrine f.:   occurs in bone weakened by an endocrine disorder.

fatigue f.:   spontaneous fracture in healthy bone resulting from fatigue or stress produced by excessive physical activity in a short period of time; seen in fibulas/tibias of young long-distance runners, the hips and heels of young military recruits, and in the metatarsals. Also called **stress f., march f.**

hoop stress f.:   involves the medial or anteromedial femoral neck and occurs during broaching of the femoral canal for a prosthesis or during the actual impaction of the prosthesis.

inflammatory f.:   occurs in association with inflammation secondary to an infection, such as syphilis.

insufficiency f.:   stress f. that occurs in bone because of its diminished volume (that is, osteopenia).

neoplastic f.:   a form of pathologic f. Presence of a tumor in bone, whether originating in the bone or metastatic from elsewhere, causes sufficient weakening to allow it to fracture spontaneously or with less trauma than it would normally take to break a healthy bone.

pathologic f.:   occurs with or without trauma where bone has been weakened by a local or sys-temic process. The most common causes are a tumor (benign or malignant), local infection, or bone cyst. This term is less widely applied to congenital disorders such as osteogenesis imperfecta, osteopetrosis, and neurofibromatosis. The term is applied more to congenital or acquired disorders such as osteomalacia, rickets, Paget disease, scurvy, and osteoporosis.

stress f.:   crack in bone from overexertion placed on bone structure of limb or metatarsals and from pull of muscle on bone. Not noticeable on initial radiograph but is on later radiographs when callus formation has taken place at the site. A bone scan will show the fracture. Also called **march f.** More recently, the term **stress reaction to bone** has been used since fracture lines often do not appear and because the term more accurately describes the condition.

DEGREE AND NATURE OF HEALING

The quality of bone healing is stated in terms of the solidarity of adhesiveness of the bone fragments. As most fractures heal, a surrounding "sleeve" of bone, or **callus,** is formed. This new bone formation is composed of cartilage, bone, blood vessels, and fibrous tissue and is often referred to in discussing bone healing. If the bone is completely healed, the term **healed** is used. Anything less is considered a *state of healing,* unless there is *a failure of progression of healing with expectation of no further healing.* This is then considered a **nonunion.**

The absence of complete union is called **ununited,** but this term by some users implies an expectation of failure to unite. In **delayed union** the speed of callus formation (fracture healing) is slower than anticipated, but this does not imply expectancy of either total healing or nonunion. A **pseudoarthrosis** is the formation of a jointlike structure at the old fracture site and is a type of nonunion. It consists of fibrocartilaginous tissue and a synovial fluid sac. If a bone unites but in abnormal position and/or alignment, the term **malunion** is used. If two bones parallel to one another unite by osseous tissue, such as the tibia/fibula or ulna/radius complex, the result is a **crossunion,** or **synostosis.**

For example, in a simple fracture of the midshaft of the radius and ulna, assume that the radius adheres to the ulna at the distal fracture site and that the radius does not heal because of angulated healing of the ulna. Such a situation can be described as a **malunited fracture** of the **midshaft** of the ulna with a nonunion of the radius and crossunion of the distal radius and ulna. When the diagnoses are listed, they might be given as (1) malunion, fracture, closed, midshaft, ulna, right, or (2) nonunion, fracture, closed, midshaft, radius, right, associated with crossunion.

Secondary union is a term that has multiple meanings. It implies delayed healing either by the eventual adhesion of granulating surfaces of bone fragments or surgical intervention late in the course of fracture healing to promote union.

Nutritional support is important in bone healing to augment medical and surgical care. Bones need mineral and protein to heal, another consideration in treatment.

INTERNATIONAL CLASSIFICATION SYSTEM AND TRAUMA REGISTRY SYSTEM

AO/ASIF (Long Bone Fractures)

For uniform description in the literature.
- The system defines bones by number (**1,** humerus; **2,** radius and ulna; **3,** femur; **4,** tibia and fibula; **5,** spine, jaw, clavicle, and scapula; **6,** pelvis and sacrum; **7,** hand; **8,** foot).
- Nature of fracture by letter (**A,** simple involving at least 90% of the cortex or extraarticular; **B,** wedge with some contact between fragments or partial articular; **C,** complete with no contact between fragments or complete articular).

- Degree of comminution by number (**A**—1, spiral; 2, oblique; 3, transverse less than 30°. **B**—1, spiral wedge; 2, bending wedge; 3, fragmented wedge. **C**—1, spiral; 2, segmental; 3, irregular).

The subgroups .1, .2, and .3 further define the complexity of each of the above groupings.

Limitation: agreement among raters.[*]

AO/ASIF (Soft Tissue Classification)

For uniform description in the literature.

Integumentary Injury (I)
Closed (C)
ICI: no skin lesion.
IC2: contusions but no skin laceration.
IC3: circumscribed degloving.
IC4: extensive closed degloving
IC5: necrosis from contusion.

Open (O)
IOI: skin breakage from inside out.
IO2: skin breakage from outside in < 5 cm, contusion at edges.
IO3: skin breakage > 5 cm, increased contusion, devitalized edge.
IO4: considerable full thickness contusion, abrasion, extensive open degloving, skin loss.

Muscle/Tendon Injury (MT)

MTI: no muscle injury.
MT2: circumscribed muscle injury, one compartment only.
MT3: circumscribed muscle injury, two compartments.
MT4: muscle defect, tendon laceration, extensive muscle contusion.

*Müller ME et al, 1991 (see Bibliography).

MT5: compartment syndrome, crush syndrome with wide injury zone.

Neurovascular injury (NV)
NV1: no neurovascular injury.

NV2: isolated nerve injury.

NV3: isolated vascular injury.

NV4: extensive segmental vascular injury.

NV5: combined neurovascular injury, subtotal and total amputation.[*]

Orthopaedic Trauma Association (Gustilo)

An alternative to the AO system was developed by Gustilio for the Orthopaedic Trauma Association to establish a uniform trauma registry. His classification system uses many of the terms that are in this chapter. However, it is highly specific as to the nature and location of associated injuries.

Reference: Gustilo RB: *The fracture classification manual.* St. Louis, Mosby, 1991.

CLASSIFICATION SYSTEMS BY GRADES, TYPES, AND MECHANISMS

The trend toward standard classification of fractures and dislocations is certainly a step forward, but such a system is designed for computer storage and is sometimes difficult to apply when viewing a fracture for the first time. It should not be forgotten that most of these specific classification systems were developed to address a specific set of circumstances. Attempting to apply them to other areas frequently leads to misinterpretation and erroneous conclusions. The authors, therefore, feel that these systems should be interpreted as meant by the original author(s). The reference is indicated at the end of the definition (see Bibliography for full reference citations).

*Müller ME et al, 1991 (see Bibliography).

Allman (Clavicle Fractures)

To define location of most common sites of occurrence and of nonunion.

Group I: fractures of middle third.

Group II: fractures distal to coracoclavicular ligament, nonunion frequent.

Group III: fractures of proximal end, nonunion and displacement rare.

Limitations: does not incorporate other factors such as degree of trauma.
Reference: Allman FL

Anderson and d'Alonzo (Odontoid Fractures of the Second Cervical Vertebra)

Based on location of fracture; to define fracture pattern likely to require surgery for healing.

Type I: avulsion fracture of tip of odontoid.

Type II: fracture at junction of odontoid to body of vertebra.

Type III: fracture line extends downward into cancellous bone of body of vertebra.

Reference: Anderson LD and d'Alonzo RT

Ashurst (Ankle Sprain/Fractures)

Based on direction or mechanism of force.

External Rotation Injuries
first degree: transsyndesmotic fracture of the fibula.

alternate first degree: rupture of the anterior tibiofibular ligament with or without spiral fracture of the proximal fibula.

second degree: rupture of the deltoid ligament.

alternate second degree: avulsion of the medial malleolus.

third degree: fracture of the entire lower end of the tibia and fibula with external rotation.

Abduction Injuries
first degree: transverse fracture of the medial malleolus at or below its base.

second degree: rupture of the deltoid ligament or fracture of the medial malleolus followed by a fracture of the distal fibula.

third degree: fracture of both lower tibia and medial malleolus lateral displacement.

Adduction Injuries
first degree: avulsion of the fibular malleolus at or below its base.

second degree: avulsion of the fibular malleolus at or below its base with medial malleolus below plafond a shear vertically into tibial shaft.

third degree: supra-malleolar fracture in both the tibia and fibula with medial displacement.

Fracture by Compression in Long Axis of Leg
first degree: isolated marginal fracture of the distal weight-bearing plate of the tibia.

second degree: comminution of the tibial plafond.

third degree: T or Y fractures (V fracture of Gosselin).

Limitations: fracture patterns overlap.
Reference: Ashurst APC.

Badelon (Lateral Condylar Fractures of the Humerus in Children)

Roentgenographic basis for stability versus displacement, which requires surgical reduction.
Type I: nondisplaced fracture that can be seen only on one view.

Type II: visible fracture line with minimal displacement.

Type III: displacement of more than 2 mm on all views.

Type IV: severe displacement with complete separation of fracture edges.

Reference: Badelon O et al.

Bado (Fractured Ulna with Dislocation of the Radial Head [Monteggia])

Based on mechanism of injury; to help define management.
Type 1:   fracture of any portion of the ulna diaphysis with anterior angulation and anterior dislocation of the radial head.

Type 2:   fracture of the ulnar diaphysis with posterior angulation and posterior or posterolateral dislocation of the radial head.

Type 3:   fracture of the ulnar metaphysis with lateral or anterolateral dislocation of the radial head.

Type 4:   proximal fracture of both bones at the same level with anterior dislocation of the radial head.

Limitations: some controversy as to relationship to treatment; types I and II have equivalents that involve dislocation radial head only (Type 1) and fractured radial head.
Reference: Bado JL

Brendt and Harty [modified]; (Fractures or Development of Osteochondritis Dissecans of the Dome of the Talus)

To define stages of "posttraumatic" necrosis of bone.
Stage I: normal x-ray but positive bone scan or change seen on magnetic resonance imaging (repeated minitrauma).

Stage II: incomplete separation of subchondral fragment (single injury event).

Stage IIA: cyst formation (repeated minitrauma).

Stage III: complete separation of fragment, which is in anatomic position (single injury event).

Stage IV: separation of fragment (single injury event).

Reference: Anderson IF

Boyd and Griffin (Extracapsular Fractures of Proximal Femur from Neck to 5 cm Distal to Lesser Trochanter)

To define surgical approach and prognosis for fractures near and around the femoral neck.

Type 1: intertrochanteric f., simple to reduce and maintain.

Type 2: intertrochanteric f. with comminution and additional coronal seen from lateral.

Type 3: subtrochanteric f. with at least one fracture line passing just distal to or through lesser trochanter.

Type 4: fractures of the trochanteric region and proximal shaft and fracture in two planes requiring two plane fixation.

Limitations: crosses over from subtrochanteric fracture type to intertrochanteric and neck fractures.
Reference: Boyd HB and Griffin LL.

Bucholtz (Pelvic Fracture Displacement)

To define fracture pattern that is likely to be stable.

Type I: nondisplaced, such as pubic fracture.

Type II: diastasis pubis, but no superior displacement.

Type III: total ring disruption with or without superior migration of segment.

Reference: Buckholtz RW.

Canale-Kelly (Talar Fractures)

Based on location of fracture and association with displacement and effect on blood supply; to define prognosis for long-term outcome with particular reference to avascular necrosis.

Type I: minimal displacement, only one source of blood supply might be disrupted.

Type II: subtalar subluxation or dislocation, two or three sources of blood supply might be affected.

Type III: body of talus dislocated from the ankle and the subtalar joint.

Type IV: fracture of talar neck associated with dislocation of the body from the ankle, or subtalar joint and additional subluxation or dislocation of the head of the talus from the talonavicular joint.

Reference: Canale ST and Kelly FB.

Chadwick and Bentley (Distal Tibia Fractures Affecting Epiphysis in Children)

Based on roentgenographic analysis; reflects the mechanism of type IV Salter fractures of the distal tibia and fibula and helps predict retardation of growth.

Group I: epiphysis not fractured.

Group 1a: abduction injury with fracture of the distal fibular shaft and lateral displacement.

Group 1b: supination/hyper–plantar flexion injury with posterior metaphyseal fragment of the tibia and posterior displacement.

Group 1c: supination/external rotation injury with large anteromedial metaphyseal component, tibia and posterior displacement.

Group 1d: adduction injury (rare), posteromedial metaphyseal fragment of the tibia with fracture of the distal fibular shaft and medial displacement.

Group II: vertical fracture through epiphysis with shift of lateral fragment.

Group III: adduction injury, Salter type I or II fibular slip with type IV medial malleolar fracture.

Reference: Chadwick CJ and Bentley G.

Colonna [Delbet] (Hip Fractures in Children)

Attributes classification to Delbet; no purpose given.

Type I: transepiphyseal separations with or without dislocation of femoral head.

Type II: transcervical fractures, displaced and nondisplaced.

Type III: cervicotrochanteric fractures, displaced and nondisplaced.

Type IV: intertrochanteric fractures.

Reference: Colonna PC.

Colton (Olecranon Fractures)

To define treatment.

Avulsion group: transverse fracture line separates a small fragment of olecranon with or without displacement.

Oblique group: primary failure being an oblique line from the trochlear notch to the distal outer ulnar shaft, degree of comminution staged a to d.

Stage a—single fracture line, displaced and nondisplaced.

Stage b—nondisplaced single central large V-shaped fragment.

Stage c—displaced single central large V-shaped fragment.

Stage d—highly comminuted central pieces of bone with displacement.

Fracture dislocation (Monteggia group): fracture line at or slightly proximal to coronoid, which may result in anterior fracture/dislocation of the elbow.

Unclassified group: high energy, highly comminuted fractures not matching the above descriptions.

Reference: Colton CL.

Dias-Tachdjian (Ankle Fractures in Children)

Uses Lauge-Hansen guidelines, foot position and direction of force in correlation with the Salter-Harris classification to plan surgical and other treatment approaches.

Supination-inversion: inversion force applied to supinated foot.

Grade I: Salter-Harris type I or II of distal fibular epiphysis.

Grade II: grade I with Salter-Harris type III or IV of tibial epiphysis.

Supination-plantar flexion: plantar flexion force on supinated foot.

Grade I: Salter-Harris type I or II of distal tibia, usually with posterior displacement.

Supination-external rotation: external rotation ankle force on fully supinated foot.

Grade I: Salter-Harris type II of distal tibia with long spiral fracture of distal tibia.

Grade II: grade I with spiral fracture of fibula.

Pronation–eversion–external rotation: a combination of eversion and external rotation force on pronated foot.

Grade I: posterolateral displacement of Salter-Harris type II tibial fracture with short oblique fibular fracture above physis.

Limitations: fractures not covered under this system include Salter-Harris type III distal tibia and triplane fracture (as described by author).

Reference: Dias LS and Tachdjian MO.

Essex-Lopresti (Os Calcis Fractures)

Based on direction of injury force (A–C superior to inferior, and D–F anterosuperior to posteroinferior); helps define method of closed and open management.

Type A: nondisplaced fracture inferior to lateral process of talus and through lateral cortex.

Type B: type A with shearing of sustentaculum tali along with one-third to one-half of the posterior facet.

Type C: type B with depression of joint and superior posterior displacement of distal portion.

Type D: affects lateral half or two-thirds of subtalar joint and fracture of the lateral cortex without displacement.

Type E: type D with superior displacement of anterior portion of calcaneus.

Type F: type E with displacement of posterior facet of calcaneus and further superior migration of anterior portion.

Reference: Essex-Lopresti P.

Evans-Wales (Intertrochanteric Fractures of Femur)

Grouped by stable or unstable and expected response to treatment.

Type I: fracture line extends upward and outward from lesser trochanter:
Undisplaced stable
Displaced reduced with stable medial apposition
Displaced unreduced with no medial apposition
Comminuted unstable with no medial apposition

Type II: reversed obliquity with line from lesser trochanter to inferior lateral cortex.

Limitations: directed at open versus closed management, which is no longer used.
Reference: Evans EM and Wales SS.

Ferkel-Cheng (Arthroscopic Classification of Osteochondral Lesions of the Talus)

To define stages of appearance and attachment of lesion to subchondral bone.

Stage A: smooth, intact, but soft or ballottable.

Stage B: rough surface.

Stage C: fibrillations or fissures.

Stage D: flap present or bone exposed.

Stage E: loose, nondisplaced fragment.

Stage F: displaced fragment.

Reference: Ferkel RD et al, 1995.

Ferkel-Sgaglione (CT Classification of Osteochondral Lesions of the Talus)

To define stages of attachment of subchondral bone.

Stage I: cystic lesion within dome of talus.

Stage IIA: cystic lesion with communication to talar dome surface.

Stage IIB: open articular surface lesion with overlying nondisplaced fragment.

Stage III: nondisplaced lesion with lucency.

Stage IV: displaced fragment.

Reference: Ferkel RD et al, 1990.

Fielding-Magliato (Subtrochanteric Fractures of Femur)

Based on distance from lesser trochanter for selection of method of surgical fixation.

Type 1: at level of lesser trochanter.

Type 2: between 2.5 and 5 cm below lesser trochanter.

Type 3: 5 to 7.5 cm below lesser trochanter.

Limitations: oblique and comminuted fractures involve more than one level, newer appliances cover a wider spectrum of conditions.
Reference: Fielding JW and Magliato HJ.

Frykman (Distal Radial and Ulnar Fractures)

Based on radial joint involvement with and without ulnar styloid fractures to define method of fixation.

Type I: radial extraarticular without ulnar styloid fracture.

Type II: radial extraarticular with ulnar styloid fracture.

Type III: radiocarpal joint only without ulnar styloid fracture.

Type IV: radiocarpal joint only with ulnar styloid fracture.

Type V: distal radioulnar joint only without ulnar styloid fracture.

Type VI: distal radioulnar joint only with ulnar styloid fracture.

Type VII: both radiocarpal and distal radioulnar joint without ulnar styloid fracture.

Type VIII: both radiocarpal and distal radioulnar joint with ulnar styloid fracture.

Reference: Frykman G.

Garden (Subcapital Fractures of Femoral Neck)

Based on AP and lateral radiographic guidelines for reduction and likelihood of avascular necrosis.

Stage 1: incomplete, impacted, head tilted in posterolateral direction.

Stage 2: complete but undisplaced.

Stage 3: complete, displaced, but fragments remain in contact.

Stage 4: fracture fragments completely displaced, no contact between fragments.

Reference: Garden RS.

Gartland (Supracondylar Fractures of the Humerus in Children)

Based on displacement; to define surgical treatment.

Type I: undisplaced.

Type II: displaced and difficult to hold with cast immobilization.

Type III: posteromedial or posterolateral displacement with difficult reduction that is hard to maintain due to periosteal stripping.

Reference: Gartland JJ.

Gustilo (Open Fractures)

Based on size of wound and soft tissue involvement; to determine fixation types and limb salvage.

Type I: clean wound < 1 cm.

Type II: laceration > 1 cm without extensive soft tissue damage, flaps, or avulsions.

Type IIIA: extensive soft tissue laceration but adequate soft tissue coverage of bone.

Type IIIB: extensive soft tissue laceration with periosteal stripping, exposed bone, usually massively contaminated.

Type IIIC: arterial injury, requires repair regardless of size of wound.

Limitations: types II and III have interobserver variation.

Reference: Gustilo RB et al.

Hawkins (Talar Neck Fractures)

Based on location of fracture and association with displacement and effect on blood supply; prognosis for long-term outcome with particular reference to avascular necrosis.

Type I: minimal displacement, only one source of blood supply might be disrupted.

Type II: subtalar subluxation or dislocation, two or three sources of blood supply might be affected.

Type III: body of talus dislocated from the ankle and the subtalar joint.

Reference: Hawkins LG.

Herbert and Fisher (Wrist Scaphoid Fractures)

To differentiate between fractures that are likely to unite in 6 to 8 weeks and those that would not; to define need for surgery.

Type A1: nondisplaced tubercle hairline fracture.

Type A2: nondisplaced hairline waist fracture.

Type B1: oblique fracture of distal third.

Type B2: displaced middle waist fracture.

Type B3: proximal pole fracture.

Type B4: fracture dislocation of carpus.

Type B5: comminuted fractures.

Type C: delayed union.

Type D1: fibrous union.

Type D2: sclerotic nonunion (pseudoarthrosis).

Limitations: type B5 and C have been deleted; D2 changed to pseudoarthrosis; D3 sclerotic pseudoarthrosis; D4 avascular necrosis.

Reference: Herbert TJ and Fisher WE. (Modified *J Bone Joint Surg* 1996;78-B:519–528).

Hohl-Moore (Tibial Plateau Fractures)

Based on pattern; designed for surgical planning.
Type 1: minimally displaced.
Type 2: local compression.
Type 3: split compression.
Type 4: total condyle.
Type 5: both condyles.

Limitations: does not take into account ligament injury.
Reference: Hohl M and Moore TM.

Ideberg (Glenoid Fractures of the Scapula)

To define mechanism and to compare surgical and nonsurgical treatment.
Type I: avulsion of the anterior margin.
Type II: transverse fracture through glenoid fossa with inferior triangular fragment displaced with the humeral head.
Type III: oblique fracture through the glenoid exiting on the midsuperior border of the scapula; often associated with acromioclavicular fracture or dislocation.
Type IV: horizontal, exiting through medial border of the blade.
Type V: type IV with a separation of the inferior half of the glenoid.

Reference: Ideberg R.

Jensen (Intertrochanteric Femur Fractures)

Modified Evans system to determine possibility of stable reduction and secondary fracture displacement.
Type I: single fracture line, nondisplaced, stable on fixation.
Type II: single fracture line, displaced, stable on fixation.
Type III: comminuted, not involving the lesser trochanter; risk of loss of reduction.

Type IV: unstable, lesser trochanteric fragment, portion of greater trochanter attached to neck; greater risk of loss of reduction.
Type V: unstable lesser and greater trochanteric fragments; greatest risk of loss of reduction.

Reference: Jensen JS.

Johansson (Femoral Fractures following Total Hip Replacement)

To define fracture pattern that is likely to require surgery for healing.
Type I: fracture proximal to tip of the prosthesis.
Type II: fracture extends from proximal shaft to point distal to tip of prosthesis.
Type III: fracture lines entirely below distal tip of prosthesis.

Reference: Johansson JE et al.

Key and Conwell (Pelvic Fractures)

Based on stability and location; to define need for stabilization.
I: fractures without break in pelvic ring.
   A: avulsion fractures.
      1: anterosuperior spine.
      2: anteroinferior spine.
      3: ischial tuberosity.
II: single break in pelvic ring.
   A: fracture of two ipsilateral rami.
   B: fracture near or subluxation of symphysis pubis.
   C: fracture near or subluxation of the sacroiliac joint.
III: double break in pelvic ring.
   A: double vertical fractures or dislocation of pubis (straddle).
   B: double vertical fractures or dislocation (Malgaigne).
   C: severe multiple fractures.

IV: fractures of the acetabulum.
- **A:**   small fragment with dislocated hip.
- **B:**   linear fracture associated with nondisplaced pelvic fracture.
- **C:**   linear fracture associated with hip joint instability.
- **D:**   fracture secondary to central dislocation of the acetabulum.

Reference: Key JA and Conwell HE.

Kilfoyle (Medial Condylar Fractures of the Humerus in Children)

To define need for closed (first two types) versus open treatment (type III).
Type I: greenstick impacted fracture on medial condylar apophyseal region, stable.
Type II: fracture through the medial condyle into the joint with little or no displacement.
Type III: intraarticular fracture of medial epicondyle with displacement and rotation.

Reference: Kilfoyle RM.

Kyle (Femoral Trochanteric Fractures)

Based on stability and displacement; to define nail-type management.
Type I: stable, undisplaced intertrochanteric fractures.
Type II: stable, displaced varus deformity with fracture of the lesser trochanter.
Type III: unstable, displaced fracture of greater trochanter with posteromedial comminution and varus deformity.
Type IV: type III with subtrochanteric component.

Limitations: designed to compare sliding versus rigid nail; other devices now available.
Reference: Kyle RF et al.

Lauge-Hansen (Ankle Fractures)

Patterns based on four principal causes; to identify surgical and other treatment approach.
supination-eversion: external or lateral rotation.
supination-adduction.
pronation-abduction.
pronation-adduction.

Limitations: interobserver disagreement; eversion a misnomer—it should be "external rotation" or "lateral rotation"; mechanism not consistent in producing specific injury.
Reference: Lauge-Hansen N.

Letts-Vincent-Gouw ("Floating Knee" Fracture in Children Involving Both Femur and Tibia)

For descriptive purposes.
Type A: both bones diaphyseal closed.
Type B: one bone metaphyseal and other diaphyseal closed.
Type C: epiphyseal and diaphyseal closed.
Type D: one open fracture.
Type E: two open fractures with major soft tissue injury.

Reference: Letts M et al.

Letournel and Judet (Acetabular Fractures)

Based on division into five basic groups (fractures of the posterior wall, posterior column, anterior wall, anterior column, and transverse fractures) to define best surgical approach for reduction.
- **A:**   posterior wall.
- **B:**   posterior column.
- **C:**   anterior wall.
- **D:**   anterior column.
- **E:**   transverse.

F: posterior column and posterior wall.
G: transverse and posterior wall.
H: T-shaped.
I: anterior and posterior hemitransverse.
J: complete, both columns.

Reference: Judet R et al.

Levine-Edwards (Axis Fracture)

Treatment based on location, displacement, and mechanism of injury.
Type I: through neural arch, no angulation, displacement to 3 mm.
Type II: through neural arch, angulation and translation.
Type IIa: through neural arch, slight or no translation but very severe angulation.
Type III: severe angulation and displacement with concomitant unilateral or bilateral facet dislocation at second and third cervical vertebrae.

Reference: Levine AM and Edwards CC.

Mallory (Femoral Shaft Fractures Occurring During Total Hip Replacement Surgery)

Based on location, prognosis, and degree of internal and external fixation required for healing.
Type I: fracture includes areas of lesser trochanter and calcar.
Type II: fracture extends beyond lesser trochanter to a point up to 4 cm proximal to the prosthetic tip.
Type III: fracture line extends below a point 4 cm above prosthetic tip.

Reference: Mallory TH et al.

Mangled Extremity Severity Score [MESS] (Degree of Injury to Soft and Hard Tissue of a Limb)

To assess the prognostic effects of injury, ischemia, shock, and age.

Skeletal/Soft Tissue
Group 1: low energy stab wounds, low caliber gun shot, simple fractures—1 point.
Group 2: medium energy, open or multiple level fractures, moderate crush injury—2 points.
Group 3: high energy, close range shotgun blast or high velocity gunshot wound—3 points.
Group 4: massive crush injury, industrial accident—4 points.

Shock Group
Group 1: normotensive; blood pressure stable at scene and during surgery—0 points.
Group 2: transient hypotension; unstable blood pressure at scene but stable when given intravenous drugs—1 point.
Group 3: prolonged hypotension; systolic blood pressure < 90 mm Hg with recovery in OR only.

Ischemia Group
Group 1: none; no signs of ischemia, pulses intact—0 points.
Group 2: mild; diminished pulses without ischemia—1 point.
Group 3: moderate; no pulse by Doppler, sluggish capillary refill and other activity, paresthesias—2 points.
Group 4: advanced; no pulse, cool, no capillary refill—3 points.

Age
Group 1: < 30 years—0 points.
Group 2: > 30–< 50 years—1 point.
Group 3: < 50 years—2 points.

Reference: Helfet DL et al.

Mason (Radial Head Fractures)

Prognosis based on displacement and comminution.
Type I: undisplaced marginal fracture.
Type II displaced segmental.
Type III: comminuted.

Type IV: comminuted with posterior elbow dislocation.

Reference: Mason ML.

Mast-Spiegel-Pappas (Distal Tibial Fractures Affecting Tibial Plafond, Pilon)

Based on mechanism of deforming load to help define a clear prognosis.

Type I: essentially malleolar fracture with large posterior plafond fragment.

Type II: spiral extension mechanism includes a spiral shaft fracture with no comminution plafond.

Type III: central compression with impaction of talus into distal tibia, graded A to C per Rüedi and Allgöwer:

  Type IIIA: cleavage fracture of articular surface without displacement.

  Type IIIB: significant fracture and dislocation of articular surface without comminution.

  Type IIIC: type IIIB with significant comminution and impaction.

Limitations: the word pilon implies impaction into a surface, which is more a posterior or rotatory displacement in types I and II.

Reference: Mast JW et al.

Mayo (Olecranon Fractures)

Surgical and closed management based on location, comminution, and stability.

Type I: undisplaced.

  IA: noncomminuted.

  IB: comminuted.

Type II: displaced, stable.

  IIA: noncomminuted.

  IIB: comminuted.

Type III: unstable.

  IA: noncomminuted.

  IB: comminuted.

Reference: Cabenela ME and Morrey BF.

Meyers-McKeever (Intercondylar Eminence Fractures of the Tibia in Children)

For surgical planning.

Type I: nondisplaced avulsion.

Type II: anterior one-third to one-half lifted with posterior rim intact.

Type III: completely displaced.

Reference: Meyers MH and McKeever FM.

Milch (Medial and Lateral Condylar Fractures of the Humerus in Children)

To define closed versus open treatment.

Type 1:   fracture line from trochlear groove to lateral superior or trochlear sulcus to medial superior; more stable on reduction (compression fracture mechanism).

Type 2:   fracture line from trochlear sulcus to lateral superior or trochlear groove to medial superior; more unstable (compression fracture–dislocation mechanism).

Reference: Milch H.

Neer (Humeral Head Fractures)

Based on location and number of fragments; to define method of treatment.

Anatomic neck: two part (neck and shaft only).

Surgical neck: below tuberosity; considered two part even if comminuted.

Greater tuberosity: may be two part, three part with anatomic neck, or four part with anatomic neck and lesser tuberosity.

Lesser tuberosity: may be two part, three part with anatomic neck, or four part with anatomic neck and greater tuberosity.

Fracture-dislocation, anterior: two part with greater tuberosity, three part with anatomic neck and greater tuberosity, four part with lesser tuberosity.

Fracture-dislocation, posterior: two part with lesser tuberosity, three part with anatomic neck, four part with greater tuberosity.

Limitations: interobserver disagreement on x-ray interpretation.
Reference: Neer CSI.

Neer-Horowitz (Proximal Humeral Physeal Fractures in Children)

Based on location.
Grade I: < 5 mm displacement.
Grade II: displaced up to one-third the width of the shaft.
Grade III: displaced from one- to two-thirds the width of the shaft.
Grade IV: displaced more than two-thirds the width of the shaft.

Reference: Neer CSI and Howrowitz BS.

Ogden (Fractures with Injury to All Bone and Cartilage Components That May Affect Growth)

To better define effects on growth, including nonphyseal growth areas.
Type I: entirely through physis.
   1A: undulates through provisional calcification of hypertrophic zone; no effect on growth.
   1B: more into degenerative cartilage zone and primary spongiosa; no effect on growth.
   1C: affects a portion of germinal layer of physis leading to bridging bar.
Type 2:   through provisional calcification and hypertrophic zone with piece of metaphysis.
   2A: attached metaphyseal fragment.
   2B: comminuted metaphyseal fragment.
   2C: shorter metaphyseal fragment that traverses most of metaphysis.
   2D: similar to type 1C; affects germinal layer of physis with growth effect.

Type 3:   fracture extends from articular surface through epiphysis up to, but not across, physis.
   3A: transverse fracture line entirely through physis.
   3B: transverse fracture line through spongiosa, leaving small portion of metaphysis with epiphysis.
   3C: local compression of physis.
   3D: nonarticular epiphysis such as ischial tuberosity.
Type 4:   fracture extends from articular surface, through epiphysis and past physis to metaphysis.
   4A: basic transepiphyseal physeal fracture.
   4B: 4A with line across portion of physis, similar to type 3.
   4C: involves nonarticular cartilaginous region such as proximal femur.
Type 5:   affects germinal layer without bony fracture.
Type 6:   involves zone of Ranvier (ring of cells at margin of physis from local contusion).
Type 7:   completely intraepiphyseal.
   7A: involves both articular cartilage and bone of secondary ossification center.
   7B: injury to cartilage growth surface on articular surface of epiphysis.
Type 8:   injury to metaphyseal growth and remodeling mechanism.
Type 9:   selective injury to diaphyseal growth mechanism, appositional.

Limitations: complexity.
Reference: Ogden JA.

Ogden (Tibial Tuberosity Fractures in Children)

Need for surgical reduction and fixation.
Type 1:   injury to most distal part of tuberosity.
   1A: mild displacement, relatively stable, possible propagation into main ossification center.

1B: separation of fragment from metaphysis with or without separation from rest of the secondary ossification center.

Type 2:   separation of entire ossification center of tuberosity with possible propagation into main ossification center of proximal end of tibia; fracture of tuberosity segment at juncture of main ossification centers of tibia and tuberosity.

2A: without comminution of ossification center.

2B: with comminution of ossification center.

Type 3:   more severe separation of fragments; propagation of fracture through main proximal tibial epiphysis into joint; disruption of articular surface under anterior attachments of medial or lateral meniscus or both.

3A: single displaced fragment.

3B: comminuted displaced fragments.

Reference: Ogden JA ct al.

Olecranon Fractures (no eponym)

Type I: involves only proximal third of articular surface or no articular surface.

Type II: involves middle third of articular surface.

Type III: may occur in conjunction with anterior displacement of the radius.

Reference: Crenshaw AH.

Pauwels (Femoral Neck Fractures)

Based on angle of fracture to define stability of fracture in management.

Type I: angle of fracture line is 30 degrees from the horizontal

Type II: angle of fracture line is 50 degrees from the horizontal

Type III: angle of fracture line is 70 degrees from the horizontal.

Reference: Pauwels F.

Pipkin (Hip Dislocations with Femoral Head Fracture)

Based on location of fracture head and neck when associated with a posterior hip dislocation (type V Epstein Thompson); to determine prognosis for long-term outcome

Type I: posterior dislocation of the hip with fracture of the femoral head caudad to fovea centralis.

Type II: posterior dislocation of the hip with fracture of the femoral head cephalad to fovea centralis.

Type III: type I or II with femoral neck fracture.

Type IV: type I, II, or III with associated acetabular fracture.

Reference: Pipkin G.

Poland (Childhood Fractures Involving Epiphysis)

Entirely descriptive, written at time of development of radiographs.

Type I: separation across physis only

Type II: separation across physis with fragment metaphysis

Type III: separation of portion of epiphysis across physis

Type IV: separation of both portions of epiphysis from physis.

Reference: Poland J.

Quénu and Küss modified (Fractures-Dislocations of Tarsometatarsal Articulation)

To determine the magnitude of soft tissue injury, displacement plane, prognosis, and treatment.

Type A: total incongruity; all five metatarsals displaced in same direction.

Type B: partial incongruity:
medial dislocation
lateral dislocation

Type C: divergent usually between first and second ray:
total—all five rays involved.
partial—some lateral rays intact.

Reference: Hardcastle PH et al.

Riseborough and Radin (Distal Humeral Intercondylar T Fractures)

Based on roentgenographic analysis to compare closed versus open treatment.

Type 1:   undisplaced fracture between capitellum and trochlea.

Type 2:   nondisplaced T or Y fracture, with fracture exiting from groove proximally between condyle and then dividing transversely or obliquely across the shaft separating the condyles from each other and the shaft; no appreciable separation or rotation on AP roentgenogram.

Type 3:   significant separation with rotational displacement of condyles.

Type 4:   severe comminution of articular surface and wide condylar separation.

Reference: Riseborough EJ and Radin EL.

Rockwood (Acromioclavicular Separations)

To determine degree of injury or need for surgical intervention.

Type I: neither acromioclavicular or coracoclavicular ligament torn.

Type II: acromioclavicular ligament torn but coracoclavicular ligament intact.

Type III: both acromioclavicular and coracoclavicular ligament torn.

Type IV: Both ligaments torn and clavicle displaced posteriorly through trapezius.

Type V: both ligaments torn and wide superior separation of the clavicle.

Type VI: both ligaments torn and distal clavicle caught inferior to coracoid and posterior to conjoined tendon.

Reference: Rockwood CA.

Rowe and Lowell (Central Fracture Dislocations of Acetabulum)

To define surgical planning and risk of complications.

Type I: undisplaced (single line or stellate).

Type II: inner wall fractures.

Type IIA: femoral head reduced under acetabular dome initially.

Type IIB: femoral head out, reduced under acetabular dome initially.

Type III: superior dome fractures.

Type IIIA: acetabulum generally congruent with femoral head.

Type IIIB: acetabulum incongruent with femoral head.

Type IV: bursting fracture (all elements of acetabulum involved).

Type IVA: fractures with congruity between femoral head and acetabular dome.

Type IVB: fractures with incongruity between femoral head and acetabular dome.

Reference: Rowe CR and Lowell JD.

Rüedi and Allgöwer (Distal Tibial Pilon Fractures)

Degree of comminution and displacement of articular fragments; to define nature of management of pilon fractures of the distal tibia.

Type A: cleavage fracture of the articular surface without major dislocation of the fragments.

Type B: significant fracture and dislocation of the articular surface without comminution.

Type C: severe comminution and impaction of tibial articular surface.

Reference: Rüedi T and Allgöwer M.

Russell-Taylor (High Proximal Femoral Fractures)

To predict effectiveness of closed nailing techniques.

Group I: does not involve piriformis fossa.

Group Ia: comminution and fracture line extends from below lesser trochanter to femoral isthmus.

Group Ib: fracture line and comminution involving area from lesser trochanter to femoral isthmus.

Group II: involvement of piriformis fossa.

Group IIa: fracture extends from lesser trochanter to isthmus with involvement of piriformis fossa (seen on lateral roentgenogram).

Group IIb: fracture extends into the piriformis fossa (seen on lateral roentgenogram) with significant medial comminution and loss of lesser trochanteric continuity.

Reference: Russell TA.

Salter-Harris (Fractures Involving the Physis in Children)

To predict growth disturbance and need for exact reduction.

Type I: fracture line across physis only.

Type II: fracture line across physis with portion through metaphysis.

Type III: fracture through physis and portion of epiphysis.

Type IV: fracture line through epiphysis, crosses physis, and out metaphysis.

Type V: crush injury to physis.

Reference: Salter RB and Harris WR.

Samilson-Preito (Degenerative Change Associated with Shoulder Dislocation)

Relating degenerative change to timing of treatment.

mild: inferior exostosis of humeral head or glenoid < 3 mm in size on AP radiograph.

moderate: inferior exostosis of humeral head or glenoid between 3 and 7 mm in size with slight joint irregularity.

severe: > 8 mm osteophyte with joint narrowing and sclerosis.

Reference: Samilson RL and Preito V.

Schatzker (Tibial Plateau and Proximal Tibial Fracture Patterns)

Based on pathoanatomic factors, etiologic factors, and therapeutic features; to determine treatment of fracture of the tibial plateau and proximal tibia.

Type I: pure cleavage.

Type II: cleavage combined with depression.

Type III: pure central depression.

Type IV: fracture of medial condyle.

Type V: bicondylar fractures.

Type VI: plateau fracture with dissociation of tibial metaphysis and diaphysis.

Limitations: type 5 could be divided into axial, laterally tilted, and medially tilted.

Reference: Schatzker J et al.

Seinsheimer (Femoral Intertrochanteric and Subtrochanteric Fractures)

Based on number of fragments and the location and configuration of fracture lines; to select method of surgical fixation.

Type I: nondisplaced or < 1 mm displacement.

Type II: two part fractures.

Type IIA: transverse.

Type IIB: spiral with lesser trochanter attached to proximal fragment.

Type IIC: spiral with lesser trochanter attached to distal fragment.

Type III: three part fractures.

Type IIIA: spiral with lesser trochanter a part of the proximal fragment.

Type IIIB: spiral with lesser trochanter a butterfly fragment.

Type IV: comminuted with four or more fragments.

Type V: subtrochanteric-intertrochanteric configuration.

Limitations: lesser trochanteric continuity and involvement of piriformis fossa a major factor of
stability.
Reference: Seinsheimer FI.

Stewart and Milford (Hip Dislocation with Associated Acetabular and Femoral Head Fracture)

For prognosis.

Grade I: simple dislocation without acetabular
fracture.

Grade II: dislocation with one or more large acetabular fractures but stable after reduction.

Grade III: explosive or blast fracture with disintegration of acetabular rim, unstable after
reduction.

Grade IV: dislocation with fracture of head or
neck of femur.

Reference: Stewart MJ and Milford LW.

Stress Injury to Bone (Stress "Fractures")

To grade relative state or level of effect on bone.

Grade 0:   positive bone scan in an asymptomatic
subject with negative radiographs. Seen only in
research surveys.

Grade I: local symptoms associated with a positive bone scan and negative radiographs.

Grade II: local symptoms with a positive bone
scan and minimal findings on radiographs.

Grade III: local symptoms with a positive bone
scan and clear evidence of bone absorption on
radiographs.

Grade IV: local symptoms with a positive bone
scan and actual bone fracture.

Thompson and Epstein (Hip Dislocation with Acetabular Fracture)

Based on size and stability of associated fractures to
determine outcome of treatment.

Type I: with or without minor fracture.

Type II: with a large single posterior acetabular
rim fracture.

Type III: with comminution of the posterior rim
with or without a major fragment.

Type IV: with fracture of the acetabular floor.

Type V: with fracture of the femoral head.

Limitations: does not take into account size and place
of femoral head fragment (see Pipkin classification).
Reference: Thompson VP and Epstein HC.

Tile (Pelvic Fractures)

Numbers based on mechanism and letters based on
vertical and rotational stability (A, stable; B, rotationally unstable and vertically stable; C, rotationally
and vertically unstable); to determine if surgical or
closed treatment is indicated.

Type AI: does not involve pelvic ring such as
avulsion fracture and fractured ilium.

Type A2:   stable pelvic ring such as low energy
fall in elderly; minimal displacement.

Type BI: "open book" or anterior compression
injury.

Type B2:   lateral compression force with ipsilateral fracture.

Type B3:   lateral compression force with contralateral fractures.

Type CI: unilateral fracture with both anterior and
posterior complex.

Type C2:   bilateral injuries.

Type C3:   vertical shear fracture with fractured
acetabulum.

Reference: Tile M.

Torode and Zieg (Pelvic Fractures in Children)

Type I: avulsion of the bony elements of the pelvis.

Type II: iliac wing fractures.

Type III: simple ring fracture including pubic rami or disruption of pubic symphysis.

Type IV: unstable ring fracture including straddle (bilateral pubic rami) fractures, pubic rami or symphysis with posterior elements or sacroiliac joint disruption, anterior fracture with acetabular fracture.

Reference: Torode I and Zieg S.

Tronzo (Intertrochanteric Fractures)

Based on reduction potential.

Type I: incomplete trochanteric fracture reduced anatomically with traction.

Type II: uncomminuted fracture of both trochanters, with or without displacement, reduced with traction; anatomic reduction usually achieved.

Type III: comminuted fracture with large lesser trochanteric fragment, posterior wall exploded, fracture line makes beak of inferior femoral neck unstable.

Type IV: comminuted and unstable disengaged trochanteric fractures with explosion of posterior wall and medial displacement of femoral neck spike.

Type V: trochanteric fracture with reverse obliquity (downward from a medial to lateral direction).

Reference: Tronzo RG.

Tscherne (Classification for Tibial Fractures with Associated Soft Tissue Injury and Extent of Contamination)

To define risk of surgical management.

Grade C0:   simple fracture configuration with little or no soft tissue injury.

Grade CI: superficial abrasion, mild to moderately severe fracture configuration.

Grade CII: deep contaminated abrasion with local damage to skin or muscle, moderately severe to severe fracture configuration.

Grade CIII: extensive contusion or crushing of the skin or destruction of the muscle, severe fracture.

Limitations: definition of severity is lacking, no vascular annotation.

Reference: Oestern HH and Tscherne H.

Watson-Jones (Tibial Tuberosity Fractures in Children)

To determine need for surgical reduction and fixation.

Type I: small fragment displaced superiorly.

Type II: larger fragment hinged upwards involving secondary center of ossification.

Type III: displaced fracture passes posteriorly and proximally across epiphyseal plate.

Limitations: does not account for potential entry of type II into knee joint.

Reference: Watson-Jones.

Weber [Danis-Weber] (Ankle Fractures)

Based on the appearance of the fibular fracture; to define direction of causative and thus reducing forces.

Type A: caused by internal rotation and adduction, produces a transverse fracture of the lateral malleolus below the plafond.

Type B: caused by external rotation resulting in an oblique fracture of the lateral malleolus.

Type C-1:   abduction injury with oblique fracture of fibula proximal to disrupted tibiofibular ligament (medial malleolus or deltoid ligament may be affected).

Type C-2:   abduction–external rotation injury with more proximal fracture of fibula and more extensive disruption of interosseous membrane (medial melleolus or deltoid ligament may be affected).

Reference: Weber BG.

Winquist-Hansen (Femoral Shaft Fractures)

Based on comminution and stability; to determine if static locking nail is necessary.

Grade I: comminuted with small piece not affecting stability.

Grade II: comminuted with $\geq$ 50% abutting major cortex sufficient to prevent rotation and shortening with good proximal and distal nail purchase.

Grade III: < 50% major cortex contact allowing rotation or shortening; requires proximal and distal crossfixation.

Grade IV: no fixed contact between major proximal and distal fragment; requires proximal and distal crossfixation.

Segmental transverse: segmental transverse allowing stability without crossfixation.

Segmental oblique and transverse: requires proximal and distal crossfixation.

Spiral: requires proximal and distal crossfixation.

Proximal transverse: requires proximal crossfixation.

Proximal oblique: requires proximal and distal crossfixation.

Proximal comminuted: requires proximal and distal crossfixation.

Distal transverse: requires distal crossfixation.

Distal oblique: requires proximal and distal crossfixation.

Distal comminuted: requires proximal and distal crossfixation.

Reference: Winquist RA and Hansen ST.

Young (Pelvic Fractures)

Radiologic assessment based on probable mechanism to recognize pattern at high risk for hemorrhage or related injury in acute setting.

LC: transverse fracture of pubic rami, ipsilateral, or posterolateral to posterior injury.

I: sacral compression on side of impact.

II: crescent (iliac wing) fracture on side of impact.

III: LC-I or LC-II injury on side of impact: contralateral open-book (APC) injury.

APC (anterior-posterior compression):   symphyseal diastasis and/or longitudinal rami fractures.

I: slight widening of pubic symphysis and/or anterior SI joint; stretched but intact SI, sacrotuberous, and sacrospinous ligaments; intact posterior SI ligaments.

II: widened anterior SI joint; disrupted anterior SI, sacrotuberous, and sacrospinous ligaments; intact SI posterior ligaments.

III: complete SI joint disruption with lateral displacement; disrupted anterior SI, sacrotuberous, sacrospinous ligaments; disrupted posterior SI ligaments.

VS (vertical shear):   symphyseal diastasis or vertical displacement anteriorly and posteriorly, usually through the SI joint, occasionally through the iliac wing and/or sacrum.

CM (combination):   combination of other injury patterns, LC/VS being the most common.

Reference: Young JWR et al.

Zickle (Subtrochanteric Fracture)

To define a method of fixation.

Type IA: short oblique fracture from above the lesser trochanter to the lower lateral shaft.

Type IB: long oblique fracture from above the lesser trochanter to the lower lateral shaft; comminution may be present.

Type IC: transverse fracture just below lesser trochanter to a point near the isthmus.

Reference: Zickle RE.

DISLOCATIONS

This section is divided into two parts: The first is a general list of terms applied to all joints, and the second is a list by specific anatomic location. Post-traumatic arthritis, recurrent dislocation, limitation of joint motion, joint mice, instability, and/or avascular necrosis may accompany various dislocation types. Hand and wrist dislocations are very complicated and, therefore, are discussed separately in Chapter 10, *The Hand and Wrist.*

General Dislocations

closed d.: one in which the skin is not broken. Formerly called **simple d.**

complete d.: one that completely separates the joint surfaces.

complicated d.: associated with surrounding tissue injuries.

consecutive d.: the luxated bone has changed its position since its first displacement.

developmental dysplasia: exists in infancy with or without dislocation of the hips. Formerly called **congenital d.**

frank d.: a complete dislocation in any area.

habitual d.: one that repeatedly recurs; usually congenital.

incomplete d.: subluxation with only slight displacement.

old d.: inflammatory changes have occurred.

open d.: one in which the skin is broken. Formerly called **compound d.**

partial d.: incomplete dislocation.

pathologic d.: results from paralysis or disease in the joint or surrounding area.

primitive d.: bones remain as originally displaced.

recent d.: there is no complicating inflammation.

recurrent d.: repetitive dislocation with or without adequate trauma.

traumatic d.: caused by serious injury.

Specific Dislocations (By Anatomy)

Cervical Dislocation
Bell-Dally d.: nontraumatic dislocation of the first cervical vertebra (atlas).

Shoulder Dislocations
A/C joint separation: acromioclavicular joint disruption and separation.

anterior shoulder d.: involves the glenohumeral joint with the humeral head displaced anteriorly and inferiorly; may be associated with one of the following:
  Bankhart lesion: seen surgically as detachment of the glenoid labrum and sometimes a bone fragment from the glenoid. **Perthes-Bankhart lesion.**
  Hill-Sachs lesion: seen radiographically as an indentation of the posteromedial humeral head, which occurred at the time of the dislocation. Also called **hatchet head deformity.**

locked scapula: rare scapulothoracic dissociation with entrapment of scapula into chest wall or with anterior displacement. Usually associated with severe neurovascular injury.

luxatio erecta: dislocation of shoulder so that the arm stands straight up over the head.

posterior shoulder d.: involves the glenohumeral joint with the humeral head displaced posteriorly.

reverse Bankhart lesion: seen surgically as a detachment of the rim of the posterior labrum from the glenoid rim.

reverse Hill-Sachs lesion: defect of anteromedial humeral head; may be seen on radiographs or at surgery.

sternoclavicular joint separation: disruption of the sternoclavicular joint.

subcoracoid d.: glenohumeral dislocation with the humeral head displaced medially.

subglenoid d.: glenohumeral dislocation with the humeral head displaced inferiorly.

Elbow Dislocations

direct injury d.:   posterior displacement of the olecranon.

divergent d.:   ulna and radius are dislocated separately.

milkmaid's d.:   dislocation of radial head superiorly and anteriorly. Also called **superior radial head d., milkmaid's elbow.**

Monteggia f.-d.:   fracture of the ulna with a radial head dislocation.

Spine Dislocations

spondylolisthesis: not a true dislocation, because it rarely occurs as a result of trauma or muscle imbalance, but is a forward displacement of one vertebral body over another; usually occurs as a result of a defect in the pars interarticularis.

spondylolysis: acute (traumatic) dissociation of pars interarticularis or posterior elements (lamina) with or without spondylolisthesis.

unilateral facet subluxation: dislocation of one of the two facets at any level; most common in the cervical region.

Hip Dislocations

anterior d.:   involves the femoral head anteriorly.

central d.:   one in which the femur jams into the acetabulum. Also called **bursting d.**

developmental dysplasia of the hip (DDH):   formerly called **congenital dysplasia of the hip (CDH), congenital d., luxatio coxae congenita.**

luxatio perinealis: dislocation of femoral head into the perineum.

Monteggia d.:   involves femoral head to near the anterosuperior spine of the ilium; hip joint dislocation.

Otto pelvis: gradual central displacement of the femur by unknown causes.

posterior d.:   femoral head slips posteriorly; more common than anterior d.

posterior f.-d.:   chip f. of the acetabulum with a posterior d. of the femoral head.

Patella (Dislocation vs. Subluxation)

One of the most common dislocations is a patellar dislocation, erroneously called a dislocated knee. The dislocated patella simply goes out of the femoral groove. A subluxation is a tendency for the patella to move partially out of the groove.

horseback rider's knee: dislocation of fibular head. Injury associated with rider hitting leg against a post.

knee d.:   slippage of the femur off the tibia. Commonly called a **true knee d.** to distinguish it from a dislocated patella.

parachute jumper's d.:   anterior dislocation of proximal fibula.

Ankle and Foot Dislocations

Chopart d.:   navicula and cuboid dislocate across talus and calcaneus (Chopart joint).

fracture-dislocation of ankle: any combination of tibial and fibular fractures resulting in a displaced talus.

Lisfranc d.:   tarsometatarsal dislocation; not to be confused with a **frank dislocation,** which denotes a complete dislocation in any area.

medial swivel d.:   navicula is displaced medially on a fracture of the midtalus, but the calcaneocuboid joint stays intact and the subtalar joint is not dislocated. The calcaneus rotates on the intact interosseous talocalcaneal ligament.

metatarsophalangeal joint d.:   occurs at the base of the toe.

Nélaton d.:   dislocation of the ankle in which the talus is forced between the end of the tibia and fibula.

Smith d.:   upward and backward dislocation of the metatarsals and medial cuneiform bone.

subastragalar d.:   separation of the calcaneus and navicular bone from the talus.

tarsal d.:   usually an ankle dislocation associated with a fracture of the neck of the talus; commonly an open injury. This term may also denote other tarsal bone dislocation such as of the cuneiform and cuboid.

SUBLUXATIONS

Subluxations are categorized by anatomic location as there are no eponymic terms.

facet s.: malalignment of opposing facet, allowing one cervical body to rotate around another.

radioulnar s.: involves the distal ulnar radial joint.

sacroiliac s.: involves the sacroiliac joint; usually associated with a pelvic fracture and other dissociations of the pelvic ring.

shoulder s.: involves the glenohumeral joint (as opposed to the acromioclavicular joint).

wrist s.: involves the proximal carpal bones on the radius and ulna.

STRAINS AND SPRAINS

The term **strain** applies to an injury of muscle or its tendon. The term **sprain** applies to ligamentous injury. However, the term *strain* is often interchanged with the word *sprain*. In part, this is because both injuries can occur at the same time, such as a low back strain. It is clear at the time of injury that there is an acute tear or stretching of a back muscle, but there can also be a concurrent injury to the ligaments or disk tissue. If the symptoms continue, the sprain component becomes more apparent because the muscle normally recovers very rapidly.

Strains are often associated with injury to muscle caused by strenuous exercise without preconditioning and are usually referred to the back region. **Sprains** and ruptures of ligaments occur in the knee, ankle joints, and, sometimes, shoulder. At the ankle, a sudden twisting motion with full weight on the side of the foot can cause a sprain. A fracture may occur as well. There are many terms for muscle, tendon, and ligament injuries as follows.

Shoulder Sprain

acromioclavicular s.: stretching of the ligaments of the acromioclavicular joint but without any disruption. Often the term **shoulder sprain** implies this specific condition, as opposed to an effect on the glenohumeral joint.

Knee Sprains

anterior cruciate s.: commonly associated with a medial collateral ligament tear, dislocated patella, or torn meniscus; may occur as an isolated injury; allows the femur to slide backward on the tibia (tibia slides forward on the femur).

lateral collateral s.: isolated injury that may be associated with rupture of the biceps femoris tendon, anterior and/or posterior cruciate ligament, and iliotibial tract; allows the joint to open laterally, and with some associated injuries allows the lateral femur to slide backward on the tibia (tibia slides forward on the femur).

medial collateral s.: occurs as a result of a clipping injury; may be associated with a cruciate ligament tear, patellar dislocation, or torn medial meniscus; allows the joint to open medially, and with some associated injuries allows the medial femur to slide backward on the tibia (tibia slides forward on the femur).

posterior cruciate s.: allows the tibia to slide backward on the femur; often seen alone; allows the femur to slide forward on the tibia (tibia slides backward on the femur).

posterior oblique s.: part of the medial collateral ligament s. or rupture complex; allows the medial femur to slide backward on the tibia (medial tibia slides forward on the femur).

Ankle Sprains

deltoid s.: commonly occurs with a fibular fracture; rarely an isolated rupture.

fibular collateral s.: general term for sprain or rupture of one or more of three ligaments on the lateral side of the ankle.

   anterior talofibular s.: most common sprain or rupture of the ankle ligaments.

   calcaneofibular s.: sprain or rupture of

middle of three lateral ankle ligaments, usu-ally associated with other injuries.

tibiofibular s.:   without rupture, there is no spread-ing of the tibia and fibula; with rupture, a diasta-sis occurs; syndesmotic sprain, high ankle sprain.

SPORTS-RELATED INJURIES

Injuries from vocational and avocational sports activities have greatly increased over the past 2 de-cades. In the United States, more than 2 million sports-related injuries occur annually. Much time and effort have been devoted to the more immediate identification and treatment of these athletic injuries, which has led to the advent of sports medicine.

Sports medicine has also had an effect on the ac-tivities themselves. Exercise as a science has opened new dimensions in health care. Improved sports equipment and design are rapidly being developed, thanks to the combined efforts of engineers and medical support personnel. Also, rule changes are of-ten made in consideration of the safety of the players.

Many sports injuries are a result of muscle and tendon overuse rather than a specific sprain or strain. Some of these conditions are so common in certain sports that they are named after the sport, for ex-ample, baseball elbow.

This terminology applies to the nonathletic pop-ulation, as well, who experience similar conditions. This may be the result of an increase in activity from a previously sedentary, nonactive lifestyle, or other factors such as degenerative joint disease. The classic example is that of tennis elbow. Many people with this problem cannot attribute it to a change in activ-ity, such as painting or tennis, but have a condition of the cervical spine that causes the muscle of the fore-arm to tighten, resulting in overuse of the tendon.

The following terms are related mostly to ath-letic injuries of the soft tissues. Fracture-related sports injuries are listed in the preceding section.

ALPSA lesion: anterior labrum of the glenoid tears during anterior shoulder dislocation and strips the glenoid periosteum, leaving labrum attached to periosteum. This gives the shoulder the arthroscopic appearance of an intact labrum (ALPSA: **a**nterior **l**abrum **p**osterior **s**uperior to **a**nterior).

archer's shoulder: recurrent posterior disloca-tion or subluxation of the shoulder.

backpack palsy: similar to Erb palsy, a brachial plexus overpull caused by a heavy pack with shoulder straps, resulting in palsy of the fifth and sixth cervical nerve muscle distribution.

baseball elbow: condition of baseball pitchers where overstress on the medial side of the elbow causes medial collateral ligament bone spurs, myositis, ulnar nerve injuries, or posterior com-partment loose bodies. Also referred to as **jave-lin thrower's elbow.**

baseball finger: acute rupture of the terminal end of the distal extensor tendon. This may be ei-ther intratendinous or bony and is a result of a di-rect axial blow to the digit. The injury causes an inability to extend the distal interphalangeal joint (extensor lag). There is usually full passive movement of the digit. Also called **mallet finger.**

basketball foot: subtalar dislocation of the foot.

BIL lesion: **b**iceps **i**nterval **l**esion seen in rotator cuff at biceps tendon and subcapularis muscle. Pain and swelling occur over intertubercular groove.

black-dot heel: small dark spot on the heel fat-pad caused by blood under the skin on the lateral side where there is repeated trauma to heel in athletic activity or shear stress in running. Also called **black heel syndrome.**

bowler's thumb: irritation of the flexor tendon of the thumb with increased nerve sensation on the lateral side caused by the repeated grasping of a large bowling ball.

boxer's f.:   fracture of the fifth metacarpal head with volar angulation. This is usually seen due to punching a wall or hard object.

breaststroker's knee: irritation of the medial

capsule of the knee, tibial collateral ligament, or patellar cartilage caused by repeated thrusts of the limbs by a breaststroke swimmer.

coach's finger: proximal interphalangeal joint dislocation in finger.

charley horse: muscle injury caused by direct contact (e.g., common soccer injury caused by contact between someone's knee thrust into the patient's thigh).

cross-over syndrome: extensor tendon inflammation at the wrist seen in kayak and canoe sports enthusiasts.

flexor origin syndrome: tendonitis originating at the flexor wad of five at the medial elbow. Also called **medial epicondylitis, reverse tennis elbow.**

football ankle: area of ill-localized pain in midmetatarsophalangeal part of foot above malleoli. X-ray changes show exostosis or loose bodies.

football finger: avulsion of the deep flexor tendon of the distal phalanx of the ring finger. Often occurs when trying to tackle an opponent by hooking the finger over the pants belt line; **ruger jerscy finger.**

gamekeeper's thumb: a traumatic rupture of the ulnar collateral ligament of the metacarpophalangeal (MCP) joint of the thumb, usually a hyperabduction injury; skier's thumb.

gobies: rock-induced skin abrasions that are observed on the fingers and dorsal surfaces of hands in rock climbers. Also known as **bouldering** and **face climbing.**

golfer's elbow: inflammation at the origin of the wrist and finger flexor muscles of the inner elbow. Also called **thrower's elbow, medial epicondylitis,** and **reverse tennis elbow.**

handlebar palsy: palsy of the muscles of the hand innervated by the ulnar nerve, caused by pressure against bicycle handlebar.

heel spur: area of inflammation at the proximal attachment of the plantar fascia; usually involves the median tubercle of the plantar surface of the calcaneus; often seen in runners and commonly

the result of excessive joint pronation. Anything that causes stress on the plantar fascia (weakened feet, structural deformity, or excessive pronation of the subtalar joint) will encourage the development of a heel spur.

hip pointer: very painful irritation of the insertion of abdominal muscles along the superior iliac crest. Pain localized here can also represent the pull of a thigh muscle in that region.

hockey player's hip: painful bone bruise of the greater trochanter caused by landing on the ice.

iliotibial band syndrome: condition seen in distance runners and other endurance athletes; pain on the lateral side of the knee just anterior to the lateral collateral ligaments due to swelling in a bursa or thickening of the distal expansion of the iliotibial band.

impingement syndrome: alludes to symptomatic compression on the rotator cuff by overhanging acromioclavicular structures, the anterolateral acromion, and acromioclavicular ligament; graded according to the **Neer staging system.**
> **Stage I:**   inflammation and edema of the rotator cuff.
> **Stage II:**   degenerative fibrosis.
> **Stage III:**   partial or full thickness tear.
> **coracoid impingement syndrome:**   specific impingement of the rotator cuff and lesser tuberosity by the coracoid process.

Jersey finger: an injury to the ring finger seen commonly in football and rugby players. This is a closed rupture of the flexor digitorum profundus (FDP). There are three types:
1. FDP retracted to the palm with total loss of blood supply.
2. FDP retracts to the PIP joint with partial loss of blood supply.
3. FDP retracts to the A4 pulley with a large bone fragment; blood supply is usually intact.

jogger's heel: irritation of the fibrous and fatty tissue covering the heel due to striking the ground surface when jogging.

jumper's knee: infrapatellar tendonitis, often seen in athletes who jump as part of that sport, for example, basketball, skiing, and volleyball.

linebacker's arm (tackler's arm): a myositis ossificans reaction in the lateral brachial muscle, usually seen in the midarm of tacklers.

Lisfranc injury: low velocity injury of tarso-metatarsal joints (Lisfranc joint) due to forced plantar flexion in rotation with or without abduction, as seen in runners and basketball players. The injury was first described as one sustained during a fall from a horse while the foot is caught in the stirrup. The injuries may be severe enough to include fractures or dislocations as opposed to a lesser sprain.

little leaguer's elbow: in children, a traction injury of the elbow on the medial epicondyle caused by prolonged pitching or throwing. Serious in that it may lead to fragmentation of the bone and disturbance of growth.

little leaguer's shoulder: traction injury to the shoulder in the growth plate of the proximal humerus that may lead to a painful shoulder and eventual deformity if throwing is continued.

muscle cramps: a sudden cramp in the hamstring and calf muscles usually during athletic activities. Occurs often in athletes because of overuse of an undertrained muscle or inadequate salt or water intake during hot weather. This term is used diversely to specify a hamstring and calf muscle spasm or a contusion to the quadriceps.

ring man shoulder: bony resorption or sclerosis at the insertion of the pectoralis major muscle of upper arm. Seen in gymnasts who use rings.

rotator cuff injury: inflammation or rupture of one or more of the tendons that lie deep in the shoulder and bridge the glenohumeral joint. This type of injury is inhibiting in pitchers and tennis players, in particular, and can be caused by excessive use, direct blow, or stretch injury.

runner's bump: prominence of the posterior heel at the point of insertion of the Achilles tendon; associated with distance running.

runner's knee: tight and tense condition of quadriceps muscle of thigh that directs pain to knee.

sailboarder's injury: stirrup-type injury that occurs when surfer falls from board with foot caught in strap, causing a forced equinus position with disruption of dorsal stabilizers at Lisfranc joint. Also found in horseback riders.

shin splints: pain in the shin that follows repeated stress such as running or walking long distances without conditioning. Describes a painful condition rather than a specific anatomic lesion. The most common causes are posterior tibial tendonitis, stress fracture of tibia, muscle strain, periostitis, periosteal avulsion, fascial hernia, stress fracture, and anterior tibial compartment syndrome with the inability of blood to reach the muscle (ischemia) because of compartmental swelling during increased activity. Also known as **medial tibial stress syndrome.**

shoulder apprehension: apprehension of the patient during shoulder abduction and external rotation due to glenohumeral subluxation (usually in patients with a previous shoulder dislocation).

shoulder pointer: a tearing of the anterior deltoid muscle leading to a distinct point of discomfort at the origin (immediate vicinity of the acromioclavicular joint) of the deltoid muscle.

SLAP lesion: **s**uperior **l**abrum from **a**nterior to **p**osterior tear that occurs along line from biceps tendon attachment to superior labrum. Condition causes shoulder pain with throwing motion.

spear tackler's spine: cervical spine injury in contact sports (e.g., football) where an individual spear tackles opponent head-on (with top of helmet). Findings may include cervical cord or brachial plexus neuropraxia or preexisting posttraumatic abnormalities. Condition may lead to posttraumatic arthritis.

surfer's knots: lower limb and foot nodular swelling with possible bony changes due to trauma and pressure from using a surfboard.

tennis elbow: inflammation of the wrist and finger extensor muscles near their origin at the elbow. Also called **lateral epicondylitis.**

tennis leg: tear of the medial head of the gastrocnemius or plantaris muscle, often seen in tennis players.

tennis toe (marathoner's toe): subungual hematoma causing a black toenail. Usually painless and requires no treatment.

turf-toe: an acute injury of the first metatarsophalangeal joint as a result of hyperextension, resulting in reduced range of motion. Classically described in football players on artificial turf but can occur in any sport.

weight-lifter's shoulder: osteolysis of the lateral aspect of the clavicle as seen in weight lifters.

whiplash: a stretch injury to the neck that includes the muscles, ligaments, and disks of the cervical spine. Caused by an acceleration (forward movement) or deceleration (backward movement) of the head as in a vehicular accident. A direct head injury may also cause a whiplash because of the resultant forces on the neck. Damage may involve minor neck ligament sprain, rupture, or subluxation (partial dislocation). This term denotes a complex of symptoms including pain and stiffness and is sometimes biomechanically inaccurate because there are many mechanisms that can produce these symptoms.

Chapter 2

Musculoskeletal Diseases and Related Terms

Basic scientific and clinical research continues to improve our understanding of many musculoskeletal diseases. Improved biochemical knowledge and imaging techniques have changed the classification of some musculoskeletal disorders. This knowledge has also added an array of "new" diseases. This edition reflects many of those changes.

The musculoskeletal reaction to bone and soft-tissue lesions can be due to many factors: bones fracture or dislocate; joints become arthritic; bursae around joints become inflamed; muscles, ligaments, and tendons become strained, stretched, weakened, or torn; muscles may spasm or atrophy; cartilage may degenerate; disks become compressed; and vascular and metabolic changes may occur that affect both bone and soft tissue. All of these areas of the musculoskeletal system can be affected temporarily or permanently.

The terms *disease* and *syndrome* are sometimes used interchangeably but to be precise they have different meanings.

A **disease** is a specific result of a pathologic condition that presents as a group of symptoms associated with physical and/or psychologic changes. A disease may be classified acute or chronic, congenital or acquired, focal or systemic, malignant or benign, and contagious or noninfectious. Diseases may also be characterized as hereditary, inflammatory, metabolic, degenerative, or idiopathic.

A **syndrome** is a group of symptoms that occur together and are associated with any morbid condition that constitutes the scenario for a specific disease.

Many diseases of the musculoskeletal system overlap into other specialties, such as neurology, neurosurgery, and vascular surgery, and the patient's symptoms often present as an orthopaedic problem. Therefore, terminology of other specialties is included as they relate to orthopaedics.

Both soft-tissue and skeletal disorders can be associated with **referred pain,** which means that the pain is felt at a site other than its origin. Pain is a perception, and as with all perceptions, illusions are possible. For example, pain can originate at the lumbar region but be felt some point in the lower limb. Referred pain can also occur with direct pressure on a spinal nerve root in the back (a form of sciatica). In most cases of a back disorder with pain perceived to be in the lower limb, actual pressure is not on a spinal nerve root. Pain in the distribution of the muscles supplied by a specific spinal nerve is called **sclerotomal** pain. Pain in the sensory distribution of a spinal nerve is called **dermatomal** pain. The distinction is important in that a dermatomic distribution of pain tends to be more distinctive of actual nerve root irritation.

The goal in the treatment of musculoskeletal diseases and conditions is to help the patient become functional and productive as quickly as possible through a conservative approach, surgery, or other measures. The musculoskeletal diseases are defined here by tissue type and anatomic location.

BONE DISEASES

Osteo-, the Greek root for bone, can be used in various combinations that include more than one root, for example, osteochondral (bone and cartilage), or in terms in which *osteo-* is preceded by other terms, for example, *polyostotic fibrous dysplasia.* The "os" terms relate to small bones (**ossicles**), especially those in the foot, and are named in Chapter 11.

Bone disease types are grouped together for purposes of identifying similar or related processes by anatomic or eponymic terms. However, eponyms that are used more frequently than the common (Greek or Latin) terms are listed separately. The bone diseases are divided as follows: *osteo-* root diseases, infectious bone diseases, tumors of bone, miscellaneous Latin and English terms, and eponymic bone diseases.

Osteo- Root Diseases

hyperosteoidosis: excess osteoid tissue due to defective mineralization (osteomalacia) and to normal but delayed mineralization; **hyperparathyroidism, hyperthyroidism, Paget d.**

ostealgia: pain within bone.

osteitis: inflammation of bone with enlargement, tenderness, dull aching; many varieties.

osteitis condensans (piriform sclerosis ilium):   increased density of the ilium near the sacroiliac joint of unknown etiology; may be associated with back pain.

osteitis deformans: disease of unknown origin resulting in bowing of long bones, and deformation of flat bones; **Paget d.**

osteitis fibrosa cystica: bone disease caused by hyperfunction of parathyroid gland; **osteoplastica.**

osteitis ossificans: an older general term denoting an inflammatory process in bone that results in increased bone density.

osteitis pubis: increased bone density seen at symphysis pubis; may be associated with pain or increased physical activity.

ostemia: abnormal congestion of blood in bone.

ostempyesis: suppuration (pus) within bone.

osteoaneurysm: aneurysm in bone.

osteoarthritis: chronic disorder of a joint with excessive erosion of the cartilage surface associated with excess bone formation at the margins of the joint and gradual loss of function because of pain and stiffness. This may be the outcome of abnormal mechanical forces, such as prior injury, a systemic disorder, or part of a generalized osteoarthritic process. When the existing condition is not caused by an inflammatory process, the more proper term is **osteoarthrosis.**

osteoarthropathy: a condition of increased bone formation at the joints; sometimes used to refer to osteoarthritis. Variations of osteoarthropathy are hypertropic, hypertrophic pulmonary, pulmonary trophic, and secondary hypertrophic.

osteoarthrosis: same as the term **arthrosis;** "a heterogeneous group of conditions that lead to joint symptoms and signs associated with defective integrity of articular cartilage, in addition to related changes to the underlying bone at the joint margins."* (Fig. 2–1)

osteoarticular: pertaining to or affecting bones and joints.

osteocachexia: chronic disease of bone resulting in the wasting of bone.

osteochondritis: inflammation of bone. Formerly called **osteochondrosis.** Osteochondritis applies to a number of conditions in which the pathologic findings and cause may vary. In children, the disease affects the ossification centers at the *pressure epiphysis* (joints) or *traction epiphysis* (e.g., the patellar tendon to the tibia or the Achilles tendon attachment to the heel). In a pressure epiphysis, an area of avascular necrosis or similar process can occur. In the absence of a clear etiologic relationship or consistent pathologic findings, the osteochondritis diseases (as specified by areas affected) can be separated into traction and pressure epiphyses as follows:

*American College of Rheumatology

FIG 2–1.
Surface of tibia following excision for total knee replacement. Joint surfaces are rough with loss of cartilage and formation of new bone and cartilage at margin (osteophytes). (Courtesy of the Orthopaedic Research Laboratory, Good Samaritan Medical Center, West Palm Beach, FL.)

Traction epiphyses

Osgood-Schlatter d.: patellar tendon to tibia.
Scheuermann d.: epiphysitis of vertebral body.
Sever d.: Achilles tendon to calcaneus.
Sindig-Larsen-Johansson d.: patellar tendon to patella.

Pressure epiphyses

Blount d.: epiphyseal plate of tibia.
Avascular necrosis types
Brailsford d.: radial head.
Burns d.: humeral trochlea.
Freiberg d.: second metatarsal head.
Haas d.: head of humerus.
Kienböck d.: lunate.
Köhler d.: midpatella.
Köhler d.: tarsal navicular.
Konig d.: femoral condyle.
Legg-Calvé-Perthes d.: femoral head.
Mauclair d.: metacarpal heads.
Panner d.: capitellum.
Thiemann d.: proximal phalanx.

osteochondrodesmodysplasia: a mucopoly-saccharide disorder associated with multiple deformities of bone, joints, and tendons; **Rotter-Erb syndrome.**

osteochondrodystrophy: dwarfing disease mainly affecting spine and hips with little or no mental disturbance; **Morquio syndrome.**

osteochondrofibroma: tumor containing elements of osteoma, chondroma, and fibroma.

osteochondrolysis: osteochondritis dissecans.

osteochondromatosis: Transformation of synovial villi into bone and cartilage masses, causing loose bodies in the joint. This condition occurs in joints affected by trauma or other degenerative diseases. A condition specifically called **synovial osteochondromatosis** and **Henderson-Jones chondromatosis.**

osteochondropathy: condition affecting bone and cartilage, marked by abnormal enchondral ossification.

osteochondrophyte: an archaic term synonymous with osteochondroma.

osteochondrosis: term being replaced by **osteochondritis;** condition in children that affects the epiphyseal and apophyseal regions where increased stress occurs.

osteochondrosis dissecans: formation of a separate center of bone and cartilage on an epiphyseal surface. The osteochondral fragment may remain in place, be absorbed and replaced slowly, or break loose and become a loose body. Multiple etiologies probably exist. This was originally believed to be an inflammatory lesion, but there is no clear evidence for this, hence the change of the term from osteochondritis to osteochondrosis. Another probable etiology is a demarcation of an area of avascular necrosis; **osteochondritis dissecans.**

osteoclasia: breaking down and absorption of bone tissue.

osteocope: syphilitic bone disease with severe pain within bone.

osteocystoma: cystic tumor in bone.

osteodiastasis: abnormal separation of bones.

osteodynia: pain in bones.

osteodystrophy: defective bone formation.

osteofibrochondrosarcoma: malignant tumor containing bone and fibrous and cartilaginous tissue.

osteofibroma: tumor containing both osseous and fibrous elements.

osteofibromatosis: formation of multiple osteofibromas.

osteofibrous dysplasia: lesion that has a histologic appearance similar to fibrous dysplasia, except that the bone is being formed by osteocytes rather than by fibrocyte-like cells; **campanacci lesion; ossifying fibroma of long bones.**

osteogenesis imperfecta: condition in which bones are abnormally brittle and subject to fractures; inherited and usually is a function of abnormal Type I collagen, **osteitis fragilitans, fragilitas ossium congenita, osteopsathyrosis idiopathica,** and **brittle bones.**

Shapiro classification system
congenita A: fractures at birth, bones radiologically abnormal.

congenita B: fractures at birth, bones radiologically normal.

tarda A: first fracture before or at walking stage, bones narrow and osteopenic.

tarda B: first fracture before or at walking stage, bones radiologically normal.

Sillence (modified)
Type IA: mild, dominant inherited, associated with blue sclerae and no skeletal deformity.

Type IB: mild, dominant inherited, associated with blue sclerae, no skeletal deformity, and dentinogenesis imperfecta.

Type II: lethal, recessive inherited, associated with multiple fractures and a short survival. **Bauze:** Lethal OI.

Type III: severe, inherited recessive, associated with progressive deformity, white or blue sclerae, and nonambulatory status. **Bauze:** Severe OI.

Type IVA: moderate, inherited dominant new mutation, associated with some deformity and white sclerae in adults. **Bauze:** Mild OI.

Type IVB: moderate, new mutation, associated with some deformity, white sclerae in adults, and dentinogenesis imperfecta.

These groups were formerly called:

osteogenesis imperfecta congenita: severe form of brittle bone disease and deformity expressing itself in infancy or even at birth; can be fatal.

osteogenesis imperfecta tarda: brittle bone disease expressing itself when child begins to walk; **Lobstein d.** or **syndrome.**

osteohalisteresis: loss or deficiency of mineral elements of bones, producing softening.

osteolipochondroma: cartilage tumor with bone and fatty elements.

osteolipoma: fatty tumor containing osseous elements.

osteolysis: dissolution of bone.

familial expansile osteolysis: an autosomal dominant bone dysplasia with general and focal skeletal changes occurring in the second decade of life. There is usually pain, osteoclastic resorption, bowing, and a tendency toward pathologic fracture. Deafness and early loss of teeth may also occur.

massive osteolysis: rare condition characterized by prevalent monostotic unilateral, localized, concentric osteolysis. **Gorham d., phantom bone d., vanishing bone d., disappearing bone d.,** *hemangiomatosis, lymphangiomatosis,* and *hemolymphangiomatosis.*

pubic osteolysis: in adults, a worrisome-appearing lesion that may be mistaken for chondrosarcoma of the pubic bone area. Characterized by progressively destructive radiographic changes, soft-tissue mass with calcification, histologic features of meta-plastic cartilage, bone formation, and granulation tissue with myxoid and angiomatoid patterns.

osteomalacia: a reduction of physical strength of bone caused by decreased mineralization of osteoid; may result from a deficiency of vitamin D, calcium, or phosphorous with or without renal disease. Osteomalacia in the child is associated with the growth deformities of rickets.

osteomesopyknosis: autosomal dominant disorder characterized by osteosclerosis similar to that in pyknodysostosis, but localized to the axial spine, pelvis, and proximal part of the long bones.

osteomyelitis: inflammation of bone marrow, cortex, tissue, and periosteum; can be caused by any organism, but usually bacteria. See Infectious Bone Diseases section.)

osteomyelodysplasia: thinning of osseous tissue of bone with increase in size of marrow cavities, accompanied by leukopenia (low white blood cell count) and fever.

osteonecrosis: death of bone tissue, usually of vascular origin.

osteoneuralgia: nerve pain in bone.

osteopathia striata: affection of bone giving distinct striped appearance on radiographs; lesions characterized by multiple condensation of cancellous bone tissue, sometimes said to be in association with osteopetrosis; **Voorhoeve d.**

osteopathy: any disease process of bone.

osteopenia: any state in which bone mass is reduced below normal. This would include conditions of osteoporosis and osteomalacia.

osteoperiostitis: inflammation of bone and periosteum.

osteopetrorickets: the association of rickets and osteopetrosis in children characterized by hypophosphatemia, hypocalcemia, widened growth plates, and increased skeletal mass.

osteopetrosis: autosomal recessive disorder of macrophage colony–stimulating factor, with ar-

eas of condensed bone within bone; **Albers-Schonberg d., osteosclerosis fragilis.**

osteophlebitis: inflammation of the veins in bone.

osteophyte: bony excrescence or osseous outgrowth, usually found around the joint area of bone. Around margins of arthritic joints, osteophytes are formed by new cartilage and bone. Around the spine and at strong ligamentous attachments, a portion of the ligament may turn to bone.

osteoplastica: inflammatory bone changes seen in cystic fibrosis.

osteopoikilosis: presence of multiple sclerotic foci in ends of long bones and scattered stippling in round and flat bones; usually without symptoms but noted on radiographs.

osteoporosis: diminution of both the mineral and matrix components of bone such that the remaining bone is normal in composition but reduced in total bone mass. The secondary cause of osteoporosis is most commonly immobilization, such as casting. Primary osteoporosis is an age-related disorder characterized by decreased bone mass and increased susceptibility to fractures in the absence of other recognizable causes of bone loss.

osteoradionecrosis: necrosis (death) of bone following irradiation.

osteosclerosis: hardening or abnormal denseness of bone.

osteosis: formation of bone tissue with infiltration of connective tissue within bone.

osteospongioma: spongy tumor of bone.

osteosynovitis: inflammation of synovial membranes and neighboring bones.

osteotabes: condition in which bone marrow cells are destroyed and marrow disappears; usually in infants.

osteothrombophlebitis: inflammation through intact bone by progressive thrombophlebitis of small venules.

osteothrombosis: blood clots or plugging of veins of bone.

parosteitis: inflammation of tissues around a bone.

parosteosis: ossification of the tissue outside the periosteum.

Infectious Bone Diseases

Osteomyelitis (Fig. 2–2) may be caused by bacteria or fungi. (Viruses have been suggested as a cause, but this has not been proved.)

- Bacteria associated with osteomyelitis
  - *Staphylococcus aureus*
  - *Streptococcus* organisms
  - *Escherichia coli*
  - *Pseudomonas* organisms
  - *Klebsiella* organisms
  - *Salmonella* organisms
  - *Neisseria gonorrhoeae*
  - *Mycobacterium tuberculosis*
- Fungal types (rare)
  - Actinomycosis
  - Blastomycosis
  - Histoplasmosis

FIG 2–2.
Different radiographic presentations of subacute osteomyelitis with classification scheme. Growth plate (physis) is below joint surface. Type IA is a punched out lucency suggestive of eosinophilic granuloma. Type IB has a sclerotic margin (not depicted) as seen in a more chronic form called Brodie's abscess. Type II has loss of metaphyseal cortical bone. Type III has loss of diaphyseal cortical bone. Type IV has onion skin layering of subperiosteal bone. Type V has an epiphyseal lesion. Type VI is an osteomyelitic lesion of the vertebral body. (From *J Am Assoc Orthop Surg,* 2:340, 1994.)

Terms Related to Osteomyelitis (Bone Infection)

acute o.:   possibly up to 6 weeks, radiographs may be negative for first 2 weeks.

chronic o.:   over 6 weeks; may last for years.

chronic multifocal o.:   multiple foci of bone infection in same period, with a fastidious, slow-growing bacterium the most likely causative agent.

chronic sclerosing o. of Garré: minimally symptomatic, long-term osteomyelitis associated with radiographic findings of densely scarred bone but not the usual abscess formation.

cloacae: in osteomyelitis, these are the openings in the infected sequestra of bone.

cystic o.:   the radiographic appearance of an aborted osteomyelitis where a fluid-filled cystic cavity remains in the bone.

iatrogenic o.:   an infection brought about by surgery or other treatment.

involucrum: bone formation around infected cortical bone.

mastocytosis: rare condition associated with accumulation of histamine-producing cells called "mastocytes" or mast cells. Painless, sclerotic bone lesions can occur.

nonsuppurative o.:   term applied to tuberculosis of bone.

primary subacute o.:   osteomyelitis that presents as localized, progressive bone pain with periods of remission. There is usually little or no systemic illness and no temperature elevation. Radiographic changes are identifiable on the first visit.

SAPHO: **s**ynovitis-**a**cne-**p**ustulosis-**h**yperostosis **o**steomyelitis syndrome related to the pustulotic arthroosteitis syndrome.

sequestrum: detached piece of dead bone from sound healthy bone during process of necrosis.

sinus: drainage tract extending from an area of infected bone to skin.

suppurative o.:   infection of bone with active production of pus; may be acute or chronic.

Tumors of Bone

A staging system for musculoskeletal tumors has gained wide acceptance and is applied to both bone and soft connective tissue. It has been adopted by the American Joint Committee Task Force on Bone Tumors. The system is based on the relationship of the following factors: grade (G), site (T), and metaphysis (M). Staging is based on the scales in Tables 2–1 and 2–2.

- Histologic grade.
    - G_0: benign.
    - G_1: low-grade malignant.
    - G_2: high-grade malignant.
- Site.
    - T_0: lesion confined within a capsule.
    - T_1: lesion has extracapsular extensions.
    - T_2: lesion extends beyond compartmental barriers.
- Metastasis.
    - M_0: no metastasis.
    - M_1: metastasis.

The term *osteogenic sarcoma* formerly defined all the bone sarcomas (e.g., osteosarcoma, chondrosarcoma, and fibrosarcoma). Currently, more specific terms are preferred.

Benign tumors of bone are classified by the type of neoplastic tissue within the lesion. Nine general categories of tumors are described in the classification system of the World Health Organization (WHO).

I. Bone-forming tumors
  1. Osteoma
  2. Osteoid osteoma
  3. Osteoblastoma
II. Cartilage-forming tumors
  1. Chondroma
  2. Osteochondroma

TABLE 2–1.

Stages of Benign Musculoskeletal Lesions

	1	2	3
Grade	G_0	G_0	G_0
Site	T_0	T_0	T_{1-2}
Metastasis	M_0	M_0	M_{1-2}
Clinical course	Latent, static, self-healing	Actively progressing, expands bone or fascia	Aggressive, invasive, breaches bone or fascia
Radiographic grade	I_A	I_B	I_C
Isotope scan	Background uptake	Increased uptake in lesion	Increased uptake beyond lesion
Angiogram	No neovascular reaction	Modest neovascular reaction	Moderate neovascular reaction
CT/MRI*	Crisp, intact margin—well-defined capsule, homogeneous	Intact margin "expansile"—thin capsule, homogeneous	Indistinct broached margin—extracapsular and/or extra-compartmental extension, nonhomogeneous

From Enneking WF: A system of staging musculoskeletal neoplasms. *Clin Orthop* 204:9–24, 1986.
*A magnetic resonance imaging (MRI) study is now used in addition to the computed tomography (CT) study.

TABLE 2–2.

Stages of Malignant Musculoskeletal Lesions*

	I_A	I_B	II_A	II_B	III_A	III_B
Grade	G_1	G_1	G_2	G_2	G_{1-2}	G_{1-2}
Site	T_1	T_2	T_1	T_2	T_1	T_2
Metastasis	M_0	M_0	M_0	M_0	M_1	M_1
Clinical course	Symptomatic, indolent growth	Symptomatic, mass, indo-lent growth	Symptomatic, rapid growth	Symptomatic, rapid growth, fixed mass, pathologic fracture	Systemic symptoms, palpable nodes, pulmonary symptoms	
Isotope scan	Increased uptake	Increased uptake	Increased uptake beyond radiographic limits	Increased uptake beyond radiographic limits	Pulmonary lesions, no increased uptake	
Radiographic grade	II	II	III	III	III	
Angiogram	Modest neovascular reaction, in-volvement of neurovascular bundle	Modest neovascular reaction, in-volvement of neurovascular bundle	Marked neovascular reaction, no involvement of neurovascular bundle	Marked neovascular reaction, in-volvement of neurovascular bundle	Hypervascular lymph nodes	
CT/MRI*†	Irregular or broached capsule but intracompart-mental	Extracompart-mental extension or location	Broached (pseudo) capsule, intracompart-mental	Broached (pseudo) capsule, extracompart-mental	Pulmonary lesions or enlarged nodes	

From Enneking WF: A system of staging musculoskeletal neoplasms, *Clin Orthop* 204:9–24, 1986. (Used by permission.)
*A magnetic resonance imaging (MRI) study is now used in addition to the computed tomography (CT) study.
†MRI is now a standard part of the radiologic evaluation.

3. Chondroblastoma
4. Chondromyxoid fibroma
III. Giant-cell tumors
IV. Marrow tumors (none)
V. Vascular tumors
   1. Hemangioma
   2. Lymphangioma
   3. Glomus tumor
VI. Other connective tissue tumors
   1. Desmoplastic fibroma
   2. Lipoma
   3. Fibrous histiocytoma
VII. Other tumors
   1. Neurilemmoma
   2. Neurofibroma
VIII. Unclassified tumors (none)
IX. Tumor-like lesions
   1. Solitary bone cyst
   2. Aneurysmal bone cyst
   3. Metaphyseal fibrous defect
   4. Eosinophilic granuloma
   5. Fibrous dysplasia
   6. Osteofibrous dysplasia
   7. Myositis ossificans
   8. Brown tumor of hyperparathyroidism
   9. Intraosseous epidermoid cyst
   10. Giant-cell (reparative) granuloma

General Terms

tumor capsule: a layer of compressed normal tissue surrounding a tumor.

tumor pseudo-capsule: a layer of compressed normal tissue and neoplastic tissue surrounding a tumor.

Bone Cell Tumors

osteoblastoma: a benign tumor composed mostly of osteoblasts, occasional giant cells, fibrovascular tissue, and new bone formation. Generally located in the spine or diaphysis of long bones.

osteoid osteoma: a benign tumor characterized by increased osteoblasts and osteoid and fibrovascular tissue. Located in the cortex of long bones. Often surrounded by a thick sclerotic border as seen both radiographically and histologically.

osteoma: benign tumor characterized by dense bone production. Usually located in the skull.

osteosarcoma: a high-grade malignant bone tumor (sarcoma) generally located in the medullary cavity of the distal femur, proximal fibia, and proximal humerus. Characterized by osteoid production by malignant osteoblasts, with variable amounts of cartilage being present.

   parosteal osteosarcoma: a low-grade malignant bone tumor characterized by osteoid formation by malignant osteoblasts. This tumor is located on the outer surface of the periosteum, without involvement of the medullary cavity. Posterior cortex of the distal femur is a common location.

   periosteal osteosarcoma: a moderate-grade malignant bone tumor located beneath the periosteum but outside the cortex characterized by osteoid production by malignant osteoblasts. These osteosarcomas contain a large amount of cartilage.

   secondary osteosarcoma: osteosarcoma that arises in preexisting pathologic bone, such as in Paget's disease or following irradiation treatment.

   telangiectatic osteosarcoma: intramedullary high-grade osteosarcoma characterized by abundant vascular changes and mesenchymal tissue in conjunction with sparse malignant osteoid production; **osteotelangiectasis.**

Cartilage Tumors

chondroblastoma (Codman tumor): benign tumor composed of chondroblasts, giant cells, and chondroid material. Calcificzation often appreciated surrounding the chondroblasts (chicken wire calcification). This tumor generally is located in the epiphysis.

chondroma: an extraosseous benign tumor that contains mature chondrocytes in a cartilage matrix often surrounded by a rim of reactive bones. Varying degrees of calcification can be appreciated on radiographs and histology.

chondromyxoid fibroma: a benign tumor composed of cartilage and myxomatous and fibrous tissue. Commonly located in the proximal tibia.

chondrosarcoma: a malignant tumor characterized by cartilage production by malignant chondrocytes.

clear cell chondrosarcoma: cartilage tumor that histologically is characterized by clear, vacuolated cells.

dedifferentiated   chondrosarcoma: malignant tumor in which a well-differentiated low-grade cartilaginous component, sometimes of long duration, is associated with a poorly differentiated noncartilagenous neoplasm of recent development and higher malignant grade.

enchondroma: an intraosseous benign tumor, similar both radiographically and histologically to a chondroma.

enchondromatosis: proliferation of multiple benign cartilaginous neoplasms within the metaphysis of several bones. It can result in thinning of the overlying cortices and distortion of length in growth. Higher risk of malignant transformation into secondary chondrosarcoma than a single enchondroma. **Ollier d.**

epiphyseal osteochondroma: development of intraosseous chondromas within the epiphysis with occasional extension beyond epiphyseal margins. May occur from infancy to adulthood. Formerly called **osteomatosis, epiphyseal exostosis, intraarticular osteochondromas, epiarticular osteochondromas, dysplasia epiphysealis hemimelica,** and **epiarticular osteochondromatous dysplasia.**

mesenchymal chondrosarcoma: tumor with well-differentiated cartilaginous component associated with highly malignant round cell component of recent development.

multiple osteochondromatosis: multiple osteochondromas located in the metaphysis of long bones and pelvis resulting in growth abnormalities, with an autosomal dominant inheritance pattern.

osteochondroma: a cartilage-capped extraosseous benign tumor with a bony stalk. Generally located in the distal femur, proximal tibia, or proximal humerus.

parosteal chondrosarcoma: malignant cartilage-producing tumor arising from the surface of the bone.

periosteal chondroma: an extraosseous benign cartilage tumor located between the periosteum and bone cortex characterized by cartilage and active chondrocytes.

secondary chondrosarcoma: usually well-differentiated cartilage malignancy occurring in a previously benign cartilage tumor, such as an osteochondroma or enchondroma.

Round Cell Tumors

eosinophilic granuloma (formally histiocytosis X):   tumor-like process in bone composed of masses of histiocytes, cholesterol, and eosinophils. Common locations include the pelvis, scapula, and diaphysis of long bones in children; *Hand-Schüller-Christian d., Letterer-Siwe d.*

Ewing's sarcoma: high-grade malignant tumor commonly presenting in children; characterized by monotonous sheets of small round cells.

Hand-Schüller-Christian d.:   one of the so-called histiocytosis X group of diseases; a complex of bony tumors caused by either accumulation of cholesterol, metabolic error, or neoplasm; characterized by eosinophilic granuloma, exophthalmos, and diabetes.

Hodgkin tumor: low-grade malignant process involving the lymphatic system, with rare 13% bone involvement characterized by Reed-Sternberg cells.

Langerhans cell histiocytosis: formerly known as histiocytosis X; a nonneoplastic condition characterized by monocyte-macrophage lineage cell infiltration of multiple organs including bone. The cause is unknown, and there are many forms of the disease with uncertain outcome. When a bony lesion occurs, it may involve one or a few **eosinophilic granulomas.** When associated with cranial disorder, diabetes, and exophthalmos, it may be **Hand-Schüller-Christian d.;** in infants with a poor prognosis associated with wasting it is called **Letterer-Siwe d.**

lymphoma: a general term for new tissue growth in the lymphatic system. There are many types.

multiple myeloma: common malignant tumor characterized by multiple plasma cell–containing bone lesions.

myeloblastoma: benign tumor of bone marrow.

plasmacytoma: uncommon malignant tumor characterized by a single focus of plasma cells in a bone. Often progresses to multiple myeloma.

primary lymphoma: distinguishes this rare malignant solitary bone tumor from the more common soft tissue or systemic presentation of lymphoma. Characterized by multiple malignant lymphocytes. A slower-growing tumor seen in adults.

Fibrous Tumors

desmoplastic fibroma of bone: an aggressive but benign fibrous tumor characterized by dense bands of collagenous tissue.

fibrosarcoma: a malignant tumor characterized by fibroblastic cells and dilated vessels. More commonly presents as a soft tissue malignancy.

malignant fibrous histiocytoma: malignant tumor consisting of pleomorphic fibrous and histiocytic cell proliferation without osteoid or chondroid production.

nonossifying fibroma: common benign fibrous tumor presenting in childhood; located in the metaphysis of long bones. Characterized by whorl patterns of spindle cells, fibrous tissue, numerous xanthoma cells, and, occasionally, giant cells.

Other Tumors

adamantinoma: a malignant epithelial tumor located in the tibia.

chordoma: a malignant tumor commonly located in the sacrum; arises from residual notochord tissue.

epithelioid sarcoma: tumor composed of a nest of epithelial-like cells but with sarcomatous activity.

giant cell tumor (osteoclastoma): benign but aggressive lesion consisting of osteoclast-like giant cells originating in the metaphysis of long bones. Expansile on radiographs without any reactive bone formation.

liposarcoma: malignant soft tissue tumor composed of lipoblasts.

rhabdomyosarcoma: a malignant tumor composed of muscle cell precursors (rhabdomyoblasts).

synovial cell sarcoma: a malignant tumor composed of tissue that resembles synovium.

synovioma: a benign tumor of the synovial membrane.

MISCELLANEOUS BONE CONDITIONS

acroosteolysis: resorption of bone that involves the distal regions of the limbs but most commonly the phalanges of the fingers.

algodystrophy syndrome: association of pain and dystrophic changes in bone.

aneurysmal bone cyst: single or multiple benign, blood-filled cysts of bone.

apophysitis: inflammation of an apophysis. Depending on the location, specific types may be referred to as:

Osgood-Schlatter d.: tibial apophysis at the insertion of the patellar tendon.

Sever d.: apophysitis of the heel bone at the insertion of the Achilles tendon.

Scheuermann d.: osteochondrosis of the vertebral epiphysis in juveniles.

aseptic necrosis: osteonecrosis (bone death) caused by vascular insult, usually at the end of a bone. In adults, the most common symptom-producing aseptic necrosis occurs in the femoral head (avascular necrosis). In children, aseptic necrosis is called epiphyseal ischemic necrosis or epiphyseal aseptic necrosis. The precise pathologic condition of these diseases is debatable; therefore, the term is used here in reference to epiphyseal osteochondritis or by area:

Assmann d.: head of first metatarsal.

Buchman d.: medial cuneiform.

Freiberg d. second metatarsal head.

Iselins d.: base of the fifth metatarsal.

Kappis d.: talus.

Kienböck d.: lunate bone of wrist.

Köhler d.: tarsal navicular; sometimes of the patella.

Lance d.: cuboid.

Legg-Calvé-Perthes d.: femoral head; *Legg-Perthes d., Perthes d., coxa plana.*

Panner d.: capitellum of the humerus.

Silverskjold d.: calcaneus.

Thiemann d.: proximal phalanges.

Wagner d.: base of the first metatarsal.

Also known as **avascular necrosis** the following are classification systems for aseptic necrosis.

International Classification (for femoral head)

Stage 0: bone biopsy results consistent with avascular necrosis; normal findings in all other tests.

Stage I: positive scintiscan and/or magnetic resonance image (MRI); lesions subdivided into medial, central, or lateral depending on location and involvement of femoral head.

I-A: < 15% involvement of femoral head.

I-B: 15% to 30% involvement of femoral head.

I-C: > 30% involvement of femoral head.

Stage II: radiographic abnormalities (mottled appearance of femoral head, osteosclerosis, cyst formation, and osteopenia); no signs of collapse of femoral head on radiographs or computerized tomography scan; positive scintiscan and MRI; no changes in acetabulum; lesions subdivided into medial, central, or lateral depending on location of involvement of femoral head.

II-A: < 15% involvement of femoral head.

II-B: 15% to 30% involvement of femoral head.

II-C: > 30% involvement of femoral head.

Stage III: crescent sign; lesions subdivided into medial, central, or lateral depending on location of involvement of femoral head.

III-A: < 15% crescent sign or < 2-mm depression of femoral head.

III-B: 15% to 30% crescent sign or 2- to 4-mm depression of femoral head.

III-C: > 30% crescent sign or 4-mm depression of femoral head.

Stage IV: Articular surface flattened radiographically and joint space shows narrowing; change in acetabulum with evidence of osteosclerosis, cyst formation, and marginal osteophytes.

Lichtman (for the lunate in the wrist)

Stage I: linear line possibly seen across lunate or no radiographic finding.

Stage II: definite density changes in lunate compared to other carpal bones.

Stage III: lunate collapse with proximal migration of capitate.

Stage IV: stage III plus degenerative changes in the carpus.

Ratcliff (for pediatric fractures of femoral head)

Type I: total head involvement.

Type II: segmental head involvement.

Type III: involvement of the fracture line to the physis.

Steinberg (for the hip) (Fig. 2–3)

Stage 0: normal radiograph, bone scan, and MRI.

Stage 1: normal radiograph; abnormal bone scan and/or MRI.

Stage II: sclerosis and/or cyst formation in femoral head.

A: mild (15% of head).

B: moderate (15% to 30%).

C: severe (> 30%).

Stage III: subchondral collapse (crescent sign) without flattening.

A: mild (15% of surface).

B: moderate (15% to 30%).

C: severe (> 30%).

Stage IV: flattening of femoral head without joint narrowing or acetabular involvement.

A: mild (15% of surface and < 2-cm depression).

B: moderate (15% to 30% of surface and 2- to 4-mm depression).

C: severe (> 30% of surface or > 4-mm depression).

Stage V: flattening of head with joint narrowing and/or acetabular involvement.

A: mild (15% of surface and < 2-cm depression).

B: moderate (15% to 30% of surface and 2- to 4-mm depression).

C: severe (> 30% of surface or > 4-mm depression).

Stage VI: advanced degenerative changes.

bone infarct: area of bone where blood supply is interrupted.

bone island: small areas of compact but microscopically normal bone that appear as 0.5- to 1-cm areas on radiographs.

bone spur: ossification of ligamentous or muscular attachment to bone. Generally applied to any bony excrescence seen on radiographs, but specifically refers to a portion of ligament or tendon that has turned to bone at the attachment to bone. The most common areas include the heel, patella, humeral epicondyles, and vertebral body margins.

brown tumor: brown-appearing lesion in bone secondary to hyperparathyroidism; **osteoclastoma.**

caisson disease: avascular necrosis of bone (and soft tissue) caused by sudden increase and release in air pressure causing infarct; **diver's disease.**

cleidocranial dysostosis: autosomal dominant condition with failure to form collar bones and portions of the skull.

condensing osteitis of the clavicle: rare and benign disorder of unknown origin affecting the medial clavicle, characteristically in women of late childbearing age. The level of discomfort varies, and radiographs reveal a slight expansion of the medial one third of the clavicle.

congenital pseudarthrosis: inborn propensity for breakdown of integrity of midshaft of tibia with formation of a false joint. There are six types:

Type I: congenital anterior bowing and defect in tibia. There may be other congenital deformities.

Type II: congenital anterior bowing and hourglass deformity of tibia. Fracture occurs usually before 2 years of age.

Type III: bone cyst forms first, then bowing or fracture.

Type IV: sclerotic bone, then fracture occurs.

Type V: dysplastic fibula. May develop pseudarthrosis of tibia or fibula.

Type VI: intraosseous neurofibroma or schwannoma may develop but usually does not result in pseudarthrosis.

cortical fibrous dysplasia (ossifying fibroma of long bone, intracortical fibrous dysplasia): benign anomaly of bone cortex, usually found in children and characterized by a cystic-appearing lesion on radiographs. Microscopically, this lesion is characterized by a

FIG 2–3.
Steinberg classification based on radiograph, x-ray, and bone scan. **A,** Stage 0; **B,** Stage I; **C,** Stage II; **D,** Stage III; **E,** Stage IV; **F,** Stage V; and **G,** Stage VI. (From *J Bone Joint Surg* 77A:35, 1995.)

fibrous replacement of cortex with some trabecular bone.

exostosis: excess bone formation, usually near a joint.

hypertrophic e.: sometimes used to describe excess bone formation in osteoarthritis.

hereditary multiple e.: autosomal dominant; multiple bony excrescences growing from cortical surfaces and forming tubular extensions roughly transverse to the long axis of bone involved; *Jaffe d.*

fibrodysplasia ossificans progressiva: inherited connective-tissue disease in which soft-tissue ossificiation leads to skeletal malformation and disability; **myositis ossificans progressiva, hyperplasia fascialis ossificans progressiva, myositis fibrosa generalista,** and **fibrositis ossificans progressiva.**

fibrogenesis imperfecta ossium: rare inherited disorder in which bone in adults is replaced with collagen-deficient tissue throughout the skeleton, resulting in multiple fractures.

giant cell reparative granuloma: common benign lesion of jaw characterized by a fibrous background within which there are scattered multinucleated giant cells. A multicentric form is seen in the small bones of the hands and feet.

heterotopic ossification: formation of normal bone at ectopic soft tissue locations. In the acquired form, abnormal bone formation usually follows trauma or surgery and will sometimes occur around joints after a closed head injury. Two rare heritable and developmental forms are fibrodysplasia ossificans and progressive osseous heteroplasia.

A system to classify ectopic ossification is often referred to as the **Brooker** classification:

Class I: islands of bone within the soft tissues about the hip.

Class II: bone spurs from the pelvis or proximal end of the femur, leaving at least 1 cm between opposing bone surfaces.

Class III: bone spurs from the pelvis or proximal end of the femur, reducing the space between opposing bone surfaces to less than 1 cm.

Class IV: apparent bone ankylosis of the hip.

Another system is the **Hamblen** classification:

Grade 0: no ossification.

Grade I: formation of new bone involving less than one third of the area of the hip occupied by the femoral head and capsule.

Grade II: formation of new bone involving between one and two thirds of the same area of the hip.

Grade III: formation of new bone involving more than two thirds of that area of the hip.

infantile cortical hyperostosis: painful hyperostosis with involvement of long bones and the mandible. This usually occurs in infants 5 months of age and younger and is associated with irritability, fever, and soft-tissue swelling.

intraosseous lipoma: rare condition of benign fatty tumor that develops in the medullary canal of a long bone.

intraosseous lipomatosis: very rare disorder of progressive systemic development of leg and foot lipomas in medullary canals, producing bone pain and pathologic fractures.

intraosseous pneumatocyst: rare benign small pocket of air that appears usually in iliac bone. No treatment is required.

longitudinal epiphyseal bracket: ossification anomaly in which an abnormal arcuate or C-shaped secondary ossificiation center brackets a tubular bone in the hand or foot.

malacoplakia: disease that usually involves the gut and has a probable infectious cause. Histiocytes respond with the formation of Michaelis-Gutmann bodies. Bone lesions are rare and can be destructive.

melorheostosis: form of osteosclerosis or hyperostosis (dense bone); linear longitudinal thickenings of the shaft of long bones, very rare, resulting in a candle wax (dripping) appearance of the bone.

milk-alkali disease: excess calcium in tissue resulting from heavy ingestion of milk and certain antacids.

myelofibrosis: replacement of bone marrow by fibrous tissue.

nonossifying fibroma: an anomaly of bone that appears in youngsters as a sharply circumscribed, eccentrically located lesion in the metaphysis of long bones; microscopically, this lesion is characterized by whorl patterns of spindle cells, fibrous tissue, numerous xanthoma cells, and, occasionally, giant cells; **fibroxanthoma, fibrous cortical defect, subcortical defect.**

ochronosis: hereditary error of protein metabolism marked by accumulation of homogentisic acid resulting in degenerative arthritis and a charactertistic blackening of cartilage.

ossifying fibroma of the jaw: fibroma of the jaw with histologic appearance of small areas of ossificiation. This is in distinction to the rare ossifying fibroma of long bones.

pachydysostosis: enlargement of fibular length resulting in bowing of the leg.

periostitis: inflammation of bone covering (periosteum); usually the result of an infection such as syphilis.

progressive diaphyseal dysplasia: neuromuscular dystrophy associated with general wasting; abnormally formed shafts of long bones; *Engelmann d.*

progressive osseous heteroplasia: heritable disease characterized by focal dermal ossification with progression to intramembranous ossification of subcutaneous fat and deeper tissues leading to ankylosis. **Hemimelic progressive osseous heteroplasia** is a very rare condition in which only one side of the body is involved.

pulmonary osteodystrophy: hypertrophic cortical bone changes occurring near joints in the long bones of patients with chronic lung disease.

pyknodysostosis: condition marked by patchy areas of thickening of the cortex of bone.

regional migratory osteoporosis: most frequently seen in middle-aged men; characterized by arthralgias of lower limb joints, severe intercurrent osteoporosis, with symptoms lasting 6 to 9 months with recovery.

rickets: failure of deposition of bone salts within the organic matrix of cartilage and bone associated with stunting of growth and bone deformities.

skeletal amyloidosis: deposition of amyloid β-microglobulin material in bone that produces bubbly appearing lesions on radiographs. Condition is associated with plasma cell dyscrasias, primary systemic amyloidosis, focal amyloidosis, and those undergoing hemodialysis for chronic renal insufficiency.

slipped capital femoral epiphysis: gradual or sudden movement of the femoral head toward a posterior and medial direction; usually occurs in preteenage children. The condition is also called **slipped capital femoral epiphysis (SCFE)** or **slipped upper femoral epiphysis (SUFE).** In America, the acronym SCFE is so common that the slang word "skiffy" is used for SCFE.

solitary fibromatosis of bone: similar to generalized fibromatosis except bone lesion is isolated to one location. Systemic symptoms do not occur.

solitary osteoma of long bone: a benign periosteal or endosteal tumor composed predominantly of cortical-type bone.

subperiosteal giant-cell reparative granuloma: self-limited condition seen in older adults characterized by subperiosteal bony lesions located in cortical bone of the diaphysis with giant cells and reparative cells with bone formation; **subperiosteal ABC, periostitis**

ossificans, florid reactive periostitis, pseudo-malignant fibroosseous tumors.

transient osteopenia: decreased bone mass usually following immobilization or injury. Most often bone mass is recovered. May be seen as a spontaneous event in the juvenile hip.

uncommitted metaphyseal lesion: benign but radiologically aggressive-appearing lesion seen in the proximal metaphysis of children, microscopically characterized by whorls of fibrous tissue, new bone, giant cells, and vascular components.

unicameral bone cyst: benign bone anomaly in which a fluid-filled cavity is seen in the metaphysis of a long bone of a child. Microscopically, the cavity is lined with fibrous stroma, curlicues of trabecular bone similar to fibrous dysplasia, and cholesterol clefts.

weaver's bottom: ischial gluteal bursitis often seen in patients with a sedentary occupation.

Eponymic Bone Diseases

Albers-Schönberg d.: osteopetrosis affecting the ends of bone; *chalk bones, thick bones, marble bones.*

Albright syndrome: precocious puberty associated with bone deformities resulting from fibrous dysplasia; **polyostotic fibrous dysplasia, Albright-McCune-Sternberg syndrome, and McCune-Albright syndrome.**

Apert d.: hereditary disease resulting in multiple deformities and mental retardation; **acrocephalosyndactylism.**

Assmann d.: avascular necrosis of the head of the first metatarsal.

Blount d.: lesion of the medial proximal tibial epiphysis causing valgus (lateral bowing) deformity of the tibia; **osteochondrosis deformans tibia, tibia vara** (Fig. 2–4).

Boeck sarcoid: condition usually affecting small bones of hands and feet with granulo-matous inflammatory reaction in lymph nodes, spleen, lungs, and liver.

Bouchard nodes: cartilaginous and bony enlargement of the proximal interphalangeal joints of fingers in degenerative joint disease.

Brailsford d.: avascular necrosis of the radial head seen in children.

Brodie abscess: chronic infection of bone resulting in a characteristic coin-sized sclerotic lesion with a lucent center.

Buchman d.: avascular necrosis of the medial cuneiform.

Burns d.: avascular necrosis of the humeral trochlea head seen in children.

Caffey d.: subperiosteal cortical defect; infantile cortical hyperostosis; self-limited process of excess bone formation seen in newborns to 2-year-olds.

Engelmann d.: primarily a disorder of intramembranous ossification that usually affects the cortext of long bones and the skull with less frequent effects on the face; **progressive diaphyseal dysplasia.**

Freiberg d.: aseptic (avascular) necrosis of the second metatarsal head.

Fröhlich adiposogenital dystrophy: slipped capital femoral epiphysis; **Babinski-Fröhlich syndrome.**

Gardner syndrome: multiple osteomas concurrent with intestinal polyps, fibromas, and epidermal cysts.

Gaucher d. (cerebroside reticulocytosis): autosomal dominant bone disorder resulting from lipid storage disease that is due to an absence of glucocerebrosidase. Excessive production of histiocytes with interference of marrow function and destruction of bone occurs. There are three clinical forms:

Type 1: Adult—chronic, nonneuronopathic form associated with hypersplenism, bone lesions, skin pigmentation, and pingueculae.

FIG 2–4.
Six stages of tibia vara as described by Langen-skiöld, age range is an average. Stage I up to three years old, medial and distal beaking; stage II between 2½ and 4 years old, depression of medial metaphysis; stage III between 4 and 6 years, fragmentation of medial epiphysis; stage IV between 5 to 10 years, enlargement of epiphysis with further depression; stage V between 9 and 11 years, cleft in epiphysis with further deformity; stage VI between 10 and 13 years, fusion of the medial epiphysis. (1995 American Academy of Orthopaedic Surgeons. Reprinted from the *Journal of the American Academy of Orthopaedic Surgeons: A Comprehensive Review* 3(6): 329 with permission.)

Type 2: Infantile—acute neuronopathic form that is manifested in infancy and is associated with severe neuronal abnormalities and early demise.

Type 3: Juvenile—subacute neuronopathic form that has the features of the adult form but with neurologic symptoms that develop in the first decade of life.

Gorham d.: rare condition characterized by monostotic, unilateral, localized, concentric osteolysis.

Haas d.: avascular necrosis of the head of the humerus seen in children.

Hajdu-Cheney syndrome: rare syndrome of resorption of bone of the distal part of the limbs with associated skeletal dysplasias.

Heberden nodes: cartilaginous and bony enlargement of the distal interphalangeal joints in osteoarthritis.

Iselins d.: avascular necrosis of the base of the fifth metatarsal.

Jaffe d.: osteoid osteoma; hereditary multiple exostosis.

Kappis d.: avascular necrosis of the talus.

Kienböck d.: aseptic necrosis affecting lunate or ilium.

Klippel-Feil syndrome: congenital bone abnormalities of neck associated with dental, scapular, and other abnormalities.

Köhler d.: aseptic necrosis of tarsal navicular (scaphoiditis) or patella.

König d.: osteochondrosis dissecans of the knee;

a separate formation of bone and cartilage segment at the joint surface.

Lance d.: avascular necrosis of the cuboid.

Legg-Calvé-Perthes d.: aseptic epiphyseal ischemic necrosis of the capital femoral epiphysis in children; **coxa plana; Perthes d.; Legg-Perthes d.**

Letterer-Siwe d.: histiocyte tumor of bone, usually fatal in infants and small children; *eosinophilic granuloma.*

Marie-Bamberger d.: hypertrophied joints resulting from lung disease.

Mauclair d.: avascular necrosis of the metacarpal heads seen in children.

Milkman syndrome: bone disease in which multiple transparent stripes are seen on radiograph.

nail-patella syndrome: autosomal dominant disorder characterized by hypoplastic patella, deformed fingernails, elbow deformities, and pelvic "horns."

Niemann-Pick d.: fatal fat storage disease affecting bone marrow in infancy, marked by absence of sphingomyelinase.

Ollier d.: enchondromatosis.

Osgood-Schlatter d.: osteochondritis affecting anterior tibial tuberosity.

Paget d.: disease of excess bone removal and replacement with deformity; seen in older periods; *osteitis deformans.*

Panner d.: aseptic necrosis; osteochondritis dissecans of capitellum of humerus.

Perthes d.: aseptic necrosis of the hips in children.

Pott d.: osteomyelitis; tuberculosis of the spine.

Scheuermann d.: osteochondritis affecting anterior vertebral body apophysis.

shepherd's crook deformity: characteristic deformity of proximal femur seen in fibrous dysplasia. The deformity has the appearance of a shepherd's crook.

Silverskjold d.: avascular necrosis of the calcaneus.

Sinding-Larsen-Johansson   d.: secondary center of ossification of inferior pole of patella.

Stewart-Morel syndrome: hyperostosis of frontal bone; **Morel syndrome.**

Thiemann d.: avascular necrosis of proximal phalanges.

Tietze syndrome: chronic inflammation of the costochondral junction of a rib or ribs, causing pain; **chondropathia tuberosa.**

Van Neck d.: nonspecific ischiopubic osteochondritis.

Volkmann deformity: congenital dislocation of the ankle due to absent or defective fibula, not to be confused with **Volkmann ischemic contracture.**

von Recklinghausen d.: congenital disease of fatty tumors, peripheral nerve tumors, areas of skin pigment changes, and other disorders; **neurofibromatosis.**

Voorhoeve d.: osteopathia striata.

Wagner d.: avascular necrosis of the base of the first metatarsal.

Waldenström d.: osteochondrosis of distal humerus at the radial site of elbow (capitellum).

MUSCLE DISEASES

Myo- (Gr. *mys*) is a combining form denoting relationship to muscle. The *myo-* root diseases are followed by miscellaneous muscle diseases, the muscular dystrophies (listed together for comparison), and other muscle disorders. Eponymic terms are included.

Myo- Root Diseases

myasthenia: lack of muscle strength; **amyosthenia.**

myasthenia gravis: syndrome of attacks of muscle weakness that are episodic and reversible; **Erb-Goldflam d.**

myatrophy: muscle wasting.

myoblastoma: tumor of striated muscle consisting of groups of granular-appearing cells resembling primitive myoblasts.

myobradia: sluggish muscle reaction to electric stimuli.

myocele: herniation and protrusion of muscle through its ruptured muscle sheath.

myocelialgia: pain in abdominal muscles.

myocelitis: inflammation of abdominal muscles.

myocellulitis: myositis with cellulitis.

myocerosis: waxy-appearing degeneration of muscle.

myoclonus: any disorder in which rapid rigidity and relaxation alternate; **myoclonia.**

myocoele: the cavity within a myotome.

myocytoma: muscle tumor.

myodegeneration: muscle degeneration.

myodemia: fatty degeneration of muscle.

myodiastasis: separation of muscle. May be congenital or traumatic.

myodynia: pain in the muscles; **myalgia, myosalgia.**

myodystonia: disorder of muscle tone.

myoedema: edema, muscle swelling.

myofascitis: inflammation of muscle and its fascia, particularly of fascial insertion of muscle into bone.

myofibroma: muscular and fibrous tumor; fibroma containing muscular elements.

myofibrosis: replacement of muscle tissue by fibrous tissue.

myogelosis: area of hardening in a muscle.

myoglobinuria: protein myoglobin that appears in urine after vigorous activity; may lead to renal shutdown.

myohypertrophia: muscular hypertrophy.

myoischemia: local deficiency of blood supply in muscle.

myokerosis: waxy degeneration of muscle tissue; **myocerosis.**

myolipoma: fatty tumor of muscle.

myolysis: disintegration of degeneration of muscle tissue.

myoma: tumor made up of muscular elements.

myomalacia: pathogenic softening of muscle.

myomatosis: formation of multiple muscle tumors.

myomelanosis: black pigmentation of a portion of muscle.

myoneuralgia: muscular nerve pain.

myoneurasthenia: relaxed state of the muscular system in neurasthenia (lack of strength due to muscle nerve supply loss).

myoneuroma: nerve tumor containing muscle tissue.

myoneurosis: any abnormal nerve condition of the muscles.

myopachynsis: hypertrophy of muscle; thickening.

myopalmus: muscle twitching.

myoparalysis: paralysis of muscle; **myoparesis.**

myopathy: any disease of the muscles.

myophagism: atrophy or wasting away of muscle tissue, with removal of tissue by inflammatory cells.

myopsychopathy: any muscular nerve affection associated with mental weakness or disorder.

myorrhexis: muscle rupture.

myosarcoma: malignant muscle tumor.

myosclerosis: hardening of muscle.

myoseism: jerky, irregular muscle contractions.

myositis: inflammation of a voluntary muscle.

myositis ossificans: ossification of muscle in response to trauma. To distinguish the traumatic form of myositis ossificans from the generalized form the term **myositis ossificans circumscripta,** proliferative myositis, is sometimes used.

myospasia: clonic contraction of muscle.

myospasm: muscle spasm.

myospasmia: disease characterized by uncontrolled muscle spasms.

myostasis: stretching of muscle.

myosteoma: bony tumor in muscle.

myosynizesis: adhesions of muscle.

myotenositis: inflammation of muscle and its tendon insertion.

myotonia: increased muscular irritability and contractility with decreased power of relaxation; tension and tonic spasm of muscle.

Miscellaneous Muscle Diseases and Conditions

amyoplasia congenita: disorder of fascia and muscle resulting in contracted joints during growth. A specific form of anthrogryposis.

amyotonia congenita: muscle disorder of the newborn, usually fatal; characterized by muscle degeneration with failure of replacement (**congenital hypotonia, Oppenheim d.**); several types including **Werdnig-Hoffmann d.** (CNS origin), rod d. (microscopic rods forming within muscle cells), and central core d., which is not fatal.

congenital myotonia: disorder found at birth, in which initiation and cessation of voluntary movement are delayed; **Thomsen d.**

delayed-onset muscle soreness (DOMS):   muscle weakness, restricted range of motion, and tenderness on palpation that occurs 24 to 48 hours after intense or prolonged muscle activity.

eosinophilia-myalgia syndrome: severe myalgia associated with elevated eosinophile count in blood in the absence of any infection. Has been felt to be associated with high doses of tryptophan.

familial periodic paralysis: disorder of muscle metabolism in which periods of partial to nearly complete paralysis occur; **myotonia intermittens.**

mitochondrial myopathy: slowly progressive muscular weakness associated with abnormal mitochondria, a cell structural component important in oxygen metabolism. The onset of symptoms is usually between birth and 10 years of age, but the disorder may not appear until adulthood.

muscle atrophy: general loss of muscle from various causes; **muscle wasting.**

muscle contracture: condition of fixed high resistance to passive stretch of a muscle resulting from fibrosis of the tissues supporting the muscles or the joints or from disorders of the muscle fibers such as trauma or a congenital disorder.

ischemic c.:   contracture and degeneration of muscle due to interference with circulation from pressure, as by a tight bandage or from injury or cold.

organic c.:   contracture that is permanent and continuous.

postpoliomyelitic c.:   any distortion of a joint following an attack of poliomyelitis.

muscle cramps: uncontrolled contraction of muscle; **charley horse.**

muscle guarding: involuntary contraction of muscle in effort to avoid pain that would be produced by moving the body part.

muscle ischemia: decreased blood supply to a muscle; can be spontaneously reversible; if not, ischemic contracture may develop.

muscle spasm: sudden contraction of muscle, usually in reflexive response to stimulus from external source, for example, back spasm caused by a herniated disk.

muscular dystrophy: group of degenerative disorders of muscle resulting in atrophy and weakness; **Erb d.**

dystrophinopathy: autosomal recessive form of muscular dystrophy due to failure of formation of dystrophin resulting in a severe form. **Duchenne muscular dystrophy,** or a less severe form, **Becker muscular dystrophy.**

pseudohypertrophic: dystrophy of shoulder girdle and sometimes pelvic girdle muscles, beginning with hypertrophy in childhood, followed by atrophy; **Erb paralysis.**

fascioscapulohumeral: marked atrophy of face, shoulder girdle, and arm muscles with autosomal dominant inheritance; **Landouzy-Dejerine disease.**

limb girdle: slow, progressive dystrophy, affecting mostly the back and pelvic muscles. There are a number of types including: **Type I:** autosomal dominant; **type IIA:** autosomal recessive with lack of calcium-activated neutral protease-3 (calpain-3); **type IIB,** autosomal recessive; **type IIC and D:** autosomal recessive lack of gamma-sarcoglycan; and **type IIE:** autosomal with lack of beta-sarcoglycan.

distal: dystrophy affecting mostly the distal muscles of the extremities and usually slowly progressive proximally.

ocular: dystrophy usually confined to the levator and other facial muscles; **progressive dystrophic ophthalmoplegia.**

myotonic dystrophy: myotonia followed eventually by atrophy of face and neck muscles, ultimately extending to muscles of trunk and extremities due to autosomal dominant lack of myotonin-protein kinase.

pyomyositis: infection of muscle where abscess forms.

rhabdomyolysis: destruction of muscle following excessive activity, crush, or compartment syndrome. Can cause renal failure due to high levels of myoglobulin in blood.

Stewart-Morel syndrome: intermittent progressive muscular rigidity; **stiff man syndrome.**

trigger points: this term has several different meanings. In general, these are specific points of muscle or muscle attachment that are very tender and related to muscle spasm. Pressure on these points may cause pain referred distal to those points. These point areas may be the result of chronic spinal disorders or caused by overuse of specific muscle groups.

CARTILAGE DISEASES

Chondro- (Gr. *chondros,* gristle or cartilage). Cartilage serves a very important function in the growing process and joint motion. Healthy cartilage is essential for normal growth.

A growth plate called the epiphysis, a cartilage layer near or outside the joint, is essential to most of the longitudinal growth of bone during childhood. Disorders of this structure can lead to dwarfism or deformity. Cartilage is not apparent on radiographs, and many cartilage diseases are not detected until sufficient degeneration to cause joint narrowing takes place. Often a disorder that affects cartilage affects bone as well, such as osteo/chondr/itis (inflammation of bone and cartilage) or osteo/chondr/oma (bone and cartilage tumor).

Since diseased cartilage cells affect the combined function of bones and joints, many cartilage disease terms are found in the sections on bone tumors and joint diseases. The cartilage-related diseases are categorized in this section as follows:

1. *Chrondro-* root diseases
2. Miscellaneous cartilage diseases
3. Abnormalities of the epiphyses
4. Mucopolysaccharidoses (proteoglycan abnormalities)

Chondro- Root Diseases

chondralgia: pain in cartilage. This is an old term since there are no nerve pain fibers in cartilage. However, the perception is that pain comes from the cartilage; **chondrodynia.**

chondritis: inflammation of cartilage.

chondrodysplasia: hereditary deforming abnormal cartilage formation; **dyschondroplasia.**

chondrodysplasia punctata: X-linked dominant or recessive disorder.

chondrodystrophia: rare condition of nutritional abnormality of cartilage development; **dwarfism.**

chondroepiphysitis: inflammation of epiphyseal cartilage.

chondrofibroma: fibroma with cartilaginous elements.

chondrolipoangioma: a well-circumscribed tumor in which there is a predominance of mature cartilage, mature blood vessels, and mature fat.

chondrolipoma: fatty tumor containing cartilaginous elements.

chondrolysis: degeneration of cartilage cells, ending in cell death.

chondromalacia: softening of cartilage, as of the patella.

chondromatosis: multiple formation of chondromas.

chondrometaplasia: condition in which cells that would normally form cartilage function abnormally.

chondromyoma: muscle tumor with cartilaginous elements.

chondromyxoma: mucous tumor of bone with cartilaginous elements.

chondromyxosarcoma: sarcoma containing cartilaginous and mucous elements.

chondronecrosis: necrosis (death) of cartilage.

chondroosteodystrophy: nutritional abnormality of bone and cartilage.

chondropathology: diseased state of cartilage.

chondropathy: disease of cartilage.

chondrophyte: excess cartilaginous growth at bone ends, at the margins of a joint.

chondroporosis: normal growth process in childhood; in adults, the formation of empty space in cartilage is a part of a disease process.

chondrosarcomatosis: multiple chondrosarcomas; abnormal tumor cartilage.

chondrosteoma: tumor made up of bone and cartilaginous tissue.

Miscellaneous Cartilage Diseases

achondroplasia: autosomal dominant disorder affecting fibroblast growth factor-3; resulting in congenital dwarfism associated with deformed long bones and misshapen epiphyses; **achondroplastic dwarfism, chondrodystrophia fetalis.**

cartilage-hair hypoplasia: autosomal recessive disorder associated with short stature and abnormal facial appearance; **McKusick-type metaphyseal chondrodysplasia.**

diastrophic dwarfism: autosomal recessive dwarfism with flattening subluxation of various epiphyses due to defect in diastrophic dysplasia sulfate transporter; **diastrophic dysplasia.**

Henderson-Jones chondromatosis: synovial formation of multiple loose pieces of cartilage within a joint, often associated with pain and swelling. The condition can spontaneously resolve with absorption of the cartilage bodies.

hypochondrodysplasia: autosomal dominant condition due to mutation of fibroblast growth factor-3, resulting in milder dwarfing than achondroplasia and normal facial appearance.

Jansen d.: autosomal dominant disease or parathyroid hormone–related peptide receptor associated with mental retardation, short limb dwarfism, exophthalmia, hypercalcemia, and long bone bowing; **metaphyseal chondrodysplasia, Jansen type.**

Maffucci syndrome: dyschondroplasia with hemangiomas, some of which have calcified walls as seen on radiographs.

Ollier d.: multiple enchondromatosis, usually unilateral benign cartilage tumors of bone.

Schmid d.:   autosomal disorder affecting type X collagen and characterized by short stature, bowed lower extremities, coxa vara, flared metaphyses, and a waddling gait; **metaphyseal chondrodysplasia, Schmid type.**

Stickler syndrome: autosomal dominant disorder of type II collagen associated with small lower jaw, nearsightedness, thin limbs, mild scoliosis, and early degenerative arthritis. In another form, type IX collagen is affected and there is no eye disorder.

synchondrosis: fusion of cartilage surfaces in a joint. This may be a disease state or a normal maturation process, depending on the location.

synoviochondromatosis: process in which the joint lining forms small nodules of cartilage, which may break loose and be free in the joint. Synonymous with **synovial osteochondromatosis** or **osteochondromatosis.**

Abnormalities of the Epiphyses

The epiphyses are the cartilaginous layers at the end of long bones at the joints responsible for growth. Any dysfunction of metabolic origin or injury can cause deformity or dwarfism such as the following.

dysplasia epiphysealis hemimelia: osteochondroma arising from an epiphysis and projecting from the articular surface. This will usually interfere with joint function.

epiphyseal hyperplasia: condition in which the epiphyses form from multiple centers and become enlarged and misshapen.

epiphysiodesis: premature fusion of the epiphysis to diaphysis. This can be due to injury or surgical intent.

epiphysiolysis: separation of an epiphysis from the shaft of the bone.

epiphysiopathy: any disease of the epiphyses.

epiphysitis: inflammation of joint cartilage or epiphyses in contrast to rest of the bone.

hatchet head shoulder: flattening of humerus seen in multiple epiphyseal dysplasia. Not to be confused with hatchet head deformity seen after an anterior shoulder dislocation.

multiple epiphyseal dysplasia: multiple irregular epiphyseal ossification centers causing enlargement and flaring. **Type I multiple epiphyseal dysplasia** is due to an autosomal dominant disorder affecting oligomeric protein of cartilage, and **type II multiple epiphyseal dysplasia** is due to an autosomal dominant disorder affecting type IX collagen; **dysplasia epiphyseal multiplex congenita.**

slipped epiphysis: subluxation or dislocation of the epiphysis from the shaft of the bone. This may not necessarily be a single traumatic event but may occur gradually.

spondyloepiphyseal dysplasia: autosomal dominant and recessive disorders of type II collagen causing a spectrum of changes including inability to ossify normal epiphyseal centers, resulting in dwarfing and/or precocious osteoarthritis, primarily in spine and hips. There are four forms: congenita (autosomal dominant); tarda (autosomal recessive); X-linked; and **Kneist dysplasia** (autosomal dominant).

spondyloepiphyseal dysplasia of Maroteaux: disorder of development of vertebrae and hips but without associated biochemical and eye changes seen in Morquio syndromE.

stippled epiphysis: radiologic sign of chondrodystrophia calcificans, a disease associated with multiple calcifications of epiphyseal cartilage. A mild form of the condition may be called **epiphyseal dysplasia.**

Mucopolysaccharidoses (Metabolic Effects)

The mucopolysaccharidoses (MPSs) are a variety of hereditable metabolic disorders of mucopolysaccharides presently called *proteoglycans.* Glycosoaminoglycan chains are sugars that contain amino and sulfate components, are attached to a protein core molecule, and are formed by posttranslational pathways in the cell. Specific enzymatic failures are responsible for the accumulation of specific chemicals. *Muco-* originally signified the gelatinous appearance of the pure aggregate of these molecules. Most disorders of mucopolysaccharide metabolism are autosomal recessive. For many types, the eponymic designations are preferred because the metabolic nomenclature is complex.

Hunter s.: similar to Hurler syndrome, but less severely deforming; sex-linked dominant inheritance affecting sulfoiduronate sulfatase; *MPS II.* There are severe and mild forms of the disease.

Hunter-Scheie s.: condition that has mixed clinical appearance of Hunter and Scheie syndrome; *MPS I H/S.*

Hurler s.: autosomal recessive severely deforming condition associated with blindness, mental retardation, and early death; due to a deficiency of alpha-L-iduronidase; *MPS I H.* Formerly called **gargoylism, lipochondrodystrophy.**

Maroteaux-Lamy s.: growth retardation, lumbar kyphosis, sternal protrusion; no mental retardation; *MPS VI.*

Morquio s.: dwarfing disease affecting mostly the spine and hips; little or no mental retardation. There are two forms that have similar clinical appearance *MPS IV A* and *MPS IV B;* **chondro-osteodystrophy.** Both types are autosomal recessive inherited disorders of beta-galactosidase.

Sanfilippo s.: four forms exist and all have profound mental retardation, hyperactivity, and relatively mild somatic manifestations—*MPS III A, MPS III B, MPS III C,* and *MPS III D.*

Scheie s.: no mental impairment but noted corneal clouding, aortic disease, and stiff joints; *MPS I S.*

Sly s.: autosomal recessive disorder of glycogen phosphorylase, which causes multiple long bone growth abnormalities associated with liver and spleen enlargement; wide spectrum of severity; *MPS VII.*

DISEASES OF (SPECIFIC) SOFT TISSUE

In addition to bone, muscle, and cartilage, other tissues surround a joint. The root terms for these tissues (*fibro-, lipo-, myxo-, muco-*) denote the relationship to certain disease processes and disorders.

Fibro- Root Diseases

Fibro- (L. *fibra,* fiber) is a combining form indicating fibrous tissue such as tendons and ligaments. Such tissue contains collagen, which is the major supportive protein of bone, tendon, cartilage, and connective tissue. This elongated, threadlike structure may be subjected to the following abnormal processes.

elastofibroma: benign tumorlike growth usually seen in the back. It is a painless, slow-growing, firm, subcutaneous mass not attached to skin, and microscopically it appears as a nonencapsulated proliferation of collagen and elastin fibers with few fibroblasts. The most common location is subscapular.

fibroma: benign fibroblastic tumor.

fibromatosis: formation of multiple fibromas. This term is used for a variety of conditions including plantar and palmar fibromatosis, neurofibromatosis, and a more aggressive and locally invasive fibromatosis.

fibrosis: proliferation of fibrous tissue as a result of reaction to a reparative process.

fibrositis: inflammation of fibrous tissue.

fibrous histiocytoma: benign tumor of bone containing fibrous stroma, xanthomatous cells, and a round and spindle cell component. There is a malignant form called *malignant fibrous histiocytoma.*

Garrod fibromatosis (Garrod pads): thickening of the skin almost always confined to the dorsal aspects of the proximal interphalangeal joints of the hand.

juvenile hyaline fibromatosis: disease that develops in early childhood and is characterized by multiple fibromatous lesions of the skin, muscle, bone and ligaments, possibly leading to joint contractures. It is not necessarily progressive; histologically, it is characterized by multiple spindle cells with an amorphous matrix or collagenous tissue.

malignant fibrous histiocytoma: highly malignant soft-tissue tumor of later adult life that is initially seen as a subcutaneous to deep muscle lesion; **malignant fibrous xanthoma, fibroxanthosarcoma, malignant giant cell tumor of soft tissue.**

monostotic fibrous dysplasia: disease of bony remodeling, causing deformity of only one bone.

polyostotic fibrous dysplasia: disease marked by fibrous tissue replacement of bone with resultant deformities and clinical appearance of café-au-lait skin pigmentation and precocious puberty; **Albright syndrome.**

neurofibroma: abnormal proliferation of nerve sheath cells; **Schwann tumor.**

periarticular fibrositis: inflammatory condition of fibrous tissue surrounding a joint.

periosteal fibroma: fibrous tumor of bone-covering tissue.

pseudosarcomatous fibromatosis: disease of extensive subcutaneous fibroma formation; **subcutaneous pseudosarcomatous fibromatosis, proliferative fasciitis.**

Lipo- Root Diseases

Lipo- (Gr. *lipos,* fat) is a combining form denoting relationship to fat and fatty tissue. There are several disease processes based on this root.

lipochondrodystrophy: lipodystrophy as it affects cartilage.

lipodystrophy: defective metabolism of fat that results in the absence of subcutaneous fat, either partial or total. May be congenital or acquired.

lipofibroma: fibrous fatty tumor.

lipoma: fatty tumor; tumor made up of fat cells.

Myxo- Root Diseases

Myxo- (Gr. *myxa,* mucus) is a combining form denoting relationship to mucus. Myxomatous cells contain mucous material that is clear in appearance. These cells are naturally found in the intervertebral disks, but when seen elsewhere they usually represent an abnormality. Myxomatous cells contain the mucopolysaccharide (proteoglycan) material, which could rupture, causing mucous cysts to form. Terms containing *myxo-* indicate the presence of this type of cell.

myxofibroma: tumor containing both fibrous and myxomatous tissue.

myxoma: tumor containing myxoid cells.

myxosarcoma: sarcoma containing myxomatous tissue.

Muco- Root Diseases

The Latin word *mucus,* for the purposes of orthopaedics, does not imply secretions but rather the association of tissues that contain certain chemicals called *mucopolysaccharides,* which, when sufficient collection of material occurs, are in the form of a clear jelly and seen in certain cysts. Elsewhere in medicine, the terms *mucus* and *mucous* relate particularly to the gut and respiratory tract.

ganglion cyst: a sac, usually 1 mm to over 5 cm in size, commonly near a joint; contains a mix of collagen, proteoglycans, and other proteins with water such that the content appears clear and gelatinous. Ganglion cysts may occur anywhere, including within bone (intraosseous ganglion) and just under the periosteum (periosteal ganglion).

mucopolysaccharidosis: any of a variety of heritable disease states resulting from abnormalities in mucopolysaccharide (sugars containing SO_4 and NH_2) metabolism. These mainly affect cartilage in terms of orthopaedic diseases and cause stunted growth.

mucous cyst: in orthopaedics, a benign cyst under the fingernail.

LIGAMENT, TENDON, BURSA, AND FASCIA DISEASES

Desmo- Root Diseases

Desmo- (Gr. *desmos,* ligament) is a combining form denoting relationship to a band, bond, or ligament. Ligaments are composed of fibrous tissue that binds the joints together. Desmogenous dysfunctions and diseases may be any of the following:

desmectasis: stretching of a ligament.

desmitis: inflammation of a ligament.

desmocytoma: now called *fibrosarcoma.*

desmodynia: pain in a ligament; **desmalgia.**

desmoid: collection of fibrous tissue occurring at the insertion of a tendon (cortical desmoid) or arising from soft tissue of an extremity. The latter is a true tumor, recurrent but not malignant; **periosteal desmoid, extraabdominal desmoid.**

desmoma: a fibroma; a benign fibrous tumor.

desmopathy: any pathologic disease of a ligament.

desmoplasia: formation and development of fibrous tissue.

desmoplastic: producing or forming adhesions.

desmorrhexis: rupture of a ligament.

desmosis: disease of connective tissue.

extraabdominal desmoid (aggressive fibromatosis): a desmoid tumor that recurs with extensions in fascial planes but with no metastasis.

Eponymic Ligamentous Diseases

Duplay d.: capsulitis of the glenohumeral joint area; **frozen shoulder.**

MGHL cord: pattern where the *m*iddle *g*lenohumeral *l*igament is cordlike and enlarged.

Pellegrini-Stieda d.: ligamentous calcification of the medial collateral ligament of the knee following trauma.

Tendo-/Teno- Root Diseases

Tendo- and *teno-* (L. *tendo;* Gr. *tenōn*) are combining forms denoting relationship to a tendon. A tendon is a fibrous cord of connective tissue in which the fibers of a muscle end and by which the muscle is attached to bone.

tendonitis: inflammation of tendons and of tendon-muscle attachments; **tenontitis, tenonitis, tenositis.**

   bicipital t.: inflammation of a biceps muscle at tendon insertion of shoulder.

   calcific t.: inflammation associated with calcium deposits in the tendon and/or bursa (i.e., subacromial or subdeltoid bursa) producing pain and tenderness and limiting motion of shoulder.

   tendonitis ossificans traumatica: development of ossification in areas of tendons due to trauma.

tenodynia: pain in a tendon; **tenontodynia.**

tenontagra: gouty affection of tendons.

tenontophyma: tumorous growth in tendon.

tenontothecitis: inflammation of a tendon sheath.

tenoperiostitis: inflammation of muscle-tendon attachment to bone, for example, tennis elbow and golfer's elbow.

tenophyte: growth or concretion in tendon.

tenositis: inflammation of a tendon.

tenostosis: ossification of a tendon.

tenosynovitis: inflammation of a tendon sheath and synovial sac; **tendosynovitis.**

Other Tendon-Related Diseases

acute calcific tendonitis: rapid onset of pain and occasionally fever associated with swelling and redness. Most commonly confused with infection. Radiographs reveal subtle soft tissue calcification. Seen most commonly in the hands and wrist, but may be seen in the shoulder, elbow, hip, or knee. Rarely seen in the small, deep anterior neck muscles. This condition may be called **acute calcific retropharyngeal tendonitis** and is important to orthopaedics because it is a benign cause of severe neck pain.

Albert achillodynia: discomfort felt around terminal segment of heel cord; **achillodynia, achillobursitis.**

de Quervain d.: tenosynovitis of the abductor pollicis longus and extensor pollicis brevis.

enthesopathy: degenerative disorders of ligaments, muscles, and tendon attachments to bone, the central structure in the disease process. **Enthesis** is the site of a tendon, ligament, or muscle attachment to bone. However, the term is more specifically applied to certain degenerative disorders of tendons such as supraspinatus and Achilles tendonitis. Since a neighboring bursa may be involved, it is sometimes called a bursitis.

enthesitis: inflammation resulting from stress on muscle or tendon that is attached to bone. There is a strong tendency toward fibrosis, calcification, and even rupture.

epicondylitis: inflammation of the tendon origins on the medial epicondyle (*golfer's elbow, thrower's elbow*) or the lateral epicondyle (*tennis elbow*).

Bursa-Related Diseases

Bursae (pl.) are closed sacs of fibrous tissue lined with synovial membrane, filled with viscid fluid, and situated in places in tissue where friction would otherwise inhibit function, such as near joints. Most disorders of bursae are part of another disease process.

bursitis: inflammation of a bursa at site of bony prominences between muscles or tendons.

> **calcific bursitis:** deposition of calcium in a bursa, usually associated with inflammation; can often be seen on a radiograph.

bursolith: calculus or concretion in a bursa.

bursopathy: any pathologic condition of bursae.

Fascia-Related Diseases

Fasciae (L. *fascia,* band) are bands of fibrous tissue that lie deep to the skin and form an investment for muscles and various organs of the body. *Retinacula* (*retinaculum,* sing.) are also thickened bands that bind muscles and tendons of distal portion of limbs into position. There are several processes that are disease related.

Dupuytren contracture: thickening and contracture of the palmar fascia of the hand resulting in flexion deformities of the fingers.

fasciitis: inflammation of fascia. Usually an anatomic structure is named when describing the location of the fasciitis, for example, plantar fasciitis, inflammation of the fascia of the sole of the foot.

nodular fasciitis: fasciitis resulting in the formation of nodules.

JOINT DISEASES (ARTHRO-, SYNOVIO-, CAPSULO-, ANKYLO-)

The joint (*arthro-*) has a smooth inner lining or fluid sac (synovium) and a strong fibrous outer connective tissue enclosure (*capsulo-*). Affections of the joint cartilage, synovium, and capsule may result in transient or permanent functional changes. When motion is severely or completely lost, **ankylosis** (an abnormal fusion of a joint) is the result. The terms in this section relate to loss of joint function or a change in appearance of the joint. Joint function depends on its surrounding tissue. Diseases or dysfunctions affecting the joint spaces are presented here.

Arthro- Root Diseases

Arthro- (Gr. *arthron,* joint) is a combining form denoting relationship to a joint, the junction where two bones meet and articulate with one another. Articulatio (Latin) is a general term for joint. The *arthro-* root diseases are as follows:

arthralgia: pain in a joint; **arthrodynia.**

arthrempyesis: infection in a joint; **arthro-empyesis.**

arthritis: pathologic inflammation of a joint; may be crippling; can become a degenerative joint disease. Various types are osteoarthritis, gouty a., rheumatoid a., septic a., traumatic a., infectious a., allergenic a., and hemophilic a.

arthrocace: infected cavity of a joint; caries.

arthrocele: swollen joint.

arthrochalasis: abnormal relaxation or flaccidity of a joint.

arthrochondritis: inflammation of the cartilages of a joint.

arthrodysplasia: deformity of various joints; hereditary condition.

arthrogryposis: nonspecific term descriptive of a congenital, progressive limitation of movement as a result of soft-tissue contractures affecting two or more joints.

arthrokatadysis: limitation of motion of the hip resulting from protrusio acetabuli (deep-shelled acetabulum).

arthrokleisis: ankylosis of a joint.

arthrolith: deposit of calculus in a joint.

arthromeningitis: synovitis; inflammation of the membranous lining of a joint.

arthroncus: joint swelling; **arthrophyma.**

arthroneuralgia: nerve pain in a joint.

arthronosos: disease of joints.

arthropathy: any joint disease.

arthrophyte: abnormal growth in a joint cavity.

arthropyosis: suppuration, or formation of pus, in a joint cavity.

arthrorheumatism: articular rheumatism.

arthrosclerosis: hardening or stiffening of a joint.

arthrosis: disease or abnormal condition of a joint.

arthrosteitis: inflammation of any bony joint structure.

arthrosynovitis: inflammation of the synovial membrane of a joint.

arthroxerosis: chronic osteoarthritis.

Other Joint Diseases and Conditions

cystic arthrosis: development of large cysts just under the bony surface of a joint. It is not clear whether this is due to cystic degeneration within the bone that leaves the articular cartilage intact or to synovial invasion from the joint. Condition progresses to degenerative arthritis. This condition is probably separate from ganglions that form within the bone and are not associated with arthritic progression.

diffuse idiopathic sclerosing hyperostosis (DISH):   excess bone formation at the margins of large joints, particularly the lumbar spine and hips.

flail joint: complete loss of ligamentous stability.

frozen shoulder: severe loss of motion in the shoulder joint resulting from inflammation of the capsule.

hemarthrosis: extravasation of blood into a joint or synovial cavity.

hydrarthrosis: accumulation of watery fluid in the joint cavity.

hypertrophic arthritis: increased bone formation around the joint, as seen on radiographs; *osteoarthritis.*

internal derangement of joint: commonly named "internal knee injuries," particularly when the precise nature of the injury is unknown.

joint mice: loose pieces of cartilage or other organic material in the joint.

pauciarticular: involving a few joints as opposed to many joints.

polyarthritis: inflammation of many joints.

pseudoarthrosis: false joints that result from nonunion of a fracture or from a pathologic bone condition.

pustulotic osteoarthropathy: pain, swelling, and radiographic findings of hypertrophy and sclerotic changes involving the sternum, ribs, and clavicle associated with the skin condition pustulosis palmaris et plantaris. The sacrum, spine, and peripheral joints may also show radiographic changes. The cause is unknown.

rice bodies: small, glistening, soft, loose bodies either in joints or bursae; *loose fibrocartilage tissue.*

suppurative arthritis: bacterial infection causing pain, swelling, tenderness, redness, and effusion; **pyarthrosis.**

synarthrosis: ankylosis and contracture; usually caused by arthritic joint disease.

villous lipomatous proliferation: rare disorder of synovial joint lining where there is fatty proliferation with the formation of numerous villous formations. The term **lipoma arborescens** was applied to this condition. Because it is not a neoplasm, the villous lipomatous proliferation term is preferred.

Eponymic Joint Diseases

Behçet syndrome: disease of undetermined etiology that may produce joint complaints predominantly in young people in the third decade of life. Marked by oral and genital ulcerations and eye and skin lesions. Often arthritis, thrombophlebitis, gastrointestinal lesions, and central nervous system lesions also occur.

Kawasaki d.: mucocutaneous lymph node syndrome in children characterized by fever, exanthomatous skin disease, and sometimes arthritis (30% to 40%).

Lyme d.: inflammatory arthritis involving usually a few joints, particularly the knees, caused by an organism that is transmitted by a tick.

Reiter syndrome: arthritis of various joints, usually associated with one or more of the triad of urethral drip, conjunctivitis, and oral mucosal lesions.

Synovio-Related Diseases

Synovial fluid, or synovia, is an alkaline viscid transparent fluid resembling egg white that is found in joint cavities, tendon sheaths, and bursae and is responsible for lubrication and nourishment of these joint structures. Synovial membrane is the inner lining of a joint, which is a two-layer membrane on a bed of fat composed of certain cells that produce synovial fluid; other cells act as phagocytes. Related disease processes are the following:

synovial cyst: accumulation of fluid in any bursa forming a firm cystic structure. The fluid often becomes gelatinous as seen in a ganglion. The contents and structures of these cysts are often indistinguishable from a ganglion. Some can communicate with a joint or tendon sheath.

    popliteal cyst: seen behind the knee, this cyst usually involves the gastrocnemius-semimembranosus bursa.

    antefemoral cyst: located in the suprapatellar area.

    anteromedial cyst: found in association with the pes anserinus bursa below the anteromedial joint line.

    tibiofibular cyst: associated with the tibiofibular joint, which in 10% of people communicates with the knee.

synovial osteochondromatosis: formation by the synovium of cartilage bodies, which develop into bone.

synoviochondromatosis: synovial formation of cartilage bodies.

synovitis: inflammation of synovial membrane, which may be associated with swelling.

Miscellaneous Synovial Diseases

pigmented villonodular synovitis: inflammation of synovium with production of pigment, giant cells, and other characteristic cell types.

villous synovitis: inflammation of joint lining, resulting in long fronds of synovium.

Capsulo-Related Diseases

The capsule is the thick fibrous tissue enclosing the cavity of the synovial joint and defines the limits of the joint; more *joint c., synovial c.* There are two related dysfunctions.

adhesive capsulitis: adhesive inflammation between joint capsule and the peripheral articular cartilage of the shoulder, obscuring the subdeltoid bursa. It produces a painful shoulder, stiffness, and may result in limited joint motion; *frozen shoulder, adhesive bursitis.*

capsulitis: inflammation of the capsule.

Ankylo-Root Diseases

The combining form *ankylo-* means bent or deformed. It was originally used to describe untreated deforming loss of joint function. Now such terms apply to joints fused congenitally or those that are aligned normally because of a surgical process. Therefore the implication of *ankylo-* is not necessarily bent or deformed but rather complete fusion or restricted motion of a joint.

ankylodactylia: adhesions of fingers or toes to one another.

ankylosis: consolidation and abnormal immobility of a joint caused by fibrous or bone tissue bridging the joint space.

> ***bony a.:*** abnormal union of bones at joint site; **true ankylosis.**

> ***extracapsular a.:*** caused by rigidity of structure exterior to joint capsule, usually a surgically implanted piece of bone.

> ***false a.:*** results from other causes not related to the abnormal union of bones comprising the joint.

> ***fibrous a.:*** caused by formation of fibrous bands within the joint.

> ***intracapsular a.:*** caused by undue rigidity of structure within the joint capsule.

> ***ligamentous a.:*** results from rigidity of ligaments.

> ***spurious a.:*** false ankylosis.

VASCULAR DISEASES AND CONDITIONS

Blood Vessels

All tissues of the body are supplied with nutrients and oxygen by blood vessels. These vessels are subject to an assortment of disease processes. The larger named arteries are usually impaired by arteriosclerosis or trauma; the larger named veins are usually impaired by trauma or thrombosis; and the smaller, unnamed vessels (on either side of the circulation) can be injured by arteriosclerosis, trauma, or systemic degenerative disorders (e.g., collagen vascular diseases). In addition to these, the heart itself can be afflicted by diseases of the arteries that feed the heart muscle, causing deterioration of the muscle (cardiomyopathy).

Trauma and arteriosclerosis (hardening of the arteries) are the two most frequent arterial conditions that are seen by the orthopaedic surgeon. However, the orthopaedist will often see a host of other vascular disorders or symptoms that influence the treatment of a musculoskeletal problem. Often, patients with these specific disease entities are referred to the peripheral vascular surgeon, and a combined effort is made to restore function. The venous and arterial disorders, collagen vascular disorders, and blood vessel tumors are considered here.

Venous Disorders

deep venous thrombosis (DVT):   blood clots in the deep venous circulation usually of the lower extremity, in the calf, thigh, or pelvis. Portions of these clots may break off and lodge in the lungs, causing pulmonary emboli. These clots in the veins eventually destroy the valves of the veins and can cause chronic problems related to venous insufficiency.

phlebitis: inflammation of a vein; may be a result of infection, inflammation, or trauma and is usually associated with thrombus in that vein (thrombophlebitis).

phlebothrombosis: clot in a vein; phlebitis with secondary thrombosis.

postphlebitic syndrome: chronic venous insufficiency of lower limbs resulting from deep venous thrombosis. Develops with loss of function of valves in veins, allowing blood to pool and cause swelling, pain, leg ulceration, and varicose veins.

pulmonary embolism (PE):   acute obstruction to circulation in lungs as a result of a clot that has migrated from the pelvic or leg veins and lodged in the lung. A life-threatening problem requiring anticoagulants and sometimes surgery.

thrombophlebitis: inflammation of a vein associated with thrombosis (blood clots) usually in the lower limbs. The clot can also become infected, becoming septic thrombophlebitis.

thrombosis: formation of a clot (thrombus) within a blood vessel that results in occlusion or stenosis of the vessel, which may cause infarction of tissue supplied by that vessel.

varices (*sing.* -ix):   enlarged and tortuous (twisted) veins or lymphatic vessels, usually of the lower limbs; many types; **varicose veins.**

venous insufficiency (reflux):   malfunction of venous valves that allow blood to flow in a retrograde (backward) direction; **postphlebitic syndrome.**

Arterial Disorders

aneurysm: thin-walled, dilated segment of a vessel wall that may be caused by degeneration from arteriosclerosis, congenital abnormality, or trauma. Complications of aneurysms include rupture, thrombosis, or breakoff of a blood clot that has collected in the aneurysm.

arterial insufficiency: inadequate blood flow to an organ or extremity frequently caused by arteriosclerotic narrowing or occlusion of the blood vessel restricting blood flow. In severe cases, necrosis and gangrene may develop, requiring amputation of a limb.

arterial occlusive disease: hardening of the arteries; **arteriosclerosis.**

arteriosclerosis: name for degenerative process that affects most blood vessels in most people (in varying degrees) and begins in early teens. Its progression is related in part to genetics, diet, smoking, and high blood pressure. It can be exacerbated by injuries such as trauma or surgery; it causes narrowing and irregular surfaces in blood vessels, where fatty plaque forms on vessel walls and occludes the blood supply, which leads to ischemia. It is the most frequent problem in arteries; **atherosclerosis.**

arteriovenous fistula (AVF):   abnormal communication between an artery and a vein; **AV fistula.** See malformation, arteriovenous.

atheroma: localized collection of arteriosclerosis (thickened arterial intima) that has degenerated.

blue toe syndrome: bluish or black tender and painful discoloration of a toe. It is the result of a localized acute ischemia of the toe caused by distal embolization of platelet aggregates or arteriosclerotic plaque, which then occludes the small end vessels. This represents a proximal embologenic source, for example, aneurysm or significant arteriosclerotic plaque.

Buerger disease: thromboangiitis obliterans: an inflammation of the arteries (and veins) in extremity causing severe ischemia; occurs usually in young smokers and is a pathologic variant of arteriosclerosis.

cerebrovascular accident (CVA): ischemia of a portion of the brain as a result of an occluded blood vessel from an embolus arising from the heart or great vessels of the neck; frequently the result of hardening of the arteries, a rupture of the blood vessel in the brain, or a tumor; **stroke.**

chilblains: breakdown of skin and swelling of the hands and feet from overexposure to cold moisture; *thermal injuries.*

claudication: inadequate blood flow to large muscle groups of lower limbs resulting from hardening of the arteries, causing pain, numbness, or heaviness in muscle groups brought on by exercise and relieved by rest; may produce similar symptoms in the upper limbs after prolonged use; *intermittent claudication.*

compartment syndrome: compromise of circulation and function of tissue within a closed space caused by increased pressure within that space, with diminished oxygenated blood supply; may be due to overexertion of leg muscles, a tight bandage, or trauma-related injury. The syndrome may self-correct or progress, with eventual muscle necrosis (ischemia), loss of arterial blood supply, nerve palsy, or loss of limb. The most commonly affected compartments are the anterior leg **(anterior compartment syndrome),** volar forearm (leading to Volkmann ischemic contracture), and anterior thigh **(rectus femoris syndrome).**

embolus (*pl.* emboli): blood clot or piece of atheromatous debris that blocks an artery or vein. Can also be made up of an air bubble, fat, portion of tumor, or piece of prosthetic material. An embolus may cause a heart attack if in the heart, a stroke if in the brain, and acute ischemia if in the lower limbs.

fibromuscular d.: poorly understood, uncommon degenerative disease of the arteries frequently affecting the renal arteries of young females. The problem causes narrowing of the vessel with weblike deformities that appear as a string of beads on an arteriogram. Can also cause aneurysm.

fistula: abnormal communication between any two structures that normally do not communicate; can be the result of trauma, arteriosclerosis, or surgical procedure. An arteriovenous fistula may be created and used for hemodialysis.

frostbite: damage to tissue resulting from exposure to cold; may lower blood supply sufficiently to cause permanent sensory loss, chronic pain, or partial limb loss.

infarct: small area of ischemic necrosis resulting from acute interruption of blood supply. This term is frequently applied to areas of the brain or heart.

ischemia: acute or chronic decreased blood flow to organ or limb caused by obstruction of inflow of arterial blood or by vasoconstriction. Acutely, the symptoms include the six p's: pain, pallor, pulselessness, paresthesias, paralysis, and poikilothermia (coldness).

kinking: bending of an artery, causing pain; result of trauma or body position.

malformation, arteriovenous (AVM): congenital arteriovenous connection often resulting in disfigurement or malfunction. Frequently seen as a discolored area on the skin, but may represent a much larger diversion of blood such that it interferes with organ function. Its continuing presence may interfere with the heart because of the large alteration in flow that it creates.

popliteal cyst: degeneration of the wall of the popliteal artery resulting in a cystic-like structure within the wall of the artery that can partially or completely obstruct the artery. This term should be called "pop art cyst" (*popliteal arterial cyst*) to avoid confusion with the more common synovial or ganglion type.

popliteal entrapment: partial or complete obstruction of popliteal artery as a result of abnormal location of adjacent medial head of the gastrocnemius muscle. May include artery, vein, and/or nerve.

rest pain: distal foot pain caused by acute or chronic arterial ischemia representing a significant decrease in blood flow, usually from hardening of the arteries. The pain is burning and sharp in nature and frequently begins by keeping the patient awake at night. May be relieved by dependent position.

rubor (dependent): dark purplish-red color to foot when foot is hung over the edge of bed. It represents maximally dilated capillary beds that are responding to decreased arterial inflow and their subsequent fill by gravity.

stroke: see cerebrovascular accident (CVA).

Sudeck atrophy: vascular reflex in a limb, caused by trauma, resulting in a red, stiff, and severely painful limb; referred to as "causalgia" when caused by trauma involving a large area or affecting a large nerve.

transient ischemic attack (TIA): transient neurologic deficit that clears within 24 hours. Usually the result of decreased blood flow to the portion of brain from a blood clot from either the heart or extracranial carotid vessels. Usually from hardening of the arteries—atheromatous plaque breaks off and lodges in the vessels of the brain or eye.

Volkmann contracture: final state of an unrelieved forearm compartment syndrome; decreased blood supply to forearm muscles resulting in muscle death, contractures of tendons to wrist and hand, and a claw-hand deformity. This usually starts out as a compartment syndrome that develops after an elbow or forearm fracture.

Collagen Vascular Disorders

Collagen vascular diseases are a series of disorders relating to the basic building blocks of the body, that is, collagen. The walls of blood vessels are made up of collagen, a type of protein seen in all connective tissue such as bone, cartilage, and tendon. Certain diseases affect the collagen, particularly in scattered blood vessels.

Through a variety of mechanisms, the immune system of the body begins to attack, thereby causing degeneration in small blood vessels and/or parts of the bony anatomy (joint capsule, synovial fluid of joint and synovium). The systemic inflammatory condition that results can be mildly inconvenient or severely disabling, or can result in death. Certain diseases such as rheumatoid arthritis affect this collagen and, as a result, interfere with the function of bones, joints, and blood vessels. The term *inflammatory joint disease* is often used to describe arthritis, but this general term is also applied to gout, pseudogout, and some other systemic causes of arthritis.

Dyscollagenoses and **systemic connectivitis** are terms specifically related to the immune connective tissue disorders of rheumatoid arthritis, systemic lupus erythematosus, Sjögren syndrome, progressive systemic sclerosis, polyarteritis nodosa, polymyositis, dermatomyositis, and eosinophilic fasciitis. This spectrum of disorders represents the effects on the different collagens of the joint lining and vascular walls.

The treatment of these disorders is often complicated and frustrating for both patient and physician. Medication frequently involves corticosteroids (antiinflammatory drugs) and nonsteroidal antiinflammatory drugs (ibuprofen, aspirin), and often drugs that directly interfere with the immune mechanism of the body (antimetabolites). **Rheumatology** is the specialty devoted to the diagnosis and treatment of these systemic conditions. A rheumatologist is an internal medical specialist. Although rheumatologists often deal with nonsystemic joint diseases, specialty training in this field equips them with the pharmacologic knowledge required to diagnose the broad spectrum of autoimmune and metabolic joint disorders.

Terms associated with these various conditions are discussed here along with a series of other miscellaneous disorders.

acrosclerosis: thickening of the skin and other soft tissues of the distal part of a limb. This is usually a part of a larger disease complex such as scleroderm or CREST syndrome.

ankylosing spondylitis: inflammatory joint disease mainly affecting the spine, hips, and pelvis. Seen most commonly in young men, this can lead to fusion of the spine with deformity, depending on the position of the spine during the fusion process. Seen in the child, the disorder is called Marie-Strümpell disease or rheumatoid spondylitis.

arteritis: inflammation of small arteries.

calcinosis circumscripta: quadrad of calcium deposits in the skin (calcinosis cutis), Raynaud phenomenon, scleroderma, and telangiectasia is seen in this collagen disease that has been considered a variant of scleroderma.

CREST syndrome (limited scleroderma): complex of *c*alcinosis of articular tissue associated with *R*aynaud phenomenon, *e*sophageal dysmotility, *s*clerodactyly, and *t*elangiectasia. This condition appears to be less aggressive than scleroderma.

dermatomyositis: idiopathic, autoimmune, inflammatory myopathy characterized by proximal limb and neck weakness. Muscles may become painful, weak, and stiff. A rash can appear on the knees, knuckles, and elbows. The pathologic findings are muscle necrosis and regeneration.

ergotism: acute or chronic effects of ergot alkaloids on the blood flow to an organ such as the brain or limbs. Ergot alkaloids are in some plants and medicines that are taken for headaches.

Felty syndrome: a combination of chronic rheumatoid arthritis, enlarged spleen, and a reduced number of granulocytes in the white blood count.

focal scleroderma: disease of unknown etiology characterized by circumscribed areas of fibrosis of the skin, subcutaneous fat, fascia, and muscle into bone. It is usually restricted to a limb and usually occurs in children and young adults; **Addison's keloid.**

intermittent hydrarthrosis: rare disorder characterized by recurrent swelling in joints with no associated problems or deformity.

Jaccoud syndrome: deformity of hands and feet as a result of recurrent episodes of rheumatic fever or lupus synovitis. Often mistaken for rheumatoid arthritis.

lupus erythematosus: disease affecting not only the joints but also heart, heart lining, and circulation in bone. It is life threatening, although a protracted mild course is possible. This disease may be called **systemic lupus erythematosus** to distinguish it from discoid lupus, a more benign process.

Marie-Strümpell d.: begins in childhood, similar to rheumatoid arthritis, usually resulting in ankylosis of the spine and involvement of the liver and spleen; **rheumatoid** or **ankylosing spondylitis.**

Mönckeberg sclerosis: calcification of the middle coat of small and medium-sized muscular arteries; **medial arteriosclerosis.**

palindromic rheumatism: recurrent acute arthritis and periarthritis with symptom-free intervals of days to months. A number of patients with this disorder develop rheumatoid arthritis.

polyarteritis nodosa: disease causing nodules in small arteries with some microscopic clotting, resulting in muscle cramps and eventual loss of muscle tone; can be severe.

progressive systemic sclerosis: spectrum of disorders that are characterized by fibrosis and degenerative changes in the skin. This includes scleroderma and CREST syndrome.

Raynaud d. or phenomenon: small arterioles of upper limbs, particularly of the fingertips, become extremely sensitive to cold, and the vessels undergo segmental spasm, interrupting blood flow to tissue; occasionally progresses to necrosis and dry gangrene in fingertips.

rheumatoid arthritis: generalized inflammatory joint disease. In children, it is called **juvenile rheumatoid arthritis** and **Still disease.** The disease may result in mild, lifelong discomfort, or it may become severely crippling; in some cases, there is associated skin nodularity. Certain laboratory studies confirm the diagnosis. (Positive rheumatoid factor.)

scleroderma: disease causing a waxy thickening of the skin and classically affecting swallowing; tends to be severely progressive.

Sjögren syndrome: a group of conditions including keratoconjunctivitis sicca (dry eyes), arthritis, dry mouth, and enlargement of the parotid glands.

vasoconstriction: narrowing of vessel lumen caused by contraction of muscular vessel walls.

vasodilatation: enlargement of vessel lumen caused by relaxing of muscular vessel wall.

vasospastic: localized intermittent contraction of a blood vessel.

Blood Vessel Tumors

hemangioendothelioma: tumor composed mostly of endothelial cells of the inner walls of capillary vessels.

hemangioma: any benign small-vessel tumor of dilated blood vessels; may be flush with the skin with a violescent, patchy discoloration or elevated like a violescent or red mole. Size may vary from 1 mm to large area of the body.

hemangiopericytoma: spindle cell tumor with a rich vascular network; arises from pericytes.

hemangiosarcoma: malignant blood vessel tumor; **angiosarcoma.**

Asscociated Vascular Conditions

acrocyanosis: mottling of the skin of the extremity not produced by major vascular occlusions. May be related to an emotional change or temperature.

atrophy: reduction in size of an anatomic structure, frequently related to disuse or decreased blood supply.

arrhythmia: abnormal rhythm of the heart.

bradycardia: abnormal slowing of heart rate, usually under 60 beats/minute.

bruit: abnormal sound on mediate auscultation over a blood vessel or the heart that indicates turbulence.

congestive heart failure: condition in which heart is unable to pump out venous blood returning to it, resulting in pooling of venous blood and accumulation of fluid in various parts of the body (lungs, legs, etc.).

cyanosis: bluish-purple discoloration of the skin or nail beds; represents decreased blood flow to that area.

hypercholesterolemia: elevated blood cholesterol level; **hypercholesteremia, hypercholesterinemia.**

hypertension: elevated blood pressure, either temporary or permanent; may be an elevation of the systolic or diastolic blood vessels or pressure.

hypotension: blood pressure below normal.

hypovolemia: loss of normal amount of circulating blood volume; could be the result of hemorrhage from trauma (or from ulcer).

hypoxia: decreased amount of oxygen in any given tissue.

myocardial infarction (MI): acute or chronic blockage of blood vessels to the heart, resulting in localized area of ischemia (heart attack).

necrosis: pathologic definition of death of tissues caused by lack of blood supply to that part.

normotensive: referring to normal blood pressure.

occlusion: closed or shut, such as an occluded artery or vein.

palpitation: sensation either by patient or examiner of irregular heartbeat.

phlegmasia cerulea dolens: an acute, rare condition that includes a nonpitting edema (swelling that cannot be indented with pressure) in the legs associated with a cyanotic mottled appearance and high muscle compartment pressures. This has been associated with the use of vena cava filters.

stasis: decrease or absence of flow in the venous circulation.

stenosis: narrowing of lumen of blood vessel; a stricture.

tachycardia: abnormal increase in heart rate, usually over 100 beats/minute in an adult.

NEUROLOGIC DISEASES

Neuro- (Gr. *neuron,* nerve) is a combining form denoting the relationship to a nerve or nerves, or to the nervous sytem in general. Of all the specialties in medicine, neurology interrelates with orthopaedics more frequently than any other. The presenting symptoms of certain neurologic disorders may be quite similar to those of some orthopaedic disorders or diseases in that they result in muscular loss, altered function, and possible deformities, particularly in growing individuals.

In orthopaedic diagnoses, the nervous system is considered in two portions, the central and the peripheral. The central portion is composed of the brain and spinal cord and their covering soft tissues. The peripheral portion is composed of all the nerves in the body. Because some diseases affect both the central and peripheral nervous systems simultaneously, discussion of both is presented in an alphabetic listing of nerve disorders, except for some eponymic terms that belong to a specific category. The same term may be defined several times in this chapter to avoid cross-referencing.

General Neurologic Diseases

amyotrophic lateral sclerosis (ALS): disease principally of the spinal cord, seen in adult life; results in loss of motor control and eventual death; **Charcot d., Lou Gehrig d.**

apoplexy: old term used to describe a stroke, a bleeding into or loss of blood supply to the brain.

apraxia: inability to perform purposeful movements where there is no sensory or motor impairment; **kinetic a., motor a.**

arachnoiditis: inflammatory disease of the covering, spiderweb-like membrane of the spinal cord and nerves. In the lumbar spine, this condition can lead to fibrosis that will bind the roots of the cauda equina.

ataxia: motor incoordination.

atonia: lack of tone or tension; relaxation, flaccidity.

axonotmesis: disruption of nerve plasma without disruption of the axon sheath, resulting in a recovery of nerve function over a period of up to 3 years.

Barre-Lieou syndrome: degenerative or arthritic changes of C3, C4, and intervertebral disks, frequently involving the 5th and 6th cervical nerves. Affects mainly middle-aged and older patients, many of whom have associated complaints of dizziness, nausea, headaches, transitory deafness, blurred vision, and loss of balance because of presumed involvement of the cervical sympathetic nervous system and the vertebral artery.

causalgia: lesion of a peripheral nerve containing sensory fibers manifested by burning pain, hypersensitivity, and paresthesias in the limb. A painful condition that occurs after trauma, infection, or vascular inflammation of extremity; associated with a fracture or dislocation with soft-tissue, nerve, and vascular injury. To distinguish this from similar disorders in which a nerve is not involved, the term causalgia has been used. The terms **reflex sympathetic dystrophy, post-traumatic reflex dystrophy, Sudeck atrophy, mimocausalgia,** and **algodystrophy** are used for those disorders in which there is a similar exaggerated response to an injury such as fracture, sprain, laceration, or other minor insult.

cerebral palsy (CP): very general term applied to central nervous system disorders found at birth or infancy that affect muscle control; can range from being almost undetectable to totally incapacitating and extremely deforming. There is mild to severe loss of motor control, which is called **diplegic CP** if it seems to affect primarily the lower extremities.

>**spastic CP:** most common form; attempts by victim to use affected muscles result in uncontrolled contractions.

>**ataxic CP:** additional elements of incoordination.

>**athetoid CP:** uncontrolled writhing movements.

>**flaccid CP:** very severe form in which muscle contractions cannot be initiated.

chorea: continuing uncontrolled jerking motions caused by brain disease; may occur as a result of rheumatic fever or other diseases; may be inherited, which is called **Huntington chorea; St. Vitus dance.**

dysautonomia: an often familial condition characterized by labile blood pressure, insensitivity to pain, abnormal gastrointestinal motility, ataxia, and spinal deformity.

dural ectasia: often seen with neurofibromatosis, thickening of the dural tissues may occur. This can lead to dissolution of the spinal elements and eventual spinal instability.

entrapment syndrome: symptoms caused by entrapment of a nerve in soft or hard tissue, for example, occipital nerve entrapment syndrome, a chronic muscle irritation of the neck, causing impingement on occipital nerve.

epilepsy: disorder of nervous system characterized by seizures in which there may be clonic and tonic muscular contractions and loss of consciousness.

>**grand mal e.:** epilepsy marked by major convulsions, usually first tonic then clonic, oscillating eyeballs, feeble pulse, stupor, and unconsciousness.

>**petit mal e.:** mild or minor attack (small seizures) of epilepsy without convulsions other than slight twitching of muscles of the face or extremities.

>**jacksonian e.:** recurrent episodes of localized convulsive seizures or spasms limited to a part of the body, without loss of consciousness.

familial dysautonomia: autosomal recessive disorder of autonomic system.

ganglioneuroma: tumor made up of ganglion cells.

glioma: tumor arising from specialized connective tissue found in brain and spinal cord.

glomus tumor: benign tumor consisting of nerve and small-vessel components. These small lesions often produce severe pain and local vascular effects. They are often found near the tips of digits of the hands and feet.

hemiplegia: paralysis of one side of the body.

Klumpke palsy (lower obstetrical palsy): palsy of the lower cervical nerve roots, C8 and T1; usually seen following an infant delivery but may be seen in adult life after trauma.

locomotor ataxia: see Tabes dorsalis.

lumbar thecoperitoneal shunt syndrome: occurs after a thecoperitoneal shunt for idiopathic communicating hydrocephalus, characterized by severe, rigid, and progressive lumbar lordosis, severe bilateral restriction of straight leg raising, and abnormalities of stance and gait.

meralgia: pain in the thigh, usually caused by irritation of lateral cutaneous nerve of the thigh.

mononeuritis multiplex: impairment of sensation, usually in the foot, where there is increased or decreased sensitivity associated with a vasculitis, usually seen in rheumatoid vasculitis.

motor neuron d.: any disease caused by destruction of the nerve cells involved in voluntary muscle function.

>**upper motor neuron d.:** any brain disorder that affects the normal pathways leading to voluntary muscle function.

lower motor neuron d.: disorder of the cells in the spinal cord, resulting in loss of motor function.

multiple sclerosis: slowly progressive disease of nervous system in which scattered areas of degeneration of the myelin occur; common in the spinal cord; cause unknown.

myopathy hand: characteristic hand dysfunction due to spinal cord injury. A loss of adduction power, extension of the ulnar two or three fingers, and an inability to grip and release rapidly with these fingers distinguishes this hand weakness from other hand dysfunctions due to peripheral nerve disorders.

neural tube defect: group of malformations of the brain and spinal cord that originate at various times during fetal development. The most commonly seen kind is meningomyelocele.

neuralgia: pain along the course of a nerve or nerves.

neuritis: inflammation of any nerve; usually painful.

neurogenic: occurring because of a nervous system disorder.

neurologic d.: any disease of the nervous system.

neurolysis: dissolution of the nerve tissue in disease process.

neuroma: this condition is not an actual tumor but is due to a tumescence in the nerve due to hypertrophy of the cells covering the inside and outside of the nerve.

  traumatic n.: neuroma caused by a complete cutting of the nerve or by sufficient injury to cause excess scarring in the nerve.

  amputation n.: a traumatic neuroma occurring after an amputation.

neuropathy: any disease of the peripheral nerves (those outside the brain and spinal cord).

neuropraxia: contusion of a nerve resulting in transient disruption of nerve function; less severe than axonotmesis or neurotmesis.

neurotmesis: complete transection of a nerve, resulting in cell death.

paralysis: loss or impairment of voluntary muscle function; palsy.

paralysis agitans: chronic nervous disease in later life marked by muscular tremor or by a peculiar gait; Parkinson disease.

paraplegia: paralysis of lower part of body or lower extremities.

paresis: incomplete loss of voluntary muscle function.

paresthesia: abnormal sensations such as numbness, burning, tickling, and crawling due to central or peripheral nerve lesions such as multiple sclerosis or locomotor ataxia.

pellagra: vitamin B_6 deficiency disease manifested by disorders of skin, alimentary tract, and nervous system.

peripheral neuropathy: diseases at or distal to the nerve root.

poliomyelitis: inflammation of gray matter of spinal cord; may result in loss of voluntary muscle control.

polyneuritis: inflammation of multiple nerves.

quadriplegia: loss of voluntary muscle function in both arms and legs.

radial tunnel syndrome (supinator syndrome): peripheral nerve syndrome due to compression of radial nerve as it passes through region between radial head and the arcade of Frohse.

radiculitis: inflammation of intradural portion of a spinal nerve root prior to its entrance into the intervertebral foramen, or of the portion between that foramen and the nerve plexus.

radiculoneuritis: inflammation of nerve root and nerve.

Rett syndrome: genetically determined disorder of the extrapyramidal system manifested by scoliosis, hip dislocation, and lower limb contractures. It expresses itself in the second year of life in girls.

syncope: fainting or swooning caused by lack of oxygen or blood flow to the brain.

syringomyelia: disorder of spinal cord, marked by abnormal cavities filled with liquid.

tabes dorsalis: severe progressive disease of the central nervous sytem, caused by syphilis and characterized by demyelination of the dorsal columns of the spinal cord; **locomotor ataxia, Duchenne d.**

taboparesis: condition in which symptoms of tabes dorsalis and general paresis are associated; **neurosyphilis.**

tic: involuntary and usually quick, repetitious contractions of a muscle or muscle groups; repeated twitching.

tic douloureux: painful affliction (neuralgia) involving the trigeminal nerve.

tremor: involuntary trembling or quivering; shaking.

vertigo: loss of equilibrium.

Eponymic Neurologic Diseases

Bell palsy: loss of function of the facial nerves.

Brown-Séquard syndrome: injury to only one side of the spinal cord, resulting in loss of motion on one side of the body and loss of sensation on the opposite side.

Charcot joint d.:   joint destruction caused by loss of normal sensation.

Charcot-Marie-Tooth d.:   spontaneous degeneration of the neuromuscular complex, most commonly peroneal nerve, but also ulnar nerve, generally starting in childhood; **Marie-Charcot-Tooth d.**

type I motor and sensory neuropathy: a slowly progressive peripheral neurologic condition of childhood that can result in recurrent dislocation of the patella, peroneal muscle atrophy, high-arched/turned-in foot, and scoliosis. This is autosomally inherited and due to a failure of normal peripheral myelin protein 22 (type 1B) or a failure of myelin protein 0 (type 1B).

type II motor and sensory neuropathy: a neuronal disorder associated with peroneal muscular atrophy. Type IIa is inherited as an autosomal dominant. Other types being defined include type IVA, an autosomal recessive, and two x-linked, one of which is associated with a disorder of connexin-32.

Dejerine d.:   spontaneous local hypertrophic interstitial neuropathy of a peripheral nerve, cause unknown.

Dejerine-Sottas syndrome (familial interstitial hypertrophic neuritis):   familial neuritis associated with high-arched feet and marked sensory changes in all limbs.

Erb palsy (upper obstetrical palsy):   to be distinguished from Erb paralysis (form of muscular dystrophy). Palsy affects muscles supplied by upper cervical nerve roots C5 and C6; usually due to a distraction injury such as a difficult infant delivery, but may occur in adult life after trauma.

Friedreich ataxia: autosomally recessive inherited disease due to lack of frataxin associated with sclerosis of the dorsal and lateral columns of the spinal cord, attended by loss of coordination; usually apparent in early childhood; can be fatal.

Guillain-Barré syndrome: viral disorder involving spinal cord, peripheral nerves, and nerve roots; recovery of lost voluntary muscle function usually occurs, but the disease can be fatal.

Morton neuroma: excessive proliferation of perineural tissue, usually at the third and fourth metatarsal heads.

Naffziger syndrome: scalenus anticus syndrome; pain in brachial plexus distribution, caused by muscle impingement.

Parkinson d.: see paralysis agitans.

Parrot pseudoparalysis: decreased movement of the extremity due to syphilitic bone covering inflammation (periostitis) in infants.

Parsonage-Andrew-Turner syndrome: condition of the brachial plexus resulting in sudden onset of pain and muscle weakness in upper limbs that may lead to muscle wasting (atrophy). Pain may occur simultaneously or after several weeks, and last 1 to 4 weeks or persist for 18 months. Cause unknown; **neuralgic amyotrophy.**

Refsum syndrome: hypertrophic neuropathy that begins in childhood and progresses with repeated remissions and reactivation consisting mostly of distal sensory and motor loss.

Roussy-Lévy syndrome (hereditary areflexic dystasia): disease of peripheral nerves that is associated with a tremor and becomes arrested at puberty.

schwannoma: neoplasm of a nerve sheath.

von Recklinghausen disease: multiple neurofibromatosis.

METABOLIC DISEASES

There are thousands of chemicals in the body. Most of them are being rapidly destroyed and replaced as part of the essential chain of events that supplies energy, growth, and normal tissue replacement. There are conditions in which some of these chemicals may accumulate or be produced in inadequate quantity for normal function. Not all metabolic diseases can be identified at birth.

Gout is a disease in which uric acid accumulates in the soft tissues and joint spaces; it usually does not occur until middle adult life. Sickle cell anemia is the result of production of the wrong kind of chemical, causing changes in the shape of red cells and a subsequent decreased oxygen supply; this disorder is usually detected in infancy.

Many such disorders of chemical production and destruction (metabolism) have been defined elsewhere in this text because of certain characteristic tissues or extremity appearances. Some terms will be redefined here, with greater emphasis placed on the metabolic aspects.

Osteopenia is a term that defines abnormally diminished bone. It may occur regionally after immobilization or be due to a systemic effect involving the entire skeleton. The term does not define the quality of the bone, but simply states that there is less of it.

Osteoporosis is a condition where the mineral and organic content is normal, but there is less bone. The most common generalized osteoporosis is associated with aging (*senile osteoporosis*). Some metabolic conditions such as the postmenopausal state and abnormal gastrointestinal absorption are associated with a generalized osteoporosis. If no specific cause is found, the condition is often referred to as *idiopathic osteoporosis*. In children it is called *juvenile osteoporosis*.

Osteomalacia describes softening of bone, resulting from vitamin D deficiency or kidney disease. Milk allergy, liver disease, excision of the ovaries, kidney disorders, and chronic intestinal problems may interfere with vitamin D metabolism, absorption of calcium, or other processes, resulting in abnormal bone formation and mineralization.

Diseases Associated with Osteomalacia

Fanconi syndrome: severe form of vitamin D–resistant rickets, often fatal, and characterized by the presence of glucose, amino acids, and other chemicals in the urine.

hyperparathyroidism: abnormal increase in the level of parathyroid hormone, resulting in loss of calcium from bones.

hypoparathyroidism: abnormal decrease in the level of parathyroid hormone, either congenital or acquired, resulting in decreased bone formation and lowered serum calcium.

hypophosphatasia: autosomal recessive inherited disease characterized by severe skeletal defects resulting from a failure of calcification of bone.

milk-alkali syndrome: osteoporosis and/or osteomalacia, usually resulting from excessive intake of milk and alkali to treat ulcer disease; changes in therapy have reduced the prevalence of this disorder.

pseudohypoparathyroidism (PHPT): deficient hormone action due to target tissue resistance. Associated with short stature, shortened metacarpals and metatarsals (particularly the fourth), obesity and rounded face, reduced intelligence, subcutaneous calcification and ossifications, and some less common bone abnormalities; *Albright hereditary osteodystrophy.* Specific forms include PHPT as a result of guanine nucleotide deficiency, parathyroid hormone (PTH) receptor abnormality, and circulating antagonists to PTH action type II with normal bone responsiveness (hypohyperparathyroidism).

renal osteodystrophy: descriptive of a specific bone resorptive pattern seen in children and adults who have chronic kidney disease.

rickets: refers to the specific appearance of stunted growth, prominent rib cartilage (rachitic rosary), skull deformity (hot cross bun skull), and bowlegs; these appear during childhood and are characteristic of a variety of disorders that lead to a failure of normal calcification of bone. In the United States, the cause is rarely nutritional, but the disease is still seen because children can be born with kidney problems that produce a bone salt loss.

vitamin D–dependent rickets (VDDR): rickets due to an autosomal recessively inherited deficiency of the vitamin D enzyme 1-alpha-hydroxylase, or due to a general tissue resistance to the vitamin D metabolite.

vitamin D–resistant rickets (VDRR): rickets marked by normal-appearing kidneys that excrete excessive phosphorus into the urine; resistant to usual vitamin D therapy but responds to very high doses of vitamin D.

Diseases Associated with Osteoporosis

Cushing d.: disease caused by increase in corticosteroids from the adrenal glands or medication; may result in a characteristic vertebral body appearance and generalized osteoporosis.

hyperthyroidism: increased thyroid hormone production and increased general metabolism; may result in osteoporosis.

hypothyroidism: decreased thyroid hormone; may result in less bone production and osteoporosis.

Other Metabolic Chromosomal Conditions

beta$_2$-microglobulin amyloidosis: intraosseous and soft-tissue deposition of beta$_2$-microglobulin seen in long-term hemodialysis patients.

Coffin-Lowry syndrome: heritable disorder characterized by pronounced mental retardation, peculiar facies, short stature, and a clumsy, broad-based gait. There are multiple skeletal abnormalities.

diabetes: disorder of insulin and sugar metabolism, resulting in high blood glucose levels. Does not necessarily cause bone disorders, but in later life causes vascular compromise to the legs, possibly leading to amputation.

Down syndrome: mongolism; the condition is produced by chromosomal abnormality; *trisomy 21.*

dyssegmental dysplasia: rare lethal form of short-limbed dwarfism with different abnormal shapes of the vertebral bodies.

Ehlers-Danlos syndrome (EDS): spectrum of disorders marked by laxity of joints, velvety skin that is soft and hyperextensible, and vessel fragility. Some of these have known specific collagen defects. Ten types have been identified and reflect a wide spectrum of severity and inheritance:

type I: gravis.

type II: mitis.

type III: benign familial hypermobility.

type IV: ecchymotic or arterial due to autosomal recessive defect in type III collagen.

type V: sex linked.

type VI: autosomal recessive defect of lysine hydroxylase with joint and ocular disorders.

type VIIA1: arthrochalasis multiplex congenita, autosomal dominant disorder in type I collagen.

type VIIA2: autosomal dominant disorder of unknown chemistry.

type VIII: periodontal form.

type IX: sex linked (abnormal copper metabolism).

type X: autosomal recessive defect in fibronectin-1.

gout: disease process in which uric acid crystals are deposited into the joint lining or inflammatory cells within the joint and soft tissue. The most common form is urate (monosodium urate monohydrate). Other forms include pyrophosphate (calcium pyrophosphate dihydrate), apatite (various calcium crystals), cholesterol, and oxalate (calcium oxalate monohydrate and dihydrate).

gouty arthritis: inflammatory joint changes associated with gout; may be associated with tophi.

gouty node: collection of uric acid crystals near joints.

hemophilia: inherited disorder of coagulation; sex-linked; repeated hemorrhages may result in bone and joint deformity.

Kashin-Beck disease: endemic in eastern Siberia and northern China and Korea; abnormalities in enchondral bone growth leading to osteoarthrosis.

Klinefelter syndrome: failure of full sexual development in males, with development of some female characteristics; results from the fertilized egg receiving both female X chromosomes and the male Y chromosome.

lipid storage disease: inherited disorder resulting in multiple problems; bone disorders are secondary to displacement of the marrow by abnormal cells, resulting in avascular necrosis of the hip or irregular patterns on radiographs; also called **lipid reticuloendotheliosis.**

lipocalcinogranulomatosis: probable metabolic-based disorder with lipid-filled histiocytes and associated tumoral calcinosis.

Marfan syndrome: autosomal dominant disorder of fibrillin-1 resulting in elastic inherited defect in elastic tissue resulting in ligamentous laxity and spiderlike fingers, with joint and vessel disorders.

Menkes kinky-hair syndrome: X-linked recessive disorder that is fatal in infancy or early childhood; associated with depigmented and kinky hair, hypertrophic gingiva, loose joints, vascular tortuosity, seizures, and severe mental retardation. Similar to types V and IX Ehlers-Danlos syndrome.

metallosis: in orthopaedics, the term is applied to conditions resulting from very tiny microscopic particles that come from internal prosthetic devices.

Milroy d.: swelling of distal parts caused by a congenital disorder in which there is a retention of lymph fluid; *familial lymphedema.*

prune belly syndrome: undescended testicles, urinary tract obstructions, and hypoplastic abdominal muscles that result in a prune belly appearance and assorted musculoskeletal abnormalities; **Eagle-Barrett syndrome.**

pseudogout: more appropriately called **calcium pyrophosphate deposition disease (CPPD).** Usually occurs after age 60. Joint symptoms are consistent with degenerative arthritis development and x-rays reveal deposition of calcium within the cartilage. Can be, but not necessarily is, associated with mineral metabolic disorders such as renal disease or hyperparathyroidism.

sickle cell anemia: autosomal recessive inherited disease that affects the shape of red cells (oat-shaped erythrocytes); the result that most concerns orthopaedists is *salmonella bone infection* in infancy and bone infarcts in adults, particularly of the hip.

Shwachman syndrome: pancreatic exocrine insufficiency associated with cyclical low white blood cell production in children. Orthopaedic conditions include profound short stature.

thalassemia: autosomal recessive inherited disease of red cell structure; may result in skeletal deformity.

tumoral calcinosis: probable metabolic disorder where there is massive accumulation of calcium phosphates, pyrophosphates, or calcium carbonates in the soft tissues, particularly around joints.

Turner syndrome: failure of development of some female characteristics in girls; results from failure of the fertilized egg to receive both female X chromosomes.

DISEASES AND CONDITIONS BY ANATOMIC AREA

The back and neck disease section is found in Chapter 9—THE SPINE.

Miscellaneous Shoulder Conditions

Buford complex: shoulder joint anatomic variance consisting of a cord-like middle glenohumeral ligament that blends with a loosely attached superior labrum. The third variance is a large sublabral hole.

hooked acromion: hooked appearance of the anterolateral acromion sometimes associated with impingement of the underlying rotator cuff. This is a condition that develops in adult life.

The appearance has been categorized into three types seen on radiographs:

type I acromion: normal flat appearance of undersurface of acromion.

type II acromion: slight hooked or roughened undersurface of acromion.

type III acromion: markedly curved appearance of undersurface of acromion.

painful arc syndrome: pain in the acromioclavicular (A/C) area on active shoulder abduction; a sign of arthritis of the A/C joint.

snapping scapula: grinding sensation felt by the patient on specific motions of the scapula. May be a sign of a prominent rib or an osteochondroma of the scapula.

winged scapula: winging of scapula and prominence of interior angle at rest or on active range of motion. May be a sign of muscle paralysis, particularly palsy of the long thoracic nerve.

Hip (Coxa) Diseases

The Latin term *coxa* refers to the part of the skeleton lateral to and including the hip joint. (Do not confuse coxa [hip] with coccyx [tailbone].) The most common adult problems of the hip are osteoarthritis, other arthropathies, and avascular necrosis. These are defined in the sections dealing with bone, cartilage, and joint disease.

acetabular rim syndrome: pain and impaired function that precede osteoarthritis in hips that are congenitally dysplastic or have superior lateral trauma to the limbus and/or bony rim.

arthrokatadysis: deep hip socket formed as a part of degenerative arthritis.

coxa breva: short hip with a small femoral head caused by premature closure of the epiphysis.

coxa magna: enlarged femoral head.

coxa plana: flat femoral head (osteochondrosis) of the capitular epiphysis of the femur; *Legg-Perthes d.*

coxa saltans (snapping hip):   snapping of the hip due to tightness of the iliotibial tract over the greater trochanter, snapping of the musculo-tendinous iliopsoas overstructures deep to it, or lesions within the hip joint, such as a labral tear.

coxa senilis: degenerative hip disease concomitant with old age; **malum coxae senilis.**

coxa valga: hip deformity in which the angle of axis of the head and neck of the femur and the axis of its shaft (neck shaft angle) is increased.

coxa vara: reduced neck shaft angle, usually caused by failure of normal bone growth; **coxa adducta.**

coxa vara luxans: fissure of neck of femur, with dislocation of the head.

coxalgia: hip pain.

coxarthrocace: fungal disease of the hip joint.

coxarthropathy: any hip joint disease.

coxarthrosis: degenerative joint disease or osteoarthritis of the hip joint.

coxitis: inflammation of the hip joint; **coxarthria, coxarthritis.**

coxotuberculosis: tuberculosis of the hip joint.

developmental dysplasia of the hip (DDH): spectrum of disorders of the hip associated with deficient development of the acetabulum. This is usually apparent at birth and may start as or progress to subluxation or dislocation of the hip. This term is now replacing the older terms **congenital hip disease, congenital hip dysplasia,** and **congenital hip dislocation.**
Crowe classification (for percent of subluxation):
Grade I: < 50%;
Grade II: 50% to 75%;
Grade III: 75% to 100%;
Grade IV: more than 100%.

Meyer dysplasia: developmental anomaly that simulates Perthes d. of the hip but presents at an earlier age and does not have the progression of hip changes seen with Perthes d.: **dysplasia epiphysealis capitus femoris.**

Namaqualand hip dysplasia: autosomal dominant condition seen in African children from 3 to 20 years of age. There is a failure of growth in the femoral epiphysis, resulting in pain associated with an early degenerative arthritis of the hip.

observation hip: group of symptoms referred to the hip that includes a limp, pain, and limited motion of the hip joint with normal radiographs. The condition is a diagnostic dilemma in that it may be due to toxic synovitis, infection, or an early avascular necrosis.

protrusio acetabuli: arthritic development of hip socket into a deep, egg-shaped appearance.

proximal focal femoral deficiency (PFFD): failure of normal formation of the thigh side of the hip; varies in severity.

windswept hips: condition seen in individuals with cerebral palsy with pelvic obliquity, scoliosis, and one hip held in adduction and the opposite hip in abduction.

Deficiencies of the Acetabulum and Femur

The Committee on the Hip, American Academy of Orthopaedic Surgeons, has developed the following classification for congenital deficiencies of the acetabulum and femur:

Acetabular Classification
1. Segmental.
   - Peripheral (rim).
     a. Anterior.
     b. Posterior.
     c. Superior.
   - Central.
2. Cavitary.
     a. Anterior.
     b. Posterior.
     c. Superior.
     d. Medial (protrusion with intact medial wall).
3. Combined segmental and cavitary.
     a. Superior segmental, superior cavitary.
     b. Medial segmental, medial cavitary (protrusion with deficient medial wall).

c. Posterior segmental, posterior cavitary.
4. Pelvic discontinuity.
5. Fusion.

Femoral Classification

segmental defect: any loss of bone in the outer cortical shell of the femur.

cavitary defect: excavation of cancellous and/or cortical bone from within, the outer cortical shell remaining unviolated.

ectasia: dilatation and/or expansion of the outer cortical shell without perforation.

intercalary: segmental defect with intact bone above and below (cortical window).

Level of Defect:

Level I: proximal to the lesser inferior trochanter.

Level II: inferior lesser trochanter to 10 cm distal.

Level III: below level II.

Knee Disorders

Genu is a Latin term for knee (pl. *genua*). It is also a general term denoting any anatomic structure that is bent like a knee. Specifically, it is the site of articulation between the femur and tibia. Knee-related problems are divided into three sections:

1. Old genu descriptive terms.
2. Joint injury.

3. Other terms specifically related to the knee but not to a specific injury.

Genu Terms

genu recurvatum: ability of the knee to bend backward; caused by trauma or general joint laxity; *back-knee.*

genu valgum: deformity in which knees are close together, with ankle space increased; *knock-knee.*

genu varum: deformity in which knees are bowed out and ankles are close in; may be associated with internal tibial torsion (ITT).

Outcome of Joint Injury

The knee is an unusual joint because it contains *ligaments* within the joint. There are also medial and lateral *menisci* (crescent-shaped cartilages) that can be damaged (Fig. 2–5). Finally, the normal motions of the knee are very complex, including two planes of rotation; therefore it is very common to see multiple injuries.

A sprained knee is often a benign injury involving only mild damage to the ligament. However, a tear of the meniscus can occur in association with a sprain. A **meniscus tear** or **torn meniscus** is commonly described by its appearance, such as a **parrot-beak tear** or a **bucket-handle tear.** In the young person, a tear is usually vertical and longitudinal to the diameter of the meniscus. In degenerative tears that appear in older people, the tear is horizontal and may

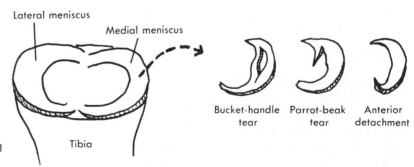

FIG 2–5.
Location of menisci and three typical derangements.

not be apparent on the superior surface of the meniscus. When the meniscus becomes fragmented, the condition is often termed a **degenerate tear** of the meniscus. The location of tears may be used to define a specific meniscus injury, for example, *posterior horn* or *anterior horn*. Meniscus injury commonly occurs as a result of a rotational injury. *Rotational instability* (rotatory or angular) is produced by rupture of specific anatomic structures. A meniscal rim can regenerate from the margin of a completely, or nearly completely, resected meniscus resulting in what is referred to as a **regenerated meniscus.** The normal up-and-down gliding mechanism of a patella may be disrupted, and the patella has a tendency to move out of its groove laterally (*subluxing patella*). A subluxing patella need not be caused by injury but does commonly occur with rotational injury. All these disorders can result in a chronic reaction in the knee, similar to the eyes' response to a foreign body. The lining of the knee becomes inflamed and may allow fluid (*effusion*) to collect. If the effusion is persistent, a *pouch,* called a *Baker cyst,* may form behind the knee.

Another outcome of knee injury is the formation of loose fragments (*loose bodies*) of meniscal cartilage or other tissue, causing inflammation (*synovitis* or *meniscitis*). The cartilage of the kneecap may become frayed (*chondromalacia patellae*). However, not all cases of chondromalacia result from injury. If the inflammation persists long enough, the patient will eventually develop *degenerative arthritis.* Often the examiner is not sure of the exact problem of the knee but suspects that something is functionally incorrect. The general term then used is *internal derangement of the knee* (IDK).

A surgically excised meniscus sometimes grows back in part (*regenerated medial meniscus*), or a portion may be left behind (*retained posterior horn*).

Other Conditions of the Knee
anterolateral rotatory instability (ALRI): the most common instability of the knee characterized by abnormal anterior displacement or subluxation of the lateral tibial plateau. It results from a tear of the anterior cruciate ligament and/or the mid-third of the lateral capsular ligament, and is determined by the Lachman test, anterior drawer sign, and flexion-rotation drawer test.

Baker cyst: sac of usually clear fluid specifically in the popliteal fossa of the knee. In the adult, it is a synovial fluid cystic extension due to intra-articular disease that results in a new synovial-lined sac in the popliteal fossa. In a child, the cyst is usually a ganglion arising from one of the tendons in the popliteal area.

bipartite patella: patella that has bony maturation occurring from two centers rather than one center, usually congenital, causing no symptoms, but may be mistaken for a fracture.

congenital dislocation: progressive anterior dislocation of the tibia caused by abnormal tissue remodeling; seen in infancy.

discoid meniscus: meniscus that is less crescentic and more "D" shaped. Often leads to symptoms in young adult life.
Watanabe classification
Type I: complete, extending across entire lateral tibial plateau.
Type II: meniscus wider than normal but some articular cartilage exposed.
Type III (Wrisberg-ligament type): deficiency of posterior tibial meniscal attachment that allows meniscus to move abnormally back and forth in joint.

flexion contracture: formation of fibrous bands that prevent complete extension of the knee.

focal fibrocartilaginous dysplasia: rare cause of unilateral genu varum (bowleg), which appears before 18 months with a cortical lucency in the proximal tibia and surrounding sclerosis. Condition is usually self-limited and resolves by age 4.

hamstrung knee: tight hamstrings during growth resulting in a slight knee flexion gait with subsequent synovitis and chondromalacia.

housemaid's knee: prepatellar bursitis: inflammation of the bursa in front of the patella.

jockey cap patella: chronic subluxating patella resulting in lateral spurring deformity.

jumper's knee: tenderness in the area of the inferior pole of the patella; usually seen in volleyball and basketball players.

megahorn meniscus: a congenitally enlarged part of either the anterior or posterior portion of the meniscus of the knee, usually the lateral side, with a variety of discoid menisci.

meniscal flounce: a normal wavy or folded pattern of the mensicus seen during arthroscopic inspection.

patella alta: a patella that is located more superior than expected, usually considered by the ratio of the length of the patella tendon to the height of the patella being greater than 1.25; **high riding patella.**

patella baja: low-riding patella with a relatively shortened patellar tendon, usually associated with knee pain.

patella clunk syndrome: a patellar snap that occurs in total joint replacement (knees) when going from flexion to extension; due to the catching of scar tissue immediately above the patella.

patellofemoral syndrome: patellar and peripatellar pain often ascribed to chondromalacia patellae, but which may be due to other disorders such as patellar malalignment.

plica syndrome: pain and/or snapping in knee due to inflammation or enlargement of a band of tissue that is present at birth and may become symptomatic in association with other conditions. There are four common plicas:

   ligamentum mucosum: in front of the anterior cruciate ligament.

   suprapatellar plica: in the suprapatellar area.

   medial shelf/medial plica: from the infrapatellar fat pad to the medial wall of the knee.

   lateral plica: from the laterial infrapatellar fat pad to the lateral synovium of the knee.

popliteal cyst: any ganglion or synovial cyst behind the knee. In adults, this is usually an outpouching of the posterior knee joint area and is a sign of chronic inflammation in the knee. In children and young adults, this may be a ganglion cyst arising from one of the tendons around the knee. Not to be confused with popliteal arterial cyst.

popliteal pterygium syndrome: severe flexion of the knee and equinus deformity of the foot associated with popliteal web extending from the ischium to the heel. Other concurrent deformities include toenail dysplasia and oral cavity abnormalities such as cleft palate or lip pits.

rhizomelic: short proximal end of a limb, such as seen in achondroplastic dwarfism.

small-patella syndrome: autosomal disorder with small patellae, pelvic girdle hypoplasia, and other skeletal anomalies.

snapping knee syndrome: the combination of dramatic popping and often intermittent locking is most commonly associated with discoid meniscus, but may also be due to other intra-articular abnormalities of the knee such as meniscal tears and enlarged bands of tissue.

snowstorm knee: formation of hundreds of brilliant, white loose bodies within the knee, usually following an earlier traumatic event.

squinting patella: patella that appears to point inward when the person is standing or walking forward. Usually a sign of femoral anteversion.

tethered patellar tendon syndrome: condition seen after total knee replacement. A large fibrous band develops behind the patella, causes pain, and interferes with joint motion.

   Type I: band oriented medial to lateral in suprapatellar region.

   Type II: band oriented vertically.

   Type III: band oriented from anterior fat pad to posterior notch.

thigh atrophy: loss of muscle tone of the quadriceps, causing dynamic instability.

Congenital Limb Absences

A standard classification accepted by the orthopaedic community is as follows.* A congenital deficiency may be at the end of a limb (terminal) or somewhere in the middle (intercalary). In addition, it may be transverse or longitudinal; the transverse deficiency is a complete across-the-limb loss, and a longitudinal deficiency leaves a longitudinal portion of the limb intact.

Terminal Transverse

acheiria: absence of the hand (carpals, metacarpals, phalanges).

acheiropodia: an extremely rare congenital absence of forearms, hands, and feet.

adactylia: absence of all five rays (metacarpals and phalanges).

amelia: complete absence of a limb.

apodia: absence of the foot.

complete aphalangia: absence of one or more phalanges from all five digits.

ectromelia: severe form of hypoplasia or actual absence of one or more long bones involving one or more limbs. This term generally includes amelia, hemimelia, and phocomelia.

hemimelia: absence of the forearm and hand or leg and foot portion of a limb.

partial hemimelia: absence of part of the forearm or leg.

Terminal Longitudinal

complete paraxial hemimelia: lengthwise loss of one side or the other of the forearm and hand or leg and foot.

incomplete paraxial hemimelia: similar to hemimelia, but a portion of affected bone remains, for example, complete absence of the ulna with a portion of the diameter of the radius intact.

*From Frantz CH, O'Rahilly R: Congenital limb deficiencies, *J Bone Joint Surg* 43(8): 1202–1224, 1961.

partial adactylia: absence of one to four rays (phalanges and metacarpals).

partial aphalangia: absence of one or more of the three phalanges from one to four digits.

Intercalary Transverse

complete phocomelia: presence of only a hand or foot.

distal phocomelia: hand directly attached to upper arm; or foot directly attached to thigh.

proximal phocomelia: presence of hand and forearm or leg and foot.

Intercalary Longitudinal

complete paraxial hemimelia: absence of radius or ulna with intact hand or absence of tibia or fibula with intact foot.

incomplete paraxial hemimelia: similar to complete hemimelia, except a portion of affected bone remains intact.

partial adactylia: absence of all or part of the first through fifth rays.

partial aphalangia: absence of the proximal or middle phalanx from one or more digits, one through five. A common deformity is a complete loss of the radius with the rest of the arm and hand being intact—intercalary complete paraxial hemimelia. Proximal focal femoral deficiency (PFFD) is an absence of a portion of the hip and/or proximal femur.

Miscellaneous Congenital Deficiencies

amniotic band syndrome: congenital presence of constricting bands that may affect trunk, limbs, and cranium; partial amputations may result.

arachnodactyly: unusually long "spidery" fingers and toes characteristically seen in patients with Marfan syndrome.

dolichostenomelia: increased length of the limb compared with that of the trunk.

fragile-X syndrome: familial form of mental retardation associated with flat feet and excessive joint laxity.

Larsen syndrome: associated skeletal abnormalities seen in infancy: dislocation of the elbows and hips, equinovarus deformities of the feet, long cylindrical fingers and shortened metacarpals, wide-spaced eyes, prominent forehead, and depressed nasal bridge.

Prader-Willi syndrome: Uncommon infantile disorder characterized by hypotonia, hypogonadism, obesity due to overeating, diabetes mellitus, delayed psychomotor development, mental deficiency, short stature, small hands and feet, hypermobile joints, and kyphosis.

rhizomelic: short proximal end of a limb, such as seen in achondroplastic dwarfism.

tibial dysplasia: complete partial absence of the tibia. These are two grading systems:

Jones, Barnes, and Lloyd-Roberts

1a: tibia not seen, hypoplastic lower femoral epiphysis.

1b: tibia not seen, normal lower femoral epiphysis.

2: distal tibia not seen.

3: proximal tibia not seen.

4: diastasis.

Kalamchi and Dawe

Type I: complete absence of the tibia.

Type II: presence of proximal tibia.

Type III: severe diastasis at ankle.

Symbols

The following symbols are used for congenital limb absences:

-: transverse

/: longitudinal

I: intercalary

T: terminal

1, 2, 3, 4, 5: denotes ray involved

⎯: when line is used above a letter, indicates the lower extremity

_: when line is used below a letter, indicates the upper extremity

Tl: tibia, complete

ti: tibia, incomplete

Fl: fibula, complete

fi: fibula, incomplete

R: radius, complete

r: radius, incomplete

U: ulna, complete

u: ulna, incomplete

ASSOCIATED DISEASE TERMINOLOGY

Diseases of the musculoskeletal system are often described by other terms relating to the disease process or some qualitative nature of the disease. These associated defined terms are given in alphabetic order.

abrasion: any superficial scraping of skin tissue or mucous membrane mechanically or through injury.

abscess: localized collection of pus in a cavity, which may form in any tissue.

acute: describes symptoms, conditions, or diseases of recent onset or recurrence that are severe or of short duration. Acute refers to the initial stage, short stage, or most severe stage of disease (e.g., acute low back strain may take a protracted course, becoming chronic, or may occur a number of times as part of a long-term chronic low back syndrome).

adenopathy: glandular swelling of the lymph nodes with morbid pathologic condition.

adhesions: tissue structures normally separated that adhere together because of inflammation or injury.

adventitious: acquired, not congenital; found out of normal place.

afebrile: without fever.

aggravated: made worse, more serious, or severe.

-agra (suffix): violent pain or seizure of acute pain.

-algia (suffix): painful.

allergy: hypersensitive state manifested by specific tissue changes after repeated exposure to particular allergens; an antibody-antigen reaction.

analgesia: loss of sensitivity to pain.

analgia: absence of pain.

anastomosis: connection of two distinct parts of cavities forming a passageway; the results of trauma or surgery. An example is the reattachment of a ruptured blood vessel after the injured portion has been removed.

anesthesia: loss of feeling or sensation of pain with or without loss of consciousness.

anomaly: malformation; a deviation from normal, usually referring to a congenital or hereditary defect.

anteflexion: abnormal forward curvature.

anteversion: forward rotation, as commonly seen in the femoral neck.

aphasia: either partial or complete, transient or permanent inability to understand or speak the spoken word as a result of a central neurologic occurrence such as stroke or injury.

aseptic: free of bacterial or fungal contamination.

asphyxia: lack of oxygen.

aspiration: withdrawal of fluids from a joint cavity, such as a bloody effusion in the knee. Also the inhalation of a liquid or solid such as the aspiration of vomit in an unconscious patient.

asthenia: lack of strength and energy.

asymmetry: dissimilarity between two corresponding parts of the body.

asymptomatic: absence of symptoms.

asynergia: disturbance of coordination.

ataxia: lack of coordination and muscle movement.

athetosis: involuntary writhing motions of the body (usually upper extremities).

atonia: lack of normal muscle tone; **atony.**

atrophy: wasting away of tissue, usually refers to muscle tissue.

atypical: irregular; appearing abnormal.

avascular: absence of adequate blood supply.

avulsion: tearing away of a part or structure from its attachment.

benign: not causing destruction of life or limb; when used in reference to tumors, denotes the absence of metastasis.

bifurcation: site at which any given structure divides in two.

bipartite: having two parts where only one is expected, for example, a bipartite patella.

bossing: rounded prominence of bone that is abnormally visible under the skin.

bruit (pronounced bru-ee): abnormal sound heard on auscultation of a blood vessel or the heart.

cachexia: systemic symptoms of malnutrition, malfunction, or debility that accompanies ill-heath or tissue breakdown.

café-au-lait: brain spots on surface of skin, often symptomatic of a systemic disease.

calcification: deposition of calcium salts either in normal bone or abnormally in soft tissue.

callosity: hardening of the epidermis because of persistent pressure.

callus: formation of new bone around a fracture site.

caries: decay and death of bone from bacterial action.

caries sicca: dry form of infection (i.e., less fluid associated with purulent material), characteristic of tuberculosis.

cellulitis: swelling and inflammation of soft tissues; may be caused by bacteria or chemical irritation.

chronic: describes symptoms, conditions, or diseases of long duration, as opposed to acute.

chylothorax: chyle (lymph duct fluid) that accumulates in the chest cavity that may occur after thoracic spine surgery with inadvertent transsection of lymph duct.

cicatrix: scar, may be formed by healing of any wound or tissue injury.

clonus: the uncontrolled spasmodic muscle jerking seen in conditions such as epilepsy or cerebral palsy. This term can refer to the spasmodic contraction of a reflex such as the ankle reflex that once elicited, continues indefinitely. When there are only several jerks in the muscle reflex, the term **unsustained clonus** is used.

-coele (suffix):   indicates a sac or cavity; *-cele.*

comatose: semiconscious state; in a coma.

congenital: present at birth.

contagious: refers to a disease or condition that can be transmitted from one person to another; communicable.

contractions: jerky movements; spasms of musculature.

contracture: permanent shortening of muscle tissue due to paralysis or spasm; loss of motion of a joint due to fibrosis of tissue around the joint.

contrecoup: a blow to one side of the body that causes damage on the other, as often seen in head injuries.

contusion: bruise of any tissue but without disruption.

convalescence: any given period of recovery.

conversion disorder: a response to psychological conflict or need manifested by unintentionally produced signs of a physical disorder where there is no known identifiable cause.

convulsion: violent involuntary contractions of voluntary muscles; paroxysm, seizure.

cramp: painful muscle spasm affecting the nerve supply to that muscle due to overexertion. Recumbency cramps are often felt in the legs and feet and occur at rest. Tonic muscle contractions can be anywhere and are associated with job-related activity. A "true" cramp is a motor unit hyperactivity that occurs at rest in the lower limbs. It is associated with motor neuron disease, fluid and electrolyte disorders, drug therapy, alcohol ingestion, or heat exposure.

crepitus: any crackling or grating sound with sensation on movement of surfaces at the joint; may indicate wearing away of cartilage.

cyanosis (adj. cyanotic):   bluish discoloration of skin resulting from abnormally low levels of oxygen in blood; the actual cause is an excessive concentration of reduced hemoglobin.

cyst: any sac, normal or abnormal, containing liquid or semisolid material.

debridement: removal of foreign material or devitalized tissue from a wound.

decalcification: loss of calcium salts from bone or soft tissue.

defervescence: period of abatement of fever.

degenerative: deterioration of quality of tissue; rarely refers to dead tissue; usually describes a state of abnormal remodeling or replacement of tissue, sometimes making it less functional.

dehiscence: splitting or separation of a part or all of a closed wound.

deossification: loss or removal of bone of osseous tissue.

derangement: displacement of position of any given anatomic part; commonly used in reference to joints.

diagnosis: identifying a disease process or the agent responsible by means of cultures, tests, surgery, or intuition (recognizing patterns of disease).

diffuse: widely distributed; used in association with symptoms or disease terms.

diverticulum: in orthopaedics, usually refers to outpouching of a joint or tendon sheath.

dowager's hump: round upper back deformity.

-dynia (suffix):   denotes pain.

dys- (prefix):   denotes defective, difficult, or painful.

dysesthesia: pinprick sensations; painful touch perception.

dysfunction: impairment of function.

dysplasia: abnormal development or replacement of tissue.

dystonia: simultaneous contraction of agonist and antagonist muscles.

dystrophy: failure of normal replacement of tissue; see osteo-, chondro-, and muscular dystrophies.

eburnation: in degenerative joint disease, changes in subchondral bone render its substance dense, smooth, and ivorylike. The bone surface becomes exposed due to complete loss of cartilage surface.

ecchymosis: extravasation of blood under the skin, as seen in a bruise.

edema: excessive accumulations of fluid in soft tissues causing swelling; may be the result of heart failure, venous insufficiency, kidney failure, or malnutrition. More specifically, in inflammation, an increase in post-capillary intraluminal pressure causes a shift in equilibrium so that fluid return is impeded and accumulates in tissues, which results in edema.

effusion: collection of fluid in a cavity such as the joint space.

emaciation: wasted condition of the body; malnutrition.

enucleation: removal, either surgically or traumatically, of a tissue, organ, or foreign body.

erosion: uneven wearing away of a surface, as seen on radiographs of diseased bones.

erythema: redness of skin, as seen in sunburn; caused by an increased blood supply (capillary congestion).

eschar: term usually restricted to skin; refers to full thickness skin graft with the formation of a hard, black, leathery, contracted material that, if removed, would reveal living tissue underneath.

esthesia: perception, feeling, sensation.

etiology: the study of all possible causes of a condition or disease, separated or related, based on what is presently known about that disease process.

exacerbation: aggravation of symptoms or increased severity of disease.

exudate: escape of fluid, cells, or cellular debris that escapes from blood vessels and deposits into soft tissues, cavities, or wounds as a result of inflammation. An exudate, in contrast to a transudate, is characterized by a high content of protein cells or solid materials derived from cells.

factitious injury: unconscious production of symptoms or actual physical injury for purposes of secondary gain, that is, attention or preferential treatment.

Fanconi anemia: radial clubhand deformity associated with dwarfism, brownish pigmentation of the skin, anomalies of the thumb, and then at 5 to 10 years of age a diminished number of all blood cells develops; **congenital pancytopenia, idiopathic refractory anemia.**

febrile: with fever.

fibrillation: involuntary contraction of small groups of muscle fibers as occurs with nerve root irritation; the fraying of a tissue such as seen in degenerative cartilage.

fissures: groove or natural division in tissue; also, ulcerlike sore.

flaccid: lacking muscle tone, whether voluntary or involuntary muscle.

flail: absence of motor control, as seen in a flail joint, may connote an abnormal mobility associated with loss of normal control such as flail chest, which is a chest crush injury.

foreign body: anything within a tissue that may lead to infection, inflammation, or scarring, requiring removal.

fretting: mechanical abrasion from relative micromotion between two surfaces. For orthopaedic appliances, this is between metal and bone or metal and cement. Microscopic particles are produced, initiating an inflammatory process that produces more loosening.

friable: tissue that is easily crumbled or separated.

fusiform: spindle shaped, tapered at ends.

gangrene: death of tissue caused by loss of blood supply (ischemia), bacterial infection, or both.

glycocalyx: extracellular polysaccharide elaborated by some bacteria that provides a binding material to internal prosthetic and fixation devices resulting in resistance to antibiotics.

granulation: reddish, moist, new tissue along edges of a healing wound.

hemorrhage: abnormal bleeding into soft tissues or a cavity; should this process form a discrete pocket of blood, it is called a hematomia; if the blood is evenly distributed in the tissue, it may appear as petechiae (very small), purpura (up to 1 cm size), or ecchymosis (larger than 1 cm).

hereditary: familial or genetic transmission of a quality or trait from parent to offspring by a gene. When the gene is inherited from the chromosome associated with the sex of the offspring, it is said to be **sex linked.** When the characteristic is inherited from the other chromosomes, it is called **autosomal.** If both chromosomes need the same gene to have the characteristic expressed, the condition is said to be **recessive.** If only one chromosome needs to carry the affected gene, the condition is called **dominant.**

herniation: abnormal protrusion of a body structure beyond its normal limits, such as disk herniation.

hibernoma: a rare, benign soft tissue tumor originating from brown fat and named for the brown appearance of fat seen in hibernating animals.

Holt-Oram syndrome: atrial septal defect or other cardiac abnormality associated with a radial clubhand deformity.

hypalgesia: diminished sensitivity to pain; hypoesthesia.

hyperalgesia: increased sensitivity to pain; hyperesthesia.

hyperextension: excessive extension of joint.

hyperglycemia: abnormally high blood glucose level increasing risk of infection.

hyperplasia: excessive increase in the number of normal cells in tissue, producing an increase in size.

hypertension: high blood pressure.

hypertonia: excessive tension of muscle or arteries.

hypertrophy: increase in size of a structure due to a functional activity such as in muscle hypertrophy.

hypoglycemia: abnormally low blood glucose level.

hypoplasia: defective or incomplete development of tissue or an organ (e.g., hypoplastic labrum; an abnormally small rim of cartilage in the shoulder joint can lead to a laxity of that joint.

hypotension: low blood pressure.

iatrogenic: adverse effects of medical or surgical treatment that could have been avoided under proper care.

idiopathic: disease process with an unknown cause.

impingement: pressure transmitted from one tissue to the next, such as nerve impingement.

induration: firmness of soft tissue caused by extravasation of fluids and/or cells from blood vessels.

infarct: local area tissue death resulting from reduced or completely obliterated blood supply.

infection: an invasion into tissue of any microorganisms (endoparasites) with an immune response by the host to the viable irritant. The terms *infection* and *inflammation* are not interchangeable. The distinction is important in that inflammation is a vascular response that may not specifically or necessarily be due to infection.

inflammation: localized increase in blood supply, resulting in small vessel dilatation and/or migration of white blood cells into the tissue. Inflammation is the normal response of living tissue to an injury with tissue alteration. The inflammatory process mobilizes the body's defense mechanism to initiate the healing process and react against any microbes that may be introduced at the site of injury with resultant heat, pain, swelling, and loss of function. Inflammation involves two basic sequences that develop separately: vascular alteration and cellular phenomena. Examples are bursitis, arthritis, and tennis elbow.

insidious: undetectable development of symptoms or disease, usually gradual in onset.

intractable: resistant to therapy, relief, cure, or control.

ischemia: insufficient blood supply to a tissue or organ.

laceration: a cut, any wound made by a sharp or blunt object.

lesion: circumscribed area of tissue altered by structural or functional disease. The word lesion describes a wound, injury, or pathologic change in tissue. A gross lesion is that visible to the naked eye.

line of demarcation: zone of inflammatory reaction separating a gangrenous area from healthy tissue.

lipping: development of excess bone at the margins of a joint, as seen in arthritis.

Loxoscelism: condition caused by a bite from a brown recluse spider. A local rash progresses to full-thickness skin death. Small hermorrhage or blister may form, surrounded by blanched skin due to ischemia. A classic description is a non-healing ulcer with red, white, and blue phenomenon.

lytic: denoting dissolution of tissue; used to refer to radiographic appearance of bone that has been displaced by some pathologic process.

maceration: softening or loss of surface tissue caused by constant exposure to moisture.

malaise: subjective feeling of being ill.

malignant: applied to neoplasms and implies the properties of anaplasia, invasion, and metastasis.

A disease resistant to treatment, resulting in eventual destruction of tissue; in tumors, implies that the tumor spreads by seeding itself in distant regions of the body or by local uncontrolled invasion.

malingering: a rare situation where an individual intentionally pretends to be ill only when being observed. This differs from **secondary gain,** where the person derives an emotional gain from believing that they are ill.

meliodosis: an infectious disease caused by *Pseudomonas pseudomallei,* which, when it affects the skeleton, may mimic tuberculosis or tumors.

mesenchymoma: neoplastic tumors in which there are at least two cells of mesenchymal derivation other than fibrous tissue; e.g., chrondro-lipoangioma (cartilage, fat, and blood vessel).

metastasis: spread of malignant cells to other organs or tissues—a malignant tumor is said to metastasize.

microgeodic d.: transient phalangeal osteolysis that presents with pain and swelling and is followed by spontaneous resolution.

morbid: the disease state; however, the term may denote ready visibility, such as "morbid anatomy."

morbidity: condition of being diseased with untoward results; could be congenital, acquired, or iatrogenic.

mucopurulent: denotes an exudate containing mucus and pus.

mucosanguineous: denotes an exudate containing mucus and blood.

myxedema: dry, waxy type of swelling associated with abnormal deposits of mucin in the skin; *nonpitting edema.*

necrosis: death of tissue or group of cells in tissue from trauma or disease.

neoplasm: abnormal new growth of tissue, either benign or malignant.

nevus: mole or birthmark.

nidus: place or source of infection or reaction.

node: confined tissue swelling or mass that can be readily seen or palpated, for example, lymph node.

nodule: small node, usually hard.

nutritional index: minimum metabolic condition required for wound healing that includes a total serum protein of at least 6.2 g/dl, serum albumin of at least 3.5 g/dl, and a total lymphocyte count of 1,500/mm^3.

obesity: abnormal accumulation of body fat.

occlusion: obstruction.

occult: hidden, not observable unless closely examined.

-odynia (suffix):   pain.

onco- (prefix):   combining form denoting relationship to swelling, mass, or tumor.

-orrhagia (suffix):   hemorrhage.

-orrhea (suffix):   discharge.

-orrhexis (suffix):   rupture.

-osis (suffix):   abnormal condition.

pectus carinatum: pigeon chest.

pectus excavatum: central depression of breast bone.

petechiae: tiny hemorrhages into the tissue; when seen in the skin, they appear as little violet dots.

phantom limb syndrome: sensations of an amputated part still being present. The perception of the phantom limb gradually shrinks to localization of sensation appropriate to the level of the stump.

-phyma (suffix):   swelling produced by exudate to subcutaneous tissue.

pleomorphic: taking on a shape that lacks description such as round, square, angular, etc. The term is often used to describe the shape of cells.

plexiform: taking on a tortuous or multiple form shape. Often used to describe the shape of a tumor.

polyps: protruding growths from mucous membranes.

procurvatum: angulation of a bone or joint that is convexed anteriorly.

prognosis: prediction of the outcome of disease or surgery.

prophylaxis: prevention of disease.

proprioception: sensibility to position, whether conscious or unconscious.

purpura: hemorrhage into the skin or other area with extravasation of blood into a congested area that is eventually resorbed.

purulent: pus-forming.

pyoderma gangrenosum: rare, destructive cutaneous lesion that starts as a painful, rapidly enlarging ulcer leading to a chronic, draining wound. Often associated with other diseases.

pyogenic: having the ability to produce pus.

pyrexia: fever.

quiescence: discontinuation of symptoms or a disease, the connotation being an expectation of the return of symptoms or disease.

rarefaction: decrease in density, usually used to refer to appearance of bone on radiograph.

recrudescence: relapse or recurrence of symptoms.

recurvatum: angulation of bone or joint that is convexed posteriorly.

regressive remodeling: removal and replacement of bone such that the replacement occurs progressively away from the original maximal border of bone, for example codfish vertebrae.

rigidus: stiffness.

rubor: redness of the skin.

rudimentary: insufficient development of a part or the development of an extra part such that no function is served by its presence; a rudimentary limb is so deficient that it serves no function, and a thirteenth rib similarly serves no function and is rudimentary.

rupture: discontinuity of tissue, usually referring to muscles and tendons.

sanguineous: bloody, as in a wound. This is in

contrast to serosanguineous fluid, which is serous fluid containing some red cells.

saponification: calcification that occurs with the breakdown of fatty acids in the avascular area of aseptic necrosis.

sarcoidosis: granulomatous disorder of unknown cause affecting mostly the skin, lungs, and eyes. The condition usually is seen in the third and fourth decade of life. When bone is involved, the disorder usually affects the hands and feet.

sebaceous: secreting a greasy substance, as in oily skin or sebaceous cyst.

sepsis: denotes the presence of infection caused by bacteria.

septicemia: bacteria in the blood. It should be noted that blood poisoning often refers to the red streaks seen in a limb that has an infection; however, this condition is more accurately a lymphangitis.

sequela (pl. sequelae): sequel that follows, that is, a morbid condition that follows the consequence of disease, meaning one pathologic condition leads to another discrete pathologic condition; for example, muscle spasticity is a sequela of cerebral palsy.

seropurulent: denotes an exudate containing both pus and serous material.

serosanguineous: denotes an exudate containing both blood and serous material.

serous: denotes an exudate that is usually yellow, fairly fluid, and possibly blood-tinged.

slough: spontaneous separation of devitalized tissue from living tissue.

somatization disorder: in some patients with chronic pain, there are recurrent somatic complaints without an apparent significant physical disorder. Physical symptoms are related to anxiety, and the patient may seek medical attention over a period of years.

spasm: sudden or violent involuntary contractions of muscle.

spastic: characterized by spasm.

splaying: to spread out, as in flatfoot deformity.

spurs: abnormal projection of bone at the margin or joints or strong ligamentous or tendinous attachments.

stenosis: stricture or narrowing of a canal or opening.

stigma: physical mark that aids in the identification of an abnormal process.

subliminal: below the threshold of sensation; weak; no muscle contractions.

supernumerary: excess number of anatomic parts, for example, six fingers on one hand.

suppurative: producing pus.

syncope: fainting.

TAR syndrome: *t*hrombocytopenia *a*genesis *r*adius; the coincidental findings of bilateral failure of formation of the radius associated with petechiae, black stools, and other signs of thrombocytopenia resulting from a failure of normal formation of platelets. This autosomal recessive disorder improves with proper support, leaving the skeletal deformity as the primary problem.

tardy: denotes delayed onset or appearance of a disease process (e.g., tardy ulnar nerve palsy, which may occur years after an elbow fracture).

tetany: symptom of a biochemical disturbance or imbalance in the body characterized by hyperactivity of sensory and motor units and marked by spasms and twitching of muscles of the hands and feet and possibly spinal muscles. Most common causes are hypocalcemia, hypokalemia, hypoparathyroidism (rare), hyperventilation, or lack of vitamin D. (Not to be confused with tetanus, an infection.)

tonus: involuntary continued contraction of a muscle after the patient has attempted voluntary relaxation.

torticollis: postural neck deformity associated with a turning and/or bending of the head and neck. May be due to congenital muscle tightness or disorders such as birth injury, psychogenic spasm, or spasm due to trauma. The term *wry-neck* is sometimes said of this condition.

toxic: poisonous.

transudate: fluid passage through a normal membrane due to imbalance in osmotic and hydrostatic forces.

trauma: any injury to tissue or psyche; can result from chemical, physical, or temporal events.

tumefaction: swelling, puffiness, edema.

tumor: a swelling, in the most generalized sense. However, the term connotes a neoplasm, that is, a new uncontrolled growth of tissue.

turgid: swollen or congested, describing a physical finding on palpation.

ulcer: penetrating disruption of mucous membrane of skin. There are two classification systems for ulcers:

Wagner
Grade 0: no open lesions
Grade 1: superficial ulcer
Grade 2: deep ulcer
Grade 3: localized osteomyelitis or abscess
Grade 4: forefoot gangrene
Grade 5: gangrene of entire foot
Depth-Ischemia
Depth
Grade 0: at risk foot, no ulcer
Grade 1: superficial ulcer, no infection
Grade 2: deep ulceration
Grade 3: extensive ulceration with exposed bone and deep infection
Ischemia
Grade A: not ischemic
Grade B: ischemia without gangrene
Grade C: partial forefoot gangrene
Grade D: complete forefoot gangrene

VATER association: acronym for a nonrandom group of occurrences that include *v*ertebral segmentation disorders and fusion, *a*nal atresia, *t*racheoesophageal fistula, *e*sophageal atresia,

and *r*adial ray defects. Other defects may occur.

vestigial: remnants of a structure that functioned in a previous stage of species or individual development.

wound: any disruption of normal tissue. A break in the skin is usually implied, but the term can be applied to a traumatic injury in which deep tissue is injured but the skin has not been broken. The International Committee of the Red Cross (ICRC) has the following classification directed at war wounds:

X Exit wound
X (cm): maximum diameter of exit wound
E Entry wound
E (cm): maximum diameter of entry wound
C Size of cavity within limb
C0: cavity will not admit two fingers at surgery
C1: cavity will admit two fingers at surgery
F Fracture
F0: no fracture
F1: simple hole in bone or insignificant comminution
F2: clinically significant comminution
V Involvement of vital structure such as viscera or major vessel
V0: no vital structure involved
V1: at least one vital structure involved
M Metallic bodies
M0: no bullet or fragments
M1: one metallic body
M2: multiple metallic bodies
Grading System
Grade 1: Sum of E+X is less than 10 with scores C0 and F0 or F1
Grade 2: Sum of E+X is less than 10 with scores C1 or F2
Grade 3: Sum of E+X is 10 or greater with scores C1 or F2

wryneck: torticollis; stiff condition of the neck caused by spastic muscle contractions.

Chapter 3

Imaging Techniques

Computerized diagnostic imaging techniques have expanded the field of radiology. Computer technology applied to radiology has contributed to diagnosing diseases more than any other method in medicine. Thus, the computer has become an indispensable tool for managing information and for recording programs from various scanning devices, which can be retrieved and read out by a central computer bank. This technology, with computer graphics and anatomic color images, gives medical specialists a more accurate diagnostic picture, has changed diagnostic procedures, and saves considerable time.

The standard radiographic technique depicts a body part as a simple two-dimensional shadow portrayed on a negative film. The new imaging technology creates two- and three-dimensional views from any angle. The types of diagnostic imaging are as follows:

- *Nuclear medicine studies*—Invasive (require an injection) tests that utilize radioisotopes; examples are positron emission tomography (PET) and bone scan (scintigraphy).
- *Magnetic resonance imaging (MRI)*—Noninvasive technology that combines radio waves and a strong magnetic field with the hydrogen atoms in the body to produce images of soft-tissue structures.
- *Ultrasound (sonography, ultrasonography), digital color Doppler, pulsed Doppler, or power Doppler*—Noninvasive forms of imaging that use a small transducer (transmitter/receiver) that is in contact with the area being examined to produce high-frequency sound waves that penetrate the area involved and reflect back to the receiver.
- *Computed axial tomography (CAT) scanning* and *radioisotope imaging (RII)*—This may be invasive (requiring intravenous injection of a radiopaque solution) or a noninvasive technique. Scans can now be obtained in a continuous helical motion and not just by a single slice at a time. These and other radiographic techniques are updated and defined in this edition.

Radiography has been an integral part of the orthopaedic examination, and the new diagnostic imaging techniques enable the orthopaedic surgeon not only to identify the anatomic site but to evaluate the physiologic conditions within and surrounding this site. Specifically, bone density, pathologic changes (necrosis of bone tissue, tumors, infections), spur formation, joint space narrowing, synovial inflammation, nerve impingements, and soft-tissue changes can be evaluated. A computer compiles vast amounts of digital data during an examination, and these data are turned into picture form. Physicians compare the many views, which can ultimately be made into a single video image. The most important contribution of imaging technology is that it enables physicians to see detailed views of the body without surgery.

The radiologist, a board-certified physician and specialist in radiology, is often consulted by the orthopaedist and other physicians to give interpretations of imaging technology and of more complicated pathologic conditions. The radiologist is assisted by qualified technologists who have learned the fundamentals of working with the radiographic and imaging equipment, developing film, and positioning patients. These specialists are challenged to meet the ever-changing technologic demands in their field to capably assist all branches of medicine.

This chapter presents the specialized terminology of radiology, new imaging technology, and its application to orthopaedics.

GENERAL RADIOLOGIC TERMS

baseline radiograph: radiograph taken at time of first examination and compared with those taken later.

catheter: a thin plastic tube inserted through the skin and into an artery or vein for the injection of contrast material in a vascular arteriography procedure; see also **femoral arteriography.**

cathode ray tube: vacuum tube that with a high enough voltage will produce x-rays.

contrast: a radiopaque medium that appears white on x-ray and can be given intravenously, intra-arterially, intrathecally, orally, rectally, or into a joint to aid visualization of internal structures; **contrast radiography, contrast study.** New **nonionic contrast agents** have been developed. Advantages over standard ionic agents are that there are fewer serious allergic reactions, meaning in patients at risk for allergic reactions, nonionic agents should be used.

echogenic: in ultrasound, giving rise to echoes of ultrasound waves. Examples are bone, metal, and air; produces white areas on the ultrasound images.

oscilloscope: instrument that displays computer data of electrical variations on the fluorescent screen of a cathode-ray tube.

Pantopaque: trade name for an iodinated oil (radiopaque contrast medium) used in a contrast radiographic procedure (i.e., myelography).

rad: measure of *radiation absorbed dose*, 100 erg/g (energy per gram).

radiograph: image produced on a film by means of ionizing radiation. **X-ray,** as in a "chest x-ray," is a commonly used synonym.

radiology: the specialized branch of medicine concerned with the diagnosis of disease utilizing ionizing (e.g., x-rays) and nonionizing (e.g., ultrasound and MRI) radiation; **roentgenology.** A **radiologist** is a specialized doctor who interprets the radiology studies.

radiolucent: permitting free passage of ionizing energy (x-ray) through an area, with dark appearance on exposed film.

radiopaque: preventing passage of ionizing energy (x-ray), thus allowing the representative area to appear light or white on exposed film; **opaque.**

roentgen (R):   unit of x- or gamma radiation exposure; 1 **gray** = 100 roentgen; 1 **centigray** = 1 roentgen.

roentgenography: the use of x-irradiation to produce either positive or negative film images or fluoroscopic images of objects; **radiography.**

scout film: general term for a radiograph prior to the injection of contrast. The purpose is to check the radiographic technique and to look for abnormalities that may be obscured once contrast is given; **scout radiograph.**

translucent: allowing some light to pass through but not clearly transparent; for example, soft tissue appears as a light shadow on a radiograph when compared with bone.

wet reading: as implied. Today, films are dried automatically and are read dry. In the past, if an immediate interpretation of the film was required, it was read while still wet. Thus, a request for an immediate interpretation is still called *wet reading.*

x-ray: electromagnetic radiation generally greater than 10 Kev in energy and less than 1 nanometer in wavelength, capable of penetrating tissue; **roentgen ray.**

ORTHOPAEDIC RADIOGRAPHIC TECHNIQUES AND PROCEDURES

arthrography: x-ray procedure showing interior outline of a joint after radiopaque medium and/or air has been injected intraarticularly; tendon, ligament, or meniscal tears can be detected in this manner; **arthrogram.**

bone densitometry: procedure for determining the relative density of bone by using several different radiographic techniques. A density gradient plate can be placed on the film at the same time radiography of the part is being performed. From this plate, a comparative density of the bone can be made, usually of the spine. Photons from a single emitting source can be used to directly measure the density of bone, such as that of the distal radius and lumbar spine. These studies can then be compared to age-matched normal values. This procedure is called **photon densitometry.**

    dual photon densitometry (DPD), dual photon absorptiometry (DPA): the use of two different emitting sources to help correct for soft-tissue density.

    dual x-ray absorptiometry (DEXA): the use of two different x-ray voltages to correct for soft-tissue density.

    quantitative computed tomography (QCT): another method of measuring bone density by using computerized tomographic images through lumbar vertebral bodies and comparing the measured density with age-matched normal values.

bone marrow pressure (BMP): measurement taken to detect bone necrosis. The pressure is taken while *intraosseous venography* and *core decompression* are performed to aid in diagnosis of ischemic necrosis of the femoral head (INFH), forming an early basis for treatment.

bursography: injection of radiopaque dye to show a bursa such as a retrocalcaneal bursa.

diskography: visualization of the cervical and lumbar intervertebral disks after direct injection of a radiopaque contrast medium into the disk; diskogram.

femoral arteriography: radiographic examination in which the femoral artery of the groin is catheterized. Through the femoral artery, the catheter can be directed to arteries throughout the body including the brain, chest, abdomen, and legs. Contrast is injected through the catheter to identify abnormalities in the arterial system or can be useful in outlining extent of a tumor; **arteriogram.** In some cases, a vascular abnormality can be treated through the catheter (e.g., by angioplasty).

fluoroscopy: direct visual radiographic procedure with the use of x-ray tube, fluoroscopic screen, and television monitor for intensification, i.e. continuous monitoring showing organ function that can be videotaped. Used in gastrointestinal studies, arthrography, and angiography.

KUB (kidneys, ureters, bladder): generally not an orthopaedic radiographic procedure but taken occasionally to study the abdominal wall and/or suspected masses.

lymphangiography: radiographic examination after introduction of radiopaque contrast medium into peripheral lymphatic vessels to determine presence of blockage or tumor in proximal lymphatic vessels.

Isovue (Iopamidol) myelography: This and Omnipaque (Iohexol) are newer water-soluble contrast agents used for myelography after injection of an iodine-based water-soluble contrast medium. The material does not have to be withdrawn after completion of the study, giving some advantages over the oil-based material that must be withdrawn.

myelography: radiographic examination with contrast medium injected into the subarachnoid space under fluoroscopy to examine the spinal cord and canal for possible disk protrusions or lesions; **myelogram.**

orthoroentgenography: for measuring limb length disparity; three separate exposures are taken of the hip (or shoulder), knee (or elbow), and the ankle (or wrist) to produce an image of the entire limb; **orthoroentgenogram.**

pneumoarthrography: injection of air into a joint before radiographic examination to determine internal outline, as in meniscal tear or other injuries and abnormalities; **pneumoarthrogram.**

roentgen stereophotogrammetry: simultaneous anterior-posterior and lateral radiographic examination performed with the examined part in a calibration cage. Radiographs can be obtained serially over time to study the progression of bony changes. Computer-driven calculations allow for the identification of three-dimensional changes as small as 2 mm. The technique is particularly useful in the study of prosthetic wear and migration over time.

scanography: for measuring leg length discrepancy, a film is moved beneath the patient for three successive exposures of the three pairs of joints, and a radiopaque scale is placed beneath the limbs so that measurements may be made from the scale of the film. A film 43 cm in length may be used rather than a film 2 to 3 times longer; **scanogram.**

sinography: radiographic examination for sinus tract infection in bone, performed after injection of water-soluble contrast medium, after saline cleanser, to determine the course of a deep draining wound; **sinogram.**

teleroentgenography: for measuring limb length disparity; radiographic examination performed with the x-ray tube 2 to 3 meters (6 to 7 ½ feet) from the plate to obtain a more parallel roentgenogram. The entire bone is visualized, but the degree of magnification (about 10%) is hard to assess; **teleroentgenogram.**

tomography: used to show detailed images of structures lying in a predetermined plane of tissue, while blurring or eliminating details of images of structures in other planes as in polytomography, planography, or zonography. It is used with radiographic magnification to detect abnormalities of the spine (laminography) or joints and in malunion fractures; **tomogram.**

ROUTINE RADIOGRAPHIC VIEWS

The number of views varies and is determined by the history and physical examination. For instance, an anteroposterior (AP) view may be unremarkable, but a lateral view may reveal a fracture or dislocation, depending on the angle of view taken. A complaint of knee pain often arises from a hip disorder, making radiographic (x-ray) views of the knee and/or hip important in diagnostic evaluation. Asymmetry of two identical bones (comparing femur to femur) can also exhibit an underlying abnormality. More than one view is usually required to diagnose the chief complaint. The terms are defined first and then given in abbreviated form by anatomic region.

Alexander v.: lateral view of scapula with shoulders protracted forward.

AP v.: anteroposterior view (x-ray beam passes from front to back).

apical v.: apex, tip, or point of subject radiographed.

apical lordotic v.: usually of the chest for the apices of the lungs, but for the clavicle if a patient's symptoms suggest an orthopaedic problem.

axillary lateral v.: for the shoulder, lateral view through axilla.

Breuerton v.: special view of the hand to search for early joint changes in rheumatoid arthritis.

Broden v.: for injuries affecting subtalar joint; lateral view of foot with a 45-degree rotation and various tilts.

Bura v.: for ulnar side of wrist; a supinated oblique view taken as an AP with 35 degrees supination.

Burnham v.: AP hyperextended view of thumb with dorsum on cassette and 15-degree cephalic tilt.

Canale v.: for the talus; an AP view with 75-degree cephalic tilt and 15-degree pronation.

carpal tunnel v.: for hook-of-hamate fracture; tangential view of volar wrist taken with wrist in dorsiflexion.

Carter-Rowe v.: view of the hip taken at a 45-degree oblique angle to determine size of bone fragment in a posterior acetabular hip fracture or other abnormality of the pelvis.

clenched fist v.: to demonstrate scapholunate instability; an AP view is taken with the fist clenched.

coned-down v.: close-up of a particular area, with radiation shielded from the rest of the patient's body.

cross-table lateral v.: for hip fracture; lateral view obtained with opposite hip in flexion.

false profile view: standing lateral x-ray of pelvis with person turned with the hip furthest from the cassette slightly posterior.

frog-leg lateral v.: AP view of hip in abduction and external rotation.

Garth v.: for acromioclavicular joint injury; apical oblique with 45-degree caudal and AP tilt.

Grashey v.: for shoulder impingement by acromion; scapular lateral with a 10-degree caudal tilt; **supraspinatus outlet v.**

Harris v.: for calcaneus; AP standing with 45-degree tilt.

Hobb v.: for sternoclavicular joint; while standing, the patient bends over end of x-ray table and cassette with hands on head, neck parallel to table, and chest about 45 degrees to table. The x-ray beam is vertical to the cassette.

Hughston v.: knee is flexed to 60 degrees, and view is obtained at a 55-degree angle to show a cartilage-osseous fracture of the femoral condyle or subluxing patella.

inlet v.: for pelvic injury; 45- to 50-degree caudad AP.

inversion ankle stress: AP view of the ankle, which is stressed in inversion to test the integrity of the lateral collateral ankle ligaments.

lateral v.: view taken side to side, left or right.

lateral monopodal stance v.: for anterior cruciate deficiency; lateral x-ray to detect posterior shift of femur on tibia.

Lowenstein v.: a frog-leg lateral.

lumbosacral series: multiple views of the lumbosacral spine to include AP, lateral, and oblique views.

Merchant v.: tangential superior to inferior patellar view taken with the knee flexed at 45 degrees; **Knuttson v.**

mortise v.: view of the ankle rotated internally until medial and lateral malleoli are parallel to film; demonstrates the talus, tibia, and fibula without superimposition, used for comparison with normal AP view and to detect joint abnormalities.

Neer transscapular v. (Neer lateral v.): posterior oblique scapular projection to help obtain a lateral view of the shoulder in trauma.

notch v.: prone view of knee with 45-degree caudal from vertical.

oblique v.: any view that is off angle from AP, PA, or lateral.

odontoid v.: specific for the odontoid process of C2 vertebra; AP view obtained with mouth open; **open-mouth v.**

outlet v.: for pelvic injury; 45-degree cephalad AP view.

PA: posteroanterior view (from back to front).

plantar axial v. of foot: offers visualization of the plantar aspect of the metatarsal heads.

prayer v.: for wrist instabilities; lateral view of

both wrists at same time with palms pressed together to bring about maximum wrist extension.

push-pull ankle stress: lateral view of the ankle, which is stressed in an attempt to evaluate the anterior talofibular ligament.

Robert v.: AP hyperextended view of thumb with dorsum on cassette.

Rosenberg v.: for osteoarthrosis knee; weight-bearing PA with knee at 45-degrees flexion.

serendipity v.: for sternoclavicular dislocation; AP view taken with patient supine and tube angled upward 40 degrees from the vertical position.

Slomann v.: for tarsal coalition; a 45-degree oblique view of the foot.

Stryker notch v.: for scapular notch; view taken with patient supine, hand on head, and camera with 10-degree cephalic tilt.

sunset v.: view of patella with knee bent at 120 degrees to permit a profile view; used for examination of patella and adjacent femoral surfaces; **sunrise v., tangential v.**

swimmer's v.: for lower cervical spine injuries; lateral view obtained with one arm held overhead while other arm is pulled down.

transthoracic lateral v.: for proximal humeral fracture or dislocation; view obtained with one arm held overhead and x-ray beam directed through chest.

trauma v.: for shoulder injuries; true AP, 45-degree oblique, and Y scapular (tangential) views.

true lateral v.: perfectly positioned lateral projection without rotation.

tunnel v.: view of tibia, fibula, and femur only with patella out of the way; a knee notch or intercondylar view; the radiographic examination is done with the tibia and fibula straight and the femur at a 45-degree angle.

von Rosen v.: view of the hips in abduction and internal rotation for determining dislocation of the hip(s) in developmental dysplasia.

West Point v.: for shoulder (glenoid) injuries; prone axillary lateral view with 25-degree lateral and posterior tilt to camera.

Y scapular v.: lateral view of scapula taken at an angle to view scapular blade such that it appears as stem of Y with coracoid and spine as the branches of the "Y."

Radiographic Views by Anatomic Region

Thoracic Region
chest: PA, lateral.

clavicle: AP, apical lordotic, tangential.

ribs:
　　anterior: PA, obliques.
　　posterior: AP, obliques.

scapula: AP, oblique, lateral.

shoulder: AP, internal rotation; AP, external rotation; axillary lateral; transthoracic lateral.

sternum: right anterior oblique, lateral.

Upper Limbs
elbow: AP, lateral, oblique.

hands/fingers: AP, lateral, oblique.

humerus: AP, lateral, transthoracic lateral.

radius/ulna: AP, lateral.

wrist: AP, lateral, oblique, AP with ulnar and radial deviation (for scaphoid fracture), carpal tunnel.

Spinal Region
C-spine: AP, lateral, both obliques, open-mouth odontoid.

coccyx: AP, lateral.

L-spine: AP, lateral, both obliques, coned-down L-5 to S-1 lateral.

pelvis: AP, inlet, outlet.

SI joints: AP, both obliques.

sacrum: AP, lateral.

T-spine: AP, lateral.

Lower Limbs

ankle: AP, lateral, and mortise oblique.

femur: AP, lateral.

foot/toes: AP, lateral, oblique.

hip: AP, frog-leg, and/or cross-table lateral.

knee: AP, lateral, tunnel, Hughston.

patella: tunnel, sunset, lateral, PA, merchant.

tibia/fibula: AP, lateral.

calcaneus: lateral, plantodorsal, axial.

Additional views requested may be views in flexion and extension, special views of the skull, "push-pull" films of hips for piston sign, and cine (movies) of x-ray images.

RADIOGRAPHIC ANGLES, LINES, SIGNS, AND METHODS

Angles

The anatomic description is taken directly from points using the intersection of two straight lines to form the angle.

acetabular angle: angle created by the intersection of a line from the inferior margin to the superior margin of the acetabulum and a line horizontal to the pelvis (connecting two inferior acetabuli; Fig. 3–1 on page 104).

acromial a.:   angle between clavicle and head of humerus.

anatomic femorotibial a. (FTA):   angle created by the intersection of lines through shaft of the tibia and shaft of the femur.

Baumann a.:   angle created by intersection of two lines drawn on an AP view of a child; one line is drawn from the medial margin of the distal humeral physeal line to the lateral margin of the lateral condylar epiphysis; and the other line is drawn in the line of the lateral condylar epiphysis. This angle is usually 11 degrees.

Böhler a.:   the two superior surfaces of the calcaneus.

carrying a.:   for the AP angle of the extended elbow, that is, the angle of the forearm when arm is extended.

CE (center edge) a.:   created by two lines drawn from the center of the femoral capital epiphysis, one line being vertical and the other extending to the acetabular edge.

Codman a.:   discrete angle at edge of the bone cortex produced by periosteal elevation and reactive bone in the area of a tumor; **Codman triangle.**

condylar-plateau a. (CPA):   angle created by the intersection of a line parallel to the tibial plateau surfaces and the distal femoral condyles.

congruence a.:   bisecting angle of the patella intersecting with vertical angle from trochlea (Fig. 3–2 on page 106).

crucial angle of Gissane: seen on lateral radiograph of foot, angle created by posterior facet of calcaneus and the superior anterolateral surface of the calcaneus.

Fowler-Phillip a.:   to measure degree of "pump bump"; angle created by intersection of a line from the posterior surface and the plantar surface of the calcaneus.

hallux valgus a.:   angle created by intersection of a longitudinal line through shaft of first metatarsal and the shaft of the proximal first phalanx.

head-shaft angle (Southwick a.):   for slipped capital femoral epiphysis; angle of femoral head physis to vertical line drawn through the femoral shaft seen on frog leg projection.

Hibb and Meary a.:   two angles created by intersection of a longitudinal line of first metatarsal and the line of the plantar surface of the calcaneus.

Hilgenreiner a.:   angle of the acetabular slope to the Y-line (horizontal line drawn through both acetabular centers); **acetabular index a.**

Kager triangle: triangular space anterior to the Achilles tendon normally visible on radiographs as a radiolucent area.

Konstram a.:   for gibbus deformity; the obtuse

FIG 3–1.
Radiographic measurements for hip dysplasia; **A,** acetabular index of depth to width; **B,** femoral head extrusion index (A/[A + B]) × 100. **C,** acetabular index expressed as angle ϕ; **D,** lateral luxation expressed as distance L; **E,** superior (vertical) subluxation expressed as distance v from inferior tip acetabulum to inferior femoral head; **F,** peak to edge distance D. (From *J Bone Joint Surg,* 77A:985, 1995.)

angle created by the intersection of the two lines drawn parallel to the surface of the superior vertebral body above and inferior surface of vertebral body below the deformed segment(s).

lateral distal femoral a.: angle of a line from the femoral head to the tibial spine to a line across the two femoral condylar surfaces; measured from lateral to vertical.

Laquesna and Deseze a.: for acetabular coverage of femoral head in developmental hip dysplasia; using a lateral x-ray view, the angle between a line seen in the shaft of the femur and from the center of the femoral head to the anterior acetabular rim; **ventral inclination a. (VCA).**

Laurin (lateral patellofemoral a.): acute angle created by intersection of line drawn from medial to lateral condylar points and a line parallel to the lateral undersurface of the patella. The angle is positive when it opens laterally.

Levine Drennan a.: angle that lies between a line drawn through the most distal points of the medial and lateral beaks of the metaphysis and a line perpendicular to the lateral cortex of the tibia; **metaphyseal-disphyseal a.**

mechanical axis: line created between the center of the femoral head and the center of the talus. In a normal knee, this axis passes close to the center of the joint; **Maquet l.**

medial proximal tibial a.: for tibial plateau slope; the angle created by a vertical tibial shaft line and a line across the tibial plateaus; measured to the medial plateau.

Merchant a.: created by intersection of two lines drawn from intracondylar apex of patella to center and a line perpendicular to plane of condyles.

Mikulicz a.: of declination formed by the neck of the femoral epiphysis and diaphysis center lines.

neck shaft a.: created by intersection of a line drawn through the femoral shaft and a line through the femoral head and neck.

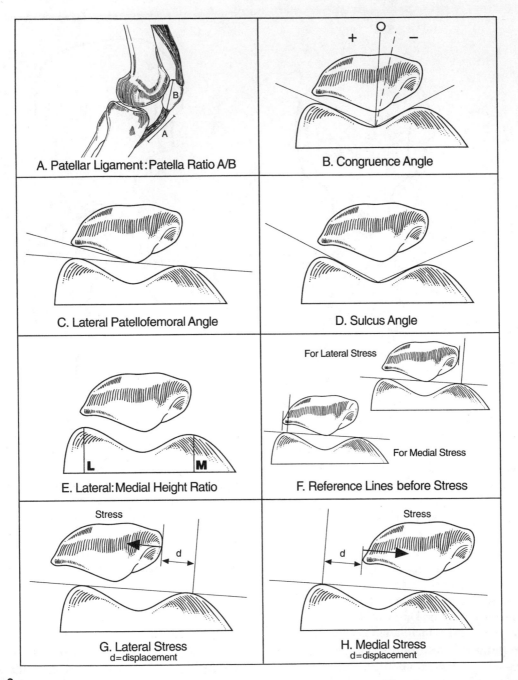

FIG 3–2.
Radiographic measurements to evaluate patellar instability. **A,** Insall-Salveti ratio, A:B, normally 0.8 to 1.2. **B,** Merchant congruence angle, normally −6 degrees (medial) and is pathologic if 16 or more degrees. **C,** Lateral patellofemoral angle open 97% of the time in asymptomatic individuals and medially or 0 degrees in recent subluxation. **D,** Sulcus angle normally 142 degrees. **E,** Lateral height:medial height normally 1.65. **F–H,** Reference lines for patella margins before and after medial and lateral stress, measuring distance d. (From *J Bone Joint Surg,* 78A:194, 1996.)

Pauwels a.: of a femoral neck fracture in reference to the horizontal line of a standing patient.

pelvic femoral a.: of inclination formed by the pelvis with line of femoral shaft.

physeal a. (physeal slope): for Legg-Perthes disease; the angle created by intersection of a line drawn vertically though the femoral shaft and the line of femoral head physis.

Q angle: made by intersection of lines drawn from anterosuperior iliac spine (ASIS) to mid-patella and from midpatella to anterior tibial tuberosity.

sacrovertebral a.: obtained by junction of lines through lateral projection of sacrum and lumbar spine.

Sharp a.: defined by intersection of lines from inferior acetabulum (bottom of teardrop) to supero-lateral acetabulum and a horizontal line.

sulcus a.: on Merchant view, lines drawn from apex of medial and lateral condyles to lowest point in groove to create this obtuse angle.

talocrural a.: angle created by intersection of lines, one drawn parallel to the tibial plafond, the other across the tips of the medial and lateral malleoli; normally 8 to 15 degrees.

Ward triangle: relatively radiolucent area of bone in the intertrochanteric area of the femur.

Lines, Indices, and Ratios

A *line* is defined as that seen or drawn directly on the film to help in the interpretation of the radiograph or an anatomic line of reference.

acetabular head quotient: for hip dysplasia; the ratio of the radius of the femoral head divided by the distance from the femoral head center to a vertical line drawn from the acetabular lip.

acetabular l.: line drawn from superolateral tip of both acetabuli for measuring femoral head or prosthetic migration.

Blackburne ratio: for a patella alta; with the knee flexed at 30 degrees, the ratio is measured A:B. *A* is the distance from the point parallel to the tibial condylar surface to the inferior weight-bearing surface of the patella. *B* is the height of the weight-bearing portion of the patella. The noncartilaginous inferior pole portion of the patella is eliminated from the measurement.

Blumensaat l.: line parallel to superior part of intercondylar notch as seen on lateral radiographs; used to judge the relative height of the patella.

canal-to-calcar isthmus ratio: for proximal femoral canal cylindrical configuration; two vertical lines are drawn from points on the inner cortex, one 10 cm from the mid–lesser trochanter and the other 3 cm from the mid–lesser trochanter. The ratio is the width of the space between these two lines at the mid–lesser trochanter divided by the width of the canal 10 cm distal to that point.

carpal height ratio: for capitate instability in the wrist; the ratio of the length of the third metacarpal to the length of the wrist from the base of the third metacarpal to the distal radius. The **revised carpal height ratio** is the width of the wrist from the base of the third metacarpal divided by the length of the capitate.

Chamberlain l.: for developmental basilar skull impression onto cervical spine; a line drawn from the posterior edge of the foramen magnum to the posterior edge of the hard palate.

demarcation (demarcation line): zone between normal and abnormal tissue, most commonly used to denote area or line of normal-appearing tissue next to gangrenous tissue in a devitalized limb. This term is also used in describing radiographic evidence of disease that shows a clear line or zone of activity.

Dorr ratio: for proximal femoral canal cylindrical configuration; width of the canal at the mid–lesser trochanter divided by the width of the canal 10 cm distal to that point.

femoral cortical index: ratio of the femoral diameter of the outer cortex to the inner cortex 10 cm distal to the mid–lesser trochanter.

femoral offset: perpendicular distance from the center line of the femoral shaft to the center of the femoral head.

fracture l.:   any line thought to be the result of a fracture.

Frankel l.:   a white line around the outer margins of the bony epiphysis, which can be seen on a bone radiograph in a patient with scurvy.

growth-arrest l.:   line of bony density seen on radiograph of a long bone. This may represent a growth-arrest scar from the growth plate as a result of stress (fracture or an illness) during a period of growth; **Harris l.**

Heuter l.:   line drawn horizontal to the medial epicondyle of the humerus, passing tip of olecranon when elbow is extended.

Insall ratio: for patella alta; with the knee flexed at 30 degrees, the ratio is the length of the patella tendon to the height of the patella. A number greater than 1.3 indicates patella alta; **Insall-Salvati ratio.**

Kohler l.:   slanted line drawn from the acetabular "tear drop" to the most lateral tangent of the pelvic ring.

lead line: radiopaque (white) thin line in the metaphysis (end region) of bones in a patient with lead poisoning.

Maquet l.:   line drawn from center of femoral head to midtalus, normally passes through middle of knee.

McGregor l.:   for developmental basilar skull impression onto cervical spine; line drawn from base of occiput to posterior edge of hard palate.

McRae l.:   for developmental basilar skull impression onto cervical spine; a line drawn from anterior to posterior edge of the foramen magnum.

medialization ratio: percentage of the horizontal radius of the cartilaginous femoral head medial to vertical line drawn from lateral tip of acetabulum, as seen on an arthrogram with the hip in the position of reduction.

Nélaton l.:   drawn from the anterosuperior iliac spine to the ischial tuberosity; normally goes through the head of the greater trochanter forming one side of Bryant triangle.

obturator/brim l.:   drawn from inner pelvic brim to midobturator foramen. Used in determining degree of femoral head or prosthetic migration.

Ogston l.:   drawn from adduction tubercle to intercondylar notch; used as a guide for transection of condyle in osteotomy for knock-knee deformity.

patella subluxation ratio: for patellar subluxation; ratio created by the distance of medial femoral condylar margin to apex of patella divided by the depth of the patella groove.

Pavlov ratio: for spinal cord space in cervical spine; ratio of vertebral body width to spinal canal diameter (Fig. 3–3).

Perkin l.:   vertical line drawn from lateral tip of acetabulum; **Ombrédanne.**

sacroiliac l.:   line drawn from both inferior sacroiliac joints, used in measuring proximal migration of femoral head or prosthesis.

FIG 3–3.
Pavlov ratio used to determine relative narrowness of cervical spinal canal, A:B, where a value 1.0 is normal and less than 0.8 indicates a developmentally narrow canal. (From *J Bone Joint Surg,* 76A:1422, 1994.)

sacroiliac/symphysis l.: horizontal line drawn from midpoint between superior symphysis pubis sacroiliac line, used in measuring proximal migration of femoral head or prosthesis.

Shenton l.: curved line seen on radiographs of a normal hip joint, formed by the top of the obturator foramen and medial femoral neck to lesser trochanter.

Spontorno index: for proximal femoral canal cylindrical configuration; outer cortical diameter at the mid–lesser trochanter divided by the width of the canal 7 cm distal to that point.

teardrop: the appearance of a teardrop found on the AP radiograph of the acetabular joint. The outer border of the teardrop is the inner border of the acetabulum. The inner border of the "drop" is the outer wall of the pelvis next to the inferior acetabulum. In grading acetabular dysplasia, the position of the teardrop is graded as A, open, when the medial line is lateral to the ilioischial line; B, when it overlaps that line; C, when it is medial to that line; and D, when the lateral border of the teardrop is medial to the ilioischial line.

Ullmann l.: line of displacement in spondylolisthesis.

Winberger l.: infraction (appearing as a radiolucent line) in the metaphysis, as seen in syphilis.

Y-line: line drawn through both triradiate cartilages at the acetabular center; **Hilgenreiner l.**

Radiographic Signs

anteater nose s.: seen in tarsal coalition; anterosuperior calcaneus has appearance of anteater nose seen on lateral radiograph.

anterior hiatal s.: seen in posterior ligament ankle instability; a lateral radiograph shows a wedge-shaped opening at the anterior dome of the talus when the foot is flexed and pushed backward.

Ashhurst s.: seen in ankle diastasis; a widening of the normal overlap of the distal anterior tubercle and fibula at the ankle joint.

bamboo spine: bamboo appearance of spine seen in ankylosing spondylitis.

cement-wedge s.: wedge-shaped area of radiographic lucency seen under tibial component, implying motion of the component.

chalk-stick fracture: appearance on a radiograph of a fracture through bone in a patient with Paget disease of bone.

choppy sea sign: an apparent but not real tear of a meniscus seen on arthrogram.

codfish vertebrae: radiographic appearance of vertebrae severely involved with osteoporosis, where the central portion is depressed secondary to collapse.

crescent s.: radiographic finding in avascular necrosis where there is a space between the subchondral plate and impacted bone of the femoral head, leaving a crescent-shaped area that is radiolucent (relatively black) on a radiograph.

Gage s.: seen in Legg-Calvé Perthes disease; a small osteoporotic segment forms a translucent "V" on the lateral side of the femoral head epiphysis; seen on AP view.

Hawkins s.: seen in avascular necrosis of the talus; zone of radiographic translucency beneath the subchondral plate of the dome of the talus.

Matev s.: seen in median nerve entrapment; a gap in the fracture callus of the medial epicondyle of the humerus.

posterior hiatal s.: anterior ligament ankle instability, a lateral radiograph with the foot pulled forward shows a wedge-shaped opening at the posterior dome of the talus.

Reimers index (migration index): for lateral acetabular deficiency; the lateral border of the femoral head to Perkin line (vertical line from lateral tip of acetabulum) divided by the width of the femoral head parallel to Hilgenreiner line (line drawn through the inferior points of both acetabuli) and multiplying by 100.

ring s.: secondary to scaphoid ligament disruption, which causes rotation of the scaphoid, giving it a ring appearance on a radiograph.

Risser s.:   for skeletal maturity, the degree of capping of the iliac apophysis from beginning (grade 1) to completion (grade 4).

rugger jersey spine: the appearance of alternate white and black zones seen on spine radiographs, frequently in patients with hyperparathyroidism or renal osteodystrophy.

scotty dog (scotch terrier) s.:   seen in spondylolysis; the oblique radiograph reveals what looks like a scotty dog. The "eye" is a pedicle seen end on; the nose, the transverse process; the collar, the lysis (fracture of the pars interarticularis); the body, the lamina; the tail, the posterior spinous process; the ears, the superior facet; and the forefoot, the inferior facet.

spur: a bony protrusion or lip at the edge of a joint, usually related to degenerative disease or osteoarthritis; **lipping, osteophyte.**

Thurston-Holland s. (corner s.):   small fragment of bone seen at margin of metaphysis just proximal to epiphysis that indicates a type II Salter fracture.

Waldenström s.:   apparent lateral displacement of femoral head seen in early Legg-Calvé-Perthes disease.

windshield wiper s.:   radiographic view outlines the shadow of a prosthesis with the appearance of a windshield wiper; with a loose internal prosthesis, there is bone absorption and formation secondary to a to-and-fro motion of the stem of the prosthesis in the shaft of the bone.

Methods

acromial profile: for impingement in the shoulder due to an anterolateral hook that develops in adults on the inferior surface of the acromion.
  Type I: flat acromial profile.
  Type II: curved acromial profile.
  Type III: hooked acromial profile.

Ahlback changes: grading system for degenerative arthritic changes seen on anteroposterior knee radiographs.

Grade 0:   normal joint space.
Grade I: joint space narrowing.
Grade II: joint space obliteration.
Grade III: minor bone attrition.
Grade IV: moderate bone attrition.
Grade V: severe bone attrition.
Grade VI: subluxation.

Bertol method: for dysplatic hips in new born infants; the ratio of two lines, one being the distance from the top of the femoral physis to central acetabular horizontal line and the other being the distance from the medial acetabular wall and superior medial femoral shaft. A ratio of 2 or greater is normal, and progressive instability produces a line ratio that progresses to 1.

bone age: in pediatric orthopaedics and radiology, refers to the predictable skeletal changes of bone that take place from infancy to adulthood. Bone age studies observe the size of bone, development of ossification centers, and outline of bones in the hand and wrist. Comparison with radiographs of normal patients at specific ages allows determination if a patient's bones are growing too rapidly or too slowly. Standard sets of radiographs are found in Greulich and Pyle (1959).

Catterall hip score: for pediatric avascular necrosis of the femoral head or Legg-Perthes disease (Fig. 3–4).
  I: no finding on AP, compression on frog-leg lateral.
  II: central compression on both AP and frog-leg lateral.
  III: lateral femoral head compression seen on AP, not covered by acetabulum, and medial femoral head is intact.
  IV: entire femoral head involved.

Cobb method: for measuring degree of curvature in scoliosis; a line is drawn across the superior vertebral plate of the superior vertebra with the greatest tilt and the inferior plate of the inferior vertebra with the greatest tilt. The intersection of these two lines creates the angle.

Edinburgh method: for dysplastic hip; radiograph obtained with a newborn's legs held paral-

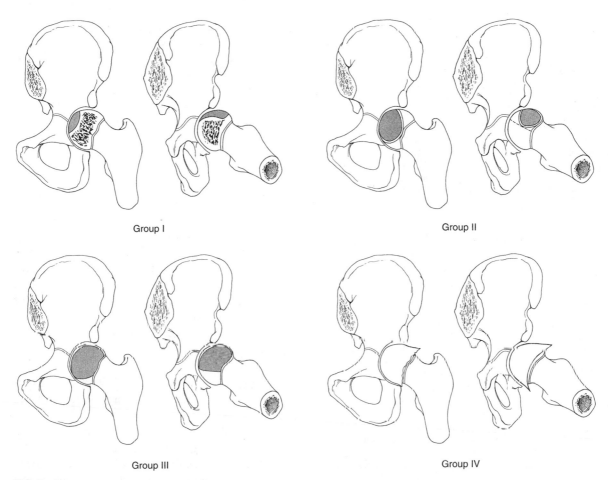

Group I

Group II

Group III

Group IV

FIG 3–4.
Catterall classification of Legg-Calvé-Perthes disease. I: anterior head only involved, no collapse; II: only anterior head with sequestrum, III: only a small part of epiphysis not involved, IV: total head involvement. (1996 American Academy of Orthopaedic Surgeons. Reprinted from the *Journal of the American Academy of Orthopaedic Surgeons: A Comprehensive Review* 4(1):9–16 with permission.)

lel with slight traction and no rotation. Proximal migration is measured by distance from superior femoral shaft to a line through the central acetabulum (inferior ilium). The gap from the lateral ischium to the most medial part of the femoral metaphysis is the index of dislocation. This gap is normally 4 mm, suspicious if over 5 mm, and diagnostic if 6 mm or more.

Fairbanks changes: a grading scale for the changes seen on the AP radiographs of osteoarthritic knees, originally used in postmeniscectomy patients seen in long-term follow-up.

Grade 0: normal.

Grade I: ridge from margin of femoral condyles.

Grade II: joint space narrowing on side of meniscectomy.

Grade III: flattening of femoral condyle.

Fergusson method: for measuring angle of degree of curvature in scoliosis, using vertical lines through spinous processes.

Ficat and Marcus: for avascular necrosis of the

FIG 3–5.
Herring classification of Legg-Calvé-Perthes disease. **A,** lateral pillar retains its height, no collapse; **B,** lateral pillar shows density changes with height loss; **C,** lateral pillar loses more than 50% of its height. (1996 American Academy of Orthopaedic Surgeons. Reprinted from the *Journal of the American Academy of Orthopaedic Surgeons: A Comprehensive Review* 4(1):9–16 with permission.)

Group A   Group B   Group C

femoral head, two similar grading scale systems are currently used.

Arlet Ficat	Marcus	
I	I	Mottled densities, may be obscure, anterosuperior weight-bearing area of femoral head.
II	II	Well-demarcated infarction, rim of increased density of bone at base of area of infarction.
III	III	Subtle flattening of femoral head or subchondral radiolucent crescent.
	IV	Pronounced collapse of avascular segment.
IV	V	Degenerative arthritis with loss of cartilage space.
	VI	Marked degenerative changes.

Gruen zones: for loosening of a femoral prosthetic component; lateral three zones are numbered from proximal to distal 1 to 3, zone 4 is at prosthetic tip, and zones 5 to 7 are from distal to proximal on the medial side, with zone 7 at the medial femoral neck.

Herring lateral pillar classification: for prognosis in Legg-Perthes disease (Fig. 3–5).
  Group A: height of pillar (lateral head above physis) normal.
  Group B: height of pillar 50% to 100% of original height.
  Group C: height of pillar < 50% of original height.

Ishihara cervical spine curve index: for spondylolytic changes in the neck; a vertical line is drawn from the base of C2 to the base of C7. The sum of the distance of the posterior vertebral bodies of C3-C6 to that vertical line is divided by that vertical line and multiplied by 100 to get the percent value.

Kellgren osteoarthritis grade:
  Grade 1: one or more osteophytes without joint space narrowing.
  Grade 2: sclerosis of the acetabulum and joint space narrowing; may be accompanied by small osteophytes.
  Grade 3: clear formation of osteophytes and narrowing of joint space.
  Grade 4: deformation of the femoral head with distinctive joint space narrowing; cyst formation in femoral head and acetabulum; both bones sclerosed. This scoring method is also used for degenerative disk in the spine.

Knee Society total knee arthroplasty roentgenographic evaluation and scoring system:[*] a system of angles and absorption at specific numerical points of prosthetic fixation to bone.

Mose concentric rings: for avascular necrosis of femoral head in children; a system using concentric rings with 2-mm separations.
  Good: both hips perfect circles.

*From Ewald FC: Knee Society total knee arthroplasty roentgenographic evaluation and scoring system, *Clin Orthop* 248:9–13, 1989.

Fair: deviation is ≤ 2 mm.
Poor: deviation > 2 mm.
Perdriolle torsimeter: for measuring spinal rotation in scoliosis; a transparent celluloid overlay is placed on radiographs to help estimate the rotation.
Salter-Thompson classification: for dividing Legg-Calvé-Perthes d. into two groups of expected outcome.
  Group A: bone underlying fracture presumed to be necrotic and any bone lateral presumed to be viable; involves approximately one half of the femoral head; similar to Catterall groups I and II.
  Group B: no evidence of an intact, visible lateral margin seen on AP radiograph; subchondral fracture extends to most lateral extent of epiphysis; similar to Catterall groups III and IV.
Severin hip dysplasia scale: for staging severity of hip deformity that may lead to dysplastic dislocation.
  Group I: normal hips.
   A: CE angle of > 19 degrees for ages 6–13 years; CE angle of > 25 degrees for ages 14 years and older.
   B: CE angle of 15–19 degrees for ages 3–13 years; CE angle 20–25 degrees for ages 14 years and older.
  Group II: moderate deformity of femoral head, neck, or acetabulum; otherwise normal joint. A and B same as Group I.
  Group III: dysplastic hip without subluxation; CE angles < 15 degrees for ages 6–13 years and < 20 degrees for ages 14 years and older.
  Group IV: subluxation.
   A: moderate, CE angle positive or equal to 0 degrees.
   B: severe, CE angle negative.
  Group V: head articulating with secondary acetabulum in the upper part of original acetabulum.
  Group VI: redislocation.

Singh index: an index of osteoporosis accomplished by a grading system using the three major trabecular patterns in the femoral intertrochanteric and head region. Grades I through VI with lowest grade being the most osteoporotic.
Stahl index: for staging lunate necrosis in wrist, uses ratio of height to width.
  Stage I: index of ≥ 45%.
  Stage II: index 30%–44%.
  Stage III: index < 30%.
Steinberg: for aseptic necrosis of the femur, Steinberg's stage II and IV are equivalent to Ficat stage III; and stage V and VI are equivalent to Ficat stage IV.
  Stage 0: normal radiograph and bone scan.
  Stage I: normal radiograph and abnormal bone scan.
  Stage II: sclerosis and/or cyst in femoral head.
   A: mild (< 20%).
   B: moderate (20%–40%).
   C: severe (> 40%).
  Stage III: subchondral collapse (crescent sign) with collapse
   A: mild (< 15%).
   B: moderate (15%–30%).
   C: severe (> 30%).
  Stage IV: head flattening with joint narrowing or acetabular change.
   A: mild (< 15% surface and 2-mm depression).
   B: moderate (15%–30% surface or 2–4-mm depression).
   C: severe (> 30% surface or > 4-mm depression).
  Stage V: flattening of head with joint narrowing and/or acetabular changes.
   A: mild.
   B: moderate.
   C: severe.
Stulberg method: system for measuring concentricity of femoral heads in Perthes disease.
Tönnis system: for hip dysplasia as seen on radiograph.

Grade 1:   dysplasia of the hip and mild subluxation.

Grade 2:   center of ossification of femoral head displaced laterally, inferior to superiolateral corner of the true acetabulum.

Grade 3:   center of ossification at level of superolateral corner of acetabulum.

Grade 4:   center of ossification proximal to the superolateral corner of acetabulum.

Waldenström: stage of healing in Legg-Calvé-Perthes disease.

Stage A: formation stage.

  1:   initial stage; epiphysis is denser, patchy, more distal, and uneven at the margins.

  2:   fragmentation stage; epiphysis in pieces, can be further divided into a mass of small granules.

Stage B: healing period; the epiphysis becomes homogeneous, evidence of diffuse and extensive revascularization.

Stage C: period of growth; normal growth and ossification of deformed femoral head.

INVASIVE AND NONINVASIVE TECHNIQUES

bone scan: a commonly employed nuclear medicine study in orthopaedics. A radioactive material (radioisotope) is attached chemically to a substance that is taken up by active bone cells. The radioisotope is then injected into a vein, and the radioactivity emitted from the bones goes to bone collagen and can be detected by a gamma camera. Usefulness of the study includes detection of infection, fractures, and metastatic lesions. A bone scan demonstrates where bone is actively being produced or destroyed, whereas a radiograph shows only where bone is present; **bone scintigraphy.**

three-phase bone scan: a modification of the routine bone scan, and applied when osteomyelitis is suspected. This scan examines the perfusion, immediate soft tissue blood pool, and delayed bone uptake; whereas, a routine bone scan examines only the delayed bone uptake phase. The advantages of the **three-phase bone scan** is that it improves the specificity of the exam for osteomyelitis. A normal perfusion phase excludes an active inflammatory process.

calcium 47:   for bone formation; an in vivo total body accretion test.

computed tomography (CT):   a computer generates a two-dimensional, cross-sectional image from a series of x-ray beams that rotate in a circular and forward motion around the patient. CT images show detailed anatomy and allow detection of differences in tissue density and shape. In orthopaedics, CT is especially useful for analyzing complicated fractures and may be performed after arthrography to aid visualization of joint pathology. With computed tomography, bone structures are clearly defined, noninvasively; tumors are located with precision; tissue is recognized as normal or abnormal; and blockages in blood vessels can be sought, invasively. The advantages of this technique are that it can be invasive or noninvasive, and it provides a sharp, detailed image. This method is best for patients who cannot tolerate rigorous radiographic examinations. **CT scan, computed axial tomography (CAT), CAT scan.**

spiral (helical) CT: the latest development in computed tomography, it allows scanning of a volume of tissue during a single breath-hold by continuous scanning as the patient is moved through the gantry. Advantages over the conventional CT are that it eliminates motion artifacts and shortens exam time. The trade-off is some loss of resolution. It is not used where high resolution is important, e.g., bone detail.

cinefluoroscopy: recorded fluoroscopic study for relative motion of bones in a joint, for example, to detect carpal instability; **videofluoroscopy, cineroentgenogram, cineradiography.**

dual photon densitometry: to estimate bone density, the part being measured is exposed to two beams of photons of different intensity. A two-dimensional picture of bone density is obtained with calculated subtraction of soft-tissue density. The results are expressed in grams of bone mineral per square centimeter.

fat saturation (fat sat, fat suppression): a technique used in MRI to suppress the signal from fat, causing it to appear black on the MR images. This technique allows pathology to be more easily identified.

gadolinium-enhanced MRI: the element gadolinium (Gd) has paramagnetic properties and is used to enhance magnetic resonance imaging. Gadolinium is especially useful in distinguishing scar tissue from disk herniation in cases of prior spine surgery. It is also useful in tumor imaging and in evaluating the blood supply to bone to exclude avascular necrosis.

gadopentetate dimeglumine: gadolinium. See **gadolinium-enhanced MRI.**

> *SPGR (spoiled grass):* image obtained with lower flip angle, giving a fat suppressed image that makes articular cartilage appear white on a magnetic resonance image.

> *STIR (short tau inversion recovery):* imaging signal acquisition that helps enhance image to detect fractures that are difficult to see on x-ray, particularly useful in occult hip fractures.

gallium scan (^{67}Ga): radioactive gallium-67 is introduced intravenously and localizes in areas of concentrated granulocytes; used to detect hidden infections, such as osteomyelitis.

gamma camera: instrument used for nuclear medicine studies. The camera contains many radiation detectors, which detect the radiation emitted from a radioisotope inside the patient's body. The camera generates an image of the whole body or of a specific area of interest (e.g., see bone scan).

indium scan (indium leukocyte scan): radioactive indium-111 is incubated with white blood cells (WBCs) taken from the patient. The indium-111 is taken up inside the WBCs, which are then injected back into the bloodstream and localize in areas of acute osteomyelitis (infection).

integrated shape imaging system (ISIS): for scoliosis; computer analysis of spinal and rib contours, may replace need for repeated radiographic evaluations.

LeukoScan: commercial term used for the method to localize infection in bone or soft tissue. Technetium-99m is attached to a monoclonal antibody that attaches to a specific cell surface protein seen only on neutrophils, the type of white cells that localize to areas of infection. It is then injected into the bloodstream.

magnetic resonance imaging (MRI): A radiographic technique in which the patient is exposed to a magnetic field. The movements of photons (water molecules), which are usually random, are aligned by the magnetic field. Radiowaves are then used to change the alignment of the protons. When the radiowaves are turned off, the protons emit a weak signal. The signals are detected and transformed into cross-sectional images. The signal decay curves of the protons as they return to their relaxed state are dependent on two factors: **T1,** (spin-lattice) longitudinal relaxation is dependent on the relationship between protons and their surrounding environment; and **T2,** (spin-spin) transverse relaxation, is the effect of spinning protons on each other. By adjusting certain imaging parameters, images can be more influenced by T1 or T2 (i.e., **T1** or **T2-weighted images**).

In orthopaedics, MRI is especially useful for diagnosing injuries to ligaments, meniscal tears, tumors, avascular necrosis, and infection. It is also useful for diagnosing fractures that are difficult to see on radiographs, such as nondisplaced fractures of the hip in the elderly. An MRI is also helpful in diagnosing diabetic feet and growth plate injuries. New methods allow for the detection of cartilage changes in osteoarthritis.

This technology has a terminology unique to the system (Fig. 3–6).

magnetic resonance spectroscopy: technique using magnetic resonance to determine the relative amounts of specific chemicals in an anatomic part. One such study is the evaluation of chemical reactions involving phosphate in the muscle. This type of evaluation helps to determine the metabolic adequacy of the muscle.

neutron radiography: technique helpful in visualizing bony tissue. A narrow beam of neutrons is passed through tissue from a nuclear reactor.

proton density: an MRI study in which the image is strongly affected by the differences in the density of protons in the tissue. Such images are usually produced with a spin-echo pulse sequence having repetition time (TR) > 600 msec and an echo time (TE) < 80 msec.

SPECT (single photon emission computerized tomography): use of a single beam emission source to make two-dimensional images revealing relative areas of bone abnormality. May be used to diagnose avascular necrosis, fractures, and infection.

strontium-85 resorption rate: a nuclear medicine in vivo study to determine bone absorption rate.

T1-weighted image: an MRI study in which the image is strongly affected by the longitudinal magnetic relaxation time, T1. Such images are usually produced with a spin-echo pulse sequence generally having repetition time (TR) < 600 msec and an echo time (TE) < 20 msec.

T2-weighted image: an MRI study in which the image is strongly affected by the transverse magnetic relaxation time, T2. Such images are usually produced with a spin-echo pulse sequence having repetition time (TR) ≥ 2000 msec and echo time (TE) ≥ 80 msec.

technetium-99m: $Tc^{99}m$ is a radioactive substance that can be chemically attached to a variety of substances for nuclear medicine imaging studies. For example, $Tc^{99}m$ can be attached to diphosphonate for imaging of bones, attached to white blood cells (WBCs) for imaging of infection, or attached to red blood cells for detection of a pulmonary embolus (blood clot to the lung); **technetium scan.**

technetium scan: see technetium-99m.

thermography: to differentiate nerve irritation, vascular disorders, and increased muscle tone; a temperature-sensitive plate displaying color gradients reveals differences in skin surface temperature.

ultrasound (ultrasound study, ultrasonography, sonography): the use of mechanical radiant energy having a 1 to 10 million MHz (megahertz = one million cycles per second) frequency to obtain images. The ultrahigh frequency sound (well beyond the upper limits of

FIG 3–6.
Cervical spinal cord as would be seen on MRI or CAT scan with myelography. The ratio of the transverse diameter to the sagittal diameter greater than 0.4 is a sign of good recovery prognosis after surgical decompression. (From *J Bone Joint Surg,* 76A:1422, 1994.)

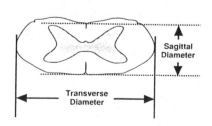

human hearing, which is 20,000 Hertz) is emitted, reflects off tissue surfaces, and is received and processed by a computer to form an image. In orthopaedics, this imaging technique is used to evaluate fluid collections, tendon and tissue abnormalities, tumors, cysts, and hemorrhages and infant hip disorders.

VASCULAR DIAGNOSTIC STUDIES

After the history and physical examination is complete, other tests may be required to diagnose abnormalities in the peripheral circulation to the limbs. These specific tests are often made in conjunction with an orthopaedic problem. These studies fall into two categories: invasive and non-invasive tests. The invasive tests are performed at the direction of vascular surgeons by radiologists.

Invasive Tests

To perform an invasive test, radiographic contrast is injected through a catheter placed into an artery or vein, and a computer-guided radiographic machine obtains an image as the iodinated contrast material courses through the vessel network. This contrast material enables visualization of any degree of narrowing (blockage) and the extent of blood flow around a blockage. Other abnormalities of vessels can also be detected. New computer technology allows vessel procedures to be performed in a short time.

angioplasty: can be performed following arteriography in which an area of narrowing has been identified. A special catheter with an inflatable balloon is placed at the area of narrowing. The balloon is inflated to open the narrowing. This procedure can treat areas of arterial narrowing that otherwise would require surgery.

arteriography: a radiographic examination in which an artery is catheterized and contrast injected to study the blood supply to an area or detect blockages of arteries. May be performed following an ultrasound study that indicates the presence of vascular compromise or in a patient with symptoms of blockage of blood vessels in the extremities. In some cases, a blockage or narrowing of an artery can be treated through the catheter (e.g., angioplasty); **arteriogram, angiogram, angiography.**

digital subtraction angiography (DSA): two-step imaging technique where radiograph is obtained of the area of interest before adding contrast medium. This first image is stored in the computer. Contrast medium that is opaque to x-ray is injected, and a second image is obtained. The opacity creates a shadow that allows visualization of blood flow. The computer subtracts the first image from the second image to produce a clear view of flowing blood and its blockages by narrowed vessels, ruptured vessels, or abnormal tissue.

venogram: a diagnostic procedure in which contrast is injected into a vein to visualize a blockage or other abnormality of the venous system; **venography, phlebography, phlebogram.**

Noninvasive Tests

These tests apply external techniques, and the body is not entered. These methods frequently provide dynamic information.

ankle-brachial index: calculated by dividing the blood pressure in the arm by the blood pressure in the ankle. Values less than 1.0 indicate decreased blood flow; **ankle-arm index.**

Doppler ultrasound (duplex or pulsed Doppler): high frequency sound waves are used to measure the speed and direction of blood within the vessels. Based on the Doppler principle, in which sound waves are reflected back at a different frequency depending on the velocity of the moving target (blood). **Color Doppler** assigns colors (usually red and blue) to blood flowing in specific directions and can be used to analyze blood flow. **Power Doppler** is a new ultrasound technique, which is more sensitive in detecting the presence of blood flow; however, it does not assess the direction of blood flow. Doppler studies are commonly used to detect narrowing of the carotid arteries and blood clots in the veins of the legs.

duplex ultrasound: provides both a two-dimensional image of the vessel and the velocity of flow. There are many uses including carotid artery stenosis, and venous blood flow to test blood clots. Duplex imaging for clots in leg veins is less invasive than venography and is the first imaging test of choice for this common clinical problem.

electrocardiogram: graphic recording of electrical activity of the heart.

plethysmography: noninvasive procedure with an instrument that measures limb flow in an artery or vein on the basis of changes in volume of part or all of the extremity. Various types employ air, water, light, or mild electric current to measure these changes.

    impedance plethysmography: instrument to measure changes in electrical impedance in a limb, which indicates changes in blood content and limb volume.

    oculoplethysmography (OPG):   noninvasive diagnostic procedure measuring carotid artery pressure indirectly by measuring blood pressure in the eyes. The medium of measurement may either be air (oculopneumoplethysmography) or water (oculohydroplethysmography).

    photoplethysmography (PPG):   noninvasive procedure with an instrument that uses light to measure blood flow to skin and thereby measure blood in larger vessels that may be occluded by arteriosclerosis.

phlebography: invasive radiographic procedure where radiopaque material is injected into a vein to visualize possible blockage or other abnormalities; **phlebogram, venography, venogram.**

pulse volume recorder (PVR):   segmental air plethysmograph to determine change in limb blood flow by change in cuff pressure.

RADIATION THERAPY

Ionizing radiation causes molecules to split when the radiation particle or wave hits the molecule. This event can cause injury to cells, particularly those that are dividing rapidly such as in tumors, the blood, and normal gastrointestinal lining.

As a result, ionizing radiation for diagnostic purposes is kept to a minimum, and treatment is made focal by a variety of techniques. The terminology listed here is restricted to techniques commonly applied to orthopaedic conditions and to some dosimetry terms.

rad (roentgen absorbed dose):   the actual energy absorbed by the local tissue, measured in ergs per gram. This is not a whole body count of absorbed dose but a number that looks at each tissue system or organ.

rem (roentgen-equivalent-man):   biologic effectiveness of radiation in a human subject. For diagnostic purposes, rad is equal to rem.

roentgen: measure of the change resulting from the exposure of air to radiation.

strontium-89 (Metastron):   treatment for metastatic bone pain. A beta-emitting radioactive material is injected intravenously. The isotope is taken up in bone and delivers the radiation to the affected areas. The effect lasts for several months.

Chapter 4

Orthopaedic Tests, Signs, and Maneuvers

Tests, signs, and maneuvers provide some of the most frequently used terms in orthopaedics. Unfortunately, the terms possess the greatest possibility for confusion because of similar names or meanings. Thus newcomers to orthopaedics meet a challenge at the very onset of their careers.

Eponyms for certain examinations vary regionally or among institutions within the same area. Such variations are a reflection of the training center's influence, where the names of prominent local physicians are frequently used for these examinations. Occasionally, the same test is given two or more names, or the name can apply to more than one test or sign. In a problem-oriented situation, eponyms are routinely used in the physical evaluation process. Familiarity with the terms and techniques enables physicians and their assistants to record and clarify an orthopaedic examination.

The physical examination is performed by using all the physical senses. The most common is a direct visual observation, although there may be some auditory findings on ausculation of the arterial pulses. Palpation, the use of hands in determining firmness, shape, and motion of a part, is also very productive. The way a patient walks (gait) or the manner in which the upper and lower limbs are used can also be informative.

A **test** may be part of the physical examination in which direct contact with the patient is made, or it may be a chemical test, radiographic examination, or other study. All tests described in this chapter will relate to the physical examination only.

A **sign** may be elucidated by a test, maneuver, or simply a visual observation, for example, a "list." It is an indication of the existence of a problem as perceived by the examiner.

A **maneuver** is a complex motion or series of movements used either as a test or treatment. It is also referred to as a method or technique.

A **phenomenon** is any sign or objective symptom, any observable occurrence or fact.

This chapter describes the physical examination by specific anatomic areas to include the neck, back, shoulder, upper limbs, hands, hips, lower limbs, knees, feet and ankles, and the neurologic, metabolic, and general examinations. The alphabetized list of tests, signs, and maneuvers is provided to assist the reader in easily identifying the proper name by specific anatomic area (in parentheses).

In addition to many new terms, a table has been included on Knee Instability Tests, an area that receives much attention. Scales and ratings, as pertains to preoperative and postoperative assessment of joints and degree of functional impairment, have been expanded to include a neurologic assessment grading system for spinal cord injury.

TESTS, SIGNS, AND MANEUVERS

Abbott method (back)
abduction sign (shoulder)
Achilles bulge sign (feet, ankles)
Achilles squeeze test (lower limb)
Addis test (lower limbs)
adduction sign (shoulder)
Adson maneuver (neck)
Allen maneuver (neck)
Allen test (hands)
Allis maneuver (hips)
Allis sign (hips)
American Shoulder and Elbow Surgeons
    (scales and ratings)
Amoss sign (back)
André Thomas sign (hands)
Anghelescu sign (back)
ankle clonus test (neurologic)
antecedent sign (general)
anterior drawer sign (feet, ankles)
anterior tibial sign (lower limb)
anvil test (neck, hips)
Apley test and sign (knees)
apprehension test (shoulder)
arthrometer test (knees)
artifact (general)
Babinski sign and reflex (back, neurologic)
Ballotment test (hands)
Barlow test (hips)
bayonet sign (knees)
Beevor sign (neurologic)
Bekhterev test (back)
bench test (back)
benediction attitude sign (hands)
benediction sign (hands)
Bouvier maneuver (hands)
bowstring sign (lower limb)
Boyes test (hands)
Bozan maneuver (hips)
bracelet test (hands)
Bragard sign (back)
British test (knees)

Brudzinski sign (neck, neurologic)
Bryant sign (shoulders)
café-au-lait (general)
Callaway test (shoulders)
camelback sign (knees)
carducci test (hands)
carpal compression test (hands)
Chaddock sign (neurologic)
Chiene test (hips)
Chvostek sign (metabolic)
circumduction maneuver (hands)
claw hand sign (hands)
Cleeman sign (lower limb)
Codman sign (shoulders)
cogwheel phenomenon, sign (general)
Coleman lateral standing block test (feet, ankles)
commemorative sign (general)
Comolli sign (shoulders)
confrontational test (hands)
contralateral straight leg raising test (back)
Coopernail sign (back)
costoclavicular maneuver (neck)
cram test (back)
Dawbarn sign (shoulders)
Dejerine sign (back)
Demianoff sign (back)
Desault sign (hips)
Destot sign (hips)
dimple sign (feet, ankle)
dimple sign (neurologic)
doll's eye sign; Cantelli sign (neurologic)
double camelback sign (knees)
drawer sign (knees)
drawer sign (load and shift t.) (shoulder)
drop arm test (shoulder)
Dugas test (shoulders)
Duchenne sign (hands)
Dupuytren sign (general)
Earle sign (hips)
Elson middle slip test (hands)
Ely test; femoral nerve stretch test (hips,
    neurologic)
Erichsen sign (back)
external rotation recurvatum test (knees)

extrinsic tightness test (hands)
fabere test; Patrick test (back)
fadire test (back)
fan sign (neurologic)
femoral nerve traction test (back)
Fick angle (angles)
finger to nose test (neurologic)
Finkelstein sign (hands)
flexion rotation drawer test (Noyes) (knees)
forced adduction test (shoulder)
Fournier test (neurologic)
Fowler maneuver (hands)
Fowler test (shoulder)
Fränkel sign (neurologic)
Froment sign (hands)
fulcrum test (shoulder)
Gaenslen sign (back)
Galeazzi sign (hips)
gear-stick sign (hips)
Goldthwait sign (back)
Gordon reflex sign (neurologic)
Gower sign (general)
grimace test (knees)
grip strength test (hands)
Guilland sign (neurologic)
Hamilton test (shoulders)
Harris-Beath footprinting mat (feet)
Hawkins impingement sign (shoulder)
Helbing sign (feet, ankles)
hemodynamics (general)
Hirschberg sign (neurologic)
Hoffmann sign (neurologic)
Homans sign (lower limbs)
Hoover test (back)
hop test (one-legged hop t.) (knee)
Hueter sign and line (general)
Hughston jerk test (knee)
Huntington sign (neurologic)
Hutchinson sign (hands)
impingement sign (shoulder)
International Classification for Surgery of the
    Hand in Tetraplegia (hands)
intrinsic tightness test (hands)
inverted radial reflex (back)

Jansen test (hips)
Jeanne sign (hands)
Jendrassik maneuver (neurologic)
Jobe test (shoulder)
Kanavel sign (hands)
Kapandji thumb opposition score (hand)
Keen sign (feet, ankles)
Kernig sign (neurologic)
Kerr sign (neurologic)
Kleinman shear test (hands)
knee instability tests (knees)
King maneuver (hips)
Kocher maneuver (shoulders)
Lachman test (knees)
Langer line (general)
Langoria sign (hips)
Lasègue sign (back)
Laugier sign (upper limbs)
Leadbetter maneuver (hips)
lead line; Burton sign (metabolic)
Leichtenstern sign (neurologic)
Léri sign (neurologic)
Lhermitte sign (neurologic)
Lichtman test (hands)
lift-off test (shoulder)
Linder sign (back)
list (back)
long tract sign (neurologic)
Lorenz sign (back)
Lovett test (hands)
Ludloff sign (hips)
McElvenny maneuver (hips)
McMurray sign; circumduction maneuver
    (knees)
Maisonneuve sign (hands)
Marie-Foix sign (feet, ankles)
masses sign (hands)
Mendel-Bekhterev sign (neurologic)
Mennell sign (back)
Meyn and Quigley maneuver (upper limbs)
Milgram test (back)
military brace maneuver (back)
Mills test (upper limbs)
Minor sign (back)

Moro reflex sign (neurologic)
Morquio sign (neurologic)
Morton test (feet, ankles)
MRC sensory grade (neurologic)
mulder sign (feet)
Murphy sign (feet, ankles)
Naffziger sign (back)
Neer impingement sign (shoulder)
Nélaton line (hips)
Neviaser test (shoulder)
no touch rule (lower limbs)
nuchocephalic reflex (neurologic)
Ober test (hips)
objective sign (general)
obturator s. (hips)
Oppenheim sign (neurologic)
Ortolani sign (hips)
overhead exercise test (neck)
paratonia (neurologic)
Parvin maneuver (upper limbs)
patellar retraction test (knees)
Payr sign (lower limbs)
pelvic rock test (back)
Phalen test and maneuver (hands)
piano key sign (hands)
Piotrowski sign (neurologic)
piston sign; Dupuytren sign (hips)
pivot-shift test (MacIntosh) (knees)
pollock sign (hands)
posterior drawer test (knees)
postural fixation (back)
pronation sign (neurologic)
prone external rotation test (knees)
pseudo-Babinski sign (neurologic)
pseudostability test (hand)
push-pull test (shoulder)
Putti sign (shoulder)
quadriceps test (general)
quadriceps active test (knees)
Queckenstedt sign (neurologic)
radialis sign; Strümpell sign (neurologic)
Raimiste sign (neurologic)
Raynaud phenomenon (general)

relocation test (shoulder)
reverse Bigelow maneuver (hips)
reverse pivot-shift (Jacob) (knees)
Romberg test and sign (neurologic)
Roux sign (hip)
Rust sign (neck)
sagittal stress test (feet, ankles)
Sarbo sign (neurologic)
scaphoid test (hands)
scapular sign of Putti (shoulder)
Schlesinger sign (lower limbs)
Schreiber maneuver (neurologic)
screw-home mechanism (feet, ankles)
Semm and Weinstein monofilament test
    (hands)
Sharp-Purser Test (neck)
Slocum test (knees)
Smith maneuver (hips)
Smith and Ross test (hand)
somatic sign (general)
Soto-Hall sign (back)
speed test (shoulder)
spilled teacup sign (hands)
spine sign (back)
sponge test (back)
Spurling test (neck)
stairs sign (neurologic)
standing apprehension test (knees)
station test (neurologic)
Stimson maneuver (hips)
straight leg raising test (back)
Strunsky sign (feet, ankles)
succinylcholine test (neurologic)
sulcus sign (shoulder)
swallow-tail sign (shoulder)
talar tilt test (feet, ankles)
tendon reflexes (neurologic)
tenodesis test (hands)
Tensilon test (metabolic)
Terri-Thomas sign (hand)
Thomas sign (hips, neurologic)
Thompson (Simmonds) test (lower limbs)
thumbnail test (knees)

thumb-to-forearm test (neurologic)

tibialis sign (neurologic)

Tinel sign; distal tingling on percussion sign (neurologic)

toe spread sign (feet, ankles)

too many toes sign (feet, ankles)

tourniquet test (lower limbs)

Trendelenburg test (hips)

tuck sign (hands)

Turyn sign (back)

two-point discrimination test (hands)

Valsalva maneuver (back)

Vanzetti sign (back)

Wartenberg sign (hands)

Watson test (hands)

Wellmerling maneuver (hips)

wet leather sign (hands)

Whitman maneuver (hips)

Wilson test (knees)

Wright maneuver (neck)

Wu sole opposition test (feet, ankles)

Yergason test (shoulders)

Zachary sensory grade (MRC) (neurologic)

Neck

Adson maneuver: for scalenus anticus syndrome, noted on obliteration of radial pulse; upper limb to be tested is held in dependent position while head is rotated to the ipsilateral shoulder while inhaling.

Allen maneuver: for same diagnosis as *Adson m.,* except the forearm is flexed at right angle with the arm extended horizontally and rotated externally at the shoulder, with the head rotated to the contralateral shoulder.

anvil test: for vertebral disorders; a closed fist striking blow on top of the head elicits pain in the vertebra(e).

costoclavicular maneuver: for thoracic outlet syndrome; pulling shoulders and chin back at the same time reduces the radial pulse when arm is by side; **military brace maneuver.**

overhead exercise test: for thoracic outlet syndrome. The hand is held overhead and making repeated fists results in immediate soreness in the forearm muscles; **Roos test.**

Rust sign: for osteomyelitis or malignant disease of the spine; the patient supports head with hands while moving body.

Sharp-Purser test: for chronic subluxation of the first on second cervical vertebra; with the patient sitting, the head is tilted forward and then backward with the examining finger on the first cervical spinous process to detect slippage.

Spurling test: for cervical spine and foraminal nerve encroachment; compression on the head with extension of the neck causes radicular pain into the upper extremities.

Wright maneuver: in thoracic outlet syndrome, raising the arm overhead obstructs the radial pulse.

Back

Abbott method: for scoliosis of the spine; traction is applied to produce overcorrection, followed by casting.

Amoss sign: for painful flexure of the spine; pain is produced when the patient places hands far behind body in bed and tries rising from supine position to sitting position.

Anghelescu sign: for testing tuberculosis of the vertebrae or other destructive processes of the spine; in the supine position the patient places weight on head and heels while lifting body upward; inability to bend the spine indicates an ongoing disease process.

Bekhterev test: for nerve root irritability in sciatica; while sitting up in bed, the patient is asked to stretch out both legs; with sciatica patient cannot sit up in bed this way but can only stretch out each leg in turn.

bench test: for nonorganic back pain. In normal hip motion, the patient should be able to bend over and touch the floor kneeling on a 12-inch high bench; not being able to implies a nonorganic (or psychologic) back pain; **Burns test.**

bowstring sign: with leg raised with knee bent in same position, pain is felt in the back of the limb pressing on the central popliteal fossa. Increased pain is sign of nerve irritability; **cram test.**

Bragard sign: for nerve or muscular involvement; with the knee stiff, the lower extremity is flexed at the hip until the patient experiences pain; the foot is then dorsiflexed. Increase in pain points to nerve involvement; no increase in pain indicates muscular involvement.

contralateral straight leg raising test: for sciatica; when the leg is flexed, the hip can also be flexed, but not when the leg is held straight. Flexing the sound thigh with the leg held straight causes pain on the affected side. **Fajersztajn crossed sciatic sign.**

Coopernail sign: for fracture of pelvis; ecchymosis of the perineum, scrotum, or labia indicates a pelvic fracture.

Dejerine sign: for herniated intervertebral disk causing radiating limb symptoms; a valsalva maneuver, such as coughing, sneezing, or straining at stool, accentuates the symptoms.

Demianoff sign: for differentiation of pain originating in the lumbosacral muscle from lumbar pain of any other origin; the pain is caused by stretching of the lumbosacral muscle.

Erichsen sign: for sacroiliac disease; when the iliac bones are sharply pressed toward each other, pain is felt in the sacroiliac area.

fabere test: for testing lower back or sacroiliac joint disorder by using a forced position of the hip; the letters stand for *f*lexion *ab*duction *e*xternal *r*otation in *e*xtension; **Patrick test, fabere test, figure of 4 test.**

fadire test: forced position of the hip causing pain; the letters stand for *f*lexion *ad*duction *i*nternal *r*otation in *e*xtension; **Patrick test, fadire sign.**

femoral nerve traction test: for radiculopathy of the second through fourth lumbar nerves; with patient prone, the knee is flexed, causing back or thigh pain.

Gaenslen sign: for sacroiliac disease; pressure on hyperextended thigh with the opposite hip held in flexion elicits pain, indicating a sacroiliac problem.

Goldthwait sign: for distinguishing lumbosacral from sacroiliac (SI) pain: with the patient supine, the leg is raised with one hand, while the examiner's other hand is placed under the patient's lower back; leverage is then applied to the side of the pelvis. If pain is felt by the patient before the lumbar spine is moved, the lesion is a sprain of the SI joint; if pain is not felt until after the lumbar spine is moved, the lesion is in the SI or lumbosacral articulation.

Hoover test: for a supposed malingering back disorder. While lying supine, the patient is asked to raise one leg with the knee straight and with the examiner holding the opposite heel. Any active effort to do this will result in pressure of the opposite heel against the examiner's hand. The lack of such effort implies malingering. Excessive pressure of the heel against the examiner's hand implies abdominal muscle weakness.

inverted radial reflex: for cervical spondylotic myelopathy (cord compression); there is spontaneous flexion of the digits when the brachialis reflex is being tested.

Lasègue sign: for sciatica; flexion of thigh upon hips is painless, and when the knee is bent, such flexion is easily made. If painless, there is no hip joint disease. If test produces pain when the knee is straightened, nerve root irritation or lower back disorder may be present. See straight leg raising test.

Linder sign: for sciatica; with the patient sitting or recumbent with outstretched legs, passive flexion of the head will cause pain in the leg or lumbar region.

list: said of a patient who leans to one side or another when standing or walking; most commonly seen in lumbar disk disease.

Lorenz sign: for ankylosing spondylitis (*Marie-Strümpell disease*); ankylotic rigidity of the spinal column, especially thoracic and lumbar segments.

Mennell sign: for spinal problems; examiner's thumb is taken over the posterosuperior spine of sacrum outward and inward for noting tenderness, which may be caused by sensitive deposits in gluteal aspect of posterosuperior spine; ligamentous strain and sensitivity.

Milgram test: for a lesion within the dural sac; while lying supine, the patient flexes both hips so that the knees are straight and both feet are lifted by only several inches. If the patient is able to hold this position without pain for 30 seconds, there is no problem within the dural sac. However, a positive test may occur for both intrathecal and extrathecal disorders.

Minor sign: for sciatica; patient rises from sitting position; supporting body on healthy side, placing hand on back, and bending affected leg, revealing pain.

Naffziger sign: for sciatica or herniated nucleus pulposus; nerve root irritation is produced by external jugular venous compression by examiner.

pelvic rock test: for sacroiliac joint disorder; forcible compression of the iliac crest toward the midline will produce pain.

postural fixation: a sign noted on range of motion of the back; any postural deformity (stiffness) noted does not reverse with range of motion.

Soto-Hall sign: for lesions in back abnormalities; with the patient supine, flexion of the spine beginning at the neck and going downward will elicit pain in the area of the lesion.

spine sign: for poliomyelitis; the patient is unable to flex the spine anteriorly because of pain.

sponge test: for detecting lesions of the spine; the examiner passes a hot sponge up and down the spine, and the patient feels pain over the lesion.

straight leg raising (SLR) test: for determining nerve root irritation; the supine patient elevates the leg straight until there is back or ipsilateral extremity pain or until the pain is increased with dorsiflexion of the foot; **Lasègue sign.**

Turyn sign: for sciatica; when examiner bends the patient's great toe dorsally, pain is felt in the gluteal region.

Valsalva maneuver: for determining nerve root irritability within the spinal canal. This maneuver is also used for many other unrelated reasons. The patient takes a deep breath and then on bearing down, such as one does when lifting a heavy object, feels pain.

Vanzetti sign: for sciatica; the pelvis is horizontal in the presence of scoliosis. In other scoliotic conditions, the pelvis is inclined as part of the deformity.

Shoulder

abduction sign: for subacromial impingement; the examiner places the shoulder in 90 degrees abduction and 30 degrees flexion and then internally rotates arm, producing pain.

adduction sign: for acromioclavicular joint disease; the shoulder is abducted 90 degrees, brought horizontally forward 90 degrees, and then flexed maximally forward, producing pain at the acromioclavicular joint.

apprehension test: for anterior subluxing or dislocating shoulder; the arm is held abducted and extended while in external rotation. The patient is apprehensive in a positive exam.

Bryant sign: for dislocation of the shoulder with lowering of the axillary folds, as noted on visual examination.

Callaway test: for dislocation of the humerus; the circumference of the affected shoulder measured over the acromion and through the axilla is greater than that on the opposite, unaffected side.

Codman sign: for rupture of the supraspinatus tendon; the arm can be passively abducted without pain, but when support of the arm is removed and the deltoid muscle contracts suddenly, pain occurs again.

Comolli sign: for scapular fracture; shortly after injury, there is triangular swelling, reproducing the shape of the body of the scapula.

Dawbarn sign: for acute subacromial bursitis; with arm hanging by side, palpation over the bursa causes pain; when the arm is abducted, pain disappears.

drawer test (load and shift test):   for shoulder instability; the patient may be sitting or lying. The scapula and clavicle is held securely in one hand, the head of the humerus in the other, the humeral head is pushed forward and backward to compare the two sides for crepitus and stability.

drop arm test: for rotator cuff tear; the patient is unable to actively control bringing the arm down from a full abducted position past 90 degrees. The arm drops at 90 degrees. This test is best performed with a local anesthetic injected into the subacromial space.

Dugas test: for dislocation of the shoulder; placing hand of affected side on opposite shoulder and bringing elbow to side of chest, a dislocation may be present if the patient's elbow will not touch side of his chest; **Dugas s.**

forced adduction test: for acromioclavicular joint arthritis; the arm is forcefully adducted across the upper chest, eliciting pain in the acromioclavicular joint.

Fowler test (push-pull test):   for anterior shoulder instability; patient lies supine, the shoulder is held in an abducted and externally rotated position using the edge of the examining surface as a fulcrum. Posterior force is then applied to the humerus. Relief of apprehension is a sign of anterior instability.

fulcrum test: for anterior-inferior shoulder instability; patient lies supine, the shoulder is held in an abducted and externally rotated position. The

arm is then further abducted and extended using the edge of the examining surface as a fulcrum.

Hamilton test: for luxated shoulder; a rod applied to the humerus can be made to touch the lateral condyle and acromion at the same time to determine a dislocation.

Hawkins impingement sign: for rotator cuff disorder; forward flexion of humerus to 90 degrees followed by horizontal adduction and internal rotation produces pain.

impingement sign: the examiner forces the shoulder into flexion and internal rotation with downward pressure on the acromion produced by the other hand. Pain is a positive sign of impingement. Subacromial injection of local anesthetic transiently relieves shoulder symptoms and eliminates impingement sign.

Jobe test: for occult anterior shoulder subluxation in throwers; patient lies supine, the shoulder is held in abducted and externally rotated position using the edge of the examining surface. Posterior force is then applied to the humerus with relief of pain; **relocation test.**

Kocher maneuver: for reducing anterior dislocations of the shoulder; done by abducting the arm, externally rotating, adduction, and then internally rotating.

lift-off test: for rupture of subscapularis muscle; weakness of internal rotation is demonstrated by inability of patient to lift hand from back.

Neer impingement sign: for rotator cuff disorder; examiner elevates humerus with one hand while depressing the scapula with the other to produce pain.

Neviaser test: for proximal triceps tendonitis; with shoulder fully adducted, tenderness over origin of triceps is increased with subsequent active elbow extension against force.

push-pull test: for anterior shoulder instability. See Fowler test.

scapular sign of Putti: for contractures about the scapula; when the arm is forcibly drawn into the chest and externally rotated the superior lateral side of the scapula wings out; **Putti sign.**

speed test: for proximal long head of biceps tendonitis; anterior proximal humeral pain created with humerus forward flexed against force while elbow is in full extension.

sulcus sign: for inferior shoulder instability; a downward longitudinal force is applied to the humerus of a resting arm. The thumb of the opposite hand can press into the lateral subacromial area, indicating a developing sulcus.

swallow-tail sign: for deltoid muscle function; extension of both arms posteriorly results in a lag on the side that has axillary nerve palsy.

Yergason test: for subluxation of the long head of the biceps tendon. While pulling distally on the elbow, the patient holds it flexed at 90 degrees with supination and forced external rotation of the shoulder against resistance by the examiner. Painful subluxation of the tendon can be palpated.

Upper Limbs

Laugler sign: for a displaced distal radial fracture; condition in which the styloid process of radius and ulna are on same level.

Meyn and Quigley maneuver: for dislocation of the elbow; the patient lies prone with the arm resting on the examining table and the elbow flexed at 90 degrees. The forearm is pulled distally while the opposite hand guides the olecranon.

Mills test: for tennis elbow; with wrist and fingers fully flexed and the forearm pronated, complete extension of the elbow is painful.

Parvin maneuver: for dislocated elbow; the patient lies prone with the arms and forearm over the edge of the examining table. Traction is applied on the wrist in a distal direction while the opposite hand pushes on the anterior distal arm in a posterior direction.

Hands

Allen test: for occlusion of radial or ulnar artery. A method of determining if radial and ulnar arteries communicate through the two palmar arches. Both arteries are occluded digitally. First one artery is released, then the other, to observe pattern of capillary refill in the hand. This can be performed with a Doppler placed on the digits during test. The test is valuable prior to an invasive procedure on the arteries at the wrist.

André Thomas sign: in low ulnar nerve palsy, in an effort to extend the fingers, flexing the wrist using the tenodesis effect will increase the claw.

Ballotment test: assesses triquetrolunate dissociation. Stabilize the lunate with one hand, the triquetrum with the other. Displace one from the other dorsally and volarly. If there is crepitus, pain, and extreme laxity, the test is positive.

benediction attitude (sign): for paralysis of the anterior interosseous branch of the median nerve; in the resting hand the index finger and thumb are held in full extension.

benediction sign: in low ulnar nerve palsy; there is metacarpophalangeal hyperextension, proximal and distal interphalangeal joint flexion in the 4th and 5th digits, and the index and middle fingers are relatively spared.

Bouvier maneuver: in low ulnar nerve palsy, passively preventing metacarpophalangeal hyperextension will allow proximal and distal interphalangeal extension.

Boyes test: for boutonnière deformity; with full extension of the PIP joint of the finger, there is decreased DIP flexion compared to the contralateral finger.

bracelet test: for early rheumatoid arthritis involving the distal radioulnar joint; compression of the lower ends of the ulna and radius elicits moderate lateral pain.

Carducci test: for boutonnière deformity; with full MP and wrist flexion there is 15 to 20 degree loss of PIP extension compared to the contralateral finger.

carpal compression test: compression of the carpal tunnel for as long as 30 seconds will produce or exacerbate symptoms of carpal tunnel syndrome. A sphygmomanometer bulb can gauge the proper pressure, about 150 mmHg.

circumduction maneuver: for the thumb; any general test or motion involving a rotation action of a group of joints; a range of motion examination.

claw hand sign: in lower ulnar nerve palsy; there is metacarpophalangeal hyperextension with proximal and distal interphalangeal flexion, and intrinsic minus posture in all palmar digits. These may be static or dynamic.

confrontational test: for hand intrinsic muscle weakness; the strength of specific muscle or muscle groups is compared by pressing the thumb or finger against opposite thumb or finger in a fashion to produce resistance against those muscles. Weakness is indicated by an inability to oppose the compared digits with equal strength (i.e., one side gives out).

Duchenne sign: in low ulnar nerve palsy with extrinsic muscles intact; the ring and little fingers will claw with metacarpophalangeal hyperextension and flexion of the middle and distal phalanges.

Elson middle slip test: for ruptured central extensor tendon slip of the proximal interphalangeal (PIP) joint, the finger is flexed to 90 degrees. If the central slip is intact, the patient can extend the PIP joint, but the distal interphalangeal (DIP) joint is flail. Otherwise, the PIP joint will not have extension power, and the DIP joint will extend while in that position.

extrinsic tightness test: to assess extrinsic extensor tendon adherence or foreshortening, passive metacarpophalangeal (MCP) joint flexion will cause MCP joint hyperextension. MCP flexion will force the proximal interphalangeal joint into extension.

Finkelstein sign: bending the thumb into the palm to determine synovitis of the abductor policis longus tendon to wrist. Passively flexing and ulnar deviating the wrist with the thumb in full opposition will elicit pain over the first dorsal extensor compartment in de Quervain disease.

Fowler maneuver: for testing rheumatoid arthritis; tight intrinsic muscles in ulnar deviation of the digits and a heavy, taut ulnar band are demonstrated when the digit is held in its normal axial relationship.

Froment sign: for ulnar nerve loss; there is paralysis of the adductor pollicis and first dorsal interosseous and second palmar interosseous. The flexor pollicis longus flexes the interphalangeal joint up to 90 degrees to effect power pinch.

grip strength test: to measure the strength of coordination of intrinsic and extrinsic finger/thumb flexors; a grip dynamometer is used.

Hutchinson s.: seen in malignant melanoma; lesion under a finger or toe nail where the pigment extends into the proximal nail fold.

International Classification for Surgery of the Hand in Tetraplegia: to determine extent of muscle capacity for intrinsic and extrinsic muscle and tendon transfers that improve hand function.

Motor Group:

0: no muscle below elbow available.

1: brachioradialis (BR) > 4+.

2: BR and extensor carpi radialis longus (ECRL) > 4+.

3: BR, ECRL, and extensor carpi radialis brevis (ECRB) > 4+.

4: BR, ECRL, ECRB, and pronator teres (PT) > 4+.

5: BR, ECRL, ECRB, PT, and flexor carpi radialis (FCR) > 4+.

6: BR, ECRL, ECRB, PT, FCR, and finger extensors > 4+.

7: BR, ECRL, ECRB, PT, FCR, finger extensors, and thumb extensors > 4+.

8: BR, ECRL, ECRB, PT, FCR, finger and thumb extensors, and partial digital flexors > 4+.

9: lacks only intrinsic muscle function.

X: exceptions.

Sensation:

O: two-point discrimination in the thumb > 10 mm.

Ocu: two-point discrimination in the thumb < 10 mm.

intrinsic tightness test: to assess adherence or contracture of intrinsic muscles with metacarpophalangeal joint passively extended. Active or passive proximal interphalangeal flexion is limited.

Jeanne sign: in ulnar nerve palsy; with adduction, pollicis dysfunction with metacarpophalangeal hyperextension will result with key pinch or gross grip.

Kanavel sign: for infection of a tendon sheath; there is a point of maximum tenderness in the palm 1 inch proximal to the base of the little finger. In pyogenic tenosynovitis, the four signs are a flexed position of the finger, symmetric fusiform enlargement of the fingers, marked tendon sheath tenderness, and pain on passive digital extension.

Kapandji thumb opposition score: for ability to oppose thumb; with fingers extended, increasing ability, to oppose from base of index to the finger tip, graded 1 to 3; 4, opposition to long finger tip; 5, opposition to ring finger tip; 6 to 8, opposition from tip of little finger to base; 9, opposition to palm distal to flexion crease; 10, opposition to palm proximal to flexion crease.

key pinch: the strength in the ability to grasp, as in holding a key; lateral pinch.

Kleinman shear test: to assess triquetrolunate disability. Stabilize the lunate with a thumb placed on the dorsum of the lunate. If the test is positive, the pisotriquetral joint is pushed dorsally from the volar side with pain, crepitus, and increased motion.

Lichtman test: in nondissociative midcarpal instability; a painful clunk is elicited with passive (and sometimes active) ulnar deviation of the wrist. The clunk occurs as the hamate reduces on the triquetrum and the entire proximal row rotates rapidly from its flexed to an extended position.

Lovett test: for boutonnière deformity; with full MP and wrist flexion there is decrease in PIP extension strength compared to the contralateral finger.

Maisonneuve sign: for Colles fracture; there is marked hyperextensibility of the hand.

masses sign: in ulnar nerve palsy; there is flattening of the metacarpal arch and hypothenar atrophy due to intrinsic dysfunction with loss of metacarpophalangeal flexion of the fifth digit.

Phalen test and maneuver: for carpal tunnel syndrome; irritation of the median nerve is determined by holding the wrist flexed or extended for 30 to 60 seconds, reproducing symptoms.

piano key sign: test for distal radioulnar joint instability; the wrist is pronated, the radius and ulna are grasped in examiner's hands, and moving each bone up and down relative to the other, a painful movement indicates instability.

Pollock sign: in high ulnar nerve palsy; inability to flex the distal interphalangeal joint of the fourth and fifth digits with paralysis of the flexor digitorum profundus to fourth and fifth digits.

prehension: the ability to grasp with the fingers and thumb.

pseudostability test: for carpal bone stability; in the normal wrist, if the hand is held in one hand and the distal forearm in the other, there is a normal anterior posterior translation. This translation is lost in carpal bone instability.

pulp pinch: the strength in the position one would use to pick up a piece of paper.

scaphoid test: for dynamic scapholunate instability; the examiner places his thumb under the scaphoid tubercle, moving wrist from ulnar to radial deviation. The scaphoid flexes against the thumbs in an upward push causing a painful clunk at the scapholunate articulation; **Watson test.**

Semm and Weinstein monofilament test: an array of nylon filaments are used to quantitate the cutaneous sensory pressure threshold. They are arranged in increasing thickness on a logarithmic scale. They will access the slowly adapting fiber receptor system (normal is 2.83).

Smith and Ross test: for boutonnière deformity; with passive MP joint and wrist flexion there is passive PIP extension if the central slip is intact and a greater than 20 degree lag if there is central slip rupture.

spilled teacup sign: in perilunate dislocation; the lunate will assume a volar flexed posture as seen on lateral radiographs. A spectrum exists from normal lunate position to complete volar dislocation of the lunate.

tenodesis test: to check structure integrity of the extrinsic extensors; extreme wrist flexion will passively extend the metacarpophalangeal joints, whereas wrist extension will allow passive digital proximal and distal interphalangeal flexion. This is due to resting tension of extrinsic extensor and flexor groups respectively.

Terri-Thomas sign: in scapholunate dissociation; there is an apparent gap between the scaphoid and lunate seen on a neutral anteroposterior wrist radiograph.

tuck sign: the puckering seen just proximal to a mass of chronically inflamed dorsal tenosynovium. This is accentuated by digital extension and commonly seen in rheumatoid arthritis.

two-point discrimination test: measures innervation density under the skin. Static two-point discrimination t. is for *slowly* adapting fibers; moving two-point discrimination t. is for *rapidly* adapting fibers. It is the ability to distinguish one point and two points with eyes closed. (Normal range is 1–5 mm.)

Wartenberg sign: for intrinsic muscle weakness of the hand; while the fingers are extended there is an inability to bring together the ring and little finger. In ulnar nerve palsy with interosseous paralysis, there is an inability to adduct the extended fifth digit to fourth digit.

Watson test: for scapholunate instability. The examiner can elicit a painful wrist click by compressing the scaphoid while the patient moves the wrist.

wet leather sign: subcutaneous palpable crepitus or squeaking with movement of tendons affected by tenosynovitis.

Hips

Allis maneuver: for reduction of anterior hip dislocation. The supine patient has the knee flexed, hip slightly flexed with longitudinal traction, and an assistant stabilizes the pelvis while applying a lateral traction force to the medial thigh. The surgeon then adducts and internally rotates the femur.

Allis sign: for femoral neck fracture; relaxation of the fascia between the crest of the ilium and the greater trochanter.

anvil test: for early hip joint disease or diseased vertebrae; a closed fist striking a blow to the sole of the foot with leg extended produces pain in the hip or vertebrae.

Barlow test: for dysplastic hip in infants; holding the symphysis pubis to sacrum with one hand, the opposite hip is flexed and an attempt is made to dislocate the hip. Pulling the hip back up or abducting the hip should produce a perceptible reduction.

Bozan maneuver: for reducing femoral neck fractures; a large swathe is placed around the crest of the ilium of the affected limb and a small swathe in the inguinal fold; traction, abduction, and internal rotation forces are then applied.

Chiene test: for determining fracture of the neck of the femur by use of a tape measure.

Desault sign: for intracapsular fracture of the hip; alternation of the arc described by rotation of the greater trochanter, which normally describes the segment of a circle, but in this fracture, rotates only as the apex of the femur rotates about its own axis.

Destot sign: in a pelvic fracture; there is the formation of a large superficial hematoma beneath the inguinal ligament and in the scrotum.

Earle sign: for pelvic fracture; bony prominence or hematoma associated with tenderness on rectal examination.

Ely test: for determining tightness of the rectus femoris, contracture of the lateral fascia of the thigh, or femoral nerve irritation; with patient in prone position, flexion of the leg on the thigh causes buttocks to arch away and leg to abduct at the hip joint.

Galeazzi sign: for congenital dislocation of the hip; the dislocated side is shorter when both thighs are flexed to 90 degrees, as demonstrated in infants; in an older patient, a curvature of the spine is produced by shortened leg.

gear-stick sign: for femoral head deformity of dysplastic hip or Legg-Calvé-Perthes disease; thigh abduction is full in flexion, but as the hip is extended with the hip abducted, there is impingement between the greater trochanter and ilium.

Jansen test: for osteoarthritis deformans of the hip; the patient is asked to cross the legs with a point just above the ankle resting on the opposite knee. If significant disease exists, this test and motion are impossible.

King maneuver: for femoral neck fracture reduction; on fracture table, the affected leg is in traction with pressure placed on the posterior thigh with internal rotation. Lateral traction with a groin sling may be added.

Langoria sign: for symptoms of intracapsular fracture of the femur; relaxation of the extensor muscles of the thigh is present.

Leadbetter maneuver: for slipped capital femoral epiphysis or femoral head fracture; injured hip is flexed to 90 degrees and manual traction applied to axis of the flexed thigh with adduction. The leg is then circumducted slowly to abduction maintaining internal rotation, and then the thigh and leg are brought down to the horizontal level.

Ludloff sign: for traumatic separation of the epiphysis of the lesser trochanter; swelling and ecchymosis are present at the base of Scarpa triangle, together with inability to raise the thigh when in a sitting position.

McElvenny maneuver: for femoral neck fracture reduction; with 36- to 45-kg traction the hip is abducted and internally rotated. Medial to inferior force is produced over the greater trochanter, and then the hip is adducted.

Nélaton line (radiographic and physical examinations): for detecting dislocation of the hip; a line from the anterosuperior iliac spine to the ischial tuberosity, which normally passes through the greater trochanter.

Ober test: for tight tensor fascia lata; with patient lying on side with hip and knee flexed, the opposite hip is extended while the knee is flexed. Inability to place the knee being tested on the table surface indicates a tight fascia lata.

obturator s.: inward rotation of the hip so that the obturator internus muscle is stretched. Results may be positive in acute appendicitis.

Ortolani sign: for congenitally dislocated hip; an audible click is heard when the hip goes into the socket as noted in infancy. If the sign is elicited, the dislocation should be corrected at that time to avoid hip dysfunction later; **Ortolani click.**

piston sign: for congenital dislocation of the head of the femur; if positive, there is up-and-down movement of the head of the femur; **Dupuytren sign.**

reverse Bigelow maneuver: for anterior dislocation of the hip, two maneuvers are done, both starting in hip flexion and abduction: In the first maneuver, while lifting the lower leg of the supine patient, there is a quick jerk on the flexed thigh; the second maneuver involves traction in the line of deformity with the hip then being adducted, sharply internally rotated, and extended.

Roux sign: in a pelvic lateral compression fracture, there is a distance between the greater trochanter and pubic spine on the affected side.

Smith maneuver: for reduction of femoral neck fractures; thigh is externally rotated and placed in traction, then fully abducted, internally rotated, and subsequently adducted.

Stimson maneuver: for posterior hip dislocation; the patient is placed prone on a table with the involved hip flexed and the opposite hip extended. With the involved knee flexed downward, pressure is applied to the calf, resulting in reduction of the dislocation.

Thomas sign: for hip joint flexion contracture; when the patient is walking, the fixed flexion of the hip can be compensated by lumbar lordosis. With the patient supine and flexing the opposite hip, the affected thigh raises off the table; **Strümpell sign, Thomas test.**

Trendelenburg test: for muscular weakness in poliomyelitis, ununited fracture of the femoral neck, rheumatoid arthritis, coxa vara, and congenital dislocations. With the patient standing, weight is removed from one extremity. If gluteal fold drops on that side, it signifies muscular weakness of the opposite weight-bearing hip; **Trendelenburg sign.**

Wellmerling maneuver: for femoral neck fracture reduction; the affected hip is overdistracted by 0.64 cm (¼ inch) in external rotation, and the foot is then internally rotated and traction released.

Whitman maneuver: for femoral neck fracture reduction; the hip is flexed and then extended with traction being applied and the normal hip abducted. The affected side is then abducted and a spica cast applied.

Lower Limbs

Achilles squeeze test: for Achilles tendon rupture; squeezing the calf muscle fails to produce plantar flexion of the ankle joint.

Addis test: for determination of leg length discrepancy; with patient in prone position, flexing the knees to 90 degrees reveals the potential discrepancies of both tibial and femoral lengths.

anterior tibial sign: for spastic paraplegia; involuntary extension of the tibialis anterior muscle when thigh is actively flexed on the abdomen.

Cleeman sign: for distal fracture of femur with overriding of the fragments; shows creasing of the skin just above the patella.

Homan's sign: pain in calf on dorsiflexion of foot (active or passive). Once considered a reliable test in diagnosing deep vein thrombophlebitis, but no longer considered valid. (See *phleboreogram,* Chapter 3.)

Payr sign: early sign of impending postoperative thrombosis, indicated by tenderness when pressure is placed over the inner side of the foot.

Schlesinger sign: for extensor spasm at the knee joint; with patient's leg held at the knee joint and flexed strongly at the hip joint, there will follow an extensor spasm at the knee joint with extreme supination of the foot.

Thompson test: compression of calf muscle with foot at rest results in ankle flexion if Achilles tendon is intact; **Simmons test, Achilles squeeze test.**

tourniquet test: for phlebitis of the leg; tourniquet is applied to the thigh and pressure gradually increased until the patient complains of pain in the calf; result is compared with the effect on the opposite leg.

Knees (Table 4–1)

anterior cruciate instability test: with the knee flexed, a supine patient extends the knee slowly

TABLE 4–1.

Knee Instability Tests

Instability	Positive Test	Deficient Structure
Medial	Valgus stress at 30 degrees	Medial collateral ligament
Lateral	Varus stress at 30 degrees	Minor lateral complex tear
Anterior	Anterior drawer at 90 degrees, neutral rotation	Anterior cruciate and partial medial and lateral collateral ligaments
Posterior	Posterior drawer at 90 degrees	Posterior cruciate, arcuate complex, posterior oblique ligament
Anteromedial	Slocum at 30 degrees external rotation accented	Medial capsular ligament Tibial collateral ligament Posterior oblique ligament Anterior cruciate ligament
Anterolateral	Slocum at 15 degrees internal rotation accented Jerk test Lateral pivot shift	Lateral capsular ligament Arcuate complex Anterior cruciate ligament
Posterolateral	Reverse pivot shift	Arcuate complex Lateral capsular ligament Popliteus tendon Some posterior cruciate ligament
Posteromedial (controversial)	Medial tibial plateau shifts posterior on stress	Tibial collateral ligament Medial capsular ligament Posterior oblique ligament Semimembranosus Anterior cruciate ligament

with the foot against the table surface; there is a sudden anterior shift of the tibia.

Apley test: for differentiating ligamentous from meniscal injury; tibial rotation on femur with traction or compression with the patient prone and knee flexed; **Apley s.**

arthrometer test: mechanical testing device for measuring anteroposterior ligament stability of the knee. The arthrometer is most often used in a physician's office to document the outcome of anterior cruciate ligament replacement surgery.

bayonet sign: lateral placement of infrapatellar tendon with a valgus knee produces a bayonet appearance in the quadriceps patellar tendon complex.

British test: for knee pain and/or injury; compression of patella during active quadriceps contraction as knee is extended elicits pain.

camelback sign: an unusually prominent infrapatellar fat pad of the knee and hypertrophy of the vastus lateralis.

double camelback sign: prominence of a high-riding patella and infrapatellar fat pad, producing the appearance of a camel back.

drawer sign: for ligamentous instability or rupture cruciate ligaments; with the patient supine and knee flexed to 90 degrees, the sign is positive if knee is not displaced abnormally in a posterior direction with knee pulled forward. Also called an **anterior drawer sign,** meaning the anterior cruciate is lax or ruptured.

external rotation recurvatum test: with the patient supine, the knee is brought from 10 degrees of flexion to maximum extension while palpating for external rotation of the tibia.

flexion rotation drawer test (Noyes): with

the knee extended and the thigh relaxed, there is anterolateral tibial subluxation. The knee is gradually flexed with reduction of the subluxation occurring at about 30 degrees of flexion.

grimace test: for knee pain or crepitus; if compression of the patella elicits pain or crepitus is noted, the patient will grimace.

hop test (one-legged hop test):   for anterior cruciate examination, patient hops forward on affected knee. Ability to do this is one sign of adequate anterior cruciate stability.

Hughston jerk test: for anterolateral instability of the knee noted by starting at 90 degrees flexion with tibia internally rotated and applying valgus force while rotating fibula medially. There is a jerk at about 20 degrees from full extension.

Lachman test: with the patient supine and the knee flexed to 20 degrees, the tibia is pulled anteriorly. A "give" reaction or mushy end point indicates a torn anterior cruciate ligament.

McMurray circumduction maneuver: for noting joint menisci tears or tags; there is cartilage clicking medially or laterally on manipulation of the knee; **McMurray s.**

"no touch" test: for checking patellar stability after total knee joint replacement or for anterior cruciate instability; with the patient supine and the knee flexed, there is a sudden anterior shift of the tibia when the patient extends the knee slowly with the foot on the surface.

patellar retraction test: for synovitis; compression of patella causes pain when the patient attempts to set the quadriceps muscles with the knee in full extension.

pivot-shift test (MacIntosh):   with the knee extended, the examiner internally rotates the leg and with a valgus stress gradually flexes the knee. There is a shift at 30 degrees to 40 degrees.

posterior drawer test: with the hips at 45 degrees and the knees flexed at 90 degrees the examiner sits on the foot and pushes the tibia backward; also with the hips and knees flexed at 90 degrees the heels are held together and the two knees observed for comparison of relative posterior sag of the tibia.

prone external rotation test: for posterior cruciate rupture knee; with the patient prone and knees flexed at 30 degrees, the test is considered positive for rupture if the foot externally rotates more than 10 degrees compared to the normal side.

quadriceps active test: with the patient supine the involved knee is flexed at 90 degrees and the foot rests on the table. With one hand, the examiner supports the thigh and palpates the relaxed quadriceps muscle; the other hand stabilizes the foot. When the patient is asked to slide the foot down the table, the proximal leg is pulled forward by the patellar tendon, indicating a posterior cruciate tear with resulting posterior sagging of the leg.

reverse pivot-shift (Jacob):   with the patient supine, the lateral tibial plateau shifts from posterior subluxation to reduction as the knee is brought from flexion to extension.

Slocum test: for rotary instability of the knee; the examiner pulls on the upper calf of a supine patient with the knees flexed 90 degrees. Then, while sitting on the patient's foot, the examiner pulls anteriorly, comparing the amount of give with the foot turned in 15 degrees neutral and turned out 30 degrees.

standing apprehension test: for anterior cruciate laxity; with patient standing and knee slightly flexed, examiner's hand holds the knee firmly with the thumb pushing the lateral femoral condyle medially, resulting in motion.

thumbnail test: for patellar fracture; fracture is felt as a sharp crevice when the examiner's thumbnail is passed over the subcutaneous surface of the patella.

Wilson test: with knee extended from 30 degrees with valgus stress and internal rotation of the foot, a click is heard in cases of osteochondritis dissecans.

Feet, Ankles

Achilles bulge sign: seen in ankle instability, a bulging Achilles tendon occurs when the foot is pulled forward while the leg is pushed backward with the knee flexed; **heel-cord sign.**

anterior drawer sign: for ankle instability; the heel is pulled forward with the leg being restrained by the opposite hand. A precise lateral radiograph is obtained with the patient supine and both the popliteal area and heel supported and 5 kg applied to the ankle.

Coleman lateral standing block test: to detect flexibility of cavovarus deformity of foot; lateral side of foot and full heel are placed on a 1-inch block, and loss of varus deformity implies flexibility.

dimple sign: for ruptured lateral collateral ligament of ankle; an anterior force is directed on the heel while a posterior force is directed on the distal leg. In the case of a ruptured ligament, a dimple will appear.

drawer sign: for lateral collateral ligament injury in the ankle, with the foot and ankle at rest and the knee flexed and the ankle flexed at 10 to 15 degree plantar flexion, the heel is pulled forward. The center of rotation is the deltoid ligament.

Harris-Beath footprinting mat: a pressure sensitive mat used to reflect the various pressure points under the foot.

Helbing sign: for flatfoot; medialward curving of the Achilles tendon as viewed from behind.

Keen sign: for Pott fracture of the fibula; if fracture exists, there is increased diameter around the malleoli area of the ankle.

Marie-Foix sign: for central nervous system disorder; withdrawal of the lower leg on transverse pressure of the tarsus or forced flexion of toes, even when the leg is incapable of voluntary movement.

Morton test: for metatarsalgia or neuroma; transverse pressure across heads of the metatarsals causes sharp pain in the forefoot.

Mulder sign: for interdigital neuroma in the foot; a palpable click can be heard on motion of the metatarsal heads.

Murphy sign: for Achilles tendon bursitis at the heel; dorsiflexion of the foot produces pain.

sagittal stress test: for ankle instability; with the knee flexed to at least 45 degrees, the foot is pulled forward while the leg is pushed backward. If the usual concavity of the Achilles tendon is flattened or reversed, the sign is positive for an instability of the anterior fibular collateral ligament.

screw-home mechanism: the small degree of external rotation that occurs as the knee is brought to the last few degrees of extension.

Strunsky sign: for detecting lesions of the anterior arch of the foot; sudden flexing of the toes is painless in a normal foot, but painful if inflammation exists in the anterior arch.

talar tilt test: with the ankle in neutral position the heel is grasped in one hand and the ankle in the other. The ankle is then supinated with maximum force. An anteroposterior radiograph may be obtained to define the talar tilt.

toe spread sign: for Morton neuroma; disproportional spreading of the toes, comparing one foot with the other.

too many toes sign: increased hindfoot, valgus, pronation, and abduction of forefoot. On clinical observation, refers to the excessive number of toes that appear laterally when foot is viewed from behind. Often indicates collapse of the medial arch and flatfoot deformity.

Wu sole opposition test: for posterior tendon rupture; a visual test that shows a defect as both feet are opposed to each other.

Neurologic Examination

ankle clonus test: used to indicate impending injury to the spinal cord during scoliosis surgery; anesthetically induced sustained ankle clonus (repeated ankle jerks that occur following a single stimulus) disappears.

Babinski reflex: for loss of brain control over lower extremities; scraping the soles causes toes to pull up; **toe sign.**

Babinski sign: for testing of first sacral nerve root pathology; an absent Achilles tendon reflex or diminished reflex as compared to the other side.

Beevor sign: for segmental nerve disease involving T5 to T12 or L1 nerve roots; the patient does an active sit-up with the arms held behind the head. In a positive examination, the umbilicus moves toward the segment that is weak.

Brudzinski sign: for meningitis; flexion of the neck forward results in flexion of the hip and knee; when passive flexion of the lower limb on one side is made, a similar movement will be seen in the opposite limb; **neck sign, contralateral sign.**

Chaddock sign: for upper motor neuron loss (brain); the big toe extends when irritating the skin in the external malleolar region; indicates lesions of the corticospinal paths; **external malleolus sign, Chaddock reflex.**

doll's eye sign: for testing normal or abnormal brain function; the normal coordinated eye motions seen when passively turning the head of an unconscious patient; **Cantelli sign.**

Ely test: for L3 and L4 nerve root irritation; flexing thigh with patient prone causes back and/or thigh pain; **femoral nerve stretch test, Ely sign.**

fan sign: for central nerve problems; stroking the sole of the foot with a needle causes toes to spread; part of Babinski reflex examination.

finger to nose test: for cerebellar disease; patient attempts to put a finger on nose and then on the examiner's finger, back and forth rapidly, any incoordination indicates positive test; **coordination extremity test.**

Fournier test: for determining ataxic gait; it is noted with the patient moving about abruptly in walking, starting, and stopping.

Fränkel sign: for tabes dorsalis; noted by diminished tonicity of muscles about the hip joint.

Gordon reflex: for loss of brain control; percussion on lateral thigh causes toes to go up rather than the normal downward motion.

Guilland sign: for meningeal irritation; when the contralateral quadriceps muscle group is pinched, there is brisk flexion at the hip and knee joint.

Hirschberg sign: for pyramidal tract disease; internal rotation and adduction of foot on rubbing inner lateral side.

Hoffmann sign: for testing digital reflex; nipping of three fingernails (index, middle, ring) produces flexion of terminal phalanx of thumb and second and third phalanx of some other finger; digital reflex.

Huntington sign: for lesions of the pyramidal tract; patient is supine, with legs hanging over the examining table, and is asked to cough; if coughing produces flexion of the thigh and extension of the leg in the paralyzed limb, a lesion is indicated.

Jendrassik maneuver: to enhance a patellar reflex; the reflex is tested when the patient hooks hands together with flexed fingers and pulls apart as hard as possible.

Kernig sign: for meningitis; in dorsal decubitus, the patient can easily and completely extend the leg; when sitting or lying down with thigh flexed upon the abdomen, the leg cannot be completely extended.

Kerr sign: for spinal cord lesions; alteration of the texture of the skin below the somatic level is used to locate level of lesions.

Leichtenstern sign: for cerebrospinal meningitis; tapping lightly on any bone of the extremities causes patient to wince suddenly.

Leri sign: for hemiplegia; passive flexion of the hand and wrist of the affected side shows no normal flexion at the elbow.

Lhermitte sign: for cervical cord injuries or unstable cervical spine; transient dysesthesia and weakness are noted in all four limbs when the patient flexes the head forward.

long tract sign: any sign that one would see in affection of either sensory or motor tracts in the spinal cord. For example, **Babinski reflex, Romberg test.**

Mendel-Bekhterev reflex: for organic hemiplegia; using a percussion hammer, the examiner notes flexion of the small toes if the dorsal surface of the cuboid bone is struck.

Moro reflex: for testing normal early neurologic development or the failure to progress neurologically; the infant is placed on a table, then the table is forcibly struck from either side, causing the infant's arms to be thrown out as in an embrace; should disappear as infancy progresses.

Morquio sign: for epidemic poliomyelitis; the supine patient resists attempts to raise trunk to a sitting position until the legs are passively flexed.

MRC sensory grade (Zachary or Medical Research Council sensory grade): for assessment of sensation of peripheral nerve after injury and/or repair.

S 0: absence of any sensory recovery.

S 1: recovery of deep cutaneous pain sensibility.

S 2: return of some superficial pain and tactile sensibility.

S 2+: recovery of touch and pain sensibility throughout the autonomous zone, but with persistent overreaction.

S 3: return of superficial pain and tactile sensibility throughout the autonomous zone with disappearance of overreaction.

S 3+: as S 3 but with good localization and some return of two-point discrimination.

S 4: return of sensibility as in S 3, with recovery of two-point discrimination.

nuchocephalic reflex: for diffuse cerebral dysfunction as in senility; when the shoulders are turned to the left or right, there is a failure of the head to turn in that direction within 0.5 seconds.

Oppenheim sign: for pyramidal tract disease; dorsal extension of the big toe is present when the medial side of the tibia is stroked in a downward direction.

paratonia: for diffuse cerebral dysfunction as in senility; the patient is asked to relax with the elbow passively flexed and extended. Intermittent opposition is abnormal.

Piotrowski sign: for organic disease of the central nervous system; percussion of tibialis muscle produces dorsiflexion and supination; **anticus sign** or **reflex.**

pronation sign: for central nervous disorders; there is a strong tendency for the forearm to pronate; **Strümpell sign.**

pseudo-Babinski sign: in poliomyelitis, the Babinski reflex is modified so only the big toe is extended, because all foot muscles except dorsiflexors of the big toe are paralyzed.

Queckenstedt sign: for detecting a block in the vertebral canal; compression of veins in the neck on one or both sides produces rapid rise in pressure of cerebral spinal fluid of a healthy person and quickly disappears. In a patient with blockage in vertebral canal, pressure of cerebrospinal fluid is little or not at all affected.

radialis sign: for nerve impairment; inability to close the fist without marked dorsal extension of the wrist; **Strümpell sign.**

Raimiste sign: for paretic condition; patient's hand and arm are held upright by examiner; a sound hand remains upright on being released, but a paretic hand flexes abruptly at the wrist.

Romberg test: for differentiation between peripheral and cerebellar ataxia; increase in clumsiness in movements and in width and uncertainty of gait when patient's eyes are closed indicate peripheral ataxia; no change indicates cerebellar type. (NOTE: Romberg sign is similar in testing but used for noting tabes dorsalis.)

Sarbó sign: for locomotor ataxia; analgesia of peroneal nerve is noted.

Schreiber maneuver: for patellar reflex testing; rubbing the inner side of the upper part of thigh enhances the reflex.

stairs sign: in locomotor ataxia; there is difficulty or failure of ability to descend stairs.

station test: for coordination disturbance; feet are planted firmly together; if the body sways, lack of coordination is indicated.

tendon reflexes: for testing continuity of normal muscle to spinal cord to muscle reflex arc. Any tendon may be so tested, but the most common are the deep tendon reflexes (DTRs):

  Achilles r.:   ankle jerk.
  quadriceps r.:   patellar tendon or knee jerk.
  biceps r.:   elbow jerk.
  triceps r.:   elbow jerk.
  mental r.:   jaw jerk or reflex.

Thomas sign: for cord lesions; pinching of the trapezius muscle causes goose bumps above the level of the cord lesion.

tibialis sign: for spastic paralysis of the lower limb; there is dorsiflexion of the foot when the thigh is drawn toward the body; **tibial phenomenon.**

Tinel sign: for noting a partial lesion or beginning regeneration of a nerve; tingling sensation of the distal end of a limb when percussion is made over the site of divided nerve as in carpal tunnel impingement on the median nerve of the hand; **formication sign, distal tingling on percussion (DTP) sign.**

Metabolic Tests

Chvostek sign: for determining low serum calcium leading to tetany; tapping the cheek near the facial nerves causes the muscles to twitch or go into spasm; **Chvostek test, Chvostek-Weiss sign, Weiss sign, Schultze-Chvostek sign.**

lead line: a blue line seen in the gums of a patient with lead poisoning; **Burton sign.**

Tensilon test: for myasthenia gravis; a chemical test for denoting muscle strength or weakness; injection of endrophonium chloride (Tensilon) will reverse the symptoms in patients whose muscle weakness is caused by myasthenia gravis.

General Observations

antecedent sign: any precursory indication of a malady.

artifact: a feature of a *test* that stimulates pathology or interference with the correct results of the test.

café-au lait: flat, hyperpigmented areas of skin with rugged "coast of Maine" borders or smooth borders. The presence of four or more café-au-lait spots with "coast of Maine" borders is seen often in von Recklingshausen disease.

cogwheel phenomenon: jerky motions produced on testing a muscle's strength; the jerks are neither rhythmic nor equal and represent malingering or protection from pain; **cogwheel sign.**

commemorative sign: any sign of a previous disease.

dimple sign: for a variety of joint dislocations; in the shoulder, when there is an anterior dislocation, there is a dimple in the deltoid below the acromion; in a posterolateral dislocation of the knee where the medial femoral condyle buttonholes, the anteromedial capsule, the skin is furrowed.

Dupuytren sign: for determining sarcomatous bone; a crackling sensation on compression of that area is noted.

Gower sign: for progressive muscular dystrophy and tabes dorsalis; abrupt intermittent oscillation of iris under light is the indication of ongoing process.

hemodynamic test: to determine the relationship of blood flow in normal as compared to diseased anatomic structures.

Hueter sign: for indication of fracture; absence of the transmission of osseous vibration in fractures as heard by a stethoscope, where the fibrous material is interposed between the fragments.

Langer line: the normal tension lines of skin commonly used to define direction of scar, as to how the scar runs with or across those lines.

objective sign: one that can be seen, heard, measured, or felt by the diagnostician to confirm or deny an ongoing symptom; **physical sign.**

quadriceps test: for hyperthyroidism or debilitating condition; while standing, the patient is asked to hold leg up and straight out; a disease is present if patient cannot maintain this position for 1 minute.

Raynaud phenomenon: pallor or blueness of fingers, toes, or nose brought about by exposure to cold and less commonly by other stresses.

somatic sign: any sign presented by trunk or limbs rather than sensory apparatus.

succinylcholine test: for differentiation of muscle power loss due to nerve injury or tendon rupture; injection of succinylcholine will produce contractions lasting several minutes when there is denervation.

thumb-to-forearm test: an index of generalized joint laxity; the examiner places the tip of the thumb on the forearm while flexing the wrist.

GAITS

A patient's walking pattern (gait) is very important in the evaluation of disorders, particularly those affecting the lower limbs. A limp is more apparent in the stance phase of walking. Of the various gait patterns, some have very specific characteristics, such as the following:

antalgic gait: due to pain in the stance phase (while walking through on the foot), the time spent on the affected side is shortened compared with that on the normal side.

Fick angle: a measure of toe in and toe out during normal gait; the angle formed by the axis of the foot and the direction of the gait.

gluteus maximus gait: due to weak or nonfunctioning hip extensor muscles, the patient thrusts the thorax posteriorly to maintain hip extension.

gluteus medius gait (abductor lurch): due to weak or nonfunctioning hip abductor muscles, the patient lurches toward the weak side to place the center of gravity over the hip; **gluteal lurch.**

slap foot (drop foot) gait: due to weak or nonfunctioning ankle dorsiflexor muscles, the foot slaps down after heel strike.

SCALES AND RATINGS

To have a reproducible presentation of the preoperative and postoperative condition of certain joints, various scales and rating systems have been developed. The scales and ratings are usually based on pain and the degree of functional impairment.

American Shoulder and Elbow Surgeons system: a five-point grading system for level of pain and four-point system for lowest to highest level of function in activities of daily living, work, and sports.

Charnley hip scale: for evaluating hip disease and postoperative results; scale uses pain, range of motion, and function for scoring.

Frankel neurological assessment: for spinal cord injury.

complete (A): no motor power below the level of the lesion.

sensory (B): no motor power but some sensation below the level of the lesion.

motor useless (C): some motor power below the level of the lesion, but of no functional use to the patient.

motor useful (D): motor power of functional use below the level of the lesion; the patient is able to walk with or without aids.

recovery (E): full motor power, normal sensation and no sphincter disturbance, although reflexes may be abnormal.

Harris hip scale: 100-point scale with 40 points for function and 60 points for pain in the hip.

Iowa hip scale: for evaluating hip disease and postoperative results; scale uses pain, range of motion, and function for scoring.

Knee Society clinical rating system: the Knee Society presented this rating system as a uniform system for research. It uses pain and physical examination for a maximum of 100 points. Function is scored by walking and use of stairs for a maximum total of 100 points.

Lynholm knee-scoring scale: knee scale incorporating pain, swelling, function, and stability.

Marshall knee-scoring scale: knee scale including symptoms, function, and examination references.

Mazur ankle rating: grading system for the ankle using pain and function as a basis for the rating.

Merle d'Aubigne and Postel hip scale: for evaluating hip disease and postoperative result; scale uses pain, range of motion, and function for scoring.

total hip arthroplasty outcome evaluation*: designed by the American Academy of Orthopaedic Surgeons for universal definition of outcome of total hip arthroplasty. Includes function, satisfaction, physical examination, complications, and radiographic examination. This form also takes into account preoperative factors.

OTHER PHYSICAL EXAMINATIONS

The portions of a physical examination that are not described as a test, sign, or maneuver include tests for ranges of motion, muscle strength and sensation, and sensory examinations. These tests are found in Chapter 12 and Appendix B.

*Liang MH, Katz JN, Phillips C, Sledge C, et al: The total hip arthroplasty form of the American Academy of Orthopaedic Surgeons, *J Bone Joint Surg [Am]* 73:639–645, 1991.

Chapter 5

Laboratory Evaluations

Prerequisites for the diagnosis of musculoskeletal complaints are a thorough history and clinical examination of the patient and, when necessary, a radiographic examination. From this information, further tests can be carefully selected.

This chapter discusses the examination of blood and its components, synovial fluid, and urine. The first section deals with those tests commonly performed as part of the routine evaluation of outpatients or preoperative patients. The next section discusses the laboratory findings of specific diseases as related to orthopaedics, taking into account that some generalized diseases result in orthopaedic problems. The definitions are designed to be comprehensive. According to accreditation and regulation, normal ranges of laboratory values must be reported with each laboratory result.

Because normal values are dependent on the geographic area, patient population, test methodology, and laboratory standardization, such values are not considered useful when published in textbooks because they are likely to be misleading. Therefore, normal values have been deleted and the initial statement or sentence in either section should be an adequate overview for those not concerned with the complete nature of the study.

Care must be exercised when using laboratory terminology, decimal points, significant figures in laboratory data, and other specific information. Forms are provided for most tests requested. Laboratory results should never be given over the telephone except in emergency situations. Requests may be emergency (stat), urgent, or routine.

A blood test may examine the quantity and type of cells, the level of chemicals in the serum, and (rarely) the chemical composition of the blood cell. For each laboratory test, the definition states what portion of blood is tested. For example, if it is a test on both cells and fluid of the blood, the phrase "whole blood" will be used. The preferred unit of volume is the liter (L).

The third and final section gives a list of laboratory abbreviations and annotation of units.

ROUTINE EVALUATIONS

CBC (Complete Blood Count)

The CBC is a series of whole blood tests to determine the quantity and other characteristics of blood cells. Some physicians prefer only a hemoglobin, hematocrit, and white count. Most laboratories use automated machines to provide all the parameters as a part of a standard report, and a limited study such as an "H&H" is not cost-effective. The comprehensive CBC may include the following tests.

Hgb (Hb, hemoglobin): the iron-carrying protein in the blood. Normal values depend on age and gender. (g/dl)

Hct, PCV (hematocrit, packed cell volume): the proportion of the red cells in whole blood expressed as a percentage.

H&H (hematocrit and hemoglobin): determination of hematocrit and hemoglobin levels only.

RBC (red blood count):   the number of red cells per unit volume of whole blood. (million cells/μl) (# cells $\times 10^{12}$/L)

MCV (mean corpuscular volume):   average volume of a red cell. May not be reliable if red cells are abnormal (i.e., sickle cell disease). (fl)

MCH (mean corpuscular hemoglobin):   the average amount of hemoglobin in each red cell. (pg)

MCHC (mean corpuscular hemoglobin concentration):   the average concentration of hemoglobin in the red cells. (g Hb/dl red cells)

WBC (white blood count):   number of white blood cells per unit volume of whole blood. (thousand cells/μl) ($\times 10^9$/L)

differential WBC (diff):   percentage of different white cell types: neutrophils (segmented [mature] and/or precursors [immature]), lymphocytes, monocytes, eosinophils, basophils, and occasionally other forms. With present laboratory technology, the differential count is usually performed automatically and may not indicate the maturity of the neutrophils. In the unusual cases where segmented neutrophils must be distinguished from more immature forms, the test may be performed by microscopic examination of the stained blood smear. ($\times 10^9$/L)

platelets (Plt):   a blood test measuring the number of platelets (thrombocytes) per volume of whole blood. Platelet counts are routinely done by machine. Platelets play an important role in hemostasis. ($\times 10^9$/L)

bone marrow biopsy: laboratory test performed on bone marrow from a medullary cavity, such as the posterior iliac crest, to determine, by microscopic examination, the adequacy and morphology of hematopoeitic cells.

Basic Chemistry Profiles

Many hospitals offer groups of chemistry tests (called profiles or panels) since these tests are frequently ordered together (e.g., serum electrolytes, hepatitis panel, renal panel, etc.). The basic components of these panels are listed below.

albumin: serum concentration of the major osmotically active component of blood. May be decreased in acute or chronic inflammation, liver disease, severe burns, or fever. (mg/dl)

ALP (serum alkaline phosphatase):   enzyme present in bone, liver, and other organs. Marked elevation over adult normal values may be seen in healthy adolescents. (U/dl, U/L)

ALT (alanine aminotransferase, formerly SGPT):   enzyme present in several organs, but generally used to assess liver disease. (U/L)

AST (aspartate aminotransferase, formerly SGOT):   enzyme present in many organs, particularly muscle and liver. Increased values may indicate damage to the organ. (U/L)

BUN (blood urea nitrogen):   a metabolic waste product usually cleared by the kidney. When increased, may indicate kidney disease. (mg/dl)

Ca, P: calcium and phosphorus (the latter as phosphate), in general, constitute the two main bone ions. The blood levels of these two ions do not necessarily denote bone problems. (mg/dl)

cholesterol: a steroid-based compound that has been associated with predisposition to coronary artery disease. The level of cholesterol is dependent on both genetic and dietary factors. Cholesterol is usually bound to a carrier lipoprotein, which comes in two primary densities: high and low. High-density lipoprotein (HDL) cholesterol appears to vary inversely with coronary artery disease—the higher the level, the lower the disease frequency. On the other hand, low-density lipoprotein (LDL) cholesterol appears to vary directly with coronary artery disease. (mg/dl)

Cr (creatinine):   a metabolic by-product usually cleared by the kidney. Increased levels may indicate kidney disease. (mg/dl)

Gamma GT (gamma-glutamyltransferase, gamma-glutamyltranspeptidase, GGTP):   serum enzyme that is frequently increased in liver disease caused by obstruction of the bile duct(s). (U/L)

LDH (lactate dehydrogenase): enzyme present in many organs. Increased values may indicate liver disease, red blood cell destruction within blood vessels, or recent heart attack (within 24–36 hours). (U/L)

total bilirubin: metabolic by-product of liver metabolism of hemoglobin. Usually an indicator of liver function. (mg/dl)

total serum protein: concentration of all proteins in the serum. (g/dl)

UA (uric acid): metabolic by-product usually elevated in cases of chronic gout. Elevated levels of uric acid are not necessarily correlated with acute attacks of gout. (mg/dl)

Urinalysis (UA; Routine and Microscopic [R&M])

The routine urinalysis includes a notation of the color turbidity (appearance), specific gravity (density with respect to that of water—tells how concentrated the urine is), pH (acidity or alkalinity), and the presence or absence of glucose, protein, bilirubin, ketone bodies, urobilinogen, and occult blood. A microscopic examination may be done on the urinary sediment, and the material seen may be described as white cells, red cells, epithelial cells, and a variety of crystals and casts (microscopic debris usually from diseased kidneys). The quantity of cells and crystals is expressed in the number of observed objects per high-power field (HPF) of the microscope, whereas the quantity of casts is expressed in the number of observed objects per low-power field (LPF).

GENERAL BLOOD AND SERUM TESTS

The general orthopaedic and related laboratory examinations and results found in this section are grouped according to similar disease processes, such as arthritis, infection, metabolic disturbances, and hematologic disorders, and also for assessment of spinal fluid and liver function.

However, these categories are not used as unit headings because the tests are often used to study a variety of problems, depending on the clinical circumstance. The orthopaedic laboratory work-up may include any or all of the following.

acid phosphatase (AcP): a serum assay test for acid phosphatase activity. Elevations are usually associated with disease of the prostate, particularly cancer. *Prostate-specific antigen (PSA)* may be increased in prostatic disease, particularly in prostatic cancer. It is still controversial whether PSA should be used to screen asymptomatic men for prostate cancer, but serial PSA levels are of value in following patients with prostate cancer after surgery or radiation. (U/L)

alanine aminotransferase (ALT, formerly SGPT): an enzyme present in several organs, but generally used to assess liver disease. (U/L)

ALP (alkaline phosphatase, alk PO4 tase): test to determine the level of this enzyme. The most common sources of high values are rapid growth or fracture healing. In any growth spurt the value may be as high as 3 times normal. Other bone disorders causing an increase in alkaline phosphatase include Paget disease, primary bone tumors, some metastatic diseases, and osteomalacia. Because elevations in alkaline phosphatase can result from liver disorders, two additional tests may be performed: (1) heating the enzyme will destroy it if it comes from the liver, and (2) abnormally high values of serum gamma glutamyltranspeptidase (gamma GT) and alanine aminotransferase (ALT) indicate liver disease. Isoenzymes of alkaline phosphatase can be measured by indicating the organ of origin. (U/L)

anti–double-stranded (native) DNA: test for antibodies against the genetic chemical information in the cell; values greater than 800 U/L are specific for systemic lupus erythematosus. (U/L)

antinuclear antibody (ANA): an immunologic screening test that reveals the presence of serum antibodies against cellular nuclear material (DNA); usually reported as positive or negative.

Elevations of ANA, especially when accompanied by the "peripheral rim" pattern of fluorescence, are associated with lupus erythematosus.

ASO (antistreptolysin O) titer: this test is done mostly on children with joint complaints who are suspected of having rheumatic fever. The most meaningful finding for this test is an increase in the values over a period of a week. The reports may be given as a tube dilution ratio, such as 1/256, or in Todd units, which is the inverse number.

blood gases: a measurement of the amount of oxygen (O_2) and carbon dioxide (CO_2) in the blood. The oxygen is usually presented with a percent saturation value, which is normally above 90%. The pH (acidity) of the blood is simultaneously determined.

C-reactive protein (CRP):   a plasma protein not affected by the presence of circulating hormones or anti-inflammatory drugs. Good indicator of inflammation and/or trauma. Correlates well with ESR (see below), but elevations appear and disappear before changes in ESR. (mg/L or μg/L)

creatine kinase (CK; creatine phosphokinase [CPK]):   an enzyme contained in many organs, principally skeletal muscle, heart muscle, and brain. In muscle disorders, particularly muscular dystrophy, it is elevated. In cases of suspected acute myocardial infarction, isoenzyme determinations help distinguish the organ of origin of the elevated enzyme level. (U/L)

creatinine: by-product of metabolism that is cleared by the kidney. A 2-hour *creatinine clearance (Ccr)* indicates how effectively the kidney is functioning as a blood filter. (mg/dl)

erythrocyte sedimentation rate (sed. rate, sedimentation rate, ESR):
   modified Westergren method: Test performed on anticoagulated whole blood to determine the speed of settling of cells in 1 hour. Three stages of sedimentation occur: initial aggregation and rouleaux formation, quick settling, and packing. The test is nonspecific, similar to determination of temperature or pulse, and a normal value is perfectly consistent with many disease states. An increased sedimentation rate may indicate certain conditions, particularly inflammation. Therefore, this test is often used in evaluating bone and joint infections and other inflammatory diseases. (mm/hr)

FBS (fasting blood sugar):   test done to detect diabetes. Blood sample must be obtained at least 12 hours after the least meal. In the past, a *glucose tolerance test (GTT)* was a 2- to 5-hour study of both the blood and urine obtained from a patient who had taken 75 g of sugar after fasting. The most efficient GTT is a fasting and 2-hour postprandial (after eating) blood glucose. If these values are sufficiently abnormal according to the expected values for that particular laboratory, diabetes mellitus can be diagnosed.

Three different sets of criteria are available for interpreting the plasma glucose levels in the GTT. These include the NDDG (National Diabetes Data Group), the WHO (World Health Organization) criteria, and age-related expected values for glucose criteria. Those values are available on request from your laboratory. There is usually little value in performing a 3- to 5-hour GTT. (mg/dl)

hemoglobin electrophoresis: a test to determine types of red cell hemoglobin. Abnormalities are present in sickle cell disease, thalassemia, and other red cell disorders. The results of this test are reported as normal or described by the specific abnormality.

HLA-B27:   an antigen on the surface of cells frequently present in patients with ankylosing spondylitis.

LE prep (lupus erythematosus preparation):   wherein blood is subjected to trauma, causing extrusion of the nuclei from leukocytes; if the LE factor is present, it causes nucleolysis that induces phagocytosis by the patient's own neutrophils, producing LE cells. A blood smear of white blood cells is inspected under the microscope for large intracellular collections of nuclear material; reported as either positive or negative. Now largely replaced by the antinuclear antibody and anti-native DNA tests.

prothrombin time (pro time, PT): a test that measures the clotting factors in the *ex*trinsic coagulation system, commonly done to monitor patients taking blood thinners as warfarin sodium (Coumadin).

> **INR (international normalizing ratio):** ratio of value of patient's prothrombin time to the mean of normal raised to the power of the international standard index.

> **activated partial thromboplastin time (APTT, PTT):** a test that measures the clotting factors in the *in*trinsic coagulation system. It is the test of choice in monitoring patients receiving heparin to retard blood clotting.

reticulocyte count: a blood cell test to determine the erythropoeitic activity, thereby helping in the classification of anemia. When observed under the microscope, only 1 of 100 red cells will normally take up a stain, indicating it is less than 24 hours old. Finding an increased number of reticulocytes means probable increased red blood cell production, usually in response to anemia. However, the percentage of reticulocytes is relative to the total red cell count, so that mathematical correction of the percent reticulocytes is necessary for proper interpretation. Some centers have moved to reporting *absolute* reticulocyte counts (reference range, 25,000–75,000 cells /μL or 25–75 $\times$ 10 9/L).

rheumatoid factor (RA factor): a serologic test to determine the presence of certain antibodies frequently seen in autoimmune diseases. The antibodies may be detected by several methods; some are more sensitive than others. The individual laboratory will interpret the importance of positive, negative, or numeric results.

salicylates: a test can be done on the blood to determine the specific levels of salicylates or on the urine as a screening test for the presence of aspirin. This can be done to follow the treatment of arthritis or in the event of an accidental overdose. Salicylate is also present in oil of wintergreen, which some people use topically for relief of muscle pain, so elevated levels do not always indicate aspirin therapy or overdose. (μg/ml)

serum lead: in cases of lead poisoning, the serum can be tested for that element specifically. Because lead is a heavy metal, a heavy metal screening test is frequently used to determine the presence of lead poisoning. Elevated lead levels can also be indirectly tested for by measuring the free red cell protoporphyrin or zinc protoporphyrin levels. (μg/dl)

serum protein electrophoresis (SPE, SPEP): a test to determine the presence and amount of particular types of serum proteins; used to detect multiple myeloma—a malignancy of the cells that produces immunoglobulin (Ig). A report of a high immunoglobulin or monoclonal pattern may indicate myeloma. An *immunoelectrophoresis* is a similar test reporting the concentrations of various immunoglobulins (IgG, IgA, and IgM) in the serum.

T3 (triiodothyronine), T4 (thyroxine), and TSH (thyroid-stimulating hormone): measures of the levels of thyroid active hormones and the pituitary hormone controlling thyroid function. There are various methods for determining these levels to help recognize hyper- and hypothyroidism. A caution in interpreting such values should be made in chronically ill patients. (ng/dl, μg/dl, μU/ml)

SERUM AND URINE TESTS FOR METABOLIC DISEASE

The following tests, as well as some urine excretion tests, are done to assess bone metabolism (i.e., bone formation and resorption). These tests are used most often for diagnosing and following therapeutic response in patients with osteoporosis, Paget disease, hyperparathyroidism, and other metabolic bone diseases. In Paget disease, patients can have either evidence of decreased bone formation or increased bone resorption. These studies are often ordered by an endocrinologist, but have interest to the orthopaedist.

Serum Tests for General Bone Turnover Markers

calcidiol (25(OH)D):   measurement of 25(OH)D, a liver metabolite of vitamin D, in the serum is a good index for determining vitamin D deficiency and intoxication, and aids in diagnosis of patients with metabolic bone diseases. It is measured by radioimmunoassay, or competition binding protein assay. (ng/ml)

calcitonin: still in development and research stage, serum calcitonin is most frequently used for the diagnosis and management of medullary thyroid carcinoma. It is measured by either radioimmunoassay or the concentration technique. (pg/ml)

calcitriol 1,25(OH)2D: still in development and research stage, measurement of **1,25(OH)2D** is used in the management of hypo- and hypercalcemic disorders; specifically, the following bone diseases: PTH gland disorders, renal failure, sarcoidosis, and for therapeutic management of treatment. It is measured by radioreceptor assay. (pg/ml)

serum calcium (Ca):   measures serum calcium concentration. Serum calcium levels are increased in hyperparathyroidism, while there is a concurrent decrease in serum phosphorus (PO_4). The phosphorus determination in parathyroid disease is dependent on renal function. Determination of calcium and phosphorus levels is commonly done as a screening measure. Many dis-

eases affect the blood levels of these two chemicals. (mg/dl)

parathyroid hormone (PTH):   measured in serum for the evaluation and differentiation of disorders of calcium metabolism. Intact PTH is measured by either immunoradiometric or immunochemiluminescent assay. (pg/dl, pmol/L)

Serum Tests for Bone Formation

bone specific alkaline phosphatase (BAP, BSAP):   determined by alkaline phosphatase isoenzyme electrophoresis; can be a useful marker for the rate of bone formation. It is usually elevated in Paget disease, and its determination can help in monitoring Paget disease patients being treated with antiresorptive therapy. (U/L, IU/L)

calcium 47:   total body accretion test. Nuclear medicine whole body in vivo study for bone formation.

osteocalcin or "bone Gla protein" (OC, ON, BGP):   a serum marker for assessment of bone formation; most abundant noncollagenous protein in bone. This test is still in the development and research stage, along with other biochemical marker tests, and is potentially useful in monitoring treatment of metabolic bone diseases. The method of the test is radioimmunoassay or immunoradiometric assay. (ng/ml)

procollagen propeptide: serum marker of osteoblastic activity measured in two chemical forms: the **carboxyterminal propeptide (c-PCP, PICP)** and the **aminoterminal propeptide (N-PCP).**

Serum Test for Bone Resorption

tartrate-resistant acid phosphatase (TRAP):   a serum test to measure bone resorption and to determine the metabolic activity of osteoclasts; specific acid phosphatase seen from active metabolic osteoclastic activity.

Urine Chemical Tests

Some minerals and other chemicals measured in blood are also measured in urine. These include calcium, phosphorus, creatinine, and uric acid. The following are indicators of bone resorption, with the exception of the mucopolysaccharides, which are an index of proteoglycan metabolic abnormalities.

pyridinoline collagen cross-links (PYD) and pyridinium collagen cross-links (PYD): these two names refer to the same urine tests used to measure cross-linked fragments of collagen that result from bone degradation.

  C-telopeptide (cross-links, C-tx): still in development and research stage; enzyme-linked immunosorbent assay is used to measure Type I Collagen degradation products in urine as a bone resorption marker. It is reported as cross-links NMOL/mmol creatinine. It is used for research applications such as to monitor effectiveness of different anti-resorptive therapies.

  N-telopeptide (NTx): still in development and research stage; quantitative measure of excretion of cross-linked N-telopeptides of Type I Collagen (NTx) is done by enzyme-linked immunosorbent assay (ELISA) as a resorption marker. NTx is reported as bone collagen equivalents/creatinine. Measurement of NTx is intended for use in predicting skeletal response to hormonal antiresorptive therapy in postmenopausal women and therapeutic monitoring of other antiresorptive therapies. (ng/ml)

  hydroxyproline (HYP): urine test that measures the degradation products of bone matrix; total fasting urinary hydroxyproline creatinine ratio is used traditionally as a marker of bone resorption. It is markedly increased in Paget disease. It is used to monitor treatment with antiresorptive drugs.

  free pyridinium cross-links: for bone resorption; these are the cross-links of Type I collagen which constitutes 90% of the organic bone matrix. **Pyridinoline (PYD)** and **deoxypyridinoline (Dpd, DPYD)** are excreted in the urine and not affected by diet. Deoxypyridinoline (Dpd) is more specific for bone metabolism. It is a useful marker to monitor therapies for metabolic bone diseases.

mucopolysaccharides: test done on the urine to determine the excretion of abnormal amounts of specific mucopolysaccharides that are seen in diseases causing dwarfism, gargoylism, mental retardation, and other congenital problems.

BACTERIOLOGIC STUDIES

acid-fast bacillus (AFB): refers to the bright red appearance of mycobacteria when stained by a special technique and observed under a microscope. A more efficient method involving fluorescence microscopy is now available.

anaerobic culture: bacterial culture grown in the absence of oxygen (obligate anaerobes), or minimal free oxygen (facultative anaerobes). Certain organisms require this environment for growth in contrast to the standard aerobic cultures grown in the presence of normal oxygen. Anaerobic bacteria, like their aerobic counterparts, can be pathogenic or nonpathogenic.

C&S (culture and sensitivity): bacteria from a wound, urine, blood, joint fluid, throat, or any other source are grown in tubes or on plates. The bacteria are identified by combinations of biochemical reactions that they can or cannot carry out. The results of bacterial cultures are usually listed by individual organism along with its antimicrobial sensitivity.

  typical bacterial species reports: the following bacterial species are frequently encountered in laboratory studies; they are listed for spelling purposes, without definitions. The terms "common flora" and "normal flora" denote the presence of normal, nonpathogenic bacteria.

Staphylococcus aureus (Staph. aureus)
Streptococcus organisms
Escherichia coli (E. coli)
Pseudomonas aeruginosa
Klebsiella pneumoniae
Salmonella organisms
Neisseria gonorrhoeae (cause of gonorrhea)
Mycobacterium tuberculosis
Mycobacterium organisms (atypical)

Common fungal organisms are:

Actinomyces
Blastomyces
Histoplasma
Coccidioides
Cryptococcus
Aspergillus
Candida

colony count (CC):   the placement of a known amount of urine on culture media; the report is usually given in number of bacterial colonies per milliliter of urine.

fluorescent treponemal antibody (FTA): serologic test for syphilis; usually interpreted as positive or negative, but may be reported in dilutions. Other tests commonly used are the VDRL (Venereal Disease Research Laboratories), STS (serologic test for syphilis), and *dark-field microscopic examination,* a direct visualization of the live syphilis organisms in penile and perineal chancre preparations. None of the above tests for syphilis is 100% perfect—each has a certain number of false positives, especially in patients with autoimmune disease. Therefore, the diagnosis should be confirmed with the "gold standard," the *treponemal inhibition test.*

Gram stain: a general stain used on microscopic slide specimens to aid in seeing various organisms and estimating their numbers. Depending on their color after the processing, they will be described as gram positive or gram negative. This aids in the initial selection of antibiotics that are likely to be useful. Also, white blood cells should be noted in sputum and wound specimens to indicate whether one is dealing with colonization (if white cells are not present) or actual infection (if they are).

OTHER SPECIAL STUDIES

cerebrospinal fluid (CSF):   a study that includes the following:
  protein: normally 45 mg/dl.
  glucose: normally two-thirds that of the serum glucose; decreased in bacterial infections.
  white blood cells: normally 0 to 3/mm^3; when an increased number of cells are present, they are divided into polys and lymphs.
  culture: some fluid is placed on a growth medium to see if any organisms are present; occasionally, a slide is made from a smear of the fluid and a Gram stain (q.v.) done directly to determine the presence of bacteria.
  india ink: the fungus *Cryptococcus neoformans* may look like white blood cells under the light microscope. If the CSF is mixed with a drop of india ink, the capsule of the fungus can be seen (it will displace the ink), and a diagnosis of cryptococcal meningitis can be made.

flow cytometry: for evaluation of tumors. A stream of single file tumor cells is passed by the path of a laser that is able to measure the relative amounts of DNA. This may help in the relative grading of the tumor cells. Also, after staining with certain antibodies, which have been linked to fluorescent chemicals, lymphocytes from patients with the acquired immunodeficiency syndrome (AIDS) can be counted by flow cytometry to determine the concentration of helper T-lymphocytes—an indication of response to therapy.

PPD (purified protein derivative): an intradermal injection of various strengths (most commonly intermediate) of inactive tubercular material is made; the reactions may be read as positive or negative 48 to 72 hours later. However, the size of the induration (firmness to touch), according to which a positive or negative result is determined, may be recorded in millimeters.

synovial fluid evaluation: evaluation of synovial fluid for the type and quantity of cells in the fluid. The normal white count of synovial fluid is considered to be 200 cells/microliter (μl) as the upper limit of normal. The leukocyte count is performed in a standard hemocytometer. In septic arthritis, the leukocyte count is almost always greater than 50,000 cells/μl. Occasionally, however, a patient with gout, pseudogout, or rheumatoid arthritis may have counts in this range. Noninflammatory synovial findings reveal a white count of up to 5,000 with less than 30% polymorphonuclear leukocytes. In inflammatory synovitis, a 2,000 to 200,000 white count can be anticipated with greater than 50% polys. In infectious or septic arthritis, greater than 90% polymorphonuclear leukocytes can be expected. In crystal-induced arthritis, the synovial cell count can be 500 to 200,000 with less than 90% polymorphonuclear leukocytes. In hemorrhagic arthritis, 50 to 10,000 white cells may be present, but fewer than 50% are polymorphonuclear leukocytes.

Gram stains are routinely performed for the detection of infectious arthritis, and, under certain circumstances, bacterial, fungal, and mycobacterial cultures are done. Viscosity may be useful; inflammation is associated with decreased viscosity. If crystals are seen, **polarized light microscopy** may be used to distinguish the two types of crystal-induced arthritis, gout and pseudogout, allowing the distinction between uric acid crystals seen in gout and calcium pyrophosphate crystals in pseudogout.

tine test: a skin test for tuberculosis. Four small pinpricks are made in the skin; 48 to 72 hours later the reaction is observed; usually reported as positive or negative.

BLOOD BANK PROCEDURES AND PRODUCTS*

Procedures

type and cross-match (T&C): red blood cell products are tested for the antigenic components on the surface of the red cells and antibody components in the serum; the most common are the ABO groups and the Rh type. There is subgrouping for the Rh factors and for many other antigenic components. For this reason each unit of red blood cells to be given to a patient must be cross-matched with the recipient's serum. Only cells in which the recipient's serum does not agglutinate or hemolyze the donor red cells can be transfused. A report is normally not given unless the request for specific blood group and type is made.

T&S (type and screen): the potential blood recipient is tested for most of the various antigenic components and antibodies likely to lead to hemolytic transfusion reaction. If the need arises for actual transfusion, cross-match is then performed, or under emergency circumstances, the blood can be released without cross-match.

direct blood: blood collected from family members and friends who meet all blood donation criteria and are serologically compatible with the intended recipient.

direct Coombs test (direct anti–human globulin test [DAT]): performed on patient's red blood cells to detect the presence of antibodies or complement components attached to the red cells. The red cells with attached antibodies or complement components usually have a shortened life.

*Prepared in part by Patrick Monaghan, PhD former Director, Blood Bank, National Naval Medical Center, Bethesda, Md.

indirect Coombs test (indirect anti–human globulin test):   performed on patient's serum to detect abnormal circulating antibodies. Presence of these atypical antibodies may cause a transfusion reaction. If present in women of childbearing age, these antibodies may cause hemolytic disease of the newborn (erythroblastosis fetalis).

isoantibodies: circulating, naturally occurring antibodies, which are usually of the IgM classification of immunoglobulins. Group O individuals usually have isoantibodies A and B in their plasma, group AB usually have neither, group A usually have anti-B, and group B usually have anti-A.

alloantibodies: circulating atypical antibodies that are the result of prior antigenic stimulation from previous transfusion of blood products, pregnancy, or some other event. The presence of these antibodies may cause a delay in locating compatible blood products.

autologous blood: the patient's own blood that has been collected for elective surgery. It can be stored in the liquid state at 39.2° F (4° C) for 21 to 35 days, or the red cell concentrate may be frozen at −112° F (−80° C) for 10 years. Since it is the patient's own blood, it is generally considered the safest blood to transfuse.

MSBOS (maximum surgical blood order schedule):   a number of hospitals are establishing limits on the quantity of blood that is usually cross-matched or typed and held for various elective surgical procedures. These limits are based on the actual quantities of blood transfused per procedure.

HB$_S$Ag: test performed on donor blood to detect the hepatitis B surface antigen. This is also necessary in preventing transmission of hepatitis to a blood recipient. Its presence is detectable in certain patients who currently have, or have previously had, clinical or subclinical hepatitis B. This test may be negative in patients with hepatitis A, hepatitis C, or hepatitis E.

anti-HBC: test performed on donor blood to detect the presence of the antibody to hepatitis C antigen. This is also necessary in preventing transmission of hepatitis to a blood recipient. Its presence is detectable in certain patients who currently have, or have previously had, clinical or subclinical hepatitis C. This test may be negative in patients with hepatitis A, hepatitis B, or hepatitis E.

anti–human immunodeficiency virus antibodies (anti-HIV):   test for antibodies to the viruses causing autoimmune deficiency syndrome (AIDS)—human immunodeficiency virus 1 and 2 (HIV-1 and HIV-2). It is performed routinely on every donated unit of blood to prevent the transmission of this disease to blood recipients. In patients, it is used to detect those who are suspected of having AIDS, although a positive test (i.e., having the antibody) is not necessarily the same as having AIDS. The screening methodology for this antibody can give falsely positive results, so each positive must be confirmed by the *Western blot* technique.

human immunodeficiency virus–1 antigen (HIV-1 antigen):   test for the actual HIV-1 virus itself. This test measures a specific molecular portion (antigen) of the virus and is used in addition to anti–HIV-1 for screening blood and blood products. Reported as positive or negative.

human immunodeficiency virus, viral load test (HIV, viral load):   quantitative test for determining the actual number of HIV particles within a patient's blood. The test utilizes polymerase chain reactive methodology to detect and measure levels of HIV RNA. The test is used to determine when to initiate drug therapy and to monitor response to therapy.

intraoperative autologous transfusion (IAT):   the intraoperative recovery of red cells for reinfusion during the course of surgery. The efficiency of this system has been improved with a *hemodilution* technique.

factor VIII and factor IX: blood coagulation factors that may be absent or substantially reduced in hemophilia A (factor VIII) or hemophilia B (factor IX). These factors and certain specially prepared blood products are available for replacement in acquired disorders of the labile coagulant system.

Blood Bank Products

red cells: the main blood component remaining after plasma and platelets have been removed from whole blood. It has the identical red cell mass as whole blood and therefore provides the same oxygen-carrying capacity in a smaller volume. The removal of plasma also reduces the risk of transfusion reaction caused by donor isoantibodies and alloantibodies. Red cell products may be stored at 39.2° F (4° C) in the blood bank as packed red blood cells. Recent technologic advances also make it possible to store this product in a frozen state at −112° F (−80° C) for 3 years. Patients who have a history of febrile reaction to bank-stored packed red cells should receive washed and thawed frozen red cell concentrates.

fresh frozen plasma (FFP):   approximately 220 to 250 ml of fresh human plasma, which contains all of the known coagulation proteins. All these coagulation proteins are maintained at 80% to 100% levels for 1 year when the plasma is frozen; used for the replacement of coagulation proteins.

platelet concentrate: contains approximately 5.5×10^{10} platelets in 30 to 50 ml of volume. One unit of platelet concentrate is that quantity fractionated from one unit (450 ml) of whole blood. The shelf-life of a unit of platelet concentrate is 5 days if the platelets are rotated and kept at room temperature. Platelet concentrates are ordinarily transfused into patients with low platelet counts who are actively bleeding.

cryoprecipitate: a blood plasma product that contains clotting factor I (fibrinogen), factor VIII (antihemophiliac factor in 10 to 25 ml of volume), and factor XIII. It is stored in a frozen state at −0.4° F (−18° C) or lower for up to 1 year; used in the treatment of classic hemophilia, von Willebrand disease, and fibrinogen replacement. Each unit (bag) of cryoprecipitate contains approximately 80 to 110 units of clotting factor VIII.

immune serum globulins: various immunoglobulins produced from sensitized individuals whose serum contains these antibodies; used for disease prophylaxis or attenuation, for example, $Rh_o(D)$. Immune globulin is given to $RH_o(D)$-negative women to prevent the sensitization to the Rh antigen and the resulting potential for Rh hemolytic disease of the newborn.

LABORATORY ABBREVIATIONS

Blood Components and Clotting

CBC: complete blood count.

Hct: hematocrit.

Hgb, Hb: hemoglobin.

H & H: hemoglobin and hematocrit.

WBC: white blood cell count.

wbc: white blood cell.

diff: differential white blood cell count.

   polys: polymorphonuclear leukocytes.
      segs: segmented neutrophils.
      nonsegs: bands, stabs, metamyelocytes, myelocytes, promyelocytes, myeloblasts.

   lymphs: lymphocytes.

   monos: monocytes.

   basos: basophils, basophilic granulocytes.

   eos: eosinophils, eosinophilic granulocytes.

   blasts: extremely immature blood cells.

RBC: red blood cell count.

rbc: red blood cell.

MCV: mean corpuscular volume.

MCH: mean corpuscular hemoglobin.

MCHC: mean corpuscular hemoglobin concentration.

Plt: platelet (thrombocyte).

T & C: type and crossmatch.

T & S: type and screen.

Rh: rhesus factor (Rh_o[D]).

ABO: blood group system comprising A, B, AB, and O blood.

FFP: fresh frozen plasma.

IAT: intraoperative autologous transfusion.

MSBOS: maximum surgical blood order schedule.

ESR: erythrocyte sedimentation rate.

LE prep: lupus erythematosus preparation.

PTT: partial thromboplastin time; (activated) **APTT.**

PT: prothrombin time.

Serum Chemistries

BAP, BSAP: bone specific alkaline phosphatase.

OC, BGP: osteocalcin or bone Gla protein.

PTH: parathyroid hormone.

TRAP: tartrate-resistant acid phosphatase.

1,25(OH)2D: calcitriol.

25(OH)D: calcidiol.

Na: sodium.

Cl: chloride.

K: potassium.

HCO_3: bicarbonate.

BUN: blood urea nitrogen.

FBS: fasting blood sugar.

GTT: glucose tolerance test.

Ca: calcium.

PO_4: phosphorus, phosphate.

Chol: cholesterol.

HDL: high-density lipoprotein.

LDL: low-density lipoprotein.

VLDL: very low-density lipoprotein.

UA: urinalysis, uric acid.

Cr: creatinine.

Alb: albumin.

AcP: acid phosphatase.

PSA: prostate-specific antigen.

PAP: prostatic acid phosphatase.

ALP: alkaline phosphatase.

Alk Ø: alkaline phosphatase.

GGTP: gamma-glutamyltranspeptidase.

AST: aspartate aminotransferase (SGOT).

ALT: alanine aminotransferase (SGPT).

SGOT: serum glutamic oxaloacetic transaminase (obs.).

SGPT: serum glutamic pyruvic transaminase (obs.).

LDH: lactate dehydrogenase.

Bili: bilirubin.

CPK: creatine phosphokinase (same as CK).

CK: creatine kinase.

SPE, SPEP: serum protein electrophoresis.

Ig: immunoglobulin. There are five classes: IgA, IgD, IgE, IgG, and IgM.

Serology

DAT: direct anti–human globulin test.

HIV: human immunodeficiency virus.

RF: rheumatoid factor assay.

ASO: anti–streptolysin O titer.

ANA: anti–nuclear antibody.

anti-DNA: anti–double-stranded (native) DNA antibody.

FTA (ABS): fluorescent treponemal antibody (absorbed).

VDRL: Venereal Disease Research Laboratory.

STS: serologic test for syphilis.

HbC: hepatitis C antigen.

HB_sAg: hepatitis B surface antigen.

HB_eAg: hepatitis B e antigen.

HB_sAb: hepatitis B surface antibody.

HB_cAb: hepatitis B core antibody.

HB$_e$Ab: hepatitis B e antibody.

HIV-1:   anti–human immunodeficiency virus 1 antibody.

HIV-2:   anti–human immunodeficiency virus 2 antibody.

ELISA: enzyme-linked immunosorbent assay.

EMIT: enzyme-multiplied immunoassay technique.

Urine

c-PCP, PICP: carboxyterminal propeptide.

C-Tx: cross-links: C-telopeptide.

DPYD, Dpd: deoxypyridinoline.

HYP: hydroxyproline.

NTx: N-telopeptide.

PYD: pyridin*oline* collagen cross-links.

PYD: pyridin*ium* collagen cross-links

UA: urinalysis.

R & M: routine and microscopic examinations.

Ccr: creatinine clearance.

pH: concentration of hydrogen ions; acidity.

Glu: glucose.

Ace: acetone.

KB: ketone bodies.

Prot: protein.

BHB: beta-hydroxybutyrate.

s.g.:   specific gravity.

spec grav: specific gravity.

spgr: specific gravity.

HPF: high-power field.

LPF: low-power field.

Other

PPD: purified protein derivative (tuberculosis skin test).

C & S: culture and sensitivity.

CC: colony count.

T$_3$:   L-triiodothyronine.

T$_4$:   L-tetraiodothyronine (thyroxine).

TSH: thyroid-stimulating hormone (also called thyrotropin).

EKG: electrocardiogram.

ECG: electrocardiogram.

AFB: acid-fast bacteria.

spec: specimen.

CSF: cerebrospinal fluid.

ANNOTATION OF UNITS

Weight

pg: picogram = 1/1,000,000,000,000 gram.

ng: nanogram = 1/1,000,000,000 gram.

μg: microgram = 1/1,000,000 gram.

mg: milligram = 1/1,000 gram.

g: gram (454 gram = 1 pound).

kg: kilogram = 1,000 gram = 2.2 pounds

Volume

fl: femtoliter = 1/1,000,000,000,000,000 liter.

μl: microliter = 1/1,000,000 liter.

ml: milliliter = 1/1,000 liter.

dl: deciliter = 1/10 liter.

L: liter = 0.943 quarts (1 quart = 1.06 liter).

Length

μm: micrometer = 1/1,000,000 meter.

μ: micron = micrometer (obs.).

mm: millimeter = 1/1,000 meter.

cm: centimeter = 1/100 meter (= 0.39 inch; 2.54 cm = 1 inch).

m: meter (= 39.37 inch).

Other

mEq: milliequivalent; 1/1,000 equivalent weight.

Eq: equivalent; 6.023×10^{23} ionic charges.

In an attempt to standardize the way medical (and other scientific) units are reported, Le Système Internationale d'Unités was developed. Among others, it makes the following specifications:

1. Omit periods in abbreviations (kg, mm, ml, mg).
2. Omit plurals (70 kg, not 70 kgs).
3. Avoid commas as a spacer in expressing large numbers. (In some countries, the comma is used as a decimal point.)
4. Compound prefixes should not be used (10^{-9} meter = nanometer, not millimicrometer ($m\mu m$)).
5. Omit the degree sign for the Kelvin temperature scale (310 K, not 310° K).
6. Multiples and submultiples are used in steps of 10^3 or 10^{-3} as follows:

Multiplier	Prefix	Abbreviation
10^3	kilo-	k
10^6	mega-	M
10^9	giga-	G
10^{12}	tera-	T
10^{-1}	deci-	d
10^{-2}	centi-	c
10^{-3}	milli-	m
10^{-6}	micro-	μ
10^{-9}	nano-	n
10^{-12}	pico-	p
10^{-15}	femto-	f
10^{-18}	atto-	a

7. Only one solidus (/) may be used when indicated "per" or a denominator: acceleration = velocity per second = m/s^2, not m/s/s.

8. When the compound unit is derived from the multiplication of two base units, a point ($\cdot$) is used to so indicate. A unit of torque is the Newton-meter, written N·m not Nm.
9. Preferred spellings are meter not metre, liter not litre, kilogram not kilogramme.

Routine Physiologic Parameters

vital signs: the easily measurable sustaining functions include temperature, pulse, respiration (rate), and blood pressure. These vital signs have been and will continue to be the major index of a patient's general progress.

height and weight: taken into consideration in an orthopaedic work-up because many back problems are related to being overweight and the stress that is placed on the vertebrae.

ECG (electrocardiogram): recorded measurement of the spontaneous electrical activity of the heart, using multiple leads to assess the heart from a variety of directions. This study is commonly obtained before surgery to give a baseline in the event of operative or postoperative cardiac complications, such as pulmonary embolus or cardiac arrest.

EEG (electroencephalogram): recorded measurement of the spontaneous electrical activity of the brain, using multiple leads placed on the head and ears. This study is obtained to detect certain seizures and brain disorders and the lack of activity when there has been severe damage leading to brain death.

Chapter 6

Casts, Splints, Dressings, and Traction

This chapter defines the materials applied and prescribed by an orthopaedist or assigned individual in the direct care of patients with fractures, dislocations, and other injuries and conditions of the musculoskeletal system. The types of cast immobilization materials are described, as are the traction devices and weights designed for hospital or home care. Some emergency stabilization devices are included at the end of the chapter.

The techniques of cast immobilization, splints, dressings, and traction devices are designed to provide an external means of support or protective covering while healing proceeds under optimal conditions. Casts are generally applied in fracture reduction and immobilization, but they are also helpful in the correction of pediatric deformities, dysplastic hip disease, scoliosis, and foot deformities such as club foot, with the goal being to maintain or obtain a correction of deformity, promote alignment following surgery, and to give support to damaged soft tissues in the healing process of fractures, dislocations, and sprains.

Because the care of the orthopaedic patient is a team approach, orthopaedists in private or group practice and in hospital settings are assisted by qualified orthopaedic nurses and technologists who are also involved in patient care. The orthopaedic nurse may choose to work in a doctor's office, outpatient clinic of a hospital, or become directly involved with inpatient management by assuming diverse responsibilities for a plan of quality care from admission to discharge. This requires not only the specialized knowledge of orthopaedic nursing but also skills in the use of traction equipment and appliances, and the ability to manage patients with this armamentarium.

Depending on educational background, training, and hospital policies, qualified nurses and technologists "scrub in" on orthopaedic surgical procedures in the operating room, clinic, or physician's office.

The National Association of Orthopaedic Nurses (NAON), founded in 1980, is the professional organization that offers a certification program to orthopaedic nurses who wish to further develop their skills in the management and care of orthopaedic patients. The NAON provides support and educational opportunities through its sponsored activities to promote continued professional development.

The National Board for Certification of Orthopaedic Technologists (NBCOT), founded in 1982, is the professional organization of orthopaedic technologists that offers a certifying examination and an ongoing program of education and training to promote skills in the practice of orthopaedic technology and to encourage professional growth in this field.

Under the supervision of the nursing staff, the technologist assists in setting up traction appliances, circ-O-lectric beds, and similar devices of care and has the shared responsibility of proper application of traction, weights, and equipment required for patient rehabilitation. Administrative tasks involve ordering supplies and equipment for the plaster rooms, examining rooms, wings, and clinics, and conferring with medical suppliers on catalog items and supplies.

The orthopaedic technologist, with training and

practice, becomes skilled in the art and science of cast application and knowledgeable about the many types needed for specific injuries and conditions. After cast application, and under a physician's directions, technologists instruct patients on care of the cast and prevention of complications. In addition, they may assist the patients in gait training (crutch-walking, ascending and descending stairs) and various home exercises after immobilization. Technologists also maintain and prepare the plaster room for specific procedures, as well as assume the clean-up duties that follow. In some orthopaedic offices, the technologist is skilled in basic orthopaedic radiographic techniques—skills that clearly enhance the team approach.

The orthopaedic specialty is so diversified that opportunities for continuing medical education for nurses and technologists are offered through the AAOS instructional courses across the country and within the specialty organizations of orthopaedics. Corporate-sponsored activities have also been instrumental in updating product designs and state-of-the-art equipment. Together, these groups seek to promote the highest standards of quality care in cooperation with orthopaedic surgeons and other members of the health care team.

The basic tools of the trade are as follows.

A **cast** is a circumferentially wrapped plaster of Paris–impregnated bandage or encasement applied to a portion of the body. Additional materials, such as fiberglass and plastics are also used instead of plaster of Paris.

A **splint** is a rigid or semirigid, noncircumferential material used to reinforce a soft dressing or to provide additional support for or immobilization of the body part being treated. The splint may be made of plaster of Paris, metal, wood, plastic, or, in an emergency, newspapers or magazines.

A **dressing** involves those materials used to cover a wound or surgical incision, a fabric with or without accessory medications or self-adhesive properties.

A **bandage** is a nonrigid, usually cotton material that holds a dressing in place or acts as the dressing by itself. It may be applied to provide padding over a body prominence under a cast. An elastic bandage provides support for a joint or soft tissue in controlling circulation.

Traction devices are any adjustable external appliances used in early treatment of fractures that suspend or deliver pull to any given part of the body.

Casting materials have improved considerably over the years; however, plaster of Paris casts are still widely used and familiar to all practitioners. These rolled crinoline bandages are impregnated with gypsum powder (calcium salt) that, when exposed to water, crystallizes. The reaction then slows to a maturation process (hardening) that takes approximately 24 hours to dry. The heat felt by the patient is the crystallization process that takes place within the cast material. To fabricate and mold plaster of Paris bandages is considered an art, and the technician soon learns the numerous techniques of application.

Fiberglass and thermoplast casts have become a popular form of treatment. They are lightweight, radiolucent, easier to apply, can tolerate moisture, and harden within 5 minutes, allowing for immediate weight-bearing. This rolled type consists of fiberglass and resin, fiberglass and plastic polymer, and polyurethane that also crystallize on exposure to water. Most fiberglass casts are long-wearing.

CAST MATERIALS

cast cutter: electrical circular oscillating saw for splitting and/or removing a cast. Long-handled cast-cutting instruments are also designed to remove small plaster casts from children.

cast padding: soft cotton wrap or synthetic wrap-around material used with a plaster or fiberglass cast.

cotton roll: material made from cotton that can be rolled as a bandage and acts as a buffer between the skin and plaster material; **Webril.**

felt padding: thick felt or feltlike material added to the undersurface of a cast to relieve pressure on local areas of bony prominences or pressure areas.

fiberglass cast: lightweight fiberglass wrap material that is impregnated with resin or another substance that polymerizes when exposed to water.

moleskin: adhesive, thin, velvet-like material used to smooth edges of casts or to buffer areas of excessive skin wear.

plaster rolls: gauze roll impregnated with plaster of Paris, which, when dipped in warm water, can be applied, rolled smoothly, and molded, becoming hard within minutes.

sheet wadding: strong, cotton material that clings to part being applied and molded to contour of that part.

stockinette: cloth stocking roll used initially in cast applications; comes in many sizes; can be covered by padding followed by firm cast material.

CAST IMMOBILIZATION

Cast immobilization involves the following anatomic areas: upper and lower limbs, cervical to chest region, and chest to lower spine. Spica casts incorporate a portion of the limb and trunk around the hip or shoulder. The various types are described below.

Body Casts

A body cast is a circumferential cast enclosing the trunk of the body and may extend from the head or upper chest to the groin or thigh. This type of cast immobilization is used in treating disorders of the cervical, thoracic, and lumbar spines such as fractures and scoliosis, or it may be applied following some types of surgery on the spine. There are several types of body casts.

flexion body c.:   chest-groin cast in which the patient is positioned so that the trunk is flexed forward; for treatment of painful lower back conditions.

extension body c.:   chest-groin cast in which the patient is positioned so that the trunk is extended backward; applied for specific fractures.

scoliosis c.:   special modification of the body cast for preoperative and postoperative treatment of scoliosis (curvature of the spine). These casts have in large part been replaced by operative fixation and prefabricated braces. Modifications of this type are:

> *Cotrel c.:*   modified scoliosis cast applied following Cotrel traction.
>
> *turnbuckle c.:*   special modification to allow changes in angle by use of turnbuckles on either side of the cast.
>
> *Risser localizer:*   specialized body cast with localizer pressing over convex side of curve.

halo c.:   for cervical fractures; a thoracic to pelvic level cast incorporating the necessary extensions used to support the posts that are attached to a metal halo skeletally affixed to the head.

Minerva jacket: cast immobilization extending along the side and in back of the head and neck, chest to hip area, incorporating a plaster of Paris headband; for fractures of the neck and in certain scoliosis problems.

Spica Casts

A spica cast immobilizes an appendage by incorporating a part of the body proximal to that appendage. The most common spica casts are hip, thumb, and shoulder spicas. They are listed by anatomic region in the following sections.

Limb Casts

Upper Limb Casts

arm cylinder c.:   long-arm cast with the elbow flexed and the wrist free.

Dehne c. (three-finger spica):   cast incorporating the thumb with a separate extension incorporating the index and middle fingers; for fractures of the navicular.

gauntlet c.: short cast extending from slightly above or proximal to the wrist to some point in the palm; usually has some outrigger to control one or more digits; for metacarpal and phalangeal fractures or dislocations.

hanging arm c.: long-arm cast that, through suspension from a sling around the neck, brings about traction of fracture fragments of the distal humerus.

long-arm c. (LAC): extends from the palm and wrist to the axilla, preventing movement at the elbow; for treatment of fractures of the forearm, elbow, and humerus.

   cotton-loader position c.: rarely used long-arm cast applied with the wrist in full pronation, flexion, and ulnar deviation; for distal radial fractures.

Munster c.: cast that comes above condyles to prevent pronation and supination, but allows some flexion/extension of the elbow; **supracondylar c.**

short-arm c. (SAC): any of a number of casts extending from the elbow to the palm or digits; commonly used for distal forearm and wrist fractures.

shoulder spica (airplane c.): cast that incorporates the upper torso and envelops a part or all of the limb in a position of abduction; for proximal humeral fractures and rotator cuff tears.

thumb spica: short- or long-arm cast that incorporates the thumb; for treatment of navicular fractures.

Lower Limb Casts

cast boot: any of a variety of commercially available strap-on boots that can often serve the function of a short-leg cast. These devices may include movable ankles, inserted for the ankle and feet, and moving ankle joints; **tibial gaiter.**

cylinder c.: cast from proximal thigh to just above the ankle; for injuries of the knee.

Delbert c.: a short-leg cast that is trimmed away from the anterior and posterior portions of the ankle and from the heel. This allows dorsiflexion and plantar flexion while maintaining lateral stability.

gel c.: semirigid paste cast, usually applied to the lower leg and foot for ankle injuries or swelling; **Unna boot.**

hip spica: cast incorporating the lower torso and extending to one or both lower limbs.

   single hip spica: cast incorporating the lower torso and entire position of only one leg; for femoral fractures.

   1½ hip spica: cast that incorporates the lower torso, the entire affected limb, and the opposite limb to just above the knee; for proximal femoral fractures and some pelvic fractures.

   double hip spica: cast incorporating both the lower torso and lower limbs, usually because of bilateral fractures of the hips, femur, and/or tibia.

   Batchelor plaster: hip spica cast that holds the hip in internal rotation but allows motion in other planes; for dysplastic hip in an infant.

   Petrie spica c. (broom-stick): specially applied cast for abduction to assist in ambulation for Legg-Perthes disease.

long-leg c. (LLC): non–weight-bearing cast extending from the upper thigh to the toes; for fractures of the tibia and fibula or ligamentous injuries of the knee.

   long-leg walking c. (LLWC): a cast from the upper thigh to the toes, with an attached rubber sole device called a walker.

Quengle c.: for flexion contracture of the knee, a two-part cast hinged at the knee level, with the lower end of the cast ending at the ankle or foot, and the above-knee portion ending at the upper thigh.

short-leg c. (SLC): non–weight-bearing cast extending from just below the knee to the toes; for injuries of the lower limb, ankle, and foot.

short-leg walking c. (SLWC): with an attached rubber walker or reinforced to accept a cast shoe; for ankle and foot injuries.

patellar tendon weight-bearing cast (PTB): also known as a **Sarmiento cast;** a short-leg cast with a walker; a special feature is the molding about the knee; for management of tibial fractures.

slipper c.: incorporating the foot up to the ankle; a rigid postoperative dressing following forefoot procedures.

toe spica: cast specifically designed to incorporate all of the great toe and a portion or all of the foot; usually after bunion surgery.

well-leg c.: casts applied to both lower limbs and then attached together; used in some rare instances for treatment of femoral fractures.

Other Cast Terms

bivalve c.: cast that is split in half (shelled) by cuts made on opposite sides of the cast to release pressure or allow removal and reapplication of the cast such as would be needed for physical therapy treatments.

Boston bivalve: cast split in half with a step cut rather than a straight line; most often done when the cast is going to be removed, often for physical therapy, and then re-applied.

univalve c.: cast split on one side to relieve pressure.

cast boot: any of a variety of commercially available strap-on boots that can often serve the function of short leg casts. These devices may include movable ankles, inserted for the ankle and feet, and moving ankle joints; **tibial gaiter, cast shoe, cast boot.**

collar and cuff: design or sling with a soft portion wrapped around the neck and a cufflike device wrapped around to support the distal forearm; for humeral fractures treated with a coaptation splint.

corrective c.: made to correct a deformity by non-surgical technique; commonly applied to club feet.

fenestrate: to cut an opening (window) in a dressing or cast to allow inspection of a part.

petaling edges: to eliminate abrasion from the edge of a cast, small vertical slits are made at the edges of the cast, and then the edges (petals) are folded out and held in place by adhesive tape, moleskin, or other material.

serial c.: any sequence of casts applied in the progressive correction of deformity.

wedge: circumferential cutting of the cast and re-application of plaster over the same cast after a manipulation has been performed to change bone position.

closing wedge: removal of a segment of plaster, with closing of that wedge by manipulation and reapplication of plaster.

opening wedge: circular cut cast that is opened by manipulation and then covered with a new layer of plaster.

window: removal of a piece of cast, usually square or rectangular, to allow inspection of a wound or relieve pressure at a specific point. Also said to "fenestrate."

DEVICES APPLIED TO CASTS

abduction bar: to help maintain hip abduction, any bar placed between two long-leg casts.

cast brace: modifications of standard casts often applied to facilitate early motion. The cast brace is designed with normal physiology in mind while still protecting the fracture site; it is molded in the manner of prosthetic-type devices. In addition, it is usually hinged at the joints to allow free motion of joints and to improve muscle recovery.

cast protectors: waterproof covers for a limb cast, allowing patient to shower or bathe.

walker (walking heel): hard rubber wedge directly incorporated into the sole of a cast to allow walking or resting the leg.

CAST COMPLICATIONS

Generally, a neurovascular and neuromuscular examination is made before, during, and after cast immobilization. However, even with close attention to treatment, the following complications can occur.

burns: applying cast material with water temperature too warm, which, when added to the crystallization process that produces heat, can produce skin burns.

constrictive edema: disruption of normal venous drainage with resulting fluid accumulation in soft tissue and swelling distal to the point of constriction caused by circulatory impairment. Severe swelling may lead to neurovascular involvement to include compartment syndrome.

decubitus ulcer: an area of breakdown of skin and/or subcutaneous tissue as a result of unrelieved pressure on a bony prominence or portion of the body resting on a firm surface for a long time. The lesions are staged as follows:

Stage I: only the dermis is involved.

Stage II: dermis and subcutaneous fat are involved.

Stage III: ulcer involves some deep fascia or muscle; bone not uncovered.

Stage IV: bone is exposed.

dropfoot: when referring to a complication of cast treatment, applies to paralysis of the peroneal nerve resulting from pressure over the fibular head with inability to dorsiflex the ankle.

muscle atrophy: loss of muscle tissue due to protracted disuse secondary to joint immobilization.

pin tract infection: direct bacterial contamination of area where pins have been used for external traction or skeletal fixation; could potentially lead to osteomyelitis.

pressure sore: breakdown of skin and/or subcutaneous tissue because of direct pressure of displaced or bunched cotton padding under cast, creating pressure lasting usually in excess of 4 hours; often caused by patient inserting object in cast to reach an area that is itching from plaster dust in cast; **decubitus ulcer.**

superior mesenteric artery syndrome: disruption of circulation to the bowel, occurs after application of body cast, results in abdominal pain, diarrhea, and, if unrecognized, severe problems; **cast syndrome.**

SPLINTS AND ACCESSORIES

This section is restricted to those splints applied in the early treatment of injury or management of postoperative conditions and their accessories.

Splints

airplane s.: removable cast or metal device used to hold the arm in abduction.

aluminum foam s.: straight, metallic foam, padded splint of various widths from ½ to 2 inches; can be used separately or in association with casts and are for hand and finger injuries.

baseball s.: prefabricated metallic splint applied to the volar forearm and hand; the palm portion of the splint positions the hand as if it were holding a baseball.

Bohler s.: for spiral phalangeal fractures of the fingers; a device designed to maintain proper position and continuous traction.

coaptation s.: two slabs of plaster that are placed on either side of the limb and held together by some outer dressing; for limb injuries.

dynamic s.: any splint device that incorporates springs, elastic bands, and other materials that produce a constant active force to help reduce a deformity or counteract deforming forces.

frog s.: aluminum foam splint for finger injuries; before application the splint has a frog-shaped appearance.

gutter s.: semicircular or U-shaped splint fashioned around the injured part, usually in metacarpal and phalangeal fractures of the ulnar side of the hand.

hairpin s.: spring-assisted splint to help gain extension in a finger injury affecting the joint.

half shell: usually refers to spica casts; the section of cast that remains after it has been bivalved and a portion removed.

long-arm s.: splint applied from the axilla to wrist or distal palm posteriorly; holds the elbow and wrist in any given position.

long-leg s.: splint extending from the thigh to the lower calf or distally to the toes.

night s.: any splint or similar device used only at night. Commonly refers to a volar splint for treatment of carpal tunnel syndrome.

pneumatic compression boot or sleeve: provides periodic compression to a limb to help prevent venous thrombosis and is often used on an uninjured limb. This is in contrast to the sequential type of pump used in lymphedema. The pneumatic sequential compression boot is another type used after knee replacement and is effective against deep vein thrombosis after lower limb surgery.

short-arm s.: splint extending from distal elbow to palm; used for advanced fracture healing or nondisplaced fractures.

short-leg s.: splint extending from the upper calf to toes for prevention of **dropfoot.**

sugar tong s.: long slab of plaster applied to the affected limb in the fashion of a sugar tong and held together with outer dressing; for injuries to the shoulder, arm, and forearm; **sugar tong cast.**

Velcro s.: commercial name becoming generic referring to splints that have two straps or surfaces that adhere to each other; these surfaces may be approximated and separated as many times as needed, and there is no loss of the original

strength of the adhesion of the two surfaces; can be used for any part of the body.

volar s.: specifies a splint applied to the anterior forearm.

universal gutter s.: wire mesh splint for lower extremity fractures.

wraparound s.: various commercially available splints that can be wrapped around a limb but are easily removable for physical therapy or wound care.

Accessories

In the area of casts, splints, and dressings, the following important aids to patient management are provided.

canes: for a painful hip; the patient is instructed to hold cane in hand opposite affected hip to transmit load through cane at the same moment that weight bearing takes place on affected extremity.

crutches: where a three-point gait is needed to relieve weight bearing on affected side, used in fractures, sprains, and after surgery. A three-point gait is where both crutches are placed on the ground simultaneously with the affected limb, decreasing body weight from three to one.

spring-loaded crutches: new type of crutch-assist that absorbs peak stress, reduces shock, and reduces fatigue in upper limbs. The down-directed weight is borne by the crutches that have energy-storing ability on weight bearing.

walkers: assistive lightweight metallic devices (usually four legged) that allow patient to apply weight bearing bilaterally when there is instability in walking. New variations in these devices include the option for a pair or quartet of wheels, hand brakes, and baskets for carrying items.

DRESSINGS

The term *dressing* may apply to any material used to cover a wound; however, when there is considerable swelling without a wound, a dressing is used to apply pressure.

General Types of Dressings

Adaptic d.:   nonadhesive mesh dressing for the direct covering of wounds.

Betadine d.:   any dressing that has been impregnated with povidone-iodine (Betadine) and then applied directly to the wound.

compression d.:   any dressing intended to apply pressure to reduce or prevent swelling or bleeding.

dry d.:   dressing that has not been impregnated with any solution.

figure eight d.:   dressing applied in the shape of an 8, as is often done for clavicular fractures; commercially prefabricated dressings, referred to as **clavicle straps,** are available.

gauze d.:   any dressing made of cheesecloth-type material, for example, Kling, Kerlix, 4 × 4.

iodoform d.:   narrow gauze strip impregnated with an iodine compound; for the treatment of open wounds.

Kerlix d.:   broad elastic gauze dressing often a part of a compression dressing.

Kling d.:   narrow gauze elastic bandage for compression.

Koch-Mason d.:   warm occlusive saline dressing placed over a limb with cellulitis.

occlusive d.:   any dressing that protects a wound from outside contamination.

packing: describes that portion of a dressing that is placed inside an open wound.

pressure d.:   dressing designed to apply pressure to a specific location.

protective d.:   any dressing that protects a wound from trauma.

saline d.:   any dressing impregnated with normal saline; for treatment of open wounds.

telfa d.:   sterile nonadherent dressing, often applied on fresh wounds or incisions.

wet-to-dry d.:   dressing that is impregnated with normal saline and allowed to dry; used as a part of open wound treatment.

Xeroform d.:   nonadherent mesh dressing applied to fresh wounds or incisions.

Other Dressing Materials

Ace bandage: nonadhesive, elastic material that is a direct compressive wrap or holds other dressings or splints in place. The trade name is now used generically.

adhesive tape: sticky nonpermeable tape used to secure local dressing.

bandage adhesive: sticky material applied to the skin to help in the application of various forms of tape; commonly used adhesive is *tincture of benzoin.*

pads: variety of bulky materials (rectangular or square) that cover large wounds; often referred to as ABD (abdominal) pads.

Specialized Dressings

Esmarch bandage: special rubber, rolled bandages used to expel blood from a limb before surgery; **Martin bandage.**

Gibney bandage: strips of adhesive tape applied in alternate directions about the ankle; for ligamentous and other injuries.

high Dye dressing: method of noncircumferential ankle taping designed to support the ankle after an inversion injury.

Kenny-Howard splint (A/C harness):   for acromioclavicular separations, a sling that supports wrist and elbow with a counterforce strap to push the clavicle down and a chest strap to hold the device in place.

low Dye dressing: taping technique for plantar faciitis.

Robert Jones bandage: layered bulk dressing applied to the lower limbs for a variety of injuries, but specifically following knee surgery or injury; **Shands dressing.**

Shands d.: composed of two layers of cast padding and two layers of elastic bandage applied to the leg and foot; for ankle sprains and nondisplaced fractures of the metatarsals.

universal hand d.: for compression or extensive injuries involving the hand and fingers; a bulky, even-pressured hand dressing composed of cotton or gauze fluffs and wrapped with gauze or other circular dressing material, leaving the fingertips exposed. Over this dressing, a cock-up splint is applied to hold the wrist in 15-degree extension. Some of these dressings are incorporated into a stockinette sling for elevation.

Velpeau d.: bandage applied to the arm and torso such that the elbow is at the side in flexion and the hand is pressed against the upper chest.

SUSPENSION, TRACTION, AND FRAMES

Suspension, traction, and frames are adjustable appliances used with pulleys, bars, weights, and other supports in the treatment of fractures with casts or splints, for scoliosis, and in the care of patients before and after surgery. This method of treatment is offered to ensure proper alignment in healing and to provide suspension or deliver pull, directly or indirectly, to bone, muscle, skin, and fascia.

Many of the parts of various suspensions and traction devices are known by the originator's name. Devices are listed by placement, each with its component. New techniques and methods of traction can be found in suppliers' catalogs, but the user should find this section helpful in deciphering why such devices are used in the care of patients. The various types of traction equipment are defined, followed by some emergency stabilization equipment.

Suspension

Suspension is the means by which a limb or part thereof is held suspended by some external device. Traction often accompanies the suspension.

balanced suspension (Fig. 6–1): suspension device that allows the patient to move the affected limb without changing the fracture position of that limb; preferred for treatment of long-bone injuries. There are two components:

Arizona universal leg support: for lower limb fracture, a balanced suspension device with adjustable anterior thigh pad and suspension support by two parallel lines from the knee and foot.

Thomas splint: originally designed to help splint fresh fractures; composed of a full ring around the thigh and two metal rods that extend down either side of the limb and are joined distally to the foot. The **half-ring Thomas splint** is the most commonly used.

FIG 6–1.
Balanced suspension. (Used with permission of Carol L. Willis.)

Most are adjustable for length and are thus called **adjustable Thomas splints.**

Pearson attachment: attached to a Thomas splint; consists of two metal rods joined distally, allowing flexion of the knee.

overhead suspension: the forearm is suspended overhead with the elbow bent; used in treatment of forearm and elbow fractures.

Traction (Fig. 6–2)

In general, traction is the pull on a limb or a part thereof. Skin traction (indirect traction) is applied by using a bandage to pull on the skin and fascia where light traction is required. Skeletal traction (direct traction), however, uses pins or wires inserted through bone and is attached to weights, pulleys, and ropes. This is applied when a longer period is needed in traction. External fixators are then attached to the traction apparatus to help in the healing process. The following devices are applied:

Barton tongs: skull tongs for cervical skeletal traction.

Böhler-Braun frame: metallic adjustable frame for support of the thigh and leg; for leg elevation and often in severe ankle fractures where os calcis traction is applied.

Bryant t. (Fig. 6–3): for infants only; an overhead suspension of leg and thigh such that the knees are extended and the thighs flexed to 90 degrees.

Buck t.: originally designed as skin traction incorporating the entire lower limb, but now describes skin traction of the leg only; generally used in knee injuries but also a temporary measure applied in hip fractures.

cervical halter t.: a cloth, halterlike sling for traction of the neck; applied when patient is sitting or lying down, continuously or intermittently; head halter traction.

Cotrel t.: combination of a sling cervical and pelvic traction used in scoliosis before surgery or casting to help straighten the back.

Crutchfield tongs: type of cranial skeletal tongs used for traction of the cervical spine.

Dunlop t.: commonly used for elbow fractures; the arm is held suspended by skin or a combination of skin and skeletal traction, with a weight applied to the lower arm.

Gardner-Wells tongs: device for immobilization of cervical spine injuries in which two sharp metal pins are screwed into the superficial layer of the skull. They are then connected to hanging weights or other traction devices for stabilization of the spine. They may also be used for definitive treatment of spine injuries.

halo-femoral t.: bed-type traction using a ring-shaped device directly affixed to the bone of the skull in conjunction with femoral skeletal traction; used in scoliosis or injury distraction.

halo-pelvic t.: ambulatory-type traction for cervical spine injuries that uses a ring-shaped device directly affixed to the bone of the skull in conjunction with pelvic skeletal pins. These are

FIG 6–2.
Traction. (Used with permission of Carol L. Willis.)

Skin traction

Skeletal traction

interconnected to hold the spine rigid when the patient is ambulatory.

Kirschner wire (K-wire):   skeletal t. where small wires are placed across bone(s) so that a traction device can be placed externally; applied to some pediatric and hand fractures.

Lyman-Smith t.:   use of olecranon pin and overhead traction for supracondylar (elbow) fractures.

Neufeld roller t.:   for fractured femur; a cast for the calf and thigh is hinged at the knee and suspended by a line to the anterior midthigh looped around a pulley and to a spring attached to the anterior midleg. The pulley for this loop is then supported by an overhead suspension with weight and a second pulley.

pelvic sling: sling encircling the hip and pelvic region in treatment of pelvic injuries; sling is suspended overhead.

pelvic t.:   cloth, girdle-type device with traction directed at the foot of the bed; for lower back disorders such as herniated disks.

Quigley t.:   for lateral malleolar and trimalleolar fractures; a stockinette is placed around the leg and ankle, with the ankle being suspended by the stockinette attached to an overhead frame.

Russell t.:   skin traction on the lower limb from thigh to ankle or knee to ankle, attached to a sling that suspends the distal thigh. This may be done with a continuous rope and a number of pulleys (simple) or with two different weights for one leg and knee suspension portion (split). Russell trac-

BRYANT'S TRACTION

Thomas splint

PEARSON ATTACHMENT

BUCK'S EXTENSION

SUSPENDED OR
FLOATING TRACTION

FIG 6–3.
Various traction devices. (From the American Orthopaedic Association: *Manual of orthopaedic surgery,* ed 5, Chicago, 1979, the Association.)

tion is often used in the elderly as a temporizing treatment for fractured hips or in the very young in treatment of femoral fractures.

semi-Fowler position: semisitting position with knees flexed; used in lower back and lumbar disk disorders.

skeletal t.:   any traction using a pin through the bone to deliver traction; for the tibia, femur, olecranon, os calcis, and metacarpal.

Steinmann pin: wide-diameter pin for heavy skeletal traction such as in the tibia or femur.

traction bow: U-shaped piece of metal for placement into a K-wire or Steinmann pin in skeletal traction.

Vinke tongs: special set of skeletal traction tongs used for skull traction in neck injuries.

well-leg t.:   bilateral casting of lower limbs with an interconnecting metal bar that allows traction on one leg to be supported by the other; for femoral fractures, it has the advantage that a patient can be moved out of bed.

90-90 t.:   usually skeletal; the patient is placed supine, with hips and knees flexed to 90 degrees such that the calf is suspended; for femoral fractures.

Frames

Frames are specialty units for an entire bed or additions to a bed.

Balkan f.:   upright metal bars based at the corners of a bed and connected by overhead metal bars that hold suspension and traction pulleys.

Bradford f.:   canvas bed suspended from rectangular poles with opening for the buttocks; split Bradford.

claw-type basic f.:   traction frame that is attached to the bed by a clawlike clamp device.

Foster f.:   special bed composed of two stretcher-like parts that, when connected, hold the patient sandwiched firmly between them, allowing the patient to be completely turned without injury to the spine; used for tuberculosis and spinal fractures or for patients with scoliosis following a Harrington instrumentation and fusion. A **Stryker frame** is a similarly constructed device.

Heffington f.:   device that attaches to a standard operating table to allow prone position of a patient for lumbar spine surgery. The table end is dropped 90 degrees with patient's hips flexed over the edge and the patient further flexed to reverse the lumbar lordosis.

IV-type basic f.:   traction frame that is attached to the bed by a device similar to that used for holding intravenous (IV) poles.

Jones abduction f.:   a special frame used on standard beds to assist in gaining hip abduction in tuberculosis, acute arthritis, and other diseases of the hip.

Watson-Jones f.:   for holding tibial fractures in surgery; a semicircular posterior-inferior thigh cuff with an attached adjustable extension that runs posterior to the leg with the knee in 90-degrees flexion. Tibial traction is maintained with a Steinmann pin.

Whitman f.:   specially constructed frame to assist in gaining spine extension; may be used when cast application is necessary.

EMERGENCY STABILIZATION

The use of emergency measures in trauma situations has saved many lives and limbs. There are many new types of equipment made for stabilization of the injured. These "temporary" measures of tamponade, fracture immobilization, and tissue protection are generally performed by trained emergency medical technicians (EMTs) and paramedics acting under the guidance of emergency room physicians. The various types of air splints should be used only by those trained in their use. The following emergency equipment may be used before the patient reaches the hospital.

air pressure splints: double-walled plastic tubes that, in the deflated state, are placed around the injured limb and are then inflated (by mouth) to bring about even pressure and immobilization.

Hare traction: metallic splint with multiple straps and a special distal traction device for use in transporting unstable lower-limb–injured patients.

inflatable splint: sometimes referred to as an **air splint,** it is a first-aid device used at the onset of injury; when blown up, this balloon-like splint provides good immobilization with even pressure. It is usually applied to the lower leg and foot, but other inflatable splints incorporate the entire arm or entire lower limb.

MAST (medical antishock trousers): pneumatic sleeve for immediate stabilization of lower limbs in cases of trauma. MAST encompasses lower limbs and abdomen to provide sufficient pressure to force blood to the central portion of the body. This provides some stabilization of shock and provides stability for pelvic, hip, and femoral fractures and aids in preventing further tissue damage. In addition to tamponading sites of bleeding, this device sometimes acts by increasing pulse and blood pressure. Its use is controversial, and it should be used carefully and briefly (if at all) to avoid prolonged muscle ischemia and MACS (MAST-associated compartment syndrome). MAST is inflated by a foot operated pump.

Neal-Robertson litter: modified spine board for transporting trauma patients with spinal injuries to the emergency room.

posterior splint: for emergency immobilization; rigid devices used for initial stabilization of upper and lower limb fractures.

Sager traction splint: for femoral fractures; emergency traction splint with a unit that measures the force of traction at the ankle. For children and adults; this device maintains fracture position and alignment without excessive pressure around the ankle or sciatic nerve injury.

spinal board: rigid board with multiple slots for straps used for head and thoracolumbar restraints; designed to transport patients in a relatively immobile state.

For further information on emergency stabilization measures, refer to Crosby LA and Lewallen DG (eds): *Emergency care and transportation of the sick and injured,* ed 6, Rosemont, Ill, 1997, American Academy of Orthopaedic Surgeons.

Chapter 7

Prosthetics and Orthotics

Prosthetists and orthotists are allied health professionals who measure, design, fabricate, and fit prostheses (artificial limbs) and orthoses (braces).

Prosthetics is the science that deals with functional and/or cosmetic restoration of all or part of a missing limb, following the directive of a physician's prescription.

Orthotics is the science that deals with orthoses designed to provide external control, correction, and support for the patient in need for nonoperative management of musculoskeletal disorders. Service in this area is also provided on a prescription basis.

The words *prosthetics* and *orthotics* may be used as nouns to describe the body of knowledge each pertains to, as in the preceding two paragraphs. The devices themselves are called protheses and orthoses. When referring to a specific device, the words *prosthetic* and *orthotic* are adjectives needing an appropriate noun.

Specialists in these areas are certified by the American Board for Certification (ABC) and titled certified prosthetist (CP) and certified orthotist (CO). A certified prosthetist-orthotist (CPO) has demonstrated proficiency in both fields during examinations by the board. Supportive personnel are assistants and technicians, with varying responsibilities and duties.

Many major institutions have ongoing prosthetic and orthotic clinics or conferences that meet as often as patient need requires. Members of the clinic team consist of a chief physician, physical and occupational therapists, a prosthetist, orthotist, rehabilitation nurse, and social worker. The clinic team approach is oriented toward management of the total patient, so although the rationale for prescription of an appropriate prosthetic or orthotic system is a prerequisite, the complete rehabilitation program is the long-range goal and responsibility of the team. Factors such as vocational retraining, if necessary, financial considerations of various phases of management, the necessity and duration of physical or occupational therapy, and a possible need for psychologic counseling are all taken into account. Perhaps most important, the patient must be made to feel comfortable in the clinical setting and be assured that the result will be as satisfactory as is realistic and attainable.

The prosthetist or orthotist is responsible for assisting with the prescription regarding components, elements of design, definitive and proper fitting of the system, and follow-up and adjustments as indicated at future visits to the clinic.

If prosthetic and orthotic practitioners are to serve patients at the highest professional level, they must maintain a program of further education to remain informed of new techniques, components, and concepts. Such programs are available through the American Academy of Orthotists and Prosthetists (AAOP). Other groups are the American Orthotics and Prosthetics Association (AOPA) and the Children's Amputee Prosthetic Program (CAPP).

This chapter was contributed in part by Wilton H. Bunch, MD, PhD, formerly Dean, College of Medicine, Professor, Department of Orthopaedic Surgery, University of South Florida, Tampa, Florida, retired; and Stephen Kramer, CPO, President, Universal Orthopedic Laboratories, Chicago, Illinois.

PROSTHESES

Prosthetic systems, or artificial limbs, are designed to replace function and/or cosmesis of a missing body part. Internal prostheses are surgically implanted devices, such as the artificial hip, and are described in Chapter 8.

Upper Limb Prostheses

An upper limb prosthesis is any external system designed for the amputee from the partial hand level distally to the interscapulothoracic forequarter level proximally.

partial hand amputation: distal to or through one or more of the phalanges or metacarpals or resection at any level of the thumb. Restore function with cosmetic individual finger replacements with fillers and/or opposition-type posts. Slightly more proximal amputation sites necessitate cosmetic gloves and wired finger fillers and/or more intricately designed opposition posts to restore function.

wrist disarticulation (WD): amputation through the wrist joint. Correct with wrist disarticulation prosthesis designed to fit over the sometimes bulbous distal end of the residual limb, retaining as much pronation and supination as possible; trimmed anteriorly to allow maximum flexion; used with cable and figure eight harness control, flexible elbow hinges, wrist unit, and terminal device.

below-elbow (BE) amputation: proximal to wrist but distal to elbow joint. Correct with below-elbow prosthesis designed to fit the residual limb, retaining pronation and supination in the longer levels and allowing maximum flexion; used with cable and figure eight harness control, flexible or rigid elbow hinges, wrist unit, and terminal device. **Münster** or **Hepp-Kuhn** prosthetic sockets make the system applicable for short to very short below-elbow amputations; they are carefully fitted proximal to the epi-

condyles at the elbow to provide adequate suspension without the aid of additional devices; sometimes limit forearm flexion because of restriction of tissue at cubital fold; used with cable and figure nine harness control, wrist unit, and terminal device.

elbow   disarticulation   (ED): amputation through the elbow joint. Correct with elbow disarticulation prosthesis with socket encompassing the residual limb and trimmed proximally at the shoulder to allow good range of motion; used with cable and figure eight harness control, external elbow hinges with lock, wrist unit, and terminal device.

above-elbow (AE) amputation: proximal to elbow joint but distal to shoulder. Correct with above-elbow prosthesis with socket extending over the acromion to support axial loading and carefully fitted at axilla; used with cable and figure eight harness, internal locking elbow, forearm lift assist, wrist unit, and terminal device.

shoulder   disarticulation   (SD): amputation through the glenohumeral joint. Correct with shoulder disarticulation prosthesis with larger socket extending from the spine posteriorly to near the xiphoid process anteriorly and fitted closely at the neck; used with cable and modified chest strap-type harness, shoulder joint or bulkhead (spacer) to allow passive positioning in abduction and adduction, passive positioning, and flexion and extension, internal locking elbow, forearm lift assist, wrist unit, and terminal device.

interscapulothoracic   forequarter   amputation: through the midsection, including resection of the scapula. Correct with cosmetic shoulder cap to restore normal appearance for clothing or forequarter prosthesis with socket similar to that used for shoulder disarticulations but differing in that an extension is usually employed going around and over the sound shoulder to provide additional suspension; used with cable, modified chest strap, and waist belt-type harnessing, excursion amplifier, shoulder joint similar to that used in shoulder disarticulations, internal locking elbow, forearm lift assist, wrist unit, and terminal device.

Upper Limb Prosthetic Components

The components of an upper limb prosthesis include any device that is a supportive or integral part of the prosthesis, including terminal devices.

control cables: steel cable traveling inside housing to move and lock mechanical joints, for example, flexion and locking of the elbow joint; also provide prehension to the terminal device. The housing is sometimes Teflon lined to reduce friction and thereby increase efficiency. Cable systems are generally lightweight, as for small children, with standard ⅛-inch or heavy-duty cable (e.g., Bowden single, dual, and triple control cables). Fig. 7–1 illustrates single control only.

elbow hinges: mechanical types of hinges to provide specific strength or allow controlled mobility. The following types are commonly used: single pivot providing mediolateral control, suspension polycentric, multiple action, sliding action step-up, and stump-activated locking. These

are all designed to provide additional forearm flexion for the very short below-elbow amputee or the patient with flexion contracture.

electrical switch control: prosthesis for the patient with shoulder disarticulation or above-elbow or forequarter amputation; uses switches to control current from a battery that operates an electrical elbow and/or hand. The switches are placed in strategic positions within the harness system, and by opening these switches the patient is able to operate the electrical elbow and/or hand. This type of system is most feasible for patients with limited excursion from causes such as contractures, higher levels of amputation, or bilateral limbs, since each position in the switch is 1/16 inch excursion—considerably less than that required to operate the standard system.

excursion amplifier sleeve: pulley and cable system used to increase efficiency in patients with limited excursion; generally used in shoulder disarticulation and forequarter systems.

flexible hinges: hinges made of Dacron tape or metal spirals to provide suspension while allowing retention of available pronation and supination.

FIG 7–1.
Control cable housing. (From *Below and above harness and control system,* Evanston, IL, 1966, Northwestern University Prosthetic-Orthotic Center.)

forearm lift assist: adjustable spring-loaded device attached to the elbow to provide initial forearm flexion; especially applicable for those with higher level amputations such as shorter above-elbow amputation and shoulder disarticulation.

Greifer prosthesis: electrically enhanced, strong-gripping hand component.

myobock system: The *myo*electrical *b*uilding-bl*ock* system includes optimal cosmetic configuration, high-wearing comfort, functional value, and easier service.

myoelectric control: sophisticated prosthesis available for the patient with wrist disarticulation, below-elbow or above-elbow amputation: uses electrodes placed over the flexor and extensor muscle groups to pick up the milliamperes of electricity emitted by a muscle during contraction. This electrical stimulus is then used to operate a switch that controls a motor in a mechanical hand or other component. Prosthetic sockets are generally self-suspended, thereby eliminating the need for any harness.

nudge control: mechanical unit that can be pressed by the chin to lock or unlock one or more joints of the prosthesis; seen in forequarter systems.

outside locking hinge: used on the elbow disarticulation system because of length of residual limb. Outside locking elbow and internal positive locking elbow hinges with 11 locking positions are used for above-elbow, shoulder disarticulation, and forequarter systems.

shoulder harness, chest straps, and waist belts: an infinite variety of Dacron, cloth, and leather materials is used to fabricate these components, which provide suspension as well as control through their attachment to cables that operate locks for various joints and provide function for the terminal device. The figure eight ring harness is one of the most common and provides suspension and control of prosthesis. The figure nine harness supplies only control, as the Münster socket provides suspension (Fig. 7–2).

terminal devices: hooks or hands affixed to the wrist unit, affording function and/or cosmesis.

> **hooks:**   lyre-shaped fingers that open in opposition to one another, achieved by forces exerted through the harness and cable systems, and close involuntarily by means of dynamic rubber bands or springs. Hooks are available in numerous sizes, generally in aluminum with plastisol covering for children, aluminum or stainless steel with neoprene lining, stainless steel with serrated inner surface such as the model 5X, and for heavy-duty tasks the 7 or 7LO types, designed to hold devices such as shovels or rakes. Although certain hooks differ, such as the Trautman Locktite and the APRL (Army Prosthetics Research Laboratory) types, most employ rubber bands or springs to close, and prehension is directly proportional to the strength and number used.

> **hands:**   there are a number of both functional and passive hands available. The mechanically functional hand provides prehension

FIG 7–2.
Cross point of harness connected by stainless steel ring. (From *Below and above elbow harness and control system,* Evanston, IL, 1966, Northwestern University Prosthetic-Orthotic Center.)

by means of springs attached to its internal parts; a cosmetic glove matched to the patient's skin color is applied externally. Passive hands, although nonfunctional, generally provide increased cosmesis.

wrist flexion unit: allows prepositioning of terminal device closer to the midline of the body; generally used for the bilateral patient.

wrist units: integral components at the distal end of the prosthesis that allow attachment, interchangeability, and pronation and supination of the terminal devices; types are standard constant friction and quick change; units are oval or round and available in different diameters.

Lower Limb Prostheses and Components (Fig. 7–3)

Lower limb prostheses are any external system designed for the amputee from the partial foot level distally to the hemipelvectomy level proximally. They are categorized as *exoskeletal* or *endoskeletal*. The exoskeletal prosthesis has a rigid outer shell that provides structural strength and cosmetic shape. The endoskeletal prosthesis has a tubular structure connecting the components and is covered by cosmetic foam. The primary components of the prosthesis are the socket, suspension system, foot, and knee unit.

Lisfranc: a disarticulation through the medial metatarsophalangeal joint or metatarsal-tarsal joints. Correct with extended steel shank in shoe to provide a place to push off and toe filler or foot plate with toe filler.

Chopart: distal to the ankle joint. Correct with distal weight-bearing socket with partial foot replacement.

Syme: through the ankle joint; results in a bulbous distal weight-bearing residual limb. Correct with a medial-opening or expandable-wall prosthesis, which facilitates application and removal. Weight bearing is distributed between the distal end and the patellar tendon. The socket is self-suspending because of the reduced circumference above the distal limb.

FIG 7–3.
A PTB exoskeletal prosthesis with supracondylar cuff and SACH foot.

transtibial: formerly called below knee (BK), it is proximal to the ankle but distal to the knee. Correct with PTB (patellar tendon-bearing) prosthesis, designed to bear weight through the patellar tendon, medial tibial flare, and other pressure tolerant areas; socket may be hard or have a soft liner. Suspension is with supracondylar cuff strap or without waist belt, sleeve, or suction. Self-suspending variations of the PTB prosthesis include the following:

joint and corset: for the patient with mediolateral instability of the knee, for a very short below-knee amputation or residual limb incapable of supporting total body weight because of conditions such as burns and skin adherent tissue. A typical prescription would be: PTB type of socket, external mechanical knee joints, thigh corset, fork strap, waist belt, and prosthetic foot.

suction socket suspension: for below knee prosthesis, a new design of suspension that incorporates a valve or silicone liner and locks in position, or incorporates a sock with silicone ring. Differs from PTB type.

supracondylar (PTB-SC): patellar tendon bearing with supracondylar cuff incorporates higher medial and lateral walls that encompass the femoral condyles. A medial wedge, either movable or built into a soft liner, is placed firmly over the medial epicondyle.

supracondylar-suprapatellar (SC-SP): similar to supracondylar but also includes a high anterior wall that encompasses the patella. This provides increased suspension and limits hyperextension of the knee.

knee disarticulation (knee bearing, K/B): amputation through the knee joint. Correct with distal weight-bearing socket. The socket is self-suspending with either a medial opening or a soft liner to facilitate donning. A Selesian belt is worn as an auxiliary suspension. There is also a polycentric (four-bar linkage) knee unit and prosthetic foot. Still in use are end-bearing leather or plastic sockets with external hinges, fork straps, and waist belts.

transfemoral: formerly called above knee (AK), it is proximal to the knee joint but distal to the hip joint. Correct with quadrilateral or narrow medial-lateral ischial containment socket prosthesis.

CAD-CAM: computer-assisted design/computer-assisted manufacturing refers to the contour of the socket and how it is modified. It is a hand-made computer-assisted method of providing a cosmetically accurate fit that can use any of the ischial containment sockets. Types are:

PTB (patellar tendon bearing) with cuff suspension.

PTBS (patellar tendon bearing suspension).

PTB-SC (patellar tendon bearing supracondylar).

PTB-SP (patellar tendon bearing suprapatellar).

SPC (suprapatellar cuff).

PTS (patellar tendon socket).

Ischial containment sockets (narrow M/L = medial-lateral; CAT-CAM = contour adducted trochanteric, controlled alignment method): an above-knee amputation socket design incorporating a narrow M/L shape, high lateral wall, and a slanted pocket for the ischium. Provides greater control of lateral forces during gait and a more even distribution of proximal weight-bearing areas.

quadrilateral ischial weight-bearing socket: wooden or plastic socket designed with a shelf to transpose weight through the ischial tuberosity; suspension may be achieved by a hip joint with a pelvic band and control belt or with a suction socket with a mechanical knee and prosthetic foot.

hip disarticulation (HD): amputation at the hip level but with the ischial tuberosity intact. Correct with plastic socket designed to transpose weight through the ischial tuberosity and related gluteal musculature, mechanical hip and knee joints, and prosthetic foot.

hemipelvectomy: amputation at hip level with ablation of the ischial tuberosity. Correct with plastic socket designed to distribute weight using remaining musculature, rib margin, cosmetic socket build-up, mechanical hip and knee joints, and prosthetic foot.

Lower Limb Prosthetic Components

foot and ankle components: allow normal gait patterns.

energy storing feet: incorporates a cushioned heel with a resilient toe lever that stores energy in stance phase and releases it at toe-off. Typically lighter than SACH foot. Varieties include: **Seattle foot, Carbon Copy II and III foot, Quantum foot.**

flex foot (Springlight): energy storing foot for high activity levels. Top lever and pylon are one continuous carbon graphite spring, similar in appearance to a ski tip.

SACH foot: *s*olid *a*nkle *c*ushioned *h*eel (wedge).

SAFE foot: *s*tationary *a*ttachment *f*lexible *e*ndoskeletal.

single axis: allows anteroposterior motion and controlled plantar flexion with dorsiflexion stop.

multiaxial: allows plantar flexion and dorsiflexion, inversion and eversion. It is the traditional SACH foot with sides to flex. Types are **Greisinger** and **Endolite.**

Multi-flex foot: like the SACH foot, but allows medial and lateral angulation.

knee components: designed to provide stability during early and middle stance phases, and bend in late stance and swing phase, as well as in kneeling and sitting.

external: most common application in knee bearing; no controlled friction.

fluid controlled (hydraulic or pneumatic): provides swing phase control for a variable rate of gait, eliminating excessive heel rise and terminal impact. Varieties include **Dupaco, Dyneplex, Daw, Otto Bock, Mauch.**

four-bar linkage: a polycentric system that creates a moving center of rotation. Inherently very stable.

Henschke-Mauch S'n'S: hydraulic unit that provides stance as well as swing phase control; **Mauch S'n'S.**

manual locking: knee automatically locks at full extension. Patient-controlled latch disengages lock for sitting.

Mauch S'n'S: hydraulic swing phase with stance phase control.

Oklahoma cable system (OKC system): cable that harnesses hip flexion into extension control of artificial knee, allowing step-over-step running.

safety: weight-activated stance control. When knee is extended and weight bearing, an adjustable braking mechanism is activated to resist flexion.

single axis: single point of rotation with constant friction to control swing phase.

below-knee suspension: used to support below-knee prostheses.

billet: connects supracondylar cuff to waist belt.

condylar cuff: mediolateral attachment to prosthesis with strap proximal to femoral condyles.

fork strap: anterolateral attachment to prosthesis connecting to waist belt.

suction: a silicone gel skin-tight liner worn directly over residual limb. Various devices are built into the liner that attach it directly to the prosthesis.

supracondylar cuff: tabs that attach mediolaterally to prosthesis with cuff strap going around knee proximally to femoral condyles.

waist belt: webbing wrapped circumferentially at pelvis with connection to billet or fork strap.

knee disarticulation suspension: fork strap and waist belt.

transfemoral suspension: used to support above-knee prostheses.

control belt: leather wrapped circumferentially at pelvis and attached to pelvic band.

hip joint: mechanical free-motion joint positioned anatomically on lateral wall of socket.

pelvic band: metal band contoured to pelvis and attached to upright of hip joint.

Selesian bandage or belt: webbing over hip on sound side with one lateral and two anterior socket attachments. Used in conjunction with a looser fitting suction socket.

shoulder harness or suspenders: webbing straps traversing shoulders with roller and cord or various attachments to socket.

suction socket: worn against the skin with no intervening liners or socks.

hip disarticulation or hemipelvectomy suspension: webbing over shoulder on sound side with anteroposterior socket attachments.

Other Components, Materials, and Techniques

cast sock: used to take negative plaster impressions; sometimes used with or in place of stump socks; especially applicable for the new below-knee amputee during volume reduction of the residual limb.

check socket: a disposable clear plastic socket used to ensure integral fit before definitive fabrication.

distal pad: injection of Silastic or an equivalent foam into end of socket of below- or above-knee systems; provides total contact distally and reduces possibility of edema.

extension aid: to assist knee extension in the above-knee prosthesis.

pylon: adjustable tubular section connecting socket and prosthetic foot (endoskeletal construction).

rigid dressing: plaster socket worn on residual limb to reduce volume.

rotator or torsion unit: component in the prosthesis designed to compensate for shear forces, thereby reducing torque and friction between the residual limb and interface of the socket.

sheath: nylon interface worn between residual limb and stump socks to reduce shear forces.

silicone gel socket insert: inner liner made of silicone gel designed to absorb shear forces. Often used for problem-fitting below-knee amputees. Also used for below-knee suction suspension.

sleeve: neoprene or latex sleeve worn over proximal portion of the prosthesis and extending onto the patient's thigh. Provides suction suspension.

socket: custom-designed receptacle into which the residual limb fits.

soft cosmetic cover: foam material covering endoskeletal components; shaped cosmetically.

soft socket insert: soft inner liner for PTB socket. Petite or silicone gel most common.

stockinette: tubular open-ended cotton or nylon material used to don suction socket, sometimes used with or in place of stump socks; especially applicable for the new above-knee amputee during volume reduction of the residual limb.

stump shrinker: elastic sleeve worn on residual limb to reduce volume.

stump sock: wool or cotton sock worn over residual limb to provide a cushion for friction between skin and socket interface. Available in various thicknesses called "plys."

total contact: intimacy between socket and residual limb, particularly at distal end, to control edema.

Specialized Systems

immediate postsurgical fitting (IPSF): procedure performed immediately after surgery; patient is fitted with plaster type of socket, adjustable pylon, and prosthetic foot. Advantages include early ambulation, more rapid stump maturity, and psychologic benefits.

intermediate (temporary): thermoplastic type of socket with adjustable pylon and prosthetic foot; intermediate phase of management used to expedite fitting, establish early ambulation, and reduce volume of residual limb prior to definitive fitting.

modular (endoskeletal): selectively applicable for below-knee or any level of proximal amputations; use socket according to prescription with adjustable pylon and foot and socket attachment plates; exterior surface is made of custom-shaped foam and covered with cosmetic material.

ORTHOSES

An orthosis is an externally applied system designed to provide control, correction, and support and to check deformity. The brace can either resist or assist motion to control deformity, to unweight a body segment and reduce the load, and to provide corrective measures.

The Task Force on Standardization of Prosthetic-Orthotic Terminology of the Committee on Prosthetic-Orthotic Education (CPOE), National Research Council, and the American Orthotic and Prosthetic Association (AOPA) have been largely responsible for the implementation of the terminology generally in use today. In an effort to enhance communication between the prescribing physician and the orthotist, the following descriptive guideline has been adopted. The standardization is based on indicating those joints and regions that the orthosis is to encompass or control. The orthosis would control the named joint by allowing free, assisted, or resisted motion. Orthosis types are:

AFO: ankle-foot.

AO: ankle.

BFO: balanced forearm.

CO: cervical.

CTLSO: cervicothoracolumbosacral.

CTO: cervicothoracic.

EO: elbow.

EWHO: elbow-wrist-hand.

FO: foot.

HKAFO: hip-knee-ankle foot.

HO: hip.

HO: hand.

KAFO: knee-ankle-foot.

KO: knee.

LSO: lumbosacral.

PPO: passive prehension.

PTBO: patellar tendon bearing.

SEWHO: shoulder-elbow-wrist-hand.

SIO: sacroiliac.

SO: shoulder.

SOMI: sternooccipital mandibular immobilizer.

TLSO: thoracolumbosacral.

TO: thoracic.

WHO: wrist-hand.

Use of the foregoing terms leaves the materials, design, and components to the discretion of the orthotist unless otherwise indicated by prescription, as demonstrated in the following typical examples.

> Prescription: AFO to provide dorsiflexion assist. (This simple prescription leaves orthotic management regarding materials for the system to be determined by the orthotist according to patient evaluation.)
>
> Prescription: AFO to provide dorsiflexion assist; double uprights, Klenzac ankle, calf band, Velcro closure, and shoe attachments.
>
> Prescription: AFO to provide dorsiflexion assist; thermoplastic fabrication.

As demonstrated this format provides the prescribing physician with various controls over the patient's management.*

Lower Limb Orthoses

Since all orthoses currently in use are too numerous to discuss, we will confine our list to those most commonly prescribed.

---

*Those individuals in need of further information in the area of orthotics would benefit from American Academy of Orthopaedic Surgeons: *Atlas of orthotics, biomechanical principles and applications,* St Louis, 1975, The CV Mosby Co.

Foot Orthoses

flexible o.:   leather, foam, or equivalent, providing longitudinal arch and/or metatarsal support; orthosis is removable from shoe.

rigid o.:   carbon composite fiberglass, and stainless steel designed to provide arch support for pes planus or other related problem; orthosis is removable from shoe; *Whitman plate, Schaeffer type,* and modifications thereof.

UCB o.:   (developed at the University of California, Berkeley) similar to the rigid type, but fabricated of thermoplastic or thermoset resin.

hallux valgus o.:   designed for day and night use; reduces bunion pain by decreasing valgus deformity (pulls toe to midline of body).

Denis Browne bar: consists of a rigid bar riveted or clamped to shoes at either end. The bar provides hip abduction, with ratchet adjustments controlling rotation; generally prescribed for treatment of clubfoot, equinovarus, pes planus, or tibial torsion. The new system allows for more independent control and leg movement with infant able to crawl because of jointed bars.

Fillauer bar: clamp-on bar to place on feet to hold leg in internal or external rotation. Attaches to shoes by a clip-on device.

Ankle Orthoses

elastic o.:   provides minimal support; helps control swelling.

rigid o.:   leather, canvas, or equivalent material provides substantial immobilization of the ankle to alleviate pain caused by motion.

Ankle-Foot Orthoses

Charcot restraint orthotic walker (CROW):   rigid orthotic with rocker bottom foot; inner aspect lined with foam with a double density custom insert for the foot portion.

floor reaction orthosis: rear-entry plastic device that allows full plantar flexion but stops at 90 degrees and thus gives good push-off from the foot component that is in the wearer's shoe.

metal o.:   fitted ¾ inch distal to head of fibula and is an integral part of the shoe; examples are single or double upright jointed ankle, free motion, limited motion, and dorsiflexion assist; used with calf band, buckle, or Velcro closure and stirrup with shoe attachments.

patellar tendon bearing (PTB) o.:   weight-bearing terminates just proximal to the patellar tendon and is fitted around the knee similar to the below-knee prosthetic socket; used with molded foot plate or ankle joints and stirrup with shoe attachments; designed to transmit body weight through the patellar tendon and medial femoral condyle to achieve controlled unloading of weight on the tibia and ankle-foot complex; anteroposteriorly sectioned proximally.

spring wire o.:   medial and lateral spring wire uprights attached to calf band proximally and the shoe distally; designed to provide dynamic dorsiflexion assist.

thermoplastic o.:   terminates at or near the apex of the gastrocnemius muscle proximally, with molded foot plate fitted into shoe distally; ambulatory, nocturnal, or combination of both; designed to control and correct specific problems of the foot-ankle complex.

Knee Orthoses

dynamic o.:   similar to static with the addition of external knee joints with or without locks to allow controlled motion.

elastic knee cage: elastic sleeve encompassing the knee; provides minimal support and stabilization. Variations are the following.

with medial and lateral contoured knee joints: similar, with the addition of joints providing some increased stabilization. Other options include medial and lateral condylar pads, adjustable anterior laces, and additional spiral control straps.

Swedish knee cage: metal and leather system allowing flexion but preventing hyperextension of the knee.

ligamentous control braces: commercially available custom-made braces designed to control special ligamentous deficiencies about the knee.

static o.: leather, thermoplastic, or equivalent; immobilizes knee in desired attitude of flexion or extension.

Knee-Ankle-Foot Orthoses

Legg-Perthes disease o.: the following are specialized systems designed for the treatment of Legg-Perthes disease.

A-frame o.: when this system is used with an extra-long bar to treat developmental dysplasia of the hips (DDH), an A-frame orthosis is sometimes incorporated to control the tendency for genu valgum (knock-knee), which may occur because of extensive hip abduction. The A-frame consists of a metal component fitted medially from the bar up both legs with calf and thigh bands and valgus control pads.

Atlanta brace: a hip abduction brace that allows ambulation without crutch assistance.

Newington o.: bilateral and similar in design to the Toronto o.; differs in that flat bars are used, and no joints are incorporated.

Salter sling: sling device that holds hip in abduction and internal rotation while the knee is held flexed.

Toronto o.: bilateral proximal high cuffs, center tubular column with universal multiaxial joints at base, outriggers with angled mounting blocks at either end to receive attachment of shoes; ambulatory system providing hip abduction and controlled rotation.

trilateral o. (Tachdjian): plastic quadrilateral socket fitted at the level of the ischium similar to that of the above-knee prosthetic socket; single upright with shoe attachments; designed to provide weight unloading, hip abduction, and internal rotation.

metal o.: fitted approximately 1½ inches inferior

to the perineum and is an integral part of the shoe; single or double upright jointed ankle, free motion, limited motion, or dorsiflexion assist calf, distal and proximal thigh bands, buckle or Velcro closures, jointed knee with or without lock, stirrup, and shoe attachments.

reciprocating gait o. (RGO): provides support to lower limbs and trunk for paraplegic patients; an orthosis that has a gear box or cable system attached to bilateral knee-ankle-foot o. and lumbosacral o., allowing a lower-level paraplegic to have a reciprocating gait.

thermoplastic o.: similar to the standard orthosis but fabricated of plastic material with molded foot plate fitted into shoe distally. This type of system has found increased acceptance because of its lighter weight and total contact fitting capabilities.

Other specialized knee ankle-foot orthoses include those designed to manage patients with neuromuscular conditions and fractures using plaster or plastic with polycentric knee joints and other sophisticated components.

Hip Orthoses

The following are specialized hip orthoses designed for treatment of developmental dysplasia of the hips (DDH) or Legg-Perthes disease.

abduction o. (Ilfeld splint): bilateral thigh cuffs of plastic, covered metal, or equivalent with adjustable bar to provide hip abduction and waist belt and/or thoracic section to maintain positioning. Some systems have additional adjustment for hip flexion control.

Barlow (Malmo) splint: for dysplastic hips in infants, an abduction flexion, external rotation splint.

Pavlik harness: a series of straps passing over the shoulders both anteriorly and posteriorly, transversing the chest and leading to the feet where they are attached to plastic booties; designed to provide hip flexion, abduction, and external rotation.

pillow (Frejka) o.: soft splint fitted between the thighs to provide hip abduction with straps over the shoulders to maintain positioning.

Scottish rite o.: pelvic band, bilateral free-motion hip joints, proximal thigh cuffs, adjustable tubular spreader bar with universal joints at inferior medial aspect of cuffs; ambulatory system providing hip abduction for treatment of Legg-Perthes disease.

thermoplastic/metal o.: custom-fabricated system designed to maintain the hips in degrees of flexion, abduction, and rotation, as prescribed.

Hip-Knee-Ankle-Foot Orthoses
The following orthoses, except for the RGO and standing frame type, are described in a unilateral application, although they can be fitted bilaterally.

cable twister o.: pelvic belt, free-motion hip and ankle joint, plastic-covered cable, connecting joints, stirrup, and shoe attachments; calf and thigh bands are incorporated as necessary; adjustable at hip and ankle to provide dynamic control of hip rotation and tibial torsion.

elastic twister o.: pelvic belt with elastic straps wrapped around leg and attached to a hook in the shoe; provides dynamic control of hip rotation and tibial torsion.

standard o.: standard, thermoplastic, metal, or combination of materials used in any of the knee-ankle-foot orthoses to which has been added a pelvic band that is static or with a mechanical hip joint for dynamic control of the pelvis.

standing frame (parapodium) orthosis: thoracic region reaches to floor, pelvic band, lateral uprights attached to platform base, which has cutouts to accept patient's shoes, uprights are generally overlapped to allow growth adjustment. Some type of control is employed for knee extension. Joints are optional at hips and knees. This system is used to achieve standing and increase awareness in the child with afflictions such as spina bifida.

Components Applicable to Lower Limb Orthoses

ankle, knee, or hip joint: mechanical axis placed anatomically to allow or control motion.

Bail knee lock: posterior spring-loaded ring extending from medial to lateral knee joints with capability of automatic locking.

calf band: metal covered with leather or equivalent fitted to the calf area on ankle-foot or knee-ankle-foot orthoses.

dial lock: may be set in varying degrees of flexion or extension to accommodate and/or reduce contractures; other comparable types.

distal thigh band: lower thigh band on knee-ankle-foot orthoses.

double-action ankle joint: anterior and posterior compartments provide infinite adjustment for solid, limited, or dynamic assist.

drop-lock ring: fitted into place at knee joint to maintain extension; may be unlocked for sitting.

extended steel shank: inserted in sole of shoe to or past metatarsal heads to more effectively use floor reaction force.

ischial weight-bearing ring or band: metal or equivalent component covered with soft material and fitted at the level of the ischial tuberosity; designed to unload weight from the lower limb; Thomas ring.

Klenzak orthosis: dorsiflexion or plantar flexion assist for ankle joint; spring-loaded dynamic assistive control of the foot.

lateral spring-loaded lock: spring-loaded ring lock with lever that dynamically locks at full extension.

limited- or free-motion ankle joint: permanently adjustable to allow motion as desired.

metal foot plate: similar to NYU insert but fabricated of stainless steel, Monel, or equivalent.

NYU (New York University) insert: metal o. using thermoplastic foot plate attached to ankle joint stirrups; provides correction of the foot and allows various shoes to be worn.

overlapped upright or growth extensions: uprights placed on top of one another to accommodate growth in children.

patellar pad: leather or equivalent; fits over patella with straps around uprights to maintain knee extension.

proximal thigh band: higher thigh band on knee-ankle-foot orthoses.

quadrilateral brim: similar to ischial weight-bearing ring but fabricated of plastic.

split stirrup: component mounted on various shoes to allow interchangeability of the orthosis.

spreader bar: attached medially to both stirrups of bilateral knee-ankle-foot orthoses to prevent uncontrolled abduction.

stirrup: attaches orthosis to upper shoe sections; has receptacles for ankle joints.

suprapatellar and infrapatellar straps: small straps above and below knee, continuing around uprights to maintain knee extension.

upright: metal, plastic, or equivalent used to connect various other components.

varus or valgus corrective ankle straps: soft, padded leather or equivalent components that wrap around the opposite side.

varus or valgus knee control pads: leather or equivalent components that wrap around an opposing upright to correct deformity.

Upper Limb Orthoses

Physiology in design considerations for hand and wrist-hand orthotic systems include the following:

1. Maintain thumb in opposition for prehension.
2. Allow for thumb abduction as may be required.
3. Maintain skeletal integrity.
4. Avoid restrictions in use of the orthosis.
5. Prevent or correct contractures.

6. Maintain wrist in the functional 25 to 35 degrees of dorsiflexion.

Because of infinite and intricate variety of systems, only a few common examples will be given.

Wrist-Hand and Hand Orthoses

basic hand splint: for muscle weakness in the hand; a dorsal splint that wraps around the ulnar, distal, and volar side of the hand and held in place with a strap around the distal wrist.

cock-up splint: one plastic section providing wrist dorsiflexion with incorporation of a C bar for prehension or a soft Velcro brace with palmar bar to dorsiflex the wrist.

externally powered tenodesis o.: through activation of a microswitch, tenodesis graft is achieved using a mechanical muscle.

Galveston metacarpal brace: for distal metacarpal fractures; an adjustable brace that provides dorsally directed pressure on the distal component of the fracture with counter pressure on the middorsum of the hand.

long opponens o.: identical to short opponens with forearm extension for wrist control.

palmar wrist splint: easily removable volar wrist splint that has molded palmar extension that helps hold thumb in functional position.

ratchet flexor tenodesis splint: wrist-hand o. to passively lock hand in a grasp position for a partially paralyzed forearm and hand.

reciprocal finger prehension: for severe paralysis of forearm and hand; this orthosis allows patients to use their good hand to adjust and set the fixed position of fingers.

safety pin o.: fitted to individual fingers to dynamically influence flexion or extension of a joint; sometimes called *finger benders*.

short opponens o.: consists of radial extension, opponens bar, palmar arch, ulnar extension, and dorsal extension; fabricated of plastic or metal. Positions hand and thumb for opposition.

tenodesis o.: for nerve paralysis; wrist-hand orthosis with connected hinge at wrist and metacarpophalangeal joint located such that extension of wrist brings about finger flexion.

wrist-driven lateral prehension o.: similar to long opponens with jointed radial side and a rod or connection between hand and forearm sections and thumb post. Wrist dorsiflexion produces a lateral prehension pattern using the mechanical axis.

Elbow Orthoses

Elbow orthoses may be static with humeral and forearm sections for immobilization, as in hand orthoses, and external joints to allow motion. Some are designed with turnbuckles or the equivalent to reduce contracture and may be static or dynamic.

dynamic hinged elbow fracture brace: orthotic device to allow graded active range of motion with dynamic support to the fracture joint structure to promote healing (Fig. 7–4A).

Santana elbow extension splint: designed to decrease flexion contractures of the elbow and to gain total maximum range of motion and strength (Fig 7–4B).

Elbow-Wrist-Hand Orthoses

These are static systems to provide immobilization. A torsion bar may be incorporated to assist in pronation or supination. They are useful to correct fractures of the forearm.

Shoulder Orthoses

Generally these are static or passive jointed systems used for positioning to correct chronic shoulder dislocation.

Shoulder-Elbow-Wrist-Hand Orthoses

static orthosis: provides controlled positioning.

airplane splint: jointed elbow and shoulder, allowing controlled flexion and rotation; glenohumeral joint permits controlled abduction; used for muscle injuries, humeral fractures, disloca-

tions, surgery involving the glenohumeral joint, and nerve injuries such as to the brachial plexus.

Components Applicable to Upper Limb Orthoses

C bar: component attached to or an integral part of the palmar arch, designed to maintain the web space between the thumb and hand.

first dorsal interosseous assist: principle similar to that of the spring swivel thumb; designed to hold the metacarpophalangeal (MP) joint of the index finger in abduction to provide opposition with the thumb.

flail-elbow hinge: used to overcome muscle deficit at the elbow. Spring assist provides flexion and locks in position for a chosen activity.

joint stabilizer: rigid component extending proximally and distally to a joint of a digit; provides stability or realignment for subluxation.

opponens bars: exert a static holding force on saddle joint of thumb. Keep thumb in palmar abduction, an optimal position for opposition.

outrigger: MP, proximal interphalangeal (PIP), or distal interphalangeal (DIP) extension assist; MP stop (lumbrical bar) positioned just proximal to the IP joints; holds MP joints in approximately 15 degrees of flexion.

spring swivel thumb: wire spring attached to radial aspect of orthosis and in turn connected to thumb ring. Patient flexes against this dynamic resistance; in a relaxed state, the thumb is held in the open position.

thumb interphalangeal (IP) extension assist: principle similar to the first dorsal interosseous assist; designed to return IP of the thumb to neutral after flexion and during prehension.

thumb post: static control for prehension achieved by rigid member encompassing thumb.

turnbuckle: adjustable component used to reduce contractures.

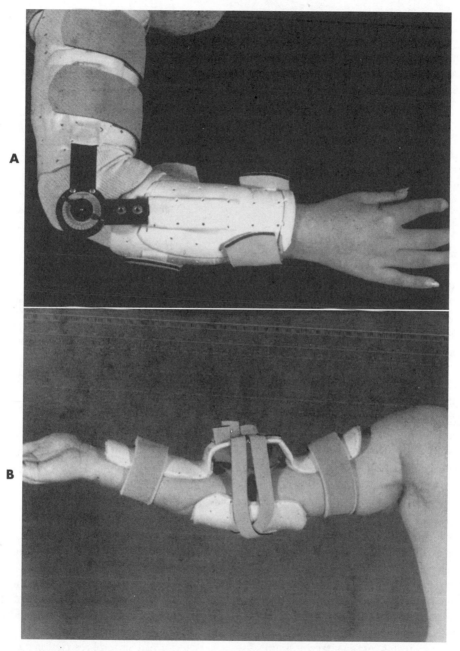

FIG 7–4.
A, Elbow orthosis: dynamic hinged elbow fracture brace. **B,** Santana elbow extension splint. (Permissions: EC Jeter, OTR, Occupational Therapy Department, National Naval Medical Center, Bethesda, MD.)

Specialized Systems for Upper Limbs

For those patients with severe involvement, external power sources are at times employed. Electrically powered or CO_2-operated artificial muscle systems are available.

Spine

Sacroiliac Orthoses

cloth binder: material encompassing appropriate region with Velcro closure.

sacroiliac belt: adjustable corset with posterior pad.

Lumbosacral Orthoses

Bennett o.:   cloth lumbar corset with reinforced frame consisting of a pelvic and thoracic band with two paravertebral uprights.

chairback o. (anteroposterior and mediolateral control):   posterior frame with lateral and posterior uprights and apron front anteriorly; control restrictions include anterior flexion, extension, and lateral flexion; used for lower back pathologic conditions, severe strain, arthritis.

lumbosacral corset: custom-fitted corset, generally having rigid paraspinal uprights.

Norton-Brown o.:   rigid low-back postoperative brace. The lateral bars extend to cover the greater trochanter to help reduce lateral bending.

surgical corset: garment encasing the torso and hips and adjustable circumferentially. Adjustment may be made anteriorly, posteriorly, laterally, or in combination. In general, the following statements apply.

  function: serves as a reminder to restrict anteroposterior and mediolateral motions; minimal unweighting of vertebral bodies and disks; restricts some rotary and twisting motions; creates intracavitary pressure system, lending support to the spinal column.

  materials: nylon, cotton, canvas, elastic, or a combination.

  fabrication: single or multiple layers.

anterior height: superior border 1 inch below xiphoid process or above lower ribs; inferior border ½ to 1 inch above symphysis pubis.

posterior height: superior border 1 inch below inferior ankle of scapula; inferior border extends to the sacrococcygeal junction or approximately the gluteal fold.

modification possibilities: posterior semirigid or rigid paraspinal uprights, posterior semirigid or rigid plate, posterior inflatable control pads, additional abdominal reinforcements with flexible stays, thoracic extension with shoulder straps and axillary loops, separate frame posteriorly, one-piece garment, special control pads for ptosis (prolapse of any organ), hernia pads, perineal straps, thigh skirt.

Williams o. (posterior and mediolateral control):   posterior frame; lateral sliding uprights with apron front anteriorly; control restrictions; extension and lateral flexion; permits free anterior flexion; used for herniated disks, severe lordosis, and situations where it is desirable to increase intervertebral space posteriorly.

Thoracic Orthoses

clavicle o.:   figure eight harness under the axilla and over the shoulder, crossing posteriorly; control restrictions: glenohumeral flexion; used for clavicular fractures.

rib belt: foam padded or elastic with Velcro closure; minimal control, reducing muscle strain; used for fractures and costochondritis.

Thoracolumbosacral Orthoses (TLSO)

anterior control (Jewett, hyperextension) o.:   anterior frame with superior and inferior pads; three-point fixation provided by additional posterior pad; control restrictions: maintains hyperextension and tends to increase lumbar lordosis; used for spondylitis, compression fractures, osteoporosis (reduction in the quality of bone or skeletal atrophy; remaining bone is normally mineralized), arthritis, spinal fusion, adolescent epiphysitis, and osteochondritis.

anteroposterior and mediolateral control (Knight-Taylor) o.: chairback-Taylor combination; posterior and lateral uprights with corset front; control restrictions: anterior flexion, extension, and lateral flexion; used for high-spinal fusion, lordosis, and osteoporosis.

anteroposterior control (Taylor) o.: posterior uprights with shoulder straps and apron front; control restrictions: anterior flexion and extension; used for kyphosis, fractures, arthritis, lordosis, carcinoma (any of the various types of malignant neoplasms derived from epithelial tissue), and after spinal surgery.

Arnold brace: brace primarily molded over the sacroiliac area with posterior support and rigid scapular thoracic support harness.

body jacket: anteroposterior sectioned, posterior or anterior opening; thermoplastic fabrication; control restrictions: general immobilization and intracavitary pressure; may be designed to provide some distraction; used for conditions such as postsurgical management of fusion, spina bifida, muscular dystrophy, and scoliosis.

Boston brace: molded brace used in scoliosis and other special disorders, for example, osteoarthritis of the dorsal and lumbar spine.

CASH o.: cruciform anterior spinal hyperextension o., a hyperextension TLSO or CTSO that allows more freedom of chest movement.

Charleston bending brace: for scoliosis, used only at night to hold the patient in maximum side bending correction.

dorsal lumbar corset: high corset with shoulder straps and paraspinal uprights; control restrictions: forward flexion, used for problems related to higher levels of amputation; see Thoracolumbosacral anterior control.

Lexan jacket: for scoliosis treatment; a prefabricated TLSO.

lumbodorsal support: lumbar corset with thoracic extension of stays and straps that go over shoulder, pass under axilla, and attach to bottom of thoracic component of the posterior stay; **dorsal lumbar o.**

New York orthopedic front-opening o.: for scoliosis treatment, a prefabricated TLSO.

Prenyl jacket: for scoliosis treatment, a prefabricated TLSO.

underarm o.: custom-fabricated or modular system; thermoplastic, generally with posterior opening; used for scoliosis. Application is most effective when apex of curve is inferior to T-10.

Wilmington jacket: used in scoliosis in circumstances in which control through the cervical spine is not essential.

Cervical Orthoses (Fig. 7–5)
Cervical orthoses are employed when immobilization is necessary due to whiplash type of injuries, fractures, and surgical fusion. The following provide minimal restrictions.

four-poster o.: same as two-poster o., but employs two bars anteriorly and two posteriorly.

A   **B**

FIG 7–5.
Cervical flexion-extension control orthosis (poster appliance). **A,** Cervical spine in slight extension with head erect. **B,** Cervical spine in flexion with chin depressed. (From American Academy of Orthopaedic Surgeons: *Atlas of orthotics,* St Louis, 1975, The CV Mosby Co.)

hard (plastic) collar (Mayo Thomas): overlapping plastic sections with Velcro closures; wraps around neck and contacts chin.

molded Thomas collar: custom-fabricated leather or plastic over modified cast.

Plastazote collar: unicellular foam, contoured to fit chin and make contact with occiput; Velcro closure. This configuration is often called a **Philadelphia** collar.

soft collar: foam with Velcro closure; wraps around neck.

wire frame collar: rounded, rectangular ring that fits under chin and onto chest, held in place by two straps supported by expansion of material on posterior neck. When optimum control and restriction are required, the following are prescribed:

> *SOMI* (sternal *o*cciput *m*andibular *i*mmobilization) o.: chin and occiput sections and sternal and posterior sections; may be fitted while patient is supine. The SOMI brace can be attached to a thermoplastic body jacket to allow control of the cervical, thoracic, and lumbar spine.

> *halo extension:* fitted bands at forehead and back of head in conjunction with a two- or four-poster device attached to a thoracolumbar or thoracolumbosacral orthosis.

> *halo traction:* skeletal immobilization traction using a pelvic plaster cast or plastic girdle; outriggers to metal ring encircling head; pins are then inserted into skull and outriggers adjusted for distraction.

two- or four-poster o. with extension to waist: body length orthosis for greater neck stability and control.

two- or four-poster o. (Dennison brace) with thoracic extension: anterior and posterior bands incorporated into the cervical orthosis.

two-poster o. (Dennison brace): for fractures and postsurgical support, a cervical brace with chest and thoracic extension; one anterior bar with chin cup and chest plate, and one posterior post with thoracic and chest plates attached by shoulder harness (straps) that can be connected to a waist circular support. A thoracic extension can be added.

Cervicothoracolumbosacral Orthoses

Milwaukee o.: leather or thermoplastic pelvic girdle, throat mold, occiput pads, neck ring, and full, connecting superstructure with control pads as necessary; used for spinal scoliosis or kyphosis.

Components and Descriptions Applicable to Spinal Systems

Beaufort seating orthosis: for trunk control in a severely disabled, sitting patient; a large bean bag full of polystyrene beads is molded to patient and then air evacuated to make a firm support.

corset front: cloth anteriorly attached to lateral uprights of spinal orthosis.

matrix seating system: for severely disabled patients; a seating system constructed from interlocking plastic components.

Milwaukee cervicothoracolumbosacral orthoses:

> *pelvic girdle:* custom-fitted section serving as foundation for orthosis.

> *superstructure:* two posterior and one anterior metal component connecting pelvic girdle and neck ring.

> *neck ring:* metal ring at neck that opens posteriorly for donning and doffing and serves as attachment for throat mold and occiput pads.

> *throat mold:* plastic or equivalent material, attached to neck ring and fitted to within 0.5 cm of throat and just below chin; limits anteroposterior motion.

> *occiput pads:* plastic or metal oblong disks fitted bilaterally to the inferior angle of the occiput bones of the head; aligned to provide slight distraction.

thoracic pad: floating pad attached to anterior and posterior uprights on same side as thoracic curve.

lumbar pad: firm foam or metal and leather incorporated into or attached near postero-superior edge of girdle on same side as thoracic curve.

axillary sling: axillary pad with webbing used to maintain alignment of neck ring.

shoulder ring: component fitted to axilla and over acromion; attached to the orthosis and used to depress an elevated shoulder.

perineal loops: straps passing between legs to reduce migration of spinal orthosis superiorly.

rotary control: modification of rigid spinal orthosis with lateral extension or sternal plate fitted bilaterally into the deltopectoral grooves to restrict rotation.

sternal attachment: component fitted to chest.

thoracic extension: component parts attached to cervical orthosis and fitted to the chest and back regions to provide increased control.

uprights: see Components and descriptions applicable to lower limb orthoses.

SHOE MODIFICATIONS

Shoe modifications are various alterations made in a shoe to complement the orthosis. On occasion, a shoe modification is prescribed by itself to correct a specific problem; for example, leg length discrepancy is treated by a shoe elevation on the shorter side, and valgus ankles may be treated with medial sole and heel wedging or medially flared heel.

orthopaedic oxford: a hard leather shoe with a leather or rubber sole; sometimes such a shoe has a steel shank (portion of shoe that lies between the floor of the shoe and the sole), with firmly constructed sides that support the foot in an upright position. This type of shoe is constructed uniformly, allowing for the addition of assistive devices.

surgical shoe or boot: a hard shoe that is constructed of thick walls, usually leather, with lacing designed to allow the shoe to be firmly tightened around the foot; generally used as part of an orthosis.

custom-molded shoes (space shoes): specially and individually constructed shoes designed to fit a patient with multiple foot deformities, as occur with rheumatoid arthritis.

Devices for Flatfeet

combined arch support: an interchangeable arch support that has both a tarsal (arch) component and a forward pad to support the metatarsal arch.

extended counter: a piece of leather extending from the inner back side of the shoe to the level of the arch, giving arch support.

medial heel wedge: small wedge of extra leather or rubber placed on the arch side of the heel.

plantar arch support: an interchangeable pad that helps support the tarsal arch.

scaphoid (navicular) pads: better known as *shoe cookies* or tarsal supports; inserted directly under the arch of the foot in the shoe.

Shaffer plate: arch support made of stainless steel; usually for adults.

Thomas heel: a heel with a curved extension for the arch side of the foot.

Whitman plate: arch support made of stainless steel; for growing feet.

Metatarsal Supports

metatarsal bars: an extra piece of rubber applied externally to the sole, providing support proximal to the metatarsal heads; used in treatment of callosities on the ball of the foot.

metatarsal pads: pads permanently placed in shoe just proximal to the ball of the foot.

metatarsal supports: interchangeable supports that have raised areas just proximal to the ball of the foot.

Devices for Insensitive Feet (Devascularized or Diabetic Neuropathies)

controlled ankle walker: plastic device incorporating a calf wrap and rigid ankle and foot plate to unweight the foot; to allow healing of an ulcer.

custom-molded shoes: see space shoes.

plastazote shoes: commercially available shoe(s) where upper is lined with plastazote as is the insole; to accommodate deformity or heel ulcers.

rocker sole modification: rigid sole attachment to reduce shear force of metatarsal heads and to prevent a healed ulcer from reulcerating.

Devices for Callosities

Budin splint: splint designed to relieve symptoms due to hammertoe deformity.

calcaneal spur pad: a heel with a special cutout center designed to redistribute the weight from a painful area of the heel.

heel pad: any soft pad inserted into the shoe to cushion the heel; used for tendonitis, heel spurs, Achilles bursitis, and similar conditions.

sole inserts: known by a variety of trade names, these inserts are made of foam rubber or other material and are designed to cushion the entire walking surface of the foot.

Special Shoes for Infants and Children

equinovarus outflare shoes: used in treatment of clubfoot condition.

normal last shoes: constructed with normal sole; term used to distinguish this from a reverse or straight last shoe.

reverse last shoes: look as if the left shoe were made for the right foot and vice versa; the side where the arch would normally be is curved out; used in treatment of clubfeet and metatarsus varus.

straight last shoes: look as if they could be worn on either foot, with a straight sole; used in treating mild forefoot problems such as metatarsus varus; incurring last.

tarsal pronator shoes: used in treatment of clubfoot condition.

torque heels: specially designed heels to make the foot turn in or out, depending on the direction of rubber slits that are arranged to cause torsion on weight bearing.

Chapter 8

Anatomy and Orthopaedic Surgery

Orthopaedic surgery is the branch of medicine that treats diseases and injuries and corrects and restores deformities of the musculoskeletal system. Surgery may be performed on bones and cartilage; muscles, tendons, and ligaments; synovia and bursa; fascia; and nerves of the upper and lower limbs, shoulder, spine, and pelvis. A general list of the types of surgery performed on these tissues is presented in Table 8–1.

Orthopaedic surgery encompasses an overwhelming number of procedures in an attempt to alter normal or abnormal anatomic structures. The five-volume *Campbell's Operative Orthopaedics* (Crenshaw AH: Campbell's operative orthopaedics, ed 9, St Louis, 1996, Mosby–Year Book, Inc) is one of the textbooks of this surgical specialty. Many of the new terms are briefly described in this chapter.

The anatomy of the musculoskeletal system is defined here to correlate with the surgery on specific tissue by anatomic area. Numerous figure illustrations are provided to enhance the understanding of anatomic structures. An associated surgical word list is included at the end of the chapter.

OSTEO- (BONE)

Anatomy of Bone

Osseous tissue (bone) constitutes the majority of the skeletal framework. It is living, hard connective tissue composed of organic (cells and matrix) and inorganic (mineral) components with submicroscopic laminations of protein and crystal layers. The matrix contains a framework of collagenous fibers that are impregnated with the mineral components, mainly in the form of apatite crystals, which give the quality of rigidity to bone. Another quality is its hematopoietic ability (i.e., to create and develop blood in the bone marrow).

If all the mineral were removed from bone, the resulting structure would be firm and pliable and have the exact shape of the mineralized bone. The process of **calcification** is not restricted to bones; it may occur in an amorphous form in tendons, bursae, and other tissues. **Ossification** is actual formation of bone tissue, which then calcifies by addition of hydroxyapatite crystals composed of calcium, phosphate, and hydroxyl ions. The following terms relate to the shape, structure, and microanatomy of bone (Fig. 8–1).

apophysis: a tubercle of bone that contributes to its growth but is the point of strong tendinous insertion rather than a part of the joint. It has no center of ossification.

articular cartilage: epiphyseal covering; thin layer of hyaline cartilage covering articular surface (ends) of bone to respond to shear forces.

bone marrow: an "organ" whose function is the manufacture (hematopoiesis) of the formed elements of blood, that is, red cells, white cells, and platelets, the most important material in the body. It is a network of connective tissue filled with blood vessels that form and develop blood corpuscles and is found in the proximal epiphyses of the humeri and femora, ribs and sternum,

TABLE 8–1.

Orthopaedic Procedures*

Prefixes/Roots: Tissue Types	Suffixes: Procedures
Osteo- (bone) 2, 4, 5, 6, 7, 8	1. -centesis: surgical puncture; perforation or tapping with aspirator, trocar, or needle
Myo- (muscle) 2, 3, 4, 5, 6, 7	
Tendo- or teno- (tendon) 3, 4, 5, 6, 7, 10	2. -clasis: surgical fracture or refracture of bones and other tissue by crushing; refracture of bone in malposition
Desmo- (ligament) 5	
Syndesmo- (ligament) 6, 7	3. -desis: binding, fixation by means of suture (tendon) or fusion (joints); not to include spine
Fascio- or fascia- (fibrous bands) 4, 5, 6, 7, 9	
Burs- (bursa, sac, pouch) 1, 4, 6, 9	4. -ectomy: excision of organ or part
Spondylo- (spine) 3, 6	5. orrhaphy: to suture or sew
Myelo- (spinal cord, meninges, bone marrow) 1, 5, 6, 9	
Lamin- (lamina) 4, 6	6. -otomy: surgical incision into a part or organ; cut into
Rachio- (spine) 1, 6	7. -plasty: to form, mold, or shape; surgical shaping or formation
Neur- (nerves) 4, 5, 6, 7, 10	
Arthro- (joint) 1, 2, 3, 4, 6, 7, 9, 10, 11	8. -synthesis: putting together, composition, surgical fastening of ends of fractured bones by sutures, rings, plates, or other mechanical means
Chondro- (cartilage) 2, 4, 6	
Synov- (synovium) 4	9. -gram: injection of contrast media for x-ray examination
Capsul- (capsule) 3, 4, 5, 6, 7	10. -lysis: dissolution of tissue; decomposition, freeing of scar or adhesions
Condyl- (condyle) 4, 6	
Aponeur- (fascial bands) 4, 5, 6	11. -oscopy: to view by a scope

*The left column (prefixes/roots) indicates the anatomy; corresponding numbers in the right column (suffixes) describe the types of surgery performed on those tissues.

and cancellous bone of vertebrae. Yellow bone marrow is found in the medullary cavity (in adults) and contains fatty marrow.

bone matrix: the intracellular substance of bone composed of osteocollagenous fibers embedded in an amorphous ground substance and inorganic salts.

calcium: a necessary mineral in combination with phosphorus to form calcium phosphate (apatite crystals), the dense, hard material of bones (and teeth); it is the most abundant mineral in the body and found in all organized tissues. Calcium is important in the function of muscles, nerves, blood coagulation, and heartbeat. Bones are a storage center for calcium.

FIG 8–1.
Composition of bone. (From Young CG, Barger JD: *Learning medical terminology step by step,* ed 3, St Louis, 1975, The CV Mosby Co.)

cambium layer: loose cellular inner layer of the periosteal tissue in the intramembranous ossification of bone.

canaliculus: communicating, narrow tubular channels between osteocytes in bone.

cancellous bone: spongy, porous, lattice-like tissue within midshaft of long bone.

condyle: prominence at the widened end of long bones and the attachment for ligaments, tendons, or muscles. Two examples are the femoral condyles, the inner and outer palpable prominences of the upper knee joint.

cortical (compact) bone: the thick outer portion of bone that surrounds the medullary (marrow) cavity.

cut-back zone: in growing bone, the zone just proximal to the epiphyseal growth plate, where the diameter of the bone is being cut back.

cutting cone: cone-appearing blood vessel as seen on longitudinal microscopic section; osteoclasts can be seen absorbing bone at the head of the cone.

diaphysis: the thick, compact, long mid-shaft of bone providing strong support.

enchondral bone: bone formed from cartilage, whether from the cartilage growth plate or from cartilage in fracture callus; **cartilage bone, substitution bone.**

endosteum: the lining of the trabecular and cortical bone that is within the medullary canal or cavity.

epiphyseal plate: the cartilage between the apophysis or epiphysis and the shaft of the bone. This cartilage is responsible for most of the longitudinal growth of the bone. Although the epiphyseal cartilage is called the growth plate, as in the previous definition, the term **epiphyseal cartilage** may also refer to the cartilage lining the joint; **growth plate, physis.**
  hypertrophic zone: zone where cells become larger.
  proliferating zone: zone of cell replication. Cells appear to be stacked like coins.
  provisional calcification: calcium appears in matrix, and beyond this point, invading blood vessels appear with bone cells on surface of calcified cartilage.
  resting zone: zone of cartilage cells with little metabolic activity and no cell division.

epiphysis: the bulbous growth end of a long bone, usually wider than the shaft and entirely cartilaginous or separated from the shaft by a cartilaginous disk. The epiphysis is a part of the bone formed from a secondary center of ossification at the ends of long bones, margins of flat bones, and at the tubercles and processes. During growth, the epiphyses are separated from the main portion of bone by cartilage, properly termed the **physis** or **epiphyseal plate.** There are two types of epiphyses:

pressure e.:   a secondary center of ossification in the articular end of a long bone with articular elements subjected to pressure.

traction e.:   a secondary center of ossification at the site of attachment of a tendon and subjected to traction. Contributes to bone shape (e.g., apophysis).

Other terms related to epiphyseal growth:

atavistic e.:   a bone that fuses naturally to another bone as in the coracoid process of the scapula.

punctum ossificationis: point of ossification (center) where bone begins to form in a specific bone or part; **ossification center.**

primary center of ossification: the first site where bone begins to form in the shaft; in a long bone, the diaphysis; **punctum ossificationis primarium.**

secondary center of ossification: a center of bone formation that appears later, on the joint side of a growth plate where the center of ossification is a part of bone that has a strong muscle attachment outside of the diaphysis; **punctum ossificationis secundarium.**

facet: a flat, platelike surface that acts as part of a joint; facets are seen in the vertebrae and in the subtalar joint of the ankle.

flat bones: bent or curved rather than flat, these bones protect viscera and other soft tissues and include the pelvis, ribs, and shoulder blade.

haversian canals: one of the minute canals running lengthwise in compact osteonal bone filled with blood vessels that are centrally enclosed and protected; part of an important system in transporting blood-borne material to widely sep-

arated bone cells. This transport system is comprised of the haversian canals, surrounding lamellae, connecting canaliculi, and lacunae. The lateral branches of these vessels are called **Volkmann canals.**

Howship lacuna: microscopic area of small depressions or grooves on the surface of bone where resorption of bone is occurring as a result of osteoclastic activity.

isthmus: narrow portion of the canal in the shaft of the bone.

lamellar bone: description of bone that, under a microscope, reveals a pattern of lamination.

line: a less prominent ridge on bone, for example, iliopectineal line; whereas, a crest is a ridge (iliac crest).

medullary canal: the canal in the center of a bone shaft containing soft, fatty marrow elements (in adults) and cancellous bone.

membranous bone: collagen model bone that is formed directly from the periosteum, without development of cartilage, and develops within a connective tissue membrane.

metaphysis: the wider portion of a long bone between the diaphysis, shaft, and the epiphysis. This portion of bone represents the most recently formed bone (growth zone) during the growth process. When fully developed, it is continuous with the epiphysis.

ossification: process of forming bone (ossifying, adj.). Other related terms include the following:

osseous: general term referring to bony matter.

ossiferous: implies that bone is being produced.

ossific: refers to the presence of bone.

osteoid: the uncalcified bony matrix (young bone).

osteoblast: a bone-forming cell; cells that produce osteoid, which is the matrix that is predominantly type I collagen and a number of bone proteins that then normally calcify with apatite crystals (hydroxyapatite).

osteoclast: bone-removing cell; these are cells derived from monocellular precursors, which under the influence of parathyroid hormone and other systemic and local substances; absorb bone in the form of multinucleated cells. The divot that is created in the bone is called a **Howship lacuna.**

osteocyte: bone cell; a living cell that has cell extensions called **canaliculi,** allowing the cell to affect the metabolism of the surrounding matrix. Osteocytes exist in both trabecular and cortical bone.

osteonal bone: a microscopic description of bone that is seen in mature adults and is composed of little tubes that look like stubby pieces of chalk, having an arteriole running down the middle. There are circular laminations of bone concentric with the artery. An **osteon** is a single unit and is barely visible to the eye.

periosteum: firm, thin, two-layered fibrous outer covering of bone; outer layer contains blood vessels; inner layer contains connective tissue cells and elastic fibers. The periosteum is important for circumferential bone growth and in bone repair because of its bone-forming cells and blood vessels that supply the osteogenic layer. The nerve endings in periosteum are responsible for the sensitivity of bone in trauma. The thin layer of multipotential cells that is immediately next to the bone is called the **cambium layer.**

sesamoid: denoting a small, round bone found in tendons (and some muscles), whose function is to increase movement in a joint by improving angle of approach of tendon into its insertion. The patella is the largest sesamoid bone in the body.

subchondral bone: bone directly under any cartilaginous surface.

trabecula: type of bone that is in small spicules, normally referred to as trabecular bone (**cancellous bone**); predominantly makes up the ends of long bones.

trabecular pattern: refers to the arrangement of the trabeculae of bone such that, when seen on radiographs or in cross-sections, there is a pattern of arches or other designs, like the spokes of a bicycle, providing the structural needs of the bone.

tubercle (small), tuberosity (large): rounded, elevated projection of bone giving attachment to a muscle or ligament; for example, ischial tuberosity or Lister's tubercle (dorsal, of radius).

Volkmann canals: found in osteonal bone; lateral passageways for transporting nutrients from the central haversian canals to bone cells (osteocytes).

woven bone: immature bone seen in very early growth and development, fracture healing, and some disease states. Also known as **wormian bone.**

> ***coarse woven bone (burlap bone):*** rapidly developing woven bone with coarse-appearing matrix.

> ***fine woven bone (linen bone):*** bone with smooth-appearing matrix but that is not lamellar.

General Surgery of Bone

bone marrow biopsy: surgical or local needle aspiration of bone marrow for microscopic inspection to determine the presence of disease affecting bone; that is, decreased cellular production or abnormal white blood cells (leukemia); usually drawn from superior iliac crest.

bone marrow transplant: a special procedure done (occasionally) in an effort to treat certain disease conditions of bone marrow. Diseased marrow is chemically destroyed and replaced (transfused) with healthy donor marrow of the same blood type. The transfused cells eventually matriculate to recipient's bone marrow where, if the transplant takes, they become established.

bone suture fixation: placement of a peg or screw device to affix a suture to bone for capsular, ligamentous, or tendon repair. Some commercial names include: TAG Wedge, STATAK, Mitek G2, Arthrex ESP, and TAG rod.

callotasis: for lengthening a bone; production of fracture and then gradual distraction using an external fixator.

closed reduction: nonsurgical manipulation of the fractured part, with return to proper position (called apposition) and alignment.

condylectomy: excision of a condyle at the joint; more specifically, removal of the round bony prominence of the articular end of bone.

condylotomy: surgical incision or division of a condyle or condyles.

corticotomy: complete transection of the cortex of a bone without transection of the intramedullary structures. This procedure is basically an osteotomy with care taken to preserve the intramedullary vessels.

diaphysectomy: removal of the shaft of bone, leaving the distal and proximal ends of bone intact.

diaplasis: reduction of a fracture or dislocation.

distraction osteogenesis: lengthening of bone with an external fixator to produce gradual distraction across growth plate.

ebonation: removal of fragments of bone from a wound.

epiphyseodesis: fusion of an epiphysis to the metaphysis of a bone by disruption of the growth plate (**epiphyseolysis**) or by metallic fixation between the epiphysis and metaphysis of bone. An **epiphyseolysis** may also occur traumatically.

fenestration: cutting a window in bone to allow drainage or access to an object covered by the bone, such as a tumor or foreign body.

open reduction: surgical incision and correction of a bone fracture under anesthesia; may or may not include internal fixation.

ostectomy: removal of a portion of bone.

osteoarthrotomy: the excision of the articular end of bone.

osteoclasis: surgical fracture or refracture of bone to bring about a change in alignment in cases of nonunion.

osteoplasty: surgical correction by shaping or formation of bone (osteorrhaphy).

osteosynthesis: surgical fixation of bone by the use of any internal mechanical means; usually done in the treatment of fractures.

periosteotomy (periostomy):   incision through the membranous covering of bone.

sequestrectomy: removal of a portion of dead bone.

synostosis: surgical fusion of any two or more bones that would otherwise be separated; may occur in a natural state as well.

Osteotomies

An osteotomy is a surgical procedure that changes the alignment of bone with or without removal of a portion of that bone. It may be considered for correction of a malaligned fracture, osteoarthritis, or other joint conditions. The following procedures are types of osteotomies.

Abbott and Gill: for bone growth asymmetry in lower limbs; a distal femoral and proximal tibial epiphyseodesis done through a medial approach. Also, proximal tibial and fibular epiphyseodesis through a lateral approach.

Amspacher and Messenbaugh: for cubitus varus with rotatory deformity of the elbow; correction of both deformities is with a distal humeral osteotomy.

Amstutz and Wilson: for congenital coxa vara.

Bailey and Dubow: for deformities of the femoral shaft; multiple osteotomies held by a telescoping intramedullary rod.

Baker and Hill: for heel valgus; lateral opening wedge osteotomy with bone allograft.

ball-and-socket o.:   dome-shaped osteotomy.

Bellemore and Barrett (modified French):   for varus deformity of elbow; lateral closing wedge osteotomy of distal humerus.

Blount: for bone growth asymmetry in the lower limbs; epiphyseal growth is arrested using staples across the growth plate.

Blount displacement o.:   for hip osteoarthritis.

Blundell Jones varus o.:   varus osteotomy of the hip for paralysis.

Borden and Gearen: for aseptic necrosis of the hip; an extracapsular transtrochanteric osteotomy.

Borden, Spencer, and Herndon: for coxa vara.

Brackett o.: ball-and-socket type for the fused hip.

Brett: of proximal tibia for genu recurvatum.

closing wedge o.: wedge cut out of bone, the open space closed, leaving a straight line.

Cole: anterior tarsal wedge for cavus deformity.

Cotton: for correction of a distal tibial deformity.

Coventry: a proximal tibial osteotomy for varus or valgus knees.

Crego: for femoral anteversion.

cuneiform: a cuneiform-shaped wedge cut in bone allowing for correction of deformities in two planes.

derotation o.: correction of rotational misalignment of a long bone.

dial o.: dome- or circular-shaped osteotomy.

Dickson: for malunion of the femoral neck.

Dimon: for intertrochanteric fractures; medial displacement of the distal fragment (**Dimon and Hughston**).

Dwyer: for clubfoot and pes cavus deformities; a lateral closing wedge osteotomy that reduces both the cavus and heel varus deformities.

Ferguson-Thompson-King-Moore o.: for long bone deformity such as malunion; a concave side resection of cortex with replacement after bone is made into chips, careful closure of the periosteum over the chips, and then closing wedge osteotomy on opposite side after sufficient callus formation has taken place.

Fish: for fixed slipped capital femoral epiphysis deformity; a cuneiform osteotomy at the base of the femoral head.

French: for cubitus varus (elbow); a closing wedge osteotomy.

Gant: open-wedge osteotomy for the fused hip.

Ganz o.: for adult acetabular dysplasia, a periacetabular osteotomy.

Ghormley: part of a hip fusion procedure.

Hass: for dislocation of the hip.

Ingram: for fusion of growth plate because of trauma; opening wedge osteotomy with concurrent insertion of fat at growth plate area.

innominate o.: of the pelvis for dislocation of the hip; two common types are **Pemberton** and **Salter.**

Irwin: for genu recurvatum; a posterior closing wedge osteotomy of the proximal tibia.

Kramer, Craig, and Noel: for fixed slipped capital femoral epiphysis deformity; osteotomy at base of femoral neck.

Langenskiöld: for fusion of growth plate; an excision of bony bridge across the epiphysis with insertion of fat. Also called coxa vara procedure.

Lorenz: for dislocation of the hip.

Lucas and Cottrell: notched rotation type of the proximal tibia.

Macewen and Shands: for congenital coxa vara.

Martin: for fixed slipped capital femoral epiphysis deformity; a closing wedge osteotomy at the base of femoral head and superior neck.

McKay: for stabilization of the hip in myelomeningocele; varus osteotomy of the proximal femur with transfer of adductors to the ischial tuberosity and external oblique muscles to the greater trochanter.

McMurray: for nonunion of the femoral neck.

Meyer-Burgdorff o.: for recurrent anterior dislocation of the shoulder; a proximal humeral osteotomy.

Moore: for long bone deformity such as a malunion; a three-quarter width wedge resection with replacement after bone is made into chips, careful closure of the periosteum over the chips, and then closed manipulation after sufficient callus formation.

Müller: for osteoarthritis of the hip; an inter-trochanteric varus osteotomy.

open-wedge o.:   straight cut made across the bone, creating angulation, and leaving an open wedge-shaped gap.

Osgood: for correction of malrotation of the femur.

Pauwels: for nonunion fracture of the femoral neck.

Pauwels-Y: for congenital coxa vara.

Phemister: for bone growth asymmetry in the lower limbs; a block of bone is fashioned at the growth plate and then rotated 90 degrees.

Platou: for femoral anteversion.

Pott eversion o.:   for correction of a distal tibial deformity.

Sarmiento: for intertrochanteric fractures; a wedge-shaped piece of bone is resected from the distal fragment to achieve a valgus osteotomy.

Sofield: multiple osteotomies of the tibia or femur for bowing deformities or nonunions.

Southwick: for slipped capital femoral epiphysis; a combination lateral and anterior trochanteric closing wedge osteotomy.

Speed: for malunion of the distal radius.

spike o.:   creation of a bony spike in a long bone to help hold the fixation of position.

Sugiuka o.:   for avascular necrosis of femoral head; the femoral head and neck are rotated to transpose the avascular area away from the weight-bearing portion of the joint.

Thompson telescoping V o.:   used in distal femoral deformities.

Weber: internal rotation osteotomy of the proximal humerus for recurrent dislocation associated with large posterior humeral head defect.

Whitman: closing wedge procedure for the fused hip.

Y-osteotomy: for cavus deformity of the foot; also referred to as **Japas osteotomy.**

Bone Grafts*

Bone grafts are used several hundred thousand times annually in the United States to aid in repair or reconstruction of the skeleton. The scope of applications is associated with congenital (skeletal hypoplasia, pseudarthrosis), developmental (scoliosis), traumatic (fractures, segmental loss), degenerative (osteoarthritis), and neoplastic (benign, malignant) disorders. Most bone grafts are autogenous, and their advantages include maximal biologic potential, histocompatibility, and no potential of transfer of disease from donor to recipient.

In general, bone grafts are removed from one site and transferred to another without direct reestablishment of the blood supply. Consequently, osteogenic cells fail to survive unless they receive sufficient nutrition by diffusion, a circumstance met only by those cells very close to the bone surface. These few surviving cells play an important role in initiation or augmentation of the early phase of bone graft incorporation.

Bone graft repair depends on local factors at and emanating from the recipient site, including ingrowth of new blood vessels and both specialized and multipotential cells required for resorption and new bone formation. The exception to dependence on local tissues occurs with immediate reanastomosis of the blood supply to the graft, often requiring microvascular techniques.

Today, tissue banks have become research centers for bone marrow, stem cell, and growth factor studies. Because all types of blood cells are produced in the bone marrow, research experiments are limitless. Bone marrow collection (harvesting) is still an important part of tissue banking, as is storage and type-matching of bone, tissue, and blood products, but greater emphasis is now being placed on biomedical research of tissue and bone marrow.

*Gary E. Friedlaender, MD, Professor and Chairman, Department of Orthopaedics and Rehabilitation. Yale University School of Medicine, New Haven, Connecticut.

General Terminology

histocompatibility: immunologic similarity or identity with respect to cell surface antigens determined by genes of the major histocompatibility complex. There can be varying degrees of histocompatibility, some consistent with successful transplantation and some incompatible with this approach unless accomplished with immunosuppression.

major histocompatibility complex: a sequence of genes that control expression of cell surface glycoproteins that are recognized as foreign when transferred into a genetically dissimilar host. Different terms are used to identify this gene complex, depending on the species, for example, human leukocyte antigen (HLA), histocompatibility-2 (H2) in mice, and rabbit leukocyte antigen (RLA).

immunosuppression: a term applied to any effort directed at lowering the body's natural immune response to foreign substances. Specifically, in transplant physiology, the use of specific chemicals to decrease the body's reaction to transplanted tissues from sources outside the body.

Nonspecific immunosuppression reduces host responses to most or all antigens and is usually caused by a systemic drug or chemical agent. Total body (or lymphoid) irradiation is another approach to nonspecific immunosuppression, useful in conjunction with bone marrow transplantation in humans and for a variety of investigational approaches in laboratory animals. Specific immunosuppression is targeted at a specific antigen or small group of related antigens, leaving responsiveness to most other foreign proteins intact. The use of monoclonal antibodies or induction of tolerance are forms of this selective approach.

implant: a synthetic device or the act of transferring into a host a synthetic device. Some include implants to reflect biologic material without cell viability.

transplant: a tissue or organ transferred from one site to another or the act of accomplishing this transfer. Some use this term to denote the transfer of viable tissue only (versus implant), and others use it to refer to any biologic material.

Classification by Species Source

allograft (allogeneic, formerly homograft): a tissue or organ transferred between genetically dissimilar members of the same species.

autograft (autogenous, autochthonous): a tissue or organ removed from one site and placed in another within the same individual.

isograft (isogeneic): a tissue or organ transplanted between genetically identical members of the same species. Synonymous with *syngraft* (**syngeneic**).

xenograft (xenogeneic, formerly heterograft): a tissue or organ transferred between species, for example, cow to human, rat to dog.

Special Procedures for Preserving Bone Grafts

Most grafts are subject to some form of long-term preservation. The most common approaches to storage include deep-freezing, freeze-drying (lyophilization), chemosterilization, and clinical extraction of proteins, or combinations of these techniques. The methods applied to long-term preservation have some impact on biologic, immunologic, and biomechanical properties, but these changes are predictable and often compatible with clinical success. Storage permits time for careful assessment of the donor graft material for potentially harmful transmissible diseases. Processing procedures may vary from one tissue bank to another. Graft material should be obtained from tissue banks that use strict processing procedures for allograft processing and donor procurement, under the guidelines of the American Association of Tissue Banks (AATB).

Some bone recovery methods are as follows:

AAA bone: a chemosterilized, autolysed antigen-extracted, and partially demineralized allogeneic preparation.

chemosterilized grafts: graft material rendered free of microbial organisms by exposure to a chemical, such as ethylene oxide, although thimerosal and alcohol have been used for bacteriostatic properties.

demineralized bone graft: one that has undergone extraction of minerals (superficially or completely) usually by exposure to hydrochloric acid.

freeze-dried grafts: the removal of water from tissue in a frozen state, the same as lyophilized. With respect to bone, usually reflects residual moisture being reduced to approximately 3% or less by weight. Tissues can be stored indefinitely at room temperature in evacuated, sealed containers until required for use. Moisture is then reconstituted by submerging the tissue in water (saline).

irradiation sterilized grafts: exposure of tissues to high-dose ionizing irradiation for the purpose of killing potential pathogens, requiring a dose between 1.5 and 5.0 megarad.

lyophilized grafts: same as freeze-dried grafts.

Revascularization of Grafts

The application of immediately revascularized *autografts* is limited by expendability of bone at the donor site, a discrete blood supply to the graft, vessels of sufficient caliber for repair (the fibula, ribs, and iliac crest represent the practical limitations), as well as microvascular expertise. This approach is especially well suited for recipient sites compromised by prior irradiation or infection, or where rapid repair is mandatory.

The incorporation of devitalized grafts occurs by a lengthy process analogous to "creeping substitution," in which the sequence of events includes revascularization of the bone, followed by resorption and new bone formation. Autografts transferred on a vascular pedicle or in which the blood flow is reestablished immediately by vascular anastomoses are incorporated rapidly by a process analogous to fracture repair.

In cases of bone *allografts,* immediate reanastomosis of blood supply is not clinically feasible because it engenders the same immunologic considerations encountered with viable solid organ transplantations, adding the requirement for substantial immunosuppression of the recipient. The following are related terms.

creeping substitution: the process by which a devascularized segment of bone in situ or a transferred bone without immediate reanastomosis of its blood supply undergoes repair, beginning with vascular invasion, followed by bone resorption and subsequent new bone formation (incorporation). This is a lengthy process that may take large cortical segments several years to incorporate, and even then, substantial portions of the graft may escape remodeling.

free-revascularized autograft: tissue transferred to a distant site along with its discrete blood supply such that direct reanastomosis of circulation can be accomplished immediately.

incorporation: a process by which recipient site factors grow into and remodel an initially devascularized bone graft. This includes invasion by blood vessels, resorption, and new bone formation. Often used interchangeably with creeping substitution with reference to grafts.

Classification of Grafts by Bone Type

cancellous g.:   a bone transplant consisting of cancellous (or medullary) tissue as opposed to cortical bone.

composite g.:   a transfer of more than one type of tissue simultaneously, such as bone and muscle transferred at the same time, or bone, muscle, and skin transferred simultaneously; must be accomplished in conjunction with reanastomosis of blood supply at the recipient site. This provides the potential advantage of repairing both bone and soft-tissue defects simultaneously.

cortical g.:   a transferred bone composed of the cortical (outer) tissue.

> **strut g.:**   cortical bone graft used to give mechanical support in the area of a cancellous bone graft.

corticocancellous g.: transferred bony tissue with both cortical and cancellous elements.

free g.: a bone graft freed of its vascular supply and soft tissue that would encumber its transfer from one location to another. This includes free revascularized autografts as well as other bone graft preparations.

intercalary g.: a segment of transferred bone without an articular surface; usually a portion of diaphysis or diaphysis plus metaphysis, with bone intercalated into bone to reestablish continuity.

intramedullary g.: graft placed in medullary canal. Also called medullary graft.

osteoarticular g.: bone graft containing an articular surface.

osteochondral g.: a transplant composed of both bone and cartilage (articular surface).

osteoperiosteal g.: bone graft taken complete with periosteal membrane coverings.

pedicle g.: tissue transferred to another site while retaining (at least temporarily) its required blood supply at the donor site, consequently limiting the distance over which a pedicle can be transferred. The recipient site vascularity can be transsected or interrupted following reestablishment of sufficient vascularity at the recipient site.

segmental g.: a portion of transferred tissue representing less than the entire anatomic part being replaced.

Classification by Shape and Bone Grafted

bone block: a bone graft that is inserted next to a joint to prevent a given direction of motion in that joint; also, a bone graft that is shaped in the form of a block and used for fusion of a joint.

chip g.: bone graft broken up into chips.

clothespin g.: coarsely shaped graft used in the spine; resembles a clothespin.

hemicylindric g.: graft cut into the shape of half a cylinder.

inlay g.: any graft that has been cut in a fusion procedure to fit the shape of the graft site.

diamond inlay: graft cut in a diamond shape with recipient site cut to receive that shape.

sliding inlay: a slot of bone cut and moved across the graft site, usually a fracture of a large bone.

massive sliding g.: large graft designed to slide when two portions of recipient bone are compressed.

morcellized g.: cortical and or cancellous bone graft that has been finely crushed before implanting.

onlay g.: graft laid directly onto the surface of recipient bone.

dual onlay g.: two strips of bone laid down on either side of the shaft.

peg g.: cylindric bone graft to be inserted into or through the medullary canal of a bone.

Eponymic Bone Graft Terms

Albee	Hey-Grooves-Kirk
Banks	Hoaglund
Boyd	Huntington
Campbell	Inclan
Codivilla	McMaster
Flanagan and Burem	Nicoli
Gillies	Phemister
Haldeman	Ryerson
Henderson	Soto-Hall
Henry	Wilson

Osteosyntheses: Internal Fixation Devices for Fracture Healing

Osteosynthesis is a surgical procedure that uses internal fixation devices, especially in the treatment of fractures. This procedure is referred to in context as open reduction and internal fixation (ORIF). It cannot be overemphasized how the orthopaedic surgeon must apply the principles of engineering to biology. The surgeon must be adept in using metal plates, nails, rods, pins, bands, screws, bolts, and staples in the correction of skeletal defects (Fig. 8–2). Pegging, pistoning, reefing, shelving, shaving down, shucking, doweling, and saucerization are a few of the shaping and engineering procedures applied within biologic

FIG 8–2.
Two internal fixation devices for hip fractures.

principles. The following internal fixation devices are used in orthopaedic surgery.

AO: abbreviation for designer of a variety of implant devices. The letters stand for *Arbeitsgemeinschaft für Osteosynthesefragen.*

ASIF: abbreviation for group that studies internal fixation systems and engineering. The letters stand for *Association for the Study of Internal Fixation.*

Asnis screw: for hip cervical fractures; a cannulated screw with reverse cutting thread.

Badgley nail: for hip fractures; an uncannulated triflanged nail with beveled proximal end that can be attached and inserted through a special side plate.

Bailey-Dubow nail: for osteogenesis imperfecta; an extensible intramedullary nail used in osteotomies.

Basile screw: for hip cervical fractures; a drill point tip screw with pronged washer to be placed over trochanter for compression.

Benoit-Gerrard: for hip fractures; a spring-loaded sliding nail plate with a proximal outside thread, smooth shaft, and a side plate; provides continuous compression.

biodegradable fixation: a variety of screws, pins, plates, and other fixation devices made of material that will be absorbed by the body. Such materials include *polyactide-glycolide copolymer (polyglactin 910).*

blade plate: general class of plate fixation devices that has a right-angle or nearly right-angle flange.

Blount plate: for fixation of hip fractures and for reconstructive procedures about the hip; a blade plate that can be bent easily to adjust to the correct shape and angle.

Blount staple: type of staple used around the knee.

Bohler nail: for hip fractures; a triflanged nail with potential use of a side plate.

Bohlman pin: for hip fractures; a threaded pin with a sharp point and smooth proximal portion.

bollard: a short, flat-headed, nail-like device that is slotted along a portion of the shaft, used in fixation of ligaments into bone.

Boyd side plate: to help stabilize trochanteric portion of hip fracture; a plate that could be placed over plate of a Jewett nail.

Brooker-Willis nail: for unstable femoral fractures; a femoral nail with distal locking screws.

Calandruccio device: a metallic device for pantalar fusions.

Calandruccio nail: for hip fractures; a sliding compression screw and plate associated with two to four smaller threaded pins through the plate and into the femoral head for extra fixation.

cancellous screw: used for trabecular problems near the joints, especially the hip.

cannulated nail/cannulated screw: general terms used for nails and screws that have a hole in the center. This hole can be used to direct the nail or screw over a guide wire.

Charnley screw: for intracapsular hip fractures and hip arthrodesis; a compression screw that slides into a barrel and attaches to a side plate.

cloverleaf nail: used in femoral shaft fractures.

Crawford-Adams pin: for hip fracture; use of small threaded pins.

cruciate screw: screw with cross-shaped head.

Delta nail: for femoral shaft fractures; a nearly triangular nail with interlocking screws.

Derby nail: for femoral shaft fracture; an intramedullary nail with wings that can be extended at the distal tip, and an antirotation washer at the proximal end.

Deyerle pin: for intracapsular hip fracture; thick, wide plate with multiple holes to permit the insertion of numerous pins parallel to one another.

dome plunger: device to facilitate injection of cement into femoral head for better fixation of sliding device.

Dooley nail: for intracapsular hip fractures; a modified Smith-Petersen nail that has an external groove around the base.

dynamic-compression plate (DCP): plate for fixation of long bone fractures and osteotomies, with plate fixation designed to allow for compression from muscle and weight-bearing forces.

dynamic hip screw (DHS): for hip fractures; a sliding screw and plate dvice.

Eggers plate and screw: used in long-bone fractures.

elastic stable intramedullary nailing (ESIN): for fixation of femoral fractures in children; insertion of a highly elastic intramedullary nail that allows early protected weight-bearing.

Elliott plate: a type of blade plate used mostly in distal femoral procedures.

encirclage: wiring or banding of bony fragments in the shaft of a bone.

Ender nail: intramedullary nail that is curved and can be used to fix intertrochanteric hip fractures through a small incision just above the knee joint; used in a condylocephalic technique.

exchange nailing: use of a larger nail after failure of fixation or union with a smaller nail.

Gamma nail: for hip fractures; a sling screw and plate device.

Gaenslen spikes: for intracapsular hip fractures; smooth spikes driven from a small incision of greater trochanter.

Garden screws: for intracapsular hip fracture; large cannulated screws usually used in pairs and inserted at varus and valgus angles.

Giebel blade plate: blade plate with two screws for fixation of proximal tibial osteotomy.

Godoy-Moreira stud-bolt: for intracapsular hip fracture; an early model compression screw with external flange and bolt.

Gore AO screw: AO cortical bone screw modified to affix a ligament replacement implant.

Gouffon pin: pointed, threaded pin used in the fixation of cervical neck fractures of the hip.

grommet: a short, flat, hollow cylinder with a head. The device fits over a screw that is considerably narrower than the inner portion of the grommet. Used for fixation of ligaments into bone.

Gross-Kemph nail: for unstable femoral shaft fractures; an interlocking nail system.

GSH (Green-Seligson-Henry) nail: for supracondylar fractures; nail inserted through intercondylar notch.

GSU nail: for distal intraarticular fracture of femur; a retrograde nail inserted through joint with nail fixed by transcortical screw.

Haboush universal nail: for intracapsular hip fractures; a fenestrated plate with a shallow "H" cross section; inserted into head and neck of femur, and outside portion bent down over lateral side of femur.

Hagie pin: used for femoral neck fractures.

Hansen pin: for intracapsular hip fractures; use of nonthreaded, wide pins.

Hansen-Street nail: used for larger bone fractures.

Hardinge expansion bolt: for intracapsular hip fractures; a hollow screw with expandable tip and short side plate for femur.

Harrington rod: used in spinal fixation for scoliosis and some fractures.

Harris nail: intramedullary nail system for intertrochanteric fractures.

Henderson lag screw: used for hip fractures.

Herbert screw: for wrist scaphoid fixation, a short screw threaded at both ends; also used in fixation of other small bone fractures or osteotomies such as bunion surgery.

Hessel/Nystrom pins: threaded pin for internal fixation of femoral neck fractures.

hex screw: hexagon head screw.

Higley side plate: for hip fractures; a side plate that could be attached superiorly for screw fixation into greater trochanter.

Holt nail: for hip fractures; a one-piece nail-plate combination, with plate fixed by Barr nuts and bolts.

hook-pin fixation: for femoral neck fractures; a hollow nail has internal hooked pins that can be deployed into the femoral head after introduction of the nail.

Howmedica compression screw: for hip fractures; wide compression screw with side plate and hexagonal shape to cross-section of shaft and barrel to prevent rotation.

Hubbard side plate: for hip fractures; a wide, long femoral side plate designed to be used with triflanged nail.

Huckstep nail: for osteotomy of femur with limb lengthening; a nail with holes for cross-screw fixation.

intramedullary nail: class of nails placed in medullary canal of long bones for midshaft fractures; includes Hansen-Street, Küntscher, Lottes, and Schneider.

Inyo nail: for fractures of the distal fibula, a tapered V-shaped nail made of malleable stainless steel.

Jewett nail: nail plate used in hip fractures.

Johansson nail: for hip fractures; a triflanged nail that is cannulated and similar to a Smith-Petersen nail.

Ken nail: 135-degree sliding nail plate used for hip fractures.

Kirschner wire (K-wire): small wire used for fixation or traction.

Klemm nail: for femoral shaft fractures; a clover-leaf intramedullary nail with provision for proximal and distal screws.

Knowles pin: used for hip fractures.

Küntscher nail (rod): original form was a cloverleaf-shaped nail for simple shaft fractures of the femur. Subsequent modifications are a curved V-shaped nail for valgus reductions of intracapsular hip fractures; a self-locking "Y" device for hip fractures where the hip nail has an open base for the passage of a cloverleaf intramedullary nail; and a device for unstable shaft fractures with interlocking proximal and distal screws.

Kurosaka screw: special screw designed for fixation of tendon attached to bone in ligament reconstruction.

lag screw: screw with threads at the tip only, used for compression.

Laing H-beam nail: for hip fractures; an H-shaped nail with an adjustable side angle plate.

Lane plate: plate for long-bone fixation.

Leinbach screw: long flexible screw, used often for olecranon fractures.

Lewis nail: intramedullary nail for metacarpal bone fixation.

limited-contact dynamic-compression plate (LC/DCP): plate for fixation of long bone fractures and osteotomies where there is only focal point of contact of the plate, with plate fixation designed to allow for compression from muscle and weight-bearing forces.

Lippman screw: for hip fractures; a threaded compression screw with a smooth shaft and threaded base with washer.

locked intramedullary osteosynthesis (LIFO): for unstable long bone fractures; a set of flexible 4 or 5 mm diameter pins with a device for proximal interlocking and fixation of two of the pins.

Lorenzo screw: bone fixation screw.

Lottes nail: used for tibial fractures.

Luck nail: several different designs for hip fractures; triflanged nail where the distal end has multiple perforations to cut off excess length, a proximal pointed nail that can accept a side plate, and a V-shaped nail-plate combination.

Lundholm screw: for hip fractures; compression screw with proximal washer and nut that could be used with or without side plate.

Mancini plate: for hip fractures; side plate with multiple-angled screw holes.

Martin screw: used in hip fractures.

Massie nail: 155-degree sliding nail used in hip fractures.

McLaughlin plate, screw: used in hip surgery.

Medoff sliding plate: for fixation of intertrochanteric and subtrochanteric femur fractures; plate is slotted to allow central portion to slide distally.

medullary rod: metallic device used in central shaft of bone.

Moe plate: for hip fractures; a long lateral plate over femoral shaft and greater trochanter fixed with multiple screws.

Moore plate (pin): used in hip surgery.

Morscher (AO-Morscher) plate: for anterior cervical fusion.

Müller plate: type of blade plate used in hip surgery.

Murphy nails: for early attempts at fixation of hip fractures; 8 to 12 penny nails inserted across fracture site.

nested nails: a general term for two nails placed side by side in the medullary canal of long bones.

Neufeld nail: for hip fractures in elderly; a V-shaped proximal end portion with short side plate.

Neufeld pin: for hip fractures; smooth rods with notches easily broken off to adjust length.

Ogden plate: for fixation of long-bone fractures associated with preexisting intramedullary devices such as rods or the stem of a prosthesis. Long metal plates have slots that are designed to accept encircling bands in locations where screws cannot be easily used.

olive wire: to help approximate a bone fragment in external skeletal fixation; a small olive-shaped expansion on a fixation wire can be pulled through the skin to the surface of the small fragment and brought against the main portion of bone.

Parham band: for oblique long-bone fractures; a metal band that can be tightened around the shaft of the bone to achieve fixation by compression.

Partridge band: for oblique long-bone fracture; a band with ribbed undersurface so that when band is tightened there might be less interference with periosteal and cortical blood flow.

PGP nail: a flexible nail used in intramedullary fixation of femoral fractures.

Phillips screw: any screw with a Phillips head.

Pidcock pin: for hip fractures; a small pin that could be passed through a hip nail and into the lateral cortex to prevent shortening.

Preston screw: for hip fractures; original screw and side plate device.

Pugh nail: 155-degree sliding nail used for hip fractures.

Putti screw: for hip fractures; a compression screw that can be attached to a flange and nut or to a Mancini plate.

Richard screw: for hip fractures; a sliding compression screw with side plate held by smaller screw to cortex.

Rush nail, rod, pin: used for major long-bone fractures.

Russell-Taylor nail: intramedullary nail for femur with slots for cross-screw fixation.

Rydell nails: for femoral neck fractures; a four-flanged spring-nail.

Sage rod: diamond-shaped rod used in forearm fractures.

Sarmiento nail: for hip fractures, an I-beam with side plate.

Schanz pins: for external skeletal fixators; screw fixation pins with proximal smooth surface for attachment to the fixation device.

Schneider nail, rod: used in femoral shaft fractures.

Seidel nail: for humeral fractures; a proximal and distal interlocking nail.

Sheffield rod: osteogenesis imperfecta; an extensible intramedullary nail used for osteotomies.

Sherman plate: used for long-bone fractures.

slide plate: used for long-bone fractures.

Smillie nail: small pin used for attachment of the osteochondral fragments in the knee.

Smith-Petersen nail: flanged nail used in hip surgery.

Smyth pin: for hip fracture; attachment of two different sized, nonparallel screws through a plate over the greater trochanter.

Steinmann pin: used in skeletal traction; of larger caliber than a K-wire.

Street medullary pin: used for large long-bone fractures.

Street nail: spit diamond nail for hip fixation.

Thompson nail: for nondisplaced intracapsular hip fractures; a Z-shaped nail.

Thornton nail: for femoral neck fractures; a three-flanged spring-nail.

tibial bolt: used for proximal and distal tibial fractures.

Tieman-Jewett nail: for hip fracture; a one-piece triflanged nail and side plate.

toggle: a small metallic cylinder with each end slightly larger than the center. Used by tying sutures around it to affix ligaments or tendons to bone.

Tronzo nail: triflanged nail used alone or with side plate.

True-Flex nail: for fixation of long bone fractures; fluted intramedullary rods.

Uppsala screw: for intracapsular hip fracture; multiple, wide, threaded screws.

Venable screw: original vitalium screw.

Veseley-Street nail: for femoral shaft fractures; a splitting of a diamond nail both distally and proximally.

Virgin screw: for hip fractures; a compression screw using a proximal washer and spring.

von Bahr screw: for femoral neck fracture; a pin threaded at the tip for multiple screw fixation.

Watson Jones nail: for hip fractures; a triflanged nail with a small proximal pin through the nail and into lateral cortex.

Weiss spring: spring device used in some spinal fusions, particularly spondylolisthesis.

Williams nail: for hip fractures; a modified Küntscher cloverleaf "Y" nail using a locking nut to secure fixation.

Williams rod: for pediatric osteogenesis imperfecta deformity or congenital pseudarthrosis of tibia; rod that is inserted through calcaneus into tibia after osteotomy.

Wilson plate: for spinal fusions.

Zickle nail: a curved 75- and 60-degree nail and screw device for femoral supracondylar fracture; or an intramedullary rod with transfixing nail for subtrochanteric fractures.

Zuelzer hook plate: commonly used in ankle fractures.

External Skeletal Fixation for Fractures

The use of external wires transfixed through bone to hold the position of a fracture is not new. Pins in plaster have been the usual method for holding bone fragments in proper position during the healing process. There has been increased use of multiple pins placed through one cortex or both cortices of bone and held by one external device. These external fixation devices are also known as **fixateurs** or **fixators.** This allows easy access to wounds, adjustment during the course of healing, and more functional use of limb involved. The devices used have increased in number and include the following.

Types by Configuration

Unilateral	Triangular
Bilateral	Semicircular
Quadrilateral	Circular

Types by Design and Manufacture

Ace-Colles	Kronner-ring
Ace-Fischer	Monticelli-Spinelli
Calandruccio	Murray

DeBasitiani   Orthofix
Denham   Rezaian
Four-bar   Roger Anderson
Ganz   Slatis
Hex-Fix   Sukhtian-Hughes
Hoffman   Videl-Adrey
Hoffman-Vital   Volkov-Oganesyan
Hughes   Wagner
Ikuta   Wasserstein
Ilizarov

Electric and Magnetic Stimulation of Fracture Healing

The use of direct electric currents and magnetic impulses in the treatment of fractures has been studied for the effect on fracture healing. In the past, the presence of nonunion (extended failure of fracture healing) has often required extensive surgical attention, including bone grafts. Electric and magnetic stimulation in treating fractures has been approved by the Food and Drug Administration for established nonunion of long bones.

capacitive coupling: application of high-frequency surface electrodes that create smaller currents that stimulate fracture healing.

direct electric stimulation: a procedure involving small voltage and amperage electric currents passed through electrodes placed immediately at the fracture site. The source of current is a battery placed external to the body or under the fat, similar to a cardiac pacemaker. For the external battery devices, the electrodes can be placed directly through the skin, eliminating the need for an incision. The limb involved is usually held in a cast.

magnetic stimulation: large magnetic coils applied externally and connected to a specific pulsating current. The home treatment device, used to control the magnetic field, is a small boxlike apparatus that is plugged into a standard 110-volt outlet; can be used up to 12 hours a day. As in electric stimulation, the affected limb is immobilized in a cast during the treatment period. Chapter 13, Musculoskeletal Research, provides more specific information on this modality of treatment (Fig 8–3).

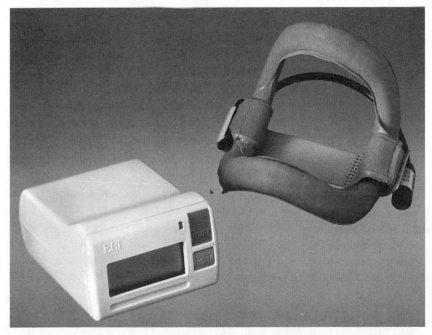

FIG 8–3.
Saddle-shaped coil signal generation device (Courtesy of EBI Medical Systems, Inc.)

Internal Prostheses

Numerous devices composed mostly of alloys and plastic have been developed to aid in joint replacement efforts. Prosthetic replacements are now available for almost every joint in the body, and even a spinal segment can now be replaced. This field continues to rapidly expand, with a constant influx of new components and the outdating of others. Therefore, some of the prostheses listed here may already be or soon will be obsolete. They are mentioned because they will still be found in some patients in the future and in their records. Chapter 13 discusses research efforts in internal prostheses.

The advent of a polymer called **methylmethacrylate** led to the development of new types of devices held firmly in place by polymers (glue). It is a cement-like substance that forms no chemical bonds but instead holds components to bones by space filling and locking effects. When applied, methylmethacrylate is soft and pliable, but it becomes very hard and firm within 15 minutes. Problems encountered with this method prompted further research and improvement in the development of joint resurfacing techniques. Although the use of methylmethacrylate is currently the preferred approach for joint replacement, new materials and methods are being researched. The various types of internal prostheses are presented here according to anatomic structure and area most subjected to the need for these devices.

Upper Limb Prostheses

Because of the special problems of fixation and the minimal occurrence of severe dysfunction in the upper limbs, there are fewer varieties of upper limb devices. However, there are total joint replacements for the shoulder (glenohumeral), elbow, wrist (including some individual carpal bones), and the fingers, including the metacarpophalangeal and interphalangeal joints. Following are the upper limb prostheses:

Bechtol p.:   for replacement of the glenohumeral joint.

biometric p.:   for replacement of interphalangeal and metacarpophalangeal joints.

Calnan-Nicole p.:   for metaphalangeal and interphalangeal joints.

capitellocondylar p.:   an unconstrained elbow prosthesis designed to allow greater supination and pronation.

Coonrad p.:   for wrist joints.

DANA (*D*esigned *A*fter *N*atural *A*natomy) total shoulder: a plastic component for glenoid associated with metallic-stemmed prosthesis for humerus.

de la Caffinière p.:   for thumb carpometacarpal joint replacement; a ball on shaft in metacarpal with plastic cup in greater multangular.

Eaton p.:   for trapezium bone replacement.

Flatt p.:   for metacarpophalangeal and interphalangeal joint replacements.

Gristina and Webb p.:   nonarticulated, semiconstrained shoulder prosthesis.

Hamas p.:   wth Silastic interface of the wrist.

Hunter rod: two-stage tendon graft procedure using a Silastic rod tendon prosthesis to preform canal for eventual transfer of tendon.

Kessler p.:   for carpometacarpal joint with a silicone arthroplasty.

Michael Reese p.:   replacement for shoulder joint involving an interlocking device.

Neer p.:   shoulder replacement prosthesis.

Niebauer p.:   for interphalangeal and metacarpophalangeal joint replacement.

Roper-Day p.:   an unconstrained metal on plastic shoulder replacement.

Smith p.:   Silastic prosthesis for interphalangeal and thumb joint replacement.

Swanson p.:   a silicone prosthesis used in the fingers, wrist, and radial head of the elbow; specifically, for the interphalangeal and metacarpophalangeal joints, the multangular, scaphoid, lunate, radial head, and great toe.

Volz p.: a single prong metal on plastic wrist prosthesis.

Elbow Prostheses

The classification of elbow prostheses is similar to that used for knee prostheses. They are generally categorized as constrained, semiconstrained, or unconstrained.

Unconstrained

Anatomic surface prosthesis	Lowe-Miller
	London
Capitellocondylar (Ewald)	Pritchard II
	Souter-Strathclyde
Ishizuki	Souter
Kudo	Wadsworth

Semiconstrained

AHSC (Arizona Health Science Center-Volz)	Pritchard-Walker
	Schlein
Coonrad	Tri-Axial
Mayo	

Constrained

Dee	Mazas
GSB (Gschwind, Scheir, and Bahler)	McKee
	Stanmore

Hip Prostheses

Straight Stem Femoral Components

These are now obsolete. The original effort to replace the hip joint was centered around femoral head replacement. One of the first femoral head components was made of acrylic attached to a metal stem (Judet). These became loose fairly rapidly, and as bone remodeling and response to stress became better understood, the devices were no longer used.

Single Femoral Component with Intramedullary Stem

It was found that there was longer fixation of the femoral head replacement if the stem was in the medullary canal. Although the cartilage on the acetabular side would often disappear over time, many of these prostheses lasted for years. Additionally, they were fairly easy to replace. These prostheses are still used in some cases for femoral head replacement in hip fractures.

Short Stem Prostheses

Bohlman	JEM Thompson
Judet	Townley-TARA
Roger Anderson	

Long Stem

Austin-Moore	Jewett
Bohlman	Matchett-Brown
Cathcart	McBride
d'Aubigne	McKeever-Collison
Dubinet	Michele
Eftekhar	Naden-Rieth
Eicher	Smith-Brown
Jaenicken and Collison	Thompson
Lippman	Valls
Jergesen	

Acetabular Side of the Hip

Cup Arthroplasty

A purposeful effort was made to stimulate the body to make new cartilage at the femoral head region. By removing the osteoarthritic surface of the femoral head and acetabulum, the cup would allow the raw exposed bony surface to form a covering of cartilage. This required extensive rehabilitative time and patient participation. It met with success in many instances.

Aufranc	Crawford-Adams	Smith-Peterson

Total Hip Replacement (THR) (Fig. 8–4)

The evolution of total hip replacement is a compliment to the efforts of biologists, clinicians, and engineers. As the concepts were tested and used, a very rapid evolution of new developments produced the subcategories of the total hip replacement. Both components are held by cement.

metal on metal: most original total hip replacements were made of metal. Fixation was secured by the use of methylmethacrylate to cement the two components in place. These prostheses had general success, but there were problems of stress fracture in the pelvis, loosening of the acetabular component, and metal fatigue.

Duff-Barclay and Scales	Ring
Gaenslen	Scarborough
McBride	Stanmore
McKee-Farrar	Urist

plastic on metal: metal wear was found to be one of the problems of the metal on metal total joint replacements. The introduction of plastic to replace the metal cup was found to give better wear characteristics. The incidence of stress fractures of the pelvis was less. Methylmethacrylate is used to secure the two components to bone.

Amstutz	Harris Design (HD two)
Amstutz (TR-28)	Howse
Aufranc-Turner	Johnston-Iowa hip
Buchholz	Ling (Exeter)
CAD	Mallory
Charnley	Matchett-Brown
Charnley-Müller	Müller
CHD	Murray and Welch-BDH
Calandruccio	Oh-Spectron
Clayton	Precision
CML	Proforma
Contour	Sarmiento (STH-2)
DF-80	Townley-horizontal
Eftkhar	platform
Freeman	Trapezoidal (T-28)
Gemini	Weller
Harris	Wilson-Burstein

metal-backed plastic on metal: the problems encountered with plastic on metal acetabular components included loosening of the acetabular component. Backing the plastic with metal seemed to protect against some of the abnormal forces and thus reduce the incidence of loosening. These metal on plastic components still require methylmethacrylate to achieve fixation.

Resurfacing Procedures

The purpose of research into resurfacing rather than replacement was to leave as much bone stock as possible. The effort that is required to remove a pre-existing total hip prosthesis often destroys a fair amount of surrounding bone. The advantage of the resurfacing procedure was that it did not require removal of the femoral head and placement of a stem with methylmethacrylate down the femoral canal. However, the acetabular cap was held with methylmethacrylate and the portion placed over the reshaped femoral head was also held with methylmethacrylate. The problem with this procedure has been an eventual loss of the femoral component because of absorption of bone. If the method did fail, replacement with other total hip devices was easier, with more bone available for fixation. Some of the techniques used are as follows:

Amstutz
Bicentric
Capello
Eicher
Freeman
Gerard
ICLH (Imperial College, London Hospital) double cup
Arthroplasty
Indiana conservative
Paltrinieri-Trentani
Salzer (uncemented ceramic double cup)
Sharrard-Trentani
TARA (*t*otal *a*rticular *r*eplacement *a*rthroplasty)
THARIES (*t*otal *h*ip *a*rticular *r*eplacement by *i*nternal *e*ccentric *s*hells)
Tillman
Wagner

Bipolar Total Hip Replacement

The bipolar total hip was designed to allow for some regeneration of the acetabular cartilage and two components of motion: one at the acetabular-prosthetic interface, and the other between the acetabular and femoral components. Although the femoral component is often fixed with methylmethacrylate, the acetabular component is not, making this a more conservative approach than the firmly fixed acetabular components. On the acetabular side, there is a plastic cup inserted into a metal cup.

Bateman	Hastings
Charnley-Hastings	Monk
Christiansen	Universal Femoral Head
Giliberty	Varikopf

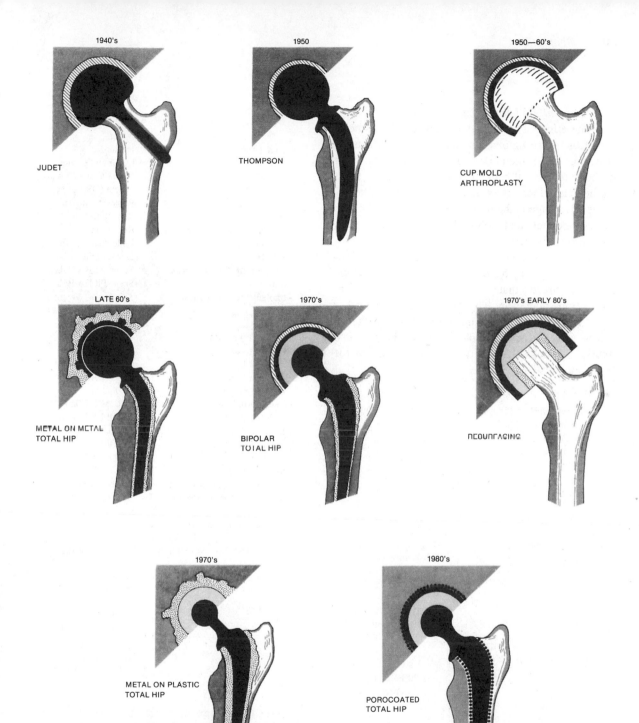

FIG 8–4.
Development of the total hip prosthesis with improvements in fixation and biological acceptance over a period of four decades. Lined areas are cartilage, grossly stippled areas are cement (methylmethacrylate), finely stippled areas are plastic, and solid black areas are metal. (Drawing by Frances Langley, USUHS.)

"Cementless" Total Hip Replacements

The effort of removing a "cemented" prosthesis can often be prodigious. Some of the early efforts involved complex metal acetabular components. With the advent of metal-backed plastic components, there has been a sudden influx of different designs. The obvious advantage is the relative ease in removal of the two components and the involvement of less bone in the removal process.

In some of the prostheses, a portion of the stem and metal cup may have a coat of scintered metallic beads or threads that produce a rough surface into which bone may grow. This is called **porocoating.**

All of the press fit and porocoated prosthetics can be used with cement. They also can be used in a hybrid fashion with one side of the joint fixed by the porocoat construct and the other by cement.

Press fit

Amstutz ATH (Anthropometric Total Hip)
Austin-Moore
Averill (normalize)
Bio-Fit
Callea and Lualdi-SCL
Capello
Corail
Deyerle-interlocking screws
Exeter-Femora
Freeman-high neck
Iowa
Itami
Jaffee
Judet
Macrofit
McCutchen
Mecring screw ring
Mittelmeier
Normalized
Norwich
Oh (Biofit)
Oh-Tifit
Osteonics
Phoenix
Precision Osteolock
Premier
Ring UPM
Self-bearing ceramic
S-ROM
Sivash
TriLock
TTAP (threaded titanium acetabular prosthesis)

Porous coated

Acetabular Cup System (ACS)
  ACS Gemini
  ACS Profile
  ACS Star
  AML Plus
  Tri-Lock
Anatomic
APR
  APR Current 1
  APR Current 2
APR Previous 1
APR Previous 2
ARC
Bias
Depuy AML (*anatomic medullary locking*)
Duraloc 100
Duraloc 300
Duraloc 400
Duraloc 500

Duraloc 1200
Duraloc Bantum
Duraloc Sector
Engh (AML)
Evolution
Flanged Revision
Gemini
Gustilo-Bias
Harris-Galante
Howmedica PCA (porocoating anatomic)
HP-Garches
Hungerford & Kenna-PCA
Impact
Implant Technology LSF
Index
Integral
Interseal Variant I
Interseal Variant II
Interseal Variant III
Interseal Variant IV
Lord-Madreporique
Lunceford, Engh and Pilliar-AML
Mallory-Head I
Mallory-Head II
McCutchen
Mecron Ring
Modular Acetabular Reconstruction System (MARS)
Omnifit
Omnifit Dual Geometry Microstructured
Omnifit PSL Microstructured
Omniflex
Opti-Fix
Opti-Fix I
Opti-Fix II
PCA
PCA Cluster
  PCA Original
  PCA Standard
Perfecta I
Perfecta II
Peri-Loc
Pilliar
Profile
Quadrant Sparing Acetabular Component (QSAC)
Ranawat/Burstein
Reflection I
Reflection V
Reflection Interfit
Roy-Camille
Secur-Fit HA PSL
Secur-Fit HA PSL X'tra Solution
S-ROM (Sivash Range of Motion)
S-ROM Arthropor I
S-ROM Arthropor II
S-ROM Arthropor III
S-ROM Arthropor Oblong
S-ROM-LS (long stem)
S-ROM-PS (primary stem)
S-ROM Super Cup
S-ROM ZZT I
S-ROM ZZT II
System 12 Osteolock
System 12 Osteolock HA
System 12 Vistalock Cluster
System 12 Vistalock Solid Back
Target
Townley
TriLock
Trilogy
Tronzo
Universal I
Universal II
Whitesides-Ortholoc

Recently, a number of prostheses have been developed to be used specifically with cement. These include:

Bantum CDH
CPT (collarless, polished, tapered)
Centraline
Exeter
VerSys

Special Hip Prosthesis

Prosthesis of antibiotic-loaded acrylic cement (PROSTALAC): facsimile of a total hip prosthesis that has a very thin polyethylene acetabular cup that is loosely cemented.

Salvage Hip Procedures

A number of custom-made devices are available for prosthetic replacement of massive acetabular and femoral bone loss. This bone loss may be a residual of prior surgical procedures or an attempt to eradicate tumors.

Kotz modular femur and tibia resection system (KMFTR): for resection of a large portion of bone about the knee joint; usually tumor resection with joint replacement; system involves interlocking section of various sizes.

saddle prosthesis: for hip replacement in circumstances where there is severe acetabular deformity; a saddle-shaped acetabular component with matching femoral component replaces hip.

Modular and Other Components

With advances in both total hip and total knee replacement, there have also been advances in the replacement of these devices. This challenging branch of orthopaedics had led to the development of interchangeable components referred to as **modular prosthetics.** Some terms referable to the various components and constructs of those components are listed below.

keel: portion of the tibial tray that has flanges that extend into the tibial metaphysis.

taper: rounded top of the femoral stem component; designed as a slightly tapered cylinder that will accept a similarly "female" shaped portion of the femoral head, which come in various sizes.

Eurotaper (12/14): taper designed with a 12-mm tip and 14-mm base.

Morse taper: specific type of taper used to accept femoral head component on the stem component.

Knee Prostheses (Fig. 8–5)

Knee prostheses are designed to replace portions or all of the knee joint. The original attempts involved solid metal to replace one side or the other of the joint. Metal with plastic interfacing, better joint mechanical design, and superior attention to detail in surgical applications have improved the relative success of knee joint replacements.

The total knee devices are listed in categories based on the degree of constraint of knee motion, that is, stability.

FIG 8–5.
Total knee prosthesis showing accumulated wear that occurred over years of use. (Courtesy of the Orthopaedic Research Laboratory, Good Samaritan Medical Center, West Palm Beach, Florida.)

unicompartmental: The unicompartmental design has evolved into a metal unicondylar component for the femur making contact with a plastic or plastic on metal tibial component. There are few patients for whom this limited procedure is appropriate. Some unicompartmental devices include:

Charnley	Manchester
Compartmental II	Modular
Geomedic (unilateral)	Oxford-meniscal
Gunston-Hult	PCA (unicompartmental)
Lotus	Robert Brigham
Lund prototype	Sevastano
MacIntosh	St. Georg sledge

bicompartmental replacement: The medial and lateral side of the joint is replaced but there is no patellar resurfacing. The breakdown of the patellar mechanism resulted in a disuse of this design.

tricompartmental: Most knee replacements entail a design that replaces both tibial-femoral surfaces as well as the patella. There are three basic categories: constrained, semiconstrained, and unconstrained.

fully constrained: The prostheses are not necessarily totally constrained. They include pure hinges, some rotating hinges, and nonhinged linked prostheses. The term **fully constrained** implies no motion and actually denotes a block of anteroposterior shifting on lateral motion. Because there is restriction in at least one plane of motion, there are forces that produce high stresses on the bone. These devices are more likely to become loose as the bone breaks down or the prosthesis itself fails. Some "fully" constrained prostheses include:

Attenborough	Stanmore
Blauth	Noiles
Constrained condylar knee (CCK)	St Georg
Endo-Model	Sheehan
Guepar	Shiers
Herbert	Spherocentric
Kenematic	Total condylar III (TC-III, TCP III)
Lacey	Walldius

semiconstrained: the degree of constraint ranges from minimal to nearly full in any given plane. This is the design of many of the current prostheses.

Cintor	LCS rotating platform (LCS rp)
Insall/Burstein	
Kinematic II	LCS substituting
Kinematic stabilizer	LCS universal APG
Low contact stress (LCS)	Robert Brigham
LCS meniscal bearing (LCS mb)	Stabilocondylar
	Total condylar (HSS)
	Whiteside

unconstrained: the most minimally constrained prosthetics with the maximal freedom of motion of the knee joint. These devices require good soft-tissue stability.

Advantim	Lubinus
AMK	Marmor
Apollo	Miller-Gallante (MG)
Anametric	Miller Gallante II
Buckholz	Modular
Cloutier	Multiradius
Concensus	Natural-knee
Continuum	NK II ultra congruent
Cruciate condylar	Ortholoc
Deane	Ortholoc II
Duocondylar	Ortholoc modular
Duopatellar	PCA
Eriksson	PFC Σ curved
Foundation	Polycentric
Freeman-Swanson	RAM
Geomedic	RMC
Geotibial retainer	Ring
Gunston	Sevastano
Gustuilo	SKI
Herbert	Synatomic
ICLH	TCCK
Johnson-Elloy accord	Townley
Kinematic	Tricon-M
Kinemax	UCI (Waugh)
LAI (Charney)	Wright
Liverpool	YIS

Patellar Implant Designs

For total knee arthroplasty, the patellar replacement can be one of three basic designs:

simple button: circular, shallow, plastic dome device that may be with or without metal backing.

fixed anatomic: anatomically shaped piece of plastic on metal backing.

rotating: an anatomically shaped piece of plastic that is attached to a metal backing in such a way that the plastic can rotate during knee motion.

There are patellar implants designed to function without replacement of other portions of the joint.

McKeever patellar resurfacing: a metallic device shaped with a medial and lateral facet.

Ankle Prostheses

The forces acting on the ankle are biplanar, yet by design, the prosthetics are monoplanar. With the highly active forces that exist across the ankle joint, there are fewer occasions for replacement of that joint. Prosthetic fixation is not as secure for these lower limb joint replacements, with loosening a continuing problem. Some replacements include the following:

Conaxial	Oregon
Conoidal	Oregon Poly II
ICLH	St Georg-Buckholz
Mayo	Smith
Newton	TPR
Odland	

ARTHRO- (JOINTS)
Anatomy of Joints (Fig. 8–6)

bursa sac: helps tendons and muscles to glide easily over bones at the joint outside the synovial fluid.

capsule: the general fibrous and ligamentous tissues that act as encasements and enclose the immediate joint area.

cartilage: the strong smooth covering at the ends of the articular surface of bone. In highly mobile joints like the wrist, fingers, and elbows this cartilage is called *hyaline*. In less mobile segments, such as the intervertebral disk, *fibrocartilage* is present.

meniscus: in the knee, a crescent-shaped fibrocartilaginous disk between the two joint surfaces. There are other menisci and meniscal-like structures in the body. The medial and lateral menisci of the knee receive the most surgical attention.

subchondral bone: named for the bone immediately next to the joint cartilage. Also called **subchondral plate.**

synovium: inner lining of a joint cavity that is a one- or two-layer cell membrane (*synovial membrane*) on a bed of fat. The synovial membrane normally produces and absorbs a clear sy-

Joint capsule
Synovial membrane
Joint cavity
Articular surfaces

FIG 8–6.
Typical structure of diarthrotic joint. (From Hilt NE, Cogburn SB: *Manual of orthopedics,* St Louis, 1980, The CV Mosby Co.)

novial fluid, which lubricates and feeds cartilage surfaces.

Types of Joints

Joints are the places of union between two or more bones. All joints are not alike in structure and fall into the following categories according to function.

ball-and-socket j.:   main points of articulation; femur to acetabulum of hip, humerus to glenoid of shoulder.

hinge j.:   located in the elbows, fingers, and knees.

immovable j.:   of orthopaedic concern, in the symphysis pubis and sacroiliac region.

synovial j.:   two bones connected by fibrous tissue (capsules) with space between them and lined with synovial membrane.

weight-bearing j.:   located in the lower spine, hips, knees, and ankles.

General Surgery of Joints

arthrectomy: excision of a joint.

arthrocentesis: needle puncture and aspiration of fluid from a joint.

arthroclasis: surgical breaking down of an ankylosis to secure free movement of a joint.

arthrodesis: a procedure to remove the cartilage of any joint to encourage bones of that joint to fuse, or grow together, where motion is not desired, for example, the spine. Also, an external fusion of a joint by means of a bone graft. The many types of arthrodeses are listed separately.

arthroereisis: a procedure to limit abnormal motion in a joint. Could be in any joint, but frequently referred to in the foot.

arthrogram: radiographic examination of the joint performed with radiopaque solution; commonly done on the shoulder, hip, and knee joints.

arthrokleisis: ankylosis of a joint by closure; production of such ankylosis.

arthrolysis: loosening adhesions in an akylosed joint to restore mobility.

arthroplasty: reconstructive surgery of a joint or joints to restore motion because of ankylosis or trauma or to prevent excessive motion. This repair and reconstruction may use silicone, metallic, or other implants.

arthroscopy (arthroendoscopy) (Fig. 8–7): a surgical examination of the interior of a joint and evaluation of joint disease by the insertion of an optic device capable of providing an external view of the internal joint area. This technique represents a major advance in orthopaedic technology during the past two decades. The optical system is fiberoptic, giving the surgeon a high-

FIG 8–7.
Arthroscope outside of sleeve that is used during surgery; close-up view of 30-degree angle for viewing difficult to see areas. (Wide-Angle Arthroscope, 4-mm diameter, 30-degree angle optic. Courtesy of Arthrex, Inc., Naples, Florida.)

resolution view of a joint, anywhere from a direct forward view to a view at 70 degrees to the end of the microscope, allowing the surgeon literally to see around corners. The arthroscopes vary in diameter from 2.7 to 5.0 mm. Miniature television cameras are attached directly to the arthroscope, allowing all operating room personnel to view the interior joint.

With the advancement of arthroscopic surgery, a wide variety of instruments has made it possible to remove synovium and plicas, repair peripheral tears, excise meniscal tissue, remove loose bodies, shave cartilage, and do many other procedures. The knee receives the most attention in arthroscopic procedures; however, the arthroscope is now used in ankle, shoulder, elbow, wrist, and other joint surgery.

arthrotomy: surgical incision into a joint for exploration and removal of joint material; usually refers to knee exploration but can apply to any joint.

arthroxesis: scraping of diseased tissue from the articular surface of bone.

Arthrodeses

Three Basic Categories of Arthrodeses

compression: a general class of arthrodeses in which the pins on either side of the joint have some external compression device; the appliance is removed after fusion takes place.

extraarticular: fusion of the joint outside the joint capsule; rarely used.

intraarticular: fusion of a joint all within its capsule, with or without intraarticular bone grafts.

Specific Arthrodeses

Abbott-Fisher-Lucas: two-stage hip fusion that includes a delayed femoral osteotomy.

Baciu and Filibiu: intraarticular ankle fusion using dowel bone graft taken from the joint to include the medial and a portion of the lateral malleolus. The graft is rotated 90 degrees and reinserted.

Badgley: intraarticular and extraarticular hip fusion, using anterior iliac crest of bone.

Blair: a tibiotalar fusion, using an anterior sliding tibial graft.

Bosworth: a method of fusing the hip following tuberculosis infection.

Brett: extraarticular shoulder fusion, using tibial graft.

Brittain: four procedures have this name: (1) intraarticular knee fusion using anterior tibial grafts, (2) extraarticular hip fusion requiring a subtrochanteric osteotomy and tibial bone graft, (3) extraarticular graft to the medial side of the humerus of shoulder, and (4) intraarticular fusion of the elbow, using two crossed intraosseous grafts.

Campbell: extraarticular fusion of the ankle and subtalar joint.

Chandler: intraarticular and extraarticular hip fusion, using the deep portion of the greater trochanter.

Charnley: intraarticular type of ankle or knee fusion, using a temporary metallic external compression clamp.

Charnley and Henderson: intraarticular and extraarticular fusion of the shoulder, using the glenoid and acromial surface abutting a split humeral head.

Chuinard and Petersen: of the ankle, using a wedge of iliac bone.

Compere and Thompson fusion: intraarticular hip fusion, using iliac crest and wing for bone graft.

Davis: intraarticular and extraarticular hip fusion, accomplished by using a live pedicle of iliac crest.

Ghormley: intraarticular and extraarticular hip fusion, using anterior iliac crest graft.

Gill: extraarticular and intraarticular fusion, using acromion bone graft from and to the shoulder.

Henderson: intraarticular and extraarticular hip fusion, using detached iliac cortical bone graft.

Hibbs: intraarticular and extraarticular hip fusion, using greater trochanter as a graft.

Horwitz and Adams: ankle fusion, using the distal fibula as a graft.

Key: knee fusion, using anterior inlay bone graft.

Kickaldy and Willis: intraarticular and extraarticular hip fusion, using iliac crest bone from the ischium to the inferior neck.

King procedure: intraarticular hip fusion, using iliac and tibial bone grafts.

Kuntscher modified: knee arthrodesis, using a bridging intramedullary rod.

Lucas and Murray: knee fusion, using patella for bone graft and held by an internal plate.

Marcus, Balourdas, Heiple: chevron-shaped tibiotalar fusion, using inlay graft taken from medial and lateral malleolus.

Müller: intraarticular shoulder fusion, using bent plates for fixation.

Potter: knee fusion, using a retrograde tibial rod and graft from the distal tibia.

Putti: (1) knee fusion, using anterior tibial graft; (2) extraarticular fusion, using the acromion of the scapula; (3) an intraarticular fusion of the shoulder.

Schneider: intraarticular hip fusion, using innominate osteotomy with greater trochanter for a bone graft.

sliding: anterior ankle fusion, using tibial bone.

Smith-Petersen: technique for fusion of the sacroiliac joint.

Stamm procedure: intraarticular hip fusion, using free iliac crest bone grafts.

Staples: intraosseous and extraosseous elbow fusion.

Steindler: intraarticular fusion of the shoulder or the elbow, using posterior bone graft.

Stewart and Harley procedure: for fusion of ankle, using lateral and medial malleoli as grafts.

Stone: intraarticular hip fusion, using a split acetabulum and bent plate from the ilium to the femoral neck.

Trumble: extraarticular hip fusion, using a tibial graft from the ischium to the femur.

Watson-Jones: intraarticular and extraarticular hip fusion, using a nail and iliac crest graft; also, a shoulder fusion, using a piece of acromion.

White: intraarticular hip arthrodesis, using posterolateral approach and iliac bone graft.

Wilson procedure: extraarticular fusion of the elbow.

Wolf blade plate: ankle arthrodesis performed with a specifically designed blade plate internal fixation device.

John C. Wilson: intraarticular and extraarticular hip fusion, using an iliac side graft.

Chondro- (Cartilage)

Cartilage (L. gristle) is a fine, glistening, resilient, *nonvascular fibrous connective* tissue that absorbs shock and facilitates the mechanics of joint motion. All mobile joint surfaces contain cartilage. *Perichondrium* is a connective tissue that covers cartilage in some places. Cartilage cells (*chondrocytes*) are widely separated and surrounded by matrix, also (*chondromucoid*) known as ground substance, composed of collagen and mucopolysaccharides. In the embryo, cartilage forms the temporary skeleton and is important to growth in providing the model in which most of the bones develop. Then, it is called ossifying or precursory cartilage.

Cartilage cannot be seen on radiographs; if open space is apparent between two bones on radiography, cartilage is present. However, if the radiograph shows two bones touching at a joint, such as the femur on the tibia, osteoarthritis and dissolution of the cartilage in that joint may have occurred.

Types of Cartilage

articular c.:   thin layer of hyaline cartilage on articular surface of bones in synovial joints; **arthrodial c.**

calcified c.:   in which granules of calcium phosphate and calcium carbonate are deposited in interstitial substance.

cellular c.: composed almost entirely of cells with little interstitial substances.

connecting c.: connects surfaces of an immovable joint; **interosseous c.**

diarthrodial c.: articular c.

elastic c.: yellow opaque flexible substance (more so than hyaline) where cells are surrounded by a territorial capsular matrix, outside of which is an interterritorial matrix containing elastic fiber networks, collagen fibers, and ground substance; **reticular c., yellow c.**

fibrocartilage: contains visible collagenic fibers with a strongly basophilic ground substance in area of chondrocytes.

floating c.: detached piece of cartilage on medial or lateral condyle of femur or on patella.

hyaline c.: somewhat elastic, semitransparent cartilage, characterized by type II collagen and proteoglycan aggrecans. Seen in movable joint surfaces and the physis (growth plate).

Surgical Procedures on Cartilage

chondrectomy: surgical removal of cartilage.

chondrodiatasis: for limb-length discrepancy; closed, gradual and progressive distraction of the growth plate by using an external bone fixation device.

chondroplasty: plastic surgery on cartilage by repair of lacerated or displaced cartilage.

chondrosternoplasty: surgical correction of funnel chest.

chondrotomy: dissection or surgical division of cartilage.

synchondrotomy: incision and division of an articulation that has no appreciable mobility and in which cartilage is the intervening connective tissue.

Capsulo- (Capsule)

A capsule is the circumferential sleeve surrounding a joint composed of a tough band of fibrous and ligamentous tissues. It may be referred to as a joint capsule or a capsular ligament.

Surgical Procedures on the Capsule

capsulectomy: excision of a joint capsule; most commonly done on the hip.

capsulodesis: imbrication of a capsule (see Chapter 10).

capsuloplasty: plastic surgery on a joint capsule.

capsulorrhaphy: suturing of a joint capsule. If used by itself, the term implies a procedure on the shoulder (glenohumeral joint) because this joint commonly has soft-tissue reconstructions.

capsulotomy: incision into a joint capsule; **capsotomy.**

Bursae

A bursa (sac or saclike cavity) is filled with viscid fluid and situated in places in tissue where friction would otherwise develop. Bursae act as cushions, relieving pressure between moving parts such as an **anserine bursa,** a goose-foot sac found between tendons of the sartorius, gracilis, and semitendinous muscles and the tibial collateral ligament. A bursal sac is easily recognized during surgery and is involved in only three procedures.

bursectomy: excision of a bursa.

bursocentesis: puncture and removal of fluid from a bursa.

bursotomy: incision into a bursa.

OTHER SPECIFIC TISSUE(S)

The entire musculoskeletal system is made up of connective tissues, that is, cell elements that establish structure and shape. Bones and joints receive the most attention in orthopaedic surgery and therefore are listed separately.

All connective tissues have, to some degree, cohesion that is supplied by a protein structure called

collagen. Collagen, in its most familiar form, is a household product, gelatin. However, when combined with other chemical and cell elements, it is the basic molecular matrix of bone, cartilage, tendons, and many other tissues. The connective tissue cells are the following.

adipose tissue: fatty tissue.

chondroblasts: cells that form cartilage.

chondroclasts: cells that remove cartilage.

chondrocytes: cartilage cells.

fibroblasts: cells that predominantly form collagen.

fibrocytes: cells seen in tendons, ligaments, and similar structures.

histiocytes: cells involved in removal of cellular or chemical debris; a type of phagocyte.

myoblasts: muscle-forming cells.

myocytes: muscle cells, voluntary (striated) and involuntary (nonstriated).

Myo- (Muscle) (Fig. 8–8)

Muscle is the contractile tissue essential for skeletal support and movement. The anatomic features of muscles with associated tissues and surgery are presented here.

Muscle fibers are composed of small bundles of cells combined to form distinct muscular units. Terms often related to muscle include actin, myocin, sarcomere, nerve spindle, motor unit, neuromuscular junction, and spindle cell.

The smooth coordinated way in which muscles work together in the execution of a movement is called **synergy** (syn- [together] plus ergon- [work]). In particular, the muscles that play the part of **synergists** during any particular movement are concerned with obviating any unwanted movement that might result from the action of the **prime movers** or **agonists.** Synergist muscles are usually classified as **corrective** if they obviate such unwanted movements, and **fixative** if they fix the point proximal to that at which the movement is taking place. **Muscle inser-**

tion is the attachment of a muscle or its tendon to the part of the skeleton that the muscle moves when it contracts. **Muscle origin** is a fixed attachment or anchor of muscle allowing a muscle to exert power when it contracts. The many muscle groups are named and illustrated in Fig. 8–8.

Surgical Procedures on Muscles

myectomy: excision of a portion of muscle.

myoclasis: intentional crushing of muscle; rare.

myomectomy (myomatectomy):   surgical removal of tumors with muscular tissue components (myoma).

myoneurectomy: surgical interruption of nerve fibers supplying specific muscles; used for patients with cerebral palsy.

myoplasty: plastic surgery on muscle in which portions of partly detached muscle are used for correction of defects or deformities.

myorrhaphy (myosuture):   muscle repair by suturation of divided muscle.

myotenontoplasty: surgical fixation of muscles and tendons.

myotenotomy: surgical division of a tendon from muscle.

myotomy: incision or dissection of muscle or muscular tissue.

Aponeuroses

Aponeurosis is the name given to the end of a muscle that becomes a tendon. This muscular component is a white, flattened, ribbon-like tendinous expansion that connects muscle with the parts it moves.

Surgical Procedures on Aponeuroses

aponeurectomy: excision of the aponeurosis.

aponeurorrhaphy: repair and suture of muscle and tendon; **fasciorrhaphy.**

aponeurotomy: surgical incision into the aponeurosis.

Cranial muscles

Facial muscles

Sternocleidomastoideus

Trapezius

Deltoideus

Pectoralis major

Biceps brachii

Serratus anterior

Linea alba

Rectus abdominis

Extensors of wrist and fingers

Flexors of wrist and fingers

Adductors of thigh

Obliquus externus

Tensor fasciae latae

Flexor retinaculum

A

Vastus lateralis

Sartorius

Rectus femoris

Vastus medialis

Patella

Patellar tendon

Gastrocnemius

Tibialis anterior

Extensor digitorum longus

Peroneus longus

Soleus

Peroneus brevis

Extensor hallucis longus tendon

Superior extensor retinaculum

ANTERIOR VIEW

FIG 8–8.

Muscular system. **A,** Anterior view. **B** (on page 220), Posterior view. (From *Mosby's medical and nursing dictionary,* ed 2, St Louis, 1986, The CV Mosby Co.)

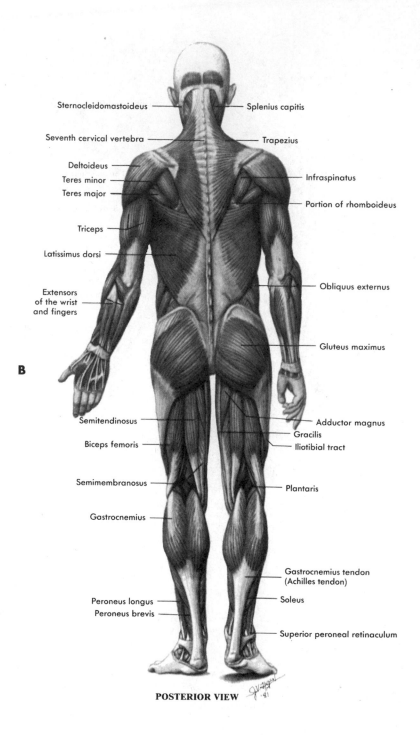

Sternocleidomastoideus

Splenius capitis

Seventh cervical vertebra

Trapezius

Deltoideus

Infraspinatus

Teres minor

Teres major

Portion of rhomboideus

Triceps

Latissimus dorsi

Extensors
of the wrist
and fingers

Obliquus externus

B

Gluteus maximus

Semitendinosus

Adductor magnus

Gracilis

Biceps femoris

Iliotibial tract

Semimembranosus

Plantaris

Gastrocnemius

Gastrocnemius tendon
(Achilles tendon)

Peroneus longus

Soleus

Peroneus brevis

Superior peroneal retinaculum

POSTERIOR VIEW

Teno- (Tendons)

The extension of muscle into a firm, fibrous cord that attaches into a bone or other firm structure is a tendon. Some muscles have a tendon at both ends, some have direct attachment to bone at one end, and a few attach directly to bone at both ends and have no tendon.

A **common tendon** serves more than one muscle; such as a **conjoined tendon** that is found in the inguinal region. The tendons that receive the most attention are the following:

Achilles t.: the common tendon of the gastrocnemius and soleus muscle inserted into the medial posterior surface of the calcaneus; **calcaneal t.** or **tendocalcaneus, heel t.**

hamstring t.: one of the tendons that bind the popliteal fossa laterally and medially. The inner hamstring includes tendons of the gracilis and sartorius muscles, and the outer hamstring is the tendon of the biceps flexor femoris muscle.

patellar t.: anterior or inferior ligamentum patellae.

Sharpey fibers: fibers of a tendon attached to bone that actually penetrate the periosteum and cortex of bone, and thus make a very strong attachment.

Surgical Procedures on Tendons

The nomenclature of surgical procedures on tendons has a certain amount of overlap, since several prefixes are used—teno-, tendo-, and tendino-. Therefore the same surgical procedure may have several forms of spelling. The preferred term for a surgical procedure is listed first, with the related term appearing after the definition.

tendon release: surgical transection of a tendon, with or without repair.

tenectomy: excision of a lesion (ganglion or xanthoma) of a tendon or of a tendon sheath.

tenodesis: tendon fixation by suturing proximal end of a tendon to the bone or by reattachment of the tendon to another site.

tenolysis: surgically freeing a tendon from adhesions; **tendolysis.**

tenomyoplasty: procedure involving repair of tendon and muscle; **tenontomyoplasty.**

tenomyotomy: excision of a portion of tendon and muscle.

tenonectomy: excision of a portion of tendon with or without excision of a portion of tendon to shorten it.

tenontomyotomy: incision into the principal tendon of a muscle, with partial or complete excision of that muscle.

tenoplasty: surgical repair of a ruptured tendon; **tendoplasty, tendinoplasty, tenontoplasty.**

tenorrhaphy: union of a divided tendon by a suture; **tenosuture, tendinosuture.**

tenosuspension: surgical repair that fashions a soft-tissue sling to hold the tendon in a specific place.

tenosynovectomy: resection or excision of excessive synovial lining within the tendon sheath.

tenotomy: incomplete or complete division of a tendon, as in clubfoot; **tendotomy.**

Desmo- (Ligaments)

Ligaments are bands of strong fibrous connective tissue that bind together the articular ends of bones and cartilage at the joints to facilitate or limit motion. Also, they give support and attachment to fascia, viscera, and muscles. An **accessory ligament** is one that supports another ligament on the lateral surface outside the joint capsule where excessive motion occurs. In the knee, elbow, and wrist the **medial, lateral,** and **collateral ligaments** provide additional support. There are many others, but the knee receives the most attention. Because ligaments tie bones together, the prefix syn- (together) is used with desmo- (ligament) for ligamentous surgery. **Syndesmosis** is the name for an articulation in which the bones are united by ligaments (e.g., the distal tibiofibular articulation).

Surgical Procedures on Ligaments

desmotomy: surgical division of a ligament or ligaments.

syndesmectomy: excision of a ligament or portion thereof.

syndesmopexy: surgical fixation of a dislocation by using the ligaments of a joint.

syndesmoplasty: ligaments sutured together.

syndesmorrhaphy: suture or repair of ligaments.

syndesmotomy: dissection or cutting of ligaments.

Fasciae

Fasciae (pronounced fash´-ē-ē) (fascia, sing.) are sheets of dense connective fibrous tissue that act as a restricting envelope for muscular components and bind groups of muscles, blood vessels, and nerves into bundles. Generally, the fascia does not play any role in the movement of joints and bones. The exception to this is the **fascia lata** of the outer thigh; this fascia has its own muscle (**tensor fascia lata**) that, when tightened, will pull through the fascia to points across the knee.

Surgical Procedures on Fasciae

fasciaplasty: plastic surgery of fascia; **fascioplasty.**

fasciectomy: excision of strips of fascia.

fasciodesis: suturing a fascia to another fascia or tendon.

fasciorrhaphy: suturing and repair of lacerated fascia; **aponeurorrhaphy.**

fasciotomy: surgical incision or transection of fascia, commonly done for forearm and leg injuries, where the pressure in the compartment surrounded by the fascia has become very high.

Neuro- (Nerves)

Nerves are cordlike structures that convey impulses between a part of the central nervous system and some other region of the body. Structural components of the nerves include epineurium, perineurium, nerve sheath, axon, Schwann cell, and myelin. **Innervation** refers to the nerve supply to any tissue. Nerves are usually named for the antomic area involved. Hilton law states that a nerve trunk that supplies any joint supplies the muscles moving that joint and the area over the skin over that joint.

Orthopaedic Surgical Procedures on Nerves

Mellesi cable graft: for neuroma excision and replacement with grafts of specific length of fascicular gap.

neurectomy: resection of a segment of a nerve.

neurolysis: destruction of a perineural adhesion by a longitudinal incision to release the nerve sheath.

neuroplasty: plastic repair of a nerve.

neurorrhaphy: suture of a severed nerve; repair.

neurotomy: division of a nerve or nerves.

neurotripsy: surgical crushing of a nerve.

rhizotomy (radicotomy, radiculectomy):   procedure dividing the nerve roots close to their origin from the spinal cord; rhizo- refers to root of the spinal cord.

VASCULAR (BLOOD VESSELS) SYSTEM* (Fig. 8–9)

There are thousands of miles of blood vessels in the human body and approximately 2000 gallons of blood per day coursing through these vessels, likened to a road map with its major arteries, tributaries, and branches. The **arteries** are the major pipelines that distribute oxygenated blood from the heart to the various organs. In each group, the main artery resembles a tree trunk that gives off numerous branches and these rebranch forming smaller vessels called **arteri-**

*James M. Salander, MD, FACS. Associate Professor of Surgery, Uniformed Services University of the Health Sciences, Bethesda, Maryland.

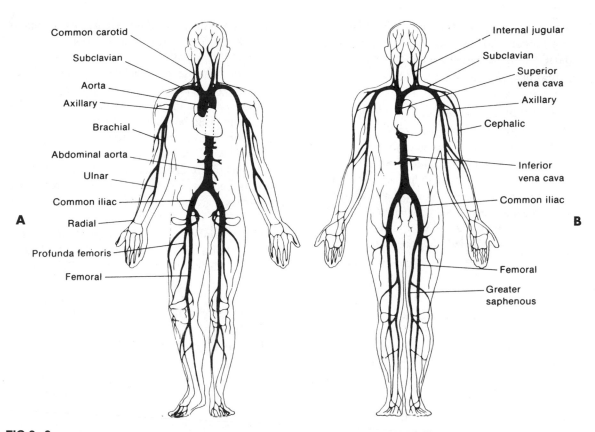

FIG 8–9.
A, The major named arteries of the body distribute oxygenated blood from the heart to the principal organs of the body. The name of each artery corresponds to the organ or region served. **B,** The major veins are named to correspond to the regions of the body they drain: Blood is returned by these veins to the heart, which pumps it through the lungs for oxygenation. (From American Academy of Orthopaedic Surgeons: *Emergency care and transportation of the sick and injured,* Chicago, 1981, The Academy.)

oles, which branch again forming microscopic vessels called **capillaries.**

The **veins** are an extension of the capillaries in that capillaries unite into vessels of increasing size to form **venules** and eventually **veins.** Their function is to carry deoxygenated blood from the various organs back to the heart. Veins differ from arteries in that they have **valves** that create a unidirectional flow. Arteries and veins often have the same name for their location in the body, for example, femoral artery and femoral vein. The following terms relate to blood vessels.

adventitia: loose outer lining of a blood vessel; outermost wall of artery.

artery: blood vessel that carries oxygenated blood away from heart on its way to various organs and tissues in the body.

arterioles: smallest vessels considered arteries (.2 mm diameter) made mostly of smooth muscle; blood flows through arterioles and moves to capillaries.

capillaries: tiny network of blood vessels supplying oxygen directly to cells of body. At this level, oxygen and other nutrients are delivered to cells, and carbon dioxide and waste materials are passed from the tissues back to the bloodstream.

cardiovascular: pertaining to blood vessels (arteries and veins) and the heart.

cerebrovascular: pertaining to blood vessel circulation of the brain and to the brain.

collateral circulation: named and unnamed secondary vessels supplying blood to an organ or extremity through indirect channels. These collateral vessels become particularly important when the main artery is damaged (occluded), for example, genicular arteries around the knee in support of an occluded popliteal artery.

diastole: filling or relaxation phase of the heart cycle.

intima: the innermost lining of the arterial wall.

lipid: one of many chemical compounds normally found in blood that are considered fats and have a relationship between the amount and kinds of lipids in the blood and hardening of the arteries.

lumen: the space inside a blood vessel, duct, or hollow viscus.

patency: refers to an open blood vessel (artery or vein) where blood is flowing.

systole: contraction phase of cardiac cycle.

vascular: pertaining to vessels. Can also refer to amount of blood supply to an organ, such as a very vascular tumor, that is, good blood supply.

vein: blood vessel that carries blood from the various organs in the body back to the heart. Veins usually have valves creating a unidirectional flow, whereas arteries do not. Small veins are then called **venules.**

Vascular Surgical Procedures (Arteries/Veins)

Peripheral vascular surgery procedures center around the treatment of disorders of the blood vessels, that is, the arteries and veins (not including the heart), and may be performed in conjunction with or-thopaedic procedures, such as the repair of a disrupted popliteal artery following knee dislocation. An understanding of peripheral vascular surgery is also necessary in diagnosing patients with vascular disease who come to the orthopaedic surgeon. For example, a patient may see an orthopaedic surgeon for a painful foot believing it to be a bony problem, only to find it is "rest pain" from occluded arteries in the thigh and calf. In this case, the patient is referred to the vascular surgeon for further evaluation and treatment. Since these two specialities overlap in diagnosis, treatment, and surgery, vascular procedures are included for reference.

Most peripheral vascular surgical procedures performed today are done to correct the problem of arteriosclerosis (hardening of the arteries). In this regard, the problems can usually be corrected by a bypass, by replacing the artery, or by cleaning it out (endarterectomy). The terms relating to blood vessel surgery follow.

aortofemoral bypass (AFB):   surgical procedure whereby the narrowing or occlusion of the abdominal aorta and iliac arteries (from arteriosclerosis) is bypassed with a graft (usually Dacron) going from just below the renal arteries down to the femoral arteries in the groins. Considered one of the bigger vascular procedures, requiring opening the abdomen (taking from 3 to 6 hours). Separate bypass grafts may be taken off the main aortofemoral graft to increase the blood supply to the kidneys, intestines, or pelvic viscera to include the male genitalia.

aortoiliac bypass: a bypass graft going from just below the renal artery down to the iliac arteries. This procedure is usually performed for abdominal aortic aneurysms (AAA).

aneurysmorrhaphy: a repair of an aneurysm in which it is left in place, but disconnected from the circulation, and a graft is sewn in its place. Following this, the aneurysm wall can either be wrapped around the graft or left in place. (Totally removing the aneurysm is rarely done since it may jeopardize adjacent organs.)

arthrectomy catheter (Simpson): a vascular procedure for a localized endarterectomy where a device is passed percutaneously or intraoperatively to an area of stenosis, using a small circular knife blade.

autogenous saphenous vein graft (ASVG): the greater saphenous vein of the lower extremity is removed and used to either bypass or replace a diseased segment of artery or vein elsewhere in the body. When the vein is removed and placed in a different location, care must be taken to ensure that the valves of the vein are either destroyed or that the vein is put in a reversed fashion so that the arterial blood will flow unimpeded.

axillofemoral bypass (AxFem): an extra-anatomic bypass whereby either Dacron or PTFE graft is used to carry blood from the axillary artery (under the arm) down to one or both common femoral arteries. This procedure is usually performed in lieu of an aortofemoral bypass because the abdomen is inaccessible resulting from infection in the abdomen, for example, infected aortofemoral graft, severe cardiac disease, or severe pulmonary disease. The patency rate for these grafts is not nearly as good as that for a usual aortofemoral bypass graft.

balloon angioplasty: a procedure usually performed by a radiologist or cardiologist using radiologic techniques whereby a balloon catheter is passed up to an area of stenosis in an artery to widen vessel, a balloon is inflated, and the area of the stenosis (stricture) is dilated. This procedure is applicable only for a short-segment isolated stenosis in large vessels, such as the common iliac or renal arteries. It is also utilized in the coronary arteries as well. The long-term benefit of this procedure is becoming more acceptable; **percutaneous transluminal angioplasty (PTA).**

carotid endarterectomy: an opening up and cleaning out of the common carotid and internal carotid artery in the neck. During this procedure, the diseased intima and portions of the media are removed to open and smooth out the channel of blood flow to the brain. The procedure removes the roughened irregular buildup of atherosclerosis and is done to prevent transient ischemic attacks (TIA) and strokes.

carotid subclavian bypass: procedure involving either vein or prosthetic material whereby a bypass graft is placed between the carotid artery and subclavian artery. It is done to improve the blood flow in the subclavian artery to the arm and hand by bringing blood up the carotid artery and down into the subclavian, bypassing a "narrowing" at the origin of the subclavian artery. (See also subclavian-carotid bypass.)

coronary artery bypass graft (CABG): procedure on the blood vessels of the heart whereby narrowed areas in the arteries leading to the heart muscle itself are bypassed with a vein graft going directly from the aorta to more distal portions of the coronary (heart) arteries. This procedure, performed by cardiac surgeons, is done while the patient is on a cardiac bypass machine.

distal bypass: procedure performed with either synthetic material or vein whereby blood is brought from either the common femoral or superficial femoral artery down to the small named blood vessels below the knee. The procedure is usually performed to prevent amputation of an extremity from severe ischemia. The patient frequently has severe pain and skin breakdown before the operation.

endarterectomy: an opening up and cleaning out of blood vessels diseased by hardening of the arteries, which begin in the intima and progress down through the media. In this procedure, the diseased intima, fatty deposits, and much of the media are removed; the roughened irregular surface of the blood vessel can produce a surface on which blood clots will collect and break off, moving downstream, or a surface on which more clot can form and occlude (close off) the artery.

end-to-end anastomosis: a joining of two vascular structures—arteries, graft and artery, or vein and artery—to bypass an occluded or damaged segment; the end of one structure is sewn to the end of the other.

end-to-side anastomosis: a joining of the end of an artery or vein or prosthetic material to the side of another vein, artery, or prosthetic material to bypass an occluded or damaged segment.

extraanatomic bypass: bypass graft in which prosthetic material or vein is used to route blood between the two arteries or two veins. The route of the graft is other than a usual anatomic position, such as axillofemoral or femoral-femoral bypass.

extracranial/intracranial bypass (ECIC): a procedure performed by neurosurgeons whereby severely narrowed or occluded blood vessels within the brain are bypassed. The usual procedure is to take the superficial temporal artery, which is a branch on the scalp, make a bone flap in the skull, and move the distal end of this artery down into the brain to supply blood flow directly into the brain.

femoral-femoral bypass (fem-fem bypass): a bypass procedure using a synthetic or vein graft material whereby one femoral artery is used to supply the blood to both lower extremities. This could be done to bypass an infection, or to provide blood flow from one undiseased iliac femoral system to another femoral system. It is considered an extraanatomic bypass.

femoral popliteal bypass (FPB): bypass graft from the femoral artery to the popliteal artery. The distal end of the graft can go to a portion of the popliteal artery above the knee or the popliteal artery below the knee. May be performed with vein or prosthetic material. It is done to correct an occluded superficial femoral artery. Indications for this procedure are claudication, rest pain, or threatened limb loss.

Greenfield filter: for lower circulatory venous embolic disorders; an umbrella-shaped metallic device that is inserted into the inferior vena cava to prevent lung emboli.

in situ bypass: instead of removing the greater saphenous vein and reversing it, it is left in place and the valve destroyed through a variety of techniques. The proximal end is sutured into the inflow artery, and the distal end of the vein is sutured into the recipient artery. The side branches of the vein are ligated in distal artery of leg. This technique provides better patency than taking the vein out and reversing its course.

laparotomy: a procedure whereby the abdomen is opened for exploration or to conduct another surgical procedure.

laser endarterectomy: technique of using a laser beam to disobliterate plaque from an artery. It can either be done intraoperatively or, in some instances, percutaneously.

limb salvage: a general category of procedures performed on a lower extremity to improve the blood supply and prevent amputation. Skin ulceration and gangrene are often present.

patch angioplasty: a local procedure whereby the artery is opened, the inside of the vessel is cleaned out and a patch of vein or prosthetic material is used to widen that area of the artery. This procedure is also done in the repair of traumatic injuries.

polytetrafluoroethylene (PTFE): (Gor-tex) a plastic graft that has gained tremendous popularity in bypassing and replacing occluded arteries throughout the body.

reversed vein bypass graft: a technique where a vein, usually the greater saphenous, is removed and used as a bypass. The small end of vein is sutured to proximal artery (inflow) and distal (large) end of vein is sutured to outflow artery. The vein must be turned around in this fashion to obviate the function of valves.

subclavian carotid bypass: bypass procedure between the subclavian artery and carotid artery to correct a severe narrowing at the origin of the common carotid artery. This allows blood to flow up the subclavian artery, along the graft, into the carotid artery, and into the brain without interrupting blood flow to the arm or hand.

thrombolytic therapy: a dissolution of thrombus in an artery or vein with urokinase or streptokinase. Has been most useful in recent thromboses, but some contraindications must be considered.

SPECIFIC ANATOMY AND SURGERY BY LOCATION

The Shoulder

Shoulder separations and shoulder dislocations are very distinct injuries and involve two different joints. Palpating the collar bone (clavicle) and working the fingers laterally, a distinct bump is felt—the acromioclavicular (A/C) joint, which is the junction between the collar bone and shoulder blade (Fig. 8–10). The acromion is the part of the shoulder blade that connects with the collar bone. Injury of this joint is often called a shoulder separation. However, a person dislocating the shoulder has disrupted the ball-and-socket joint between the arm and the shoulder blade (glenohumeral joint). The orthopaedist may not be able to feel this joint dislocation under the numerous muscles, but its presence is apparent through pain and an inability to place the arm behind the back or raise it over the head.

Anatomy
Bones

axilla: armpit.

clavicle (cleido-): collar bone.
> *acromioclavicular joint:* between clavicle and scapula.
> *sternoclavicular joint:* at the junction of the clavicle and breast bone.

humerus: arm bone between the shoulder and elbow.
> *anatomic neck:* point of attachment of shoulder capsule (humerus).
> *biceps groove:* groove for the long head of the biceps muscle; **bicipital groove.**

> *greater and lesser tuberosity:* points of attachment for the rotator cuff.
> *humeral head:* half circle-shaped portion of the humerus for the shoulder joint.
> *surgical neck* most common point of fracture of the humerus.

rhomboid fossa: an inconsistent feature on the medial side of the clavicle. It is the attachment of the costoclavicular or rhomboid ligament and has importance only because it may be mistaken for a tumor.

scapula: shoulder blade.
> *acromion process:* outermost tip of the shoulder.
> *coracoid:* knob of bone attached to the anterior scapula just medial to the shoulder.
> *glenoid fossa:* saucer-shaped depression of the scapula that has direct contact with the humerus and glenohumeral joint.
> *glenoid labrum:* ring of fibrocartilage of connective tissue attached to rim of margin of glenoidal cavity of shoulder blade to increase its depth.
> *spine:* outcropping portion of the posterosuperior scapula.
> *spinoglenoid notch:* small fingernail-sized V-shaped groove in the superior border of the scapula through which the suprascapular nerve courses.

Muscles Around the Shoulder

coracobrachialis: from the coracoid of the scapula to the inner distal humerus; pulls the arm across the midline.

deltoid: triangular muscle arising from the acromion that attaches to the lateral arm; elevates, flexes, and extends the arm.

infraspinatus: from the posterior upper scapula to the posterior superior humerus; externally rotates the arm.

latissimus dorsi: from the lower thoracic and lumbar spine to the anterior upper humerus; pulls

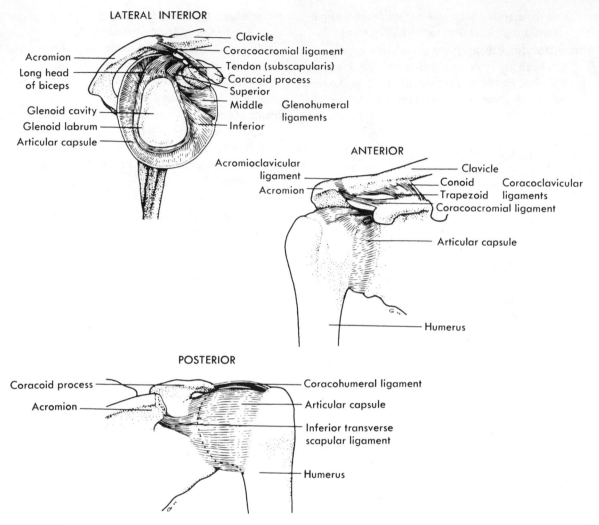

LATERAL INTERIOR

Clavicle
Coracoacromial ligament
Acromion
Tendon (subscapularis)
Long head
of biceps
Coracoid process
Superior
Glenoid cavity
Middle
Glenohumeral
ligaments
Glenoid labrum
Inferior
Articular capsule

ANTERIOR

Acromioclavicular
ligament
Acromion
Clavicle
Conoid
Coracoclavicular
Trapezoid
ligaments
Coracoacromial ligament

Articular capsule

Humerus

POSTERIOR

Coracoid process
Coracohumeral ligament
Acromion
Articular capsule
Inferior transverse
scapular ligament
Humerus

FIG 8–10.
Shoulder joints. (From Hilt NE, Cogburn SB: *Manual of orthopaedics,* St Louis, 1980, The CV Mosby Co.)

the arm down and helps depress the humeral head.

levator scapula: from central midneck to the superior medial scapula; controls scapular elevation and rotation.

pectoralis major and minor: from the clavicle (major) and coracoid (minor) to the anterior chest wall; pulls the scapula forward.

rhomboideus major and minor: from the midline of the thoracic spine to the medial scapula; pulls the scapula back toward the midline.

rotator cuff: arrangement of four muscles from the scapula to the humerus, which, with the capsule and glenoid labrum (a cartilaginous margin of the joint), hold the shoulder together. The muscles of the rotator cuff are supraspinatus, infraspinatus, teres minor, and subscapularis.

serratus anterior: from the medial scapula to the chest anteriorly; holds the scapula into the body during shoulder motions.

shoulder girdle: a general term for the soft tissue around the glenohumeral joint.

sternocleidomastoid: from the base of the skull to the sternum and medial clavicle; turns head and flexes the neck.

subscapularis: from the anterior scapula to the lesser tuberosity; strong internal rotator of the shoulder.

supraspinatus: from the top of the scapular spine to the greater tuberosity of the humerus; abducts the arm and depresses the humeral head.

teres major and minor: from the lateral scapula to the humerus; pulls the arm in with the minor externally rotated as a part of the rotator cuff.

trapezius: kite-shaped muscle from the base of the neck to lower spine to scapular spine; controls scapular motion.

Ligaments Around the Shoulder Region

At the sternoclavicular joint, the **sternoclavicular l.**

At the acromioclavicular joint, the **acromioclavicular l.** and **coracoclavicular l.** (the **conoid** and **trapezoid l.**).

At the glenohumeral joint:

anteroinferior glenohumeral l.:   lower of the three anterior glenohumeral l.

anteromedial glenohumeral l.:   most substantial of the three glenohumeral l.

anterosuperior glenohumeral l.:   most superior of the three glenohumeral l.

conjoined tendon: the common origin of two tendons from the coracoid process of the scapula leading to the arm and forearm. In surgery it is detached temporarily to gain access to the shoulder joint.

coracohumeral l.:   starting at coracoid and crossing over humeral head.

glenoid labrum: meniscus-like rim of cartilage that deepens the glenohumeral joint.

rotator interval: area of thin tissue under coracohumeral l. and between the subscapularis and supraspinatus tendons.

transverse humeral l.:   covering long head of biceps tendon over the bicipital groove.

Main Arteries, Veins, and Branches around the Shoulder

axillary artery: a continuum of the subclavian artery in the axillary area that branches into highest thoracic, lateral thoracic, anterior humeral circumflex, posterior humeral circumflex, thoracoacromial, and subscapularis.

brachial artery: a continuum of the axillary artery and main artery of the arm. The branches are listed in the Arm and Forearm section.

cephalic vein: large vein between the deltoid and pectoralis muscles.

subclavian and axillary vein: the continuous vessel running alongside the subclavian and axillary arteries. The branches are not consistent and are rarely described in orthopaedic procedures.

subclavian artery: main artery from the chest leading down through the arm that branches into internal thoracic, vertebral, thyrocervical, transcervical, superior intercostal, and suprascapular.

Nerves

anterior thoracic n.:   from the lateral cord, supplies the pectoral muscles.

axillary n.:   arising from the posterior cord, supplies the upper arm, particularly the deltoid and teres minor.

brachial plexus: a large complex of nerves from the lower cervical and upper thoracic (C-5 to T-2) spinal segments. This nerve plexus includes:

Superior, medial, and inferior *trunk*
Anterior and posterior *division*
Medial, lateral, and posterior *cord*
Lower and upper subscapular nerve

Musculocutaneous nerve
Radial nerve
Ulnar nerve
Dorsal scapular nerve
Axillary nerve
Medial nerve
Scapular nerve
Long thoracic nerve

dorsal scapular n.:   from the fifth nerve root, supplies the rhomboids.

long thoracic n. (nerve of Bell):   from the fifth, sixth, and seventh cervical root, supplies the serratus anterior.

lower scapular n.:   from the posterior cord, supplies the lower scapular and teres major muscles.

median n.:   from the lateral and medial cord, supplies the finger and wrist flexors, except the fourth and fifth profundus and flexor carpi ulnaris, and the thumb intrinsics, except the adductor.

musculocutaneous n.:   from the lateral cord, supplies the biceps coracobrachialis, brachialis, and lateral cutaneous nerve of the forearm.

radial n.:   from the posterior cord, supplies the triceps, anconeus, supinator, and hand and wrist extensors.

suprascapular n.:   from the superior trunk, supplies the supraspinatus and infraspinatus.

thoracodorsal n.:   from the posterior cord, supplies the latissimus dorsi muscle.

ulnar n.:   from the medial cord, supplies the fourth and fifth profundus and flexor carpi ulnaris along with the hand intrinsics including the thumb adductor, but not the other thumb intrinsics.

upper subscapular n.:   from the posterior cord, supplies the subscapularis muscle.

Surgery of the Shoulder
Eponyms
The following list of eponyms for surgical procedures is arranged according to the area of injury or deformity. In most instances, the arthroplasties can be referred to as capsulorrhaphies of the shoulder.

Arthroplasties for Acromioclavicular Separations
Bosworth
Dewar and Barrington
Mumford-Gurd
Neviaser

Arthroplasties for Anterior Shoulder Dislocations

Bankart	Magnuson-Stack
Bristow	Nicola
Cubbins	Putti-Platt
de Toit and Roux	Speed
Eden-Hybbinette	Trillat

Arthroplasties for Posterior Shoulder Dislocations
McLaughlin
Scott
Wilson and McKeever

For High-Riding Scapulae (Sprengel Deformity)
Chang and Farahvar
Green
Inclan-Ober
Robinson
Schrock
Woodward

Arthrodeses for Shoulder Stabilization

Brittain	Steindler
Gill	Watson-Jones
Putti	

Muscle Transfers for Paralysis of Scapula

Chaves	His-Haas
Chaves-Rapp	Whitman
DeWar and Harris	Saha
Dickson	Vastamäki
Henry	

Posterior Bone Block Elbow
Boyd
Putti
Putti-Scaglietti

Shoulder Procedures

acromionectomy: excision of all or part of the acromion, usually in cases of rotator cuff injuries.

acromioplasty: repair or partial removal of the acromion.

Armstrong p.: for rotator cuff impingement; resection of entire acromion.

Bankart p.: capsular repair in the glenoid for chronic anterior dislocation of the shoulder.

Bateman p.: for paralysis of the deltoid; a trapezius muscle transfer to the greater tuberosity.

Bosworth p.: screw fixation of the clavicle to the coracoid for acromioclavicular separations.

Boyd and Sisk p.: for stabilization of recurrent posterior shoulder dislocation; transfer of long head of biceps to posterior glenoid.

Braun p.: for partial ankylosis of the shoulder; open tenotomy of the subscapularis. Also, for painful shoulder in stroke patients; section of subscapularis and pectoralis major tendons.

brisement p.: a closed manipulation of a stiff shoulder.

Bristow p. (Bristow-Laterjet p.): coracoid process transfer for chronic anterior dislocation of the shoulder.

Brittain p.: extraarticular fusion of the shoulder.

Brooks and Saddon p.: for paralysis of biceps; transfer of pectoralis major tendon to biceps.

Bunnell p.: for paralysis of elbow flexion; transfer of triceps anterior to radial tuberosity. Also, for paralysis, biceps transfer of sternocleidomastoid to long head of biceps.

Burrows p.: for dislocation of sternoclavicular joint; use of subclavian muscle to hold reduction.

Chaves-Rapp p.: for long thoracic nerve palsy; transfer of the pectoralis major to inferior scapula.

clavicectomy: excision of all or part of the clavicle.

clavicotomy: surgical division of the collar bone.

Cofield p.: for rotator cuff tear; resection of distal clavicle, acromioplasty, and V-Y repair of rotator cuff or subscapularis substitution.

Copeland and Howard p.: for shoulder paralytic instability; fusion of scapula to ribs using tibial cortical grafts.

costectomy: excision of part or all of a rib for purposes of either a bone graft or approach to thorax.

costotransversectomy: excision of the transverse process of a vertebra and the neighboring rib for approach to the spine or cord.

Cubbins p.: passage of the coracohumeral ligament through the humeral head for an old anterior dislocation of the shoulder.

Das Gupta p.: technique of excision of scapula.

Debeyre p.: for repair of rotator cuff tear; superior approach to supraspinatus to advance tendon.

Dewar and Barrington p.: transfer of the coracoid tip to the clavicle for acromioclavicular separations.

du Toit and Roux p.: a stapling procedure of the anterior shoulder capsule for chronic anterior dislocation of the shoulder.

Eden-Hybbinette p.: a bone block to the anterior glenoid for chronic anterior dislocation of the shoulder.

Eden-Lange p.: for spinal accessory nerve palsy; transfer of levator scapulae, rhomboid major, and rhomboid minor.

Eyler p.: for paralysis of elbow flexor; transfer of flexor wad of five proximally on humerus facilitated with tendon fascia lata graft.

Fairbanks and Sever p.: for internal rotation and adduction contraction of shoulder; resection of tendinous portion of pectoralis major and minor, coracobrachialis, and short and long head of the biceps.

Gill p.: intraarticular and extraarticular fusion of the shoulder.

girdle resection: various resections of proximal humerus and/or scapula in an attempt to preserve the shoulder in ablative tumor surgery.

Green p.:   soft-tissue release and repair for high-riding scapulae.

Harmon p.:   for partial paralysis of deltoid; transfer of posterior origin to anterior part.

His-Haas p.:   for long thoracic nerve palsy; transfer of teres major from humerus to chest wall.

Hitchcock p.:   tenodesis of long head of biceps into biceps groove.

Hovanian p.:   for paralysis of biceps; transfer of latissimus dorsi to radial tuberosity. Also, for triceps weakness; transfer of latissimus dorsi to triceps muscle.

Inclan-Ober p.:   soft-tissue release and repair for high-riding scapulae.

Janecki and Nelson p.:   for scapular malignancy; radical resection that includes a portion of the clavicle, proximal humerus, and entire scapula.

Jobe and Kvitne p.:   for recurrent anterior dislocating shoulder; a criss-cross and overlapping imbrication of capsule to help recreate a labrum.

Kristiansen and Kofoed p.:   for proximal humeral fractures; percutaneous pin is used to reduce fracture, and an external fixation is then applied.

L'Episcopo Zachary p.:   for internal rotation and adduction contracture of the shoulder; resection of anterior capsule and tendon of pectoralis major with transfer of triceps and latissimus dorsi tendon.

Magnuson-Stack p.:   stapling of the subscapularis for chronic anterior dislocation of the shoulder.

Marcove, Lewis, Horos p.:   for scapular malignancy; radical resection that includes a portion of the clavicle, proximal humerus, and entire scapula.

McKeever p.:   for open fixation of clavicle fracture, using a threaded wire.

McLaughlin p.:   for rotator cuff injury of shoulder, a technique of repair; a transfer of the subscapularis into a hatchet head deformity of the humerus for old posterior dislocation of the shoulder.

McShane, Leinberry, and Fenlin p.:   for rotator cuff impingement; excision of 50% of the inferior surface of the anterolateral acromion.

Moberg p.:   for paralysis of triceps; posterior transfer of deltoid.

B.H. Moore p.:   for muscle imbalance in shoulder caused by stroke; posterior transfer of part of deltoid muscle.

J.R. Moore p.:   for posterior dislocation of humeral head in stroke; multiple anterior tendon and anterior capsule resection with bone graft to glenoid.

Mumford-Gurd p.:   resection of the distal clavicle for a chronic acromioclavicular separation.

Neer p.:   for recurrent multidirectional anterior dislocating shoulder; capsular lateral advancement with superior placement of distal flap.

Neviaser p.:   transfer of the coracoacromial ligament to the clavicle for acromioclavicular separation. Also a Knowles pin fixation of the clavicle, especially for nonunion of a fracture.

Nicola p.:   transfer of the long head of the biceps tendon through humeral head for chronic anterior shoulder dislocation.

Ober and Barr p.:   for weakness of triceps; transfer of brachioradialis.

O'Brien p.:   for multidirectional anterior dislocating shoulder, superior and inferior placement of laterally based flaps in capsular repair.

Phelps: for tumor; technique of partial resection of the scapula.

Putti p.:   fusion of the shoulder by two different methods.

Putti-Platt p.:   subscapularis muscle and capsular repair for chronic anterior dislocation of the shoulder.

Rockwood p.: for chronic acromioclavicular separation; resection of distal clavicle and repair with acromioclavicular ligament, and 12-week fixation with a lag screw to coracoid.

Roger p. for paralytic internal rotation deformity of the shoulder; a proximal derotation osteotomy of the humerus.

Rowe and Zarins p.: for chronic anterior shoulder dislocation; open reduction and fixation by a number of temporary means including sling.

Saha p.: for paralysis of deltoid; transfer of trapezius and distal acromion to humerus below greater tuberosity. Also, for paralysis of subscapularis; transfer of two superior digitations of serratus anterior or transfer of pectoralis minor. Also, for paralysis of supraspinatus; a transfer of levator scapulae or sternocleidomastoid. Also, for paralysis of infraspinatus or subscapularis; a transfer of latissimus dorsi or teres major.

scapulectomy: excision of all or part of the scapula.

Schrock p.: soft-tissue release and repair for high-riding scapulae.

Scott p.: wedge bone block procedure for chronic posterior dislocation of the shoulder.

Speed p.: ligamentous repair for sternoclavicular joint separations. Also, for chronic dislocation elbow; reduction and stabilization, using a folded expansion of triceps muscle.

Spira p.: for paralysis biceps; transfer of pectoralis minor.

Steindler p.: intraarticular fusion of the shoulder.

Stewart p.: for acromioclavicular joint separation; resection of distal clavicle with repair of coracoacromial ligament.

Swafford and Lichtman p.: for suprascapular nerve entrapment; release of ligamentous tissue at the suprascapular notch.

Tikhoff-Linberg p.: for scapular malignancy; radical resection that includes a portion of the clavicle, proximal humerus, and entire scapula.

Trillat p.: for anterior shoulder dislocation; osteotomy of coracoid with attachment to glenoid to act as bone block.

Watson-Jones p.: shoulder fusion using a piece of acromion.

Weaver and Dunn p.: for acromioclavicular separation; transfer of coracoacromial ligament to distal clavicle.

Weber osteotomy: for recurrent shoulder dislocations associated with large posterior humeral head defects; internal rotation osteotomy of proximal humerus.

Whitman p.: for long thoracic nerve palsy; stabilization of scapula with fascial strips attached to spinous processes.

Wilson and McKeever p.: K-wire (Kirschner wire) fixation after open reduction of an old posterior shoulder dislocation.

Woodward p.: soft-tissue release and repair for high-riding scapulae.

Zeir p.: for long thoracic nerve palsy; pectoralis minor transferred to scapula using a tensor fascia lata graft.

ARM AND FOREARM

Specifically, the arm is the portion of the upper limb between the shoulder and the elbow, and the forearm is between the elbow and the wrist. Most surgical procedures on the arm and forearm are of a general type, that is, nerve and vessel repairs and fracture fixations. Most forearm tendon transfers are considered in Chapter 10, The Hand.

Anatomy

Bones

humerus: the humerus, the arm bone, extends from the shoulder to the elbow (Fig. 8–11).

capitellum: provides articulation with the radial head.

FIG 8-11.
Right humerus. **A,** Anterior view. **B,** Posterior view. (From Seeley RR, Stephens TD, Tate P: *Anatomy and physiology,* St Louis, 1989, Times Mirror/Mosby College Publishing.)

epitrochlea: medial epicondyle.

medial and lateral epicondyles: large prominences on either side of the elbow.

olecranon fossa: thin portion of the bone with an opening above the elbow joint.

spiral groove: groove in the bone for the radial nerve.

trochlea: provides articulation with the ulna.

radius (Fig. 8-12):   The radius is the bone on the thumb side of the forearm.

biceps tuberosity: point of insertion of biceps tendon.

Lister tubercle: a prominence on the distal dorsum of the radius.

radial head: the articular portion of the radius to the elbow.

FIG 8–12.
Ulna and radius of the right forearm. (From Seeley RR, Stephens TD, Tate P: *Anatomy and physiology,* St Louis, 1989, Times Mirror/Mosby College Publishing.)

styloid process: the distalmost portion of radius.

ulna (Fig. 8–12): The ulna is the bone of the forearm on the little finger side of the wrist, prominent at the elbow.

coronoid process: anterior part of the ulna at the elbow joint at the brachialis insertion.

olecranon: prominent ulnar portion at the elbow.

styloid process: the distalmost portion of the ulna, prominent on turning the wrist downward.

Muscles of the arm

arcade of Struthers: a fibrous expansion of the medial distal triceps muscle; a potential area of entrapment for the ulnar nerve.

biceps m.: a two-belly muscle that flexes the elbow; extends from the scapula to the radius.

brachialis m.: flexes the elbow from the arm to the ulna.

coracobrachialis m.: pulls the arm in and up; extends from the scapula to the arm.

rotator cuff: see under Shoulder anatomy.

triceps m.: a three-belly muscle that extends the elbow; its origin is at the scapula, down the arm to the ulna.

Muscles of the Forearm

Many muscles of the forearm that affect hand function are discussed in Chapter 10. Others that relate to forearm function are the following.

aconeus: small muscle on the ulnar side of the elbow.

extensor wad of three: muscles that extend the wrist and flex the elbow.

brachioradialis muscle: located on the lateral side of the forearm; helps flex the elbow.

extensor carpi radialis brevis: short muscle that extends the wrist.

extensor carpi radialis longus: long muscle that extends the wrist.

flexor wad of five: muscles that flex the wrist and fingers and pronate the forearm-flexor carpi ulnaris, palmaris longus, flexor digitorum superficialis, pronator teres, and flexor carpi radialis; see Chapter 10.

pronator quadratus: flat muscle at the distal forearm that turns the palm down in pronation.

supinator muscle: located at the proximal forearm; brings the palm up in supination.

Blood Vessels (Fig. 8–13)

basilic vein: branches upward and laterally from ulnar side of forearm to front of elbow, winding around ulnar border of forearm to join the brachial vein which becomes the axillary vein.

brachial artery: main artery of the arm that divides at the elbow into the radial and ulnar arteries.

brachial vein: branches off axillary.

cephalic vein: branches off from an axillary artery and vein on radial side; runs upward and medially to front of elbow and winds around and enters the axillary vein.

median cephalic vein: near elbow area (where blood is drawn).

median basilic vein: near elbow area.

profundus: deep anterior brachial artery of the arm.

radial artery: one that travels deep into the muscle on the thumb side of the forearm.

FIG 8–13.
Blood vessels of the upper limb. **A,** Veins of the upper limb—the subclavian vein and its tributaries. The major veins draining the superficial structures of the limb are the cephalic and basilic veins. The brachial veins drain the deep structures. Blood vessels of the upper limb. **B,** Arteries of the upper limb—the brachiocephalic, subclavian, axillary, and brachial arteries and their branches. (From Seeley RR, Stephens TD, Tate P: *Anatomy and physiology,* St Louis, 1989, Times Mirror/Mosby College Publishing.)

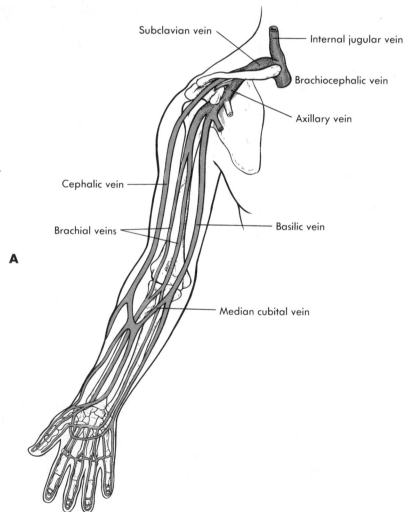

Subclavian vein

Internal jugular vein

Brachiocephalic vein

Axillary vein

Cephalic vein

Basilic vein

Brachial veins

A

Median cubital vein

radial vein: branches off from cephalic vein.

ulnar artery: one that travels deep into the muscle on the little finger side of the anterior forearm.

Other Blood Vessels
Elbow
Ulnar collateral
Anterior and posterior ulnar recurrent
Anterior and posterior radial recurrent

Forearm
Anterior and posterior interosseous

Nerves
The nerves leading to the forearm and hand are all listed in the section on shoulder anatomy. Some specific branches to the arm and forearm are listed here.

anterior interosseous n.: branch of the median nerve; supplies the deep index finger and thumb flexor and pronator quadratus.

cutaneous n. of the arm (brachial cutaneous nerve): posterior, medial, and lateral.

cutaneous n. of the forearm (antebrachial

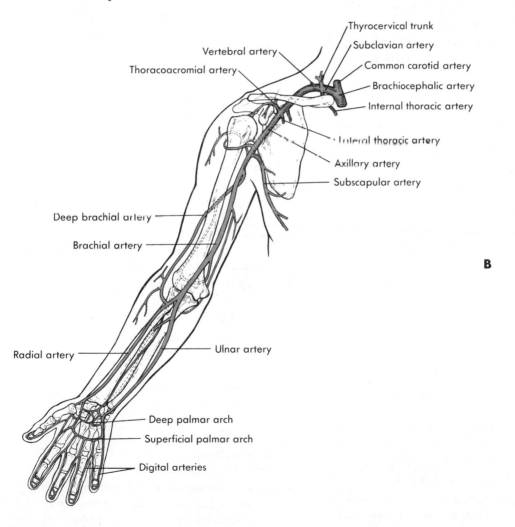

Thyrocervical trunk
Subclavian artery
Common carotid artery
Brachiocephalic artery
Internal thoracic artery
Internal thoracic artery
Axillary artery
Subscapular artery

Vertebral artery
Thoracoacromial artery

Deep brachial artery
Brachial artery

Radial artery
Ulnar artery

Deep palmar arch
Superficial palmar arch
Digital arteries

B

cutaneous nerve): posterior, medial, and lateral.

posterior interosseous n.: branch of radial nerve that passes through supinator muscle and then supplies some of the deep muscles of the posterior forearm.

superficial radial n.: does not go through supinator; supplies no muscles, but supplies sensation for the dorsal radial side of the hand and thumb.

Ligaments

cubital tunnel (arcade of Struthers): expansion of fibers from medial epicondyle to proximal dorsum of forearm; is a potential source of entrapment of ulnar nerve.

interosseous membrane: thick, fibrous tissue between most of the length of the radius and ulna.

laceratus fibrosus: expansion of fibers of the biceps tendon at the elbow; becomes an important structure in some injuries.

oblique ligament: a part of the radial collateral ligament of the elbow.

orbicular ligament: surrounding the radial head and holding it to the ulna at the elbow.

Osborne fascia: covering fascia over the ulna nerve between the medial humeral epicondyle and the olecranon.

ulnar and radial collateral ligament: on the medial and lateral side of the elbow.

Surgery of the Arm and Forearm

Amspacher and Messenbaugh p.: for malunion of humeral fracture; a distal rotation osteotomy.

Aronson and Prager: for supracondylar fracture in children; percutaneous pin fixation.

arthrodeses of the elbow: two procedures are Staples and Steindler arthrodeses.

Baumgard and Schwartz p.: for lateral epicondylitis; percutaneous or small open incision release of origin of extensor carpi ulnaris and extensor carpi radialis brevis and longus.

Blount p.: for supination deformity of forearm; closed osteoclasis of both bones of forearm setting at 45 to 90 degrees of pronation.

Bosworth p.: resection of a portion of the radial head ligament and muscle attachment for tennis elbow.

Bowers "hemi" resection: for radioulnar joint arthritis; resection of distal radial side of ulna with interposition of fascia.

Boyd and Anderson p.: for biceps distal tendon rupture; a method of reattachment.

Boyd and McLeod p.: for tennis elbow; excision of a part of the orbicular ligament.

Brady and Jewett p.: for proximal cross-union of radius and ulna; resection of radial head and 4-week screw fixation to separate radius and ulna.

Campbell p.: for arthritic radial capitellar joint; resection of capitellum and radial head with imbrication of capsule over bone. Also for malunited Colles fracture; resection of distal ulnar side of ulna to use as graft correcting radial deformity.

Campbell and Akbarnia p.: for tumor of distal radius; resection of distal radius with replacement using tibial bone graft.

De Rosa and Graziano p.: for varus deformity in elbow; closing step cut osteotomy of distal humerus.

Ellis p.: for reduction of intraarticular volarly displaced wrist fracture; a technique of screw plate fixation.

Feldon wafer resection: for radioulnar joint arthritis; resection of thin portion of bone and joint of distal ulna, preserving the styloid.

Fernandez p.: for dorsal and radial shortening of a radius fracture; dorsal wedge resection with radial replacement to correct both deformities.

Flynn p.: for nonunion or delayed union of minimally displaced lateral condylar fractures in children; open reduction, peg bone graft and fixation.

Fowles p.: for chronic posterior dislocation of elbow; a posterolateral approach with detachment of all tight structures and possible V-Y plasty of triceps.

French p.: for malunion ulna; distal ulnar osteotomy with screw and wire fixation.

Froimson and Oh (keyhole) p.: for chronic tendonitis of long head of biceps; a keyhole is fashioned in the bicipital groove and then used to insert a knotted portion of biceps tendon.

Gaille p.: for recurrent anterior dislocation shoulder; use of fascia lata graft to replace anterior capsule.

Gill p.: for nonunion of ulna; a massive sliding graft technique.

Hall and Pankovich p.: for mid-humeral fracture; use of multiple small Ender nails in antegrade or retrograde fashion.

Hassman, Brunn, and Neer p.: for recurrent elbow dislocation; plastic repair of lateral capsuloligamentous structures.

Hirayama p.: for chronic dislocation of the radial head with ulnar deformity in a child; osteotomy of the proximal ulna.

Hitchcock p.: for rupture of the long head of biceps; a method of reattachment.

Hovanian p.: for restoring elbow flexion; transfer of latissimus dorsi to olecranon.

Hohmann p.: for tennis elbow.

Kapel p.: triceps and biceps tendon formed into ligaments for a chronic dislocated elbow.

Liebolt p.: for subluxing distal radial/ulnar joint; using tendon graft.

MacAusland p.: arthroplasty of the elbow for a recurrent dislocation.

Manktelow; Ikuta p.: for loss of forearm flexor muscle mass; free neurovascular pedicle transfer of pectoralis major.

McKeever and Buck p.: for olecranon fracture with adequate remaining joint surface; excision of olecranon fragment and reattachment of triceps mechanism.

Milch p.: for radial shortening; an ulnar shortening by step cut resection of distal shaft of ulna. Also, for pronation deformity; an osteotomy of distal ulna with fixation in supinated position. Also humeral osteotomy for cubitus valgus deformity.

Milch shortening osteotomy: for radioulnar joint arthritis; resection of circular section of distal ulnar shaft with plate fixation and resultant shortening of ulna.

Mital p.: for spastic muscle contracture of elbow; Z-plasty of biceps tendon and release of brachialis sheath and joint capsule.

Mizuno, Hirohata, and Kashiwagi p.: for displaced distal humeral epiphysis; posterior open reduction and pin fixation.

Nirschl p.: for chronic lateral epicondylitis; excision of hypercapsular tendon segment of extensor carpi radialus brevis and decortication of anterolateral condyle.

Osborne and Cotterill p.: capsular reefing for a chronic dislocated elbow.

Outerbridge-Kashiwagi p.: for osteoarthritis of the elbow; debridement arthroplasty using posterior approach and fenestration of olecranon fossa.

Reichenheim-King p.: transplantation of the biceps tendon into the coronoid process for a chronic dislocated elbow.

Sauve-Kapandji p.: distal radioulnar joint arthritis; fusion of distal radius and ulna with creation of an ulnar pseudoarthrosis proximal to the fusion.

Sherk and Probst p.: for proximal humeral epiphyseal fracture; reduction and percutaneous pinning.

J.S. Speed p.: for old dislocation radial head; fashioning of sling from a portion of triceps expansion.

Speed and Boyd p.: for irreducible Monteggia fracture; reconstruction of orbicular ligament and plating of ulnar fracture.

Spittler p.: for forearm amputations; a biceps muscle cineplasty.

Steindler flexorplasty: transfer of the flexor wad of five muscles in the elbow to a higher level for loss of voluntary elbow flexion; **Eyler flexorplasty** is a variation of this procedure.

Stewart p.: for radial navicular arthritis; excision of radial styloid.

Weber-Vasey p.: for comminuted olecranon fracture; combined use of bent pin and figure eight wire fixation.

Wilson p.: for extraarticular ankylosis of elbow in flexion; release of anterior structures with Z-plasty of biceps tendon.

Zancolli p.: for supination deformity of forearm; suturing of biceps tendon after lengthening.

(The anatomy and surgery of the hand and wrist are found in Chapter 10.)

PELVIS AND HIPS

The pelvis is a large basinlike structure that supports the lower abdominal viscera, contains the birth canal, and acts as a weight-bearing bridge between the spine and the lower extremities. It is often referred to as the **pelvic girdle.** It is composed of a bilateral set of three bones that are completely fused and are on either side of the sacrum. The largest and uppermost bone is the ilium, the lowermost and strongest is the ischium, and the anteriormost is the pubis. In the outer center of these fused bones is the hip socket, called the acetabulum, the "true" anatomic hip and socket for the ball-and-socket joint.

Most hip surgical procedures involve structures immediately neighboring the acetabulum. The anatomic structures involving the pelvis that are occasionally encountered in hip procedures are listed first, followed by anatomic structures directly related to hip procedures.

Anatomy of the Pelvis

Bones

ala of the ilium: the outer flair of the ilium; resembles a wing.

anterior inferior iliac spine: prominence in the deep ilium just above the hip is origin of rectus femorus.

arcuate ligament: arcuate, meaning arch-shaped. The arcuate line of the pelvis is the iliac continuation of the iliopectineal line; the arched inferior edge of the posterior layer of the rectus sheath.

calcar: a spur. **Calcar femorale** is a bundle of cancellous laminae of bone in the neck of the femur, serving to strengthen it.

greater sciatic notch: the large notch on the posterior surface of the ilium below the postero-inferior iliac spine where the sciatic nerve exits.

gluteal lines: refers to the three curved lines across the outer surface of the ilium, anteriorly, posteriorly, and inferiorly.

iliac crest: the outer uppermost margins of the ilium, two of the four iliac spines arise from the crest; the **anterior superior iliac spine** is the origin of the oblique abdominal muscles and sartorius; the **posterior superior iliac spine** is a part of the origin of the gluteus maximus.

iliopectineal line: a ridge inside the pelvis that denotes the entrance into the birth canal, with a concave inner surface called the **iliac fossa.**

ilium: wide platelike bone that forms the top of the pelvis just below the waistline; generally referred to as "the hips."

inferior pubic ramus: lower portion of the pubic bone.

innominate bone: composed of three fused bony subunits, called the ilium, pubis, and ischium, that are attached to the sacrum and coccyx to form the pelvis.

ischial spine: prominence of bone of strong ligamentous attachment above the tuberosity; main significance is in obstetrics.

ischial tuberosity: the prominent, hard portion of bone at the base of the ischium, felt when sitting erect.

ischium: a U-shaped bone of the lower part of the pelvis, which forms a ring.

obturator foramen: refers to the large opening of the innominate bone almost entirely occluded by the obturator membrane. It is the two muscles that cover the large opening of the anterior pelvis; also pertains to the nerves and vessels penetrating this orifice. Formed in adult life when the ischium and pubis become a solid bony continuum, producing a hole or ring that is the largest foramen in the body.

pelvic girdle: a general term that denotes the entire bilateral bony pelvis; the ring that the pelvis makes with its articulation to the sacrum (sacroiliac joint) is called the **pelvic ring.**

posterior inferior iliac spine: prominence of posterior inferior ilium away from sacrum; attachment of ligaments.

pubis (pubic bone): the anterior increased shape of bone of the pelvis, which meets its counterpart from the other side at a point called the **symphysis pubis.**

sacroiliac: joint space between the sacrum and the two ilia; junction of the pelvis to the spine.

superior pubic ramus: top portion of the pubic bone.

symphysis pubis: the junction of the two pubic bones just above the genital area.

Muscles

Most of the pelvic muscles affect the hip or abdominal motion and are described in this section. However, those muscles of the lower abdominal wall surrounding the bladder, uterus, and rectum are sometimes encountered in orthopaedic procedures; they are the levator ani, pubococcygeal, transverse urethral, and cremaster (in scrotum).

sphincter ani: muscle that controls defecation; loss of control of this muscle is a serious sign of herniated disk disease.

Ligaments

anterior sacroiliac l.: large ligament between the sacrum and the ilium.

Poupart inguinal l.: anterior ligament at the groin fold from the anterosuperior iliac spine to the pubic tubercle.

sacrospinous l.: from iliac spine to sacrum.

sacrotuberous l.: ligament from the sacrum to the ischial tuberosity; small sacrosciatic.

Blood Vessels

Most large blood vessels within the pelvis are not encountered in orthopaedic practice. The aorta divides into the common iliac arteries at about the level of the fourth lumbar vertebra. Branches within the pelvis include the hypogastric, superior and inferior gluteal, iliac (which becomes the femoral to the inguinal ligament), and pudendal.

Nerves

cluneal n.: inferolateral, inferomedial, and superior sensory nerves of the buttocks and thighs.

lumbar plexus: arises from the second through fourth lumbar vertebrae, with two major nerves.
> *femoral nerve:* arises from L-2, L-3, and L-4 and supplies most of the knee extensors.
> *obturator nerve:* arises from L-2, L-3, and L-4 and supplies many of the thigh adductors.

pudendal n.: arising from just below the sacral plexus, traveling along the ischium (Alcock canal), and supplying the lower pelvic muscles that do not affect hip motion but affect sexual function.

sciatic n.: the large nerve developed by the sacral plexus supplying the hip rotators, knee flexors, and entire leg and foot muscles, as well as most of the sensation.

sciatic plexus: the major plexus of nerves arising in the pelvic area to include nerves from L-4 and L-5 and nerves of the first three sacral levels. Major injuries or disorders of this plexus are rare, but it is important to understand that this plexus forms the sciatic nerve, which eventually becomes the tibial and common peroneal nerves. Most "sciatica" is actually a nerve root irritation in the spinal column.

Miscellaneous Terms

inguinal: refers to the area of the groin. The precise line is from the anterosuperior iliac spine to the pubis; this is the line of the natural fold of skin in the groin. Terms relating to the area include inguinal nerve, hypogastric nerve, ilio-inguinal nerve, and inguinal canal.

peritoneum: inner membrane lining of the abdominal cavity.

Anatomy of the Hip

The average person refers to the prominent part of the pelvis that flares out just below the waistline (iliac crest) as the "hip." However, the hip portion of the pelvis is the lesser part of the entire pelvic mass; it is 5 inches below the iliac crest and is called the acetabulum, or "true" hip. The three bones of the pelvis merge to form the cup-shaped depression of the hip joint, which holds the femoral head in place. The proximal femur (thigh bone) and its components are described here as the major elements of the hip function and not as part of the lower extremities.

Bones

acetabulum: cup-shaped depression in the mid–outer pelvis known as the hip; this is the socket of the ball-and-socket joint of the hip.

acetabular notch: a cup-shaped defect in the lateral iliac wall above the acetabulum seen in infants who go on to progressive hip dysplasia.

   fovea centralis: central depression in the center of the acetabulum and origin of the ligamentum teres.

   posterior lip: posterior part of the acetabulum, which sometimes breaks off in a dislocation of the hip.

   superior dome: the weight-bearing portion of the acetabulum.

triradiate cartilage: structure present only during growth; the meeting point of the ischium, ilium, and pubis.

digital fossa: a deep depression on the inner surface of the greater trochanter; the site of the insertion of the obturator externus and posterior aspect of the superior border of the greater trochanter.

femoral head: the ball and topmost part of the ball-and-socket joint of the hip; in a growing child may be referred to as the **capital epiphysis.**

femoral neck: the area below the femoral head where the bone narrows into a tubelike structure about 2 inches long.

femur: as related to the hip, is considered the upper, proximal 4-inch segment of bone.

greater and lesser trochanters: part of the femur just distal to the neck where the bone widens into two large prominences, the lower, smaller, and medial of which is the lesser trochanter; the greater trochanter is the larger, lateral prominence. In thin persons the greater trochanter can be felt at about the level of the palm of the hands when the arms are resting by the sides. It is often used as a landmark in physical and x-ray examinations.

intertrochanteric: refers to any region between the two trochanters; a large number of fractures of the hip occur in this region.

piriformis fossa: small, shallow depression located at the tip of the greater trochanter; site of insertion of the piriformis tendon.

subtrochanteric: refers to the widened part of the shaft just below the lesser trochanter.

Muscles

adductors: a group of five muscles that pulls the thigh inward (adduction); these include the **adductor magnus, adductor longus, adductor brevis, pectineus,** and **gracilis muscles.**

external and internal rotators: a group of muscles originating at the pelvis around the hip, helping to control internal and external rotation;

these muscles are the internal and external **obturator gemelli** (**superior** and **inferior gemellus**), **quadratus femoris,** and **piriformis.**

gluteus maximus m.: the large buttock muscle that helps to extend the hip.

gluteus medius and minimus muscles: the deeper significant muscles that abduct the hip and prevent a waddling gait.

iliopsoas m.: a combination of the iliacus and psoas muscles arising from the anterior back and inserting into the lesser trochanter. These large hip flexors are often involved in hip reconstructive procedures.

rectus femoris m.: anterior thigh muscle of the quadriceps group; attaches across the hip joint.

sartorius m.: the muscle stretching from the anterolateral pelvis (anterosuperior iliac spine) to the medial tibia, crossing two joints; it enables the person to assume a cross legged position.

tensor fascia lata m.: the most lateral hip abductor muscle.

Ligament

Bigelow ligament (anterior iliofemoral ligament): major ligamentous expansion of the capsule covering the femoral neck.

ligamentum teres: the round ligament between the middle of the femoral head and the center of the acetabulum (fovea centralis).

Arteries

femoral a.: the major artery from the point of exit from the pelvis to the point of exit behind the knee. Near the hip, it gives off a branch called the **deep femoral (profundus) artery.** The lateral circumflex artery arises from the lateral deep profundus and supplies the lateral and anterior femoral neck. This is the major blood supplier to the femoral head in late childhood and adult life. A branch of the femoral artery is the **medial circumflex artery,** which arises from the deep femoral artery and supplies the posterior femoral head in early childhood.

inferior gluteal a.: large artery from the internal iliac artery within the pelvis; supplies the gluteus medius and minimus.

obturator a.: a branch from within the pelvis that supplies some of the adductor muscles after exiting through the obturator foramen.

superior gluteal a.: a large artery from the internal iliac artery within the pelvis supplying the gluteus maximus and lesser muscles outside the pelvis.

Nerves

All three nerves supplying the thigh and leg also supply the hip. As a result many patients with hip problems complain of thigh, calf, and even foot pain. The large nerves passing near the hip are the following.

femoral n.: supplies sensation to the anterior thigh, medial leg, and the muscle for knee extension.

obturator n.: supplies sensation to the medial side of the thigh and the muscles for pulling the thigh inward (adducting).

sciatic n.: supplies sensation to the posterior thigh and hip extensors; the more distal branches (common peroneal and posterior tibial) are discussed under nerves of the lower limbs.

Surgery of the Pelvis and Hips

Most of the surgery performed on the hip is directed toward making the hip a mobile, painless, weight-bearing joint. Surgical procedures designed to remodel the hip or replace the parts involved are described in this section. Surgical procedures to fuse the hip or to change the direction of alignment of the femur or pelvis are defined in the following sections.

Hip Arthroplasty

A hip arthroplasty is a procedure designed to directly change the contour of or to replace the hip joint (acetabulum) and/or femoral head. This term is so general that it includes most procedures for developmental dysplasia of the hips (DDH) and all procedures that involve prosthetic replacement. For example, the term **total hip arthroplasty** is used often to denote the total joint replacement procedure. Nonprosthetic procedures are listed first.

shelf procedure: a bending of the outer acetabulum (hip joint) so it more completely covers the femoral head. This is commonly done for DDH where the acetabulum is not well rounded and allows the femoral head to displace. It is necessary, in many instances, to reduce the hip and then perform a shelf procedure, using a bone graft to maintain a new position of the lateral acetabulum. Some types of operative shelf procedures are listed. This term specifically means the creation of a bony shelf at the edge of the acetabulum. However, femoral head coverage is sometimes accomplished by pelvic osteotomy with or without the addition of a bone graft to create a shelf.

Albee	Hay-Groves
Bosworth	Lance
Chiari	Lowman
Colonna	Pemberton
Eppright Wagner	Salter
Frank Dickson	Steel
Ghormley	Sutherland
Gill (Type I, II, III)	Weston
Hall Kalamchi	Wiberg

capsular arthroplasty: many procedures for a dislocation of the hip involve soft tissue manipulation only and include curetting of the acetabulum and muscle transfers but do not involve bony osteotomies such as are seen in the shelf procedures. One of these procedures is the **Colonna capsular arthroplasty.**

cup arthroplasty: surgical remodeling of the femoral head and the acetabular socket with the insertion of a metal cup. This procedure is usually reserved for younger persons with severe deforming diseases of the hip after trauma; **mold arthroplasty.**

femoral head prosthesis: insertion into the femoral shaft of a metallic or synthetic component that resembles the femoral head. In present usage, it replaces the femoral head in an older person who has a normal acetabulum but a recent fracture of the hip.

total hip arthroplasty (low friction arthroplasty: a joint replacement involving an internal prosthesis by removing the diseased joint and replacing the acetabular component with either metal or plastic materials and a metal prosthesis of the femoral segment. This type of procedure is usually reserved for older individuals who are suffering from osteoarthritis, avascular necrosis, or other degenerative diseases of the hip. See Internal Prostheses for a description of the many types used.

Closed Hip Reduction Procedures for Developmental Dysplasia of the Hip (DDH)

These are manipulations in an infant or child to reduce a dislocated hip. The method of reduction, followed by the casted position after reduction, varies.

Crego: use of skeletal traction until a closed manipulation with minimal force becomes possible.

Lange: positioning the hip in abduction, internal rotation, and extension after a closed reduction.

Lorenz: both a method of reduction and the frog-leg position cast applied following the reduction.

Ridlon: method of reducing a congenitally dislocated hip and then using a Lorenz cast.

Wingfield frame: used in a gradual method of closed reduction.

Open Hip Reduction

An open hip reduction is a procedure that, when listed by itself, implies the need to reduce a hip under direct surgical vision but with minimal reconstruction of the capsule. Some open techniques include **Calandriello, Ferguson, Howorth, Scaglietti,** and **Somerville.**

Iliopsoas Transfers

This strong hip flexor is sometimes transferred to act as a hip abductor in conditions of muscle imbalance and hip dislocation. Two such procedures are the **Mustard** and the **Sharrard.**

Osteotomies

The osteotomies of the hip are listed here for reference, but some are defined more fully in this chapter under Osteotomy.

Amstutz and Wilson	MacEwen and
Blount	Shands
Blundell Jones	McCarroll
Borden, Spencer, and	McMurray
Herndon	Müller
Brackett	Osgood
Chiari	Pauwels
derotation	Pauwels Y
dial	Pemberton
Dimon	Platou
Gant	Salter (innominate)
Ghormley	Sarmiento
Hass	Schanz
Irwin	Schede
Langenskiöld	Southwick
Lloyd-Roberts	Steel-triradiate
Lorenz	Sutherland-Greenfield
	Whitman

Arthrodeses

The arthrodeses are listed for reference but some are defined more fully under General Surgery of Joints.

Abbott	Ghormley
Abbott-Fisher-Lucas	Henderson
Albee	Hibbs
Badgley	Kickaldy and Willis
Blair	Schneider
Brittain	Stamm
Chandler	Trumble
Davis	Watson-Jones
Gant	John C. Wilson

Other Pelvic and Hip Procedures

acetabuloplasty: any surgical remodeling of the cup side of the hip joint.

Asnis p.: for mild chronic slipped capital femoral epiphysis; fixation with a cannulated screw.

Baxter and D'Astous p.: for hip contracture in myelomeningocele; resection of proximal femur and interposition of muscle mass.

Bleck p.: for excessive hip internal rotation when walking; a recession of the iliacus and psoas tendon to anterior capsule of hip.

Campbell p.: for abdominal and hip flexion contracture; excision of a part of the anterior ilium after a soft tissue release.

Canale p.: for mild chronic slipped capital femoral epiphysis; cannulated screw fixation.

Castle and Schneider p.: for spastic cerebral palsy hip dislocation; interposition of muscles over joint following resection of femur proximal to subtrochanteric line.

Chandler p.: for hip adduction gait; intrapelvic obturator neurectomy.

Couch, DeRosa, and Throop p.: for hip adduction gait; transfer of the adductor tendon to ischial tuberosity.

coxotomy: surgical opening of the hip joint.

Dimon and Hughston p.: for comminuted intertrochanteric hip fracture; a method of reduction with valgus placement and use of a high angle nail.

Dunn p.: for displaced slipped capital femoral epiphysis, removal of "hump" and fusion of epiphysis.

Fish p.: for chronic slipped capital femoral epiphysis; resection of dome-shaped wedge at femoral head.

Girdlestone resection: excision of the femoral head and neck for a fractured intertrochanteric hip joint and other diseases.

Graber-Duvernay p.: boring holes leading to the center of the femoral head for the purpose of promoting circulation.

Hardinge p.: splitting gluteus medius and respecting anterior portion of that muscle with part of vastus lateralis.

hebosteotomy: incision into the pubis; hebotomy.

Heyman-Herndon p.: for displaced slipped capital femoral epiphysis, a shortening of the femoral neck with correction of deformity.

ischiectomy: surgical excision and removal of a part of the ischium.

ischiohebotomy: surgical division of the ischiopubic ramus and ascending ramus of the pubis.

ischiopubiotomy: incision into the ischial pubic junction.

Karakousis and Vezeridis p.:   for malignancy of pelvis; resection of hemipelvis and head of femur, preserving neurovascular structures.

King and Richards p.:   for posterior acetabular fracture; oblique screw fixation.

Kramer, Craig, and Noel p.:   for chronic slipped capital femoral epiphysis; osteotomy and wedge resection at base of femoral neck.

Legg p.:   for paralysis of gluteus maximus; posterior portion of tensor fascia lata muscle is transferred to a more posterior position.

Lyden p.:   for mild chronic slipped capital femoral epiphysis; use of cannulated screw; **Lehman p.**

Lynne and Katcheria p.:   for spastic cerebral palsy subluxation of hip; ipsilateral iliac crest used as a graft in pelvic osteotomy.

Martin p.:   for chronic, severe slipped capital femoral epiphysis; a closed-wedge osteotomy at base of femoral head.

Matta and Saucedo p.:   for sacral fracture; reduction and fixation with posterior screws placed lateral to medial.

McCarty p.:   for chordoma of sacrum; resection of a portion of sacrum.

Menson and Scheck p.:   for osteoarthritis of the hip; release of the pericapsular muscles. Also called **"hanging hip"** procedure.

Morrisay p.:   for mild chronic slipped capital femoral epiphysis; percutaneous single screw fixation.

Ober-Barr p.:   for paralysis of gluteus maximus; a fascia lata graft still attached to fascia lata and flap transferred to erector spinae m.

pubiotomy: surgical incision and division in the pubic bone.

Radley, Liebig, and Brown p.:   for malignancy of ischium; resection of tuberosity and lower portion of pubis.

Root p.:   for spastic cerebral palsy with tight hip adductors; transfer of adductors to ischial tuberosity.

Root and Siegel p.:   for valgus and internal rotation deformity of hip; varus derotational osteotomy of proximal femur.

Sarmiento p.:   for intertrochanteric fracture of the hip; use of osteotomy cut in the distal fragment to achieve valgus nail plate fixation.

Selig p.:   for hip adducted gait; intrapelvic obturator neurectomy.

Soutter p.:   for abdominal and hip flexion contracture; release of the soft tissues about the iliac crest.

Staheli p.:   for developmental hip dysplasia; shelf procedure using iliac crest bone graft for buttress.

Stee p.:   for spastic cerebral palsy internal rotation and flexion hip deformity; transfer of gluteus medius to vastus intermedius.

Stener and Gunterberg p.:   for chordoma of sacrum; resecting portion of sacrum.

Sutherland p.:   for internal rotation deformity of the hip; transfer of semitendinosus and semimembranosus to lateral posterior septa of thigh.

Taylor, Townsend, and Corlett p.:   technique of vascularized free iliac crest graft.

Thomas, Thompson, and Straub p.:   for gluteus medius paralysis; transfer of external abdominal oblique to the tensor fascia lata.

trochanteric slide: an osteotomy of the outer portion of the greater trochanter done from an anterior direction so that it and the attachment of the gluteus medius and vastus lateralis can be retracted posteriorly as a single flap and then replanted with wire fixation following a hip procedure.

trochanterplasty: surgical excision of a ridge of bone to form a new femoral neck.

Veleanu, Rosianu, and Ionescu p.:   for hip

adduction gait; combination of adductor tenotomy and obturator neurectomy.

Ward, Thompson, and Vandergriend p.: for vertical shear fracture of pelvis; posterior iliac to sacral screw fixation after reduction.

Webb p.: for separation of symphysis pubis; two-screw and plate fixation after reduction.

Weber, Brunner, and Freuler p.: for displaced hip fracture in children; cancellous screw fixation after initial fixation with Kirschner wires; **Boitzy p.**

THE LOWER LIMBS

Anatomy

Bones

adductor tubercle (adductor tuberosity): the knobby prominence of the medial femoral condyle, which is easily felt by pressing on the medial side of the knee 5 cm above the joint.

anterior and posterior tibial spines: little prominences of bone inside the knee joint; attachment for the anterior and posterior cruciate ligaments.

anterior tibial tubercle: the large knob just below the anterior knee joint; the point of insertion for the quadriceps (knee extensors) muscles.

Chaput tubercle: the anterolateral tubercle of the distal tibia at the ankle joint for the strong attachment of the anterior tibiofibular ligament; **tubercle of Tillaux-Chaput.**

femoral condyles: the two prominences at the distal end of the femur, called the medial and lateral femoral condyles. The space between the condyles, called the **intercondylar notch,** contains the cruciate ligaments within the knee.

femur (Fig. 8–14): thigh bone; largest bone in the body.

fibula (Fig. 8–16): the smaller bone on the lateral side between the knee and ankle.

fibular facet (proximal tibiofibular facet): the flat portion of bone on the lateral side of the proximal tibia for articulation with the fibula.

fibular neck: narrow part of the fibula just below the proximal enlargement of the bone.

Gerdy tubercle: prominence of bone superior and lateral to the anterior tibial tuberosity; used as reference point in some knee surgery.

lateral malleolus: the distal end of the fibula, which is the outer prominence of the ankle.

linea aspera: a line of prominent bone on the lateral side of femur in the posterior proximal and middle femur for insertion of the gluteus maximus.

medial malleolus: the large prominence on the inner side of the ankle and part of the tibia.

patella (Fig. 8–15): the kneecap, a round to ovoid bone within the quadriceps (knee extensor) tendon. It has a posterior cartilaginous surface for articulation with the femoral condyles known as the **medial** and **lateral facets.**

posterior malleolus: a structure that cannot be seen or felt but is the posterior joint aspect of the tibia. It may fracture by itself or, more commonly, in association with other ankle fractures.

tibia (Fig. 8–16): the large leg bone on the medial side between the knee and ankle.

tibial plateau: the surface that articulates with the femur; may be subdivided into the medial and lateral plateaus.

trochlea: the groove that holds the patella in line on the distal femoral joint surface.

Muscles

adductor m.: the medial muscle of the thigh responsible for pulling the thigh toward the midline.

hamstring m.: three posterior thigh muscles, originating mostly at the pelvis and posterior femur, that help flex the knee. They are given this common name because when they reach the knee joint they are mostly tendinous. The three hamstring muscles are:

FIG 8–14.
Right femur. **A,** Anterior view. **B,** Posterior view. (From Seeley RR, Stephens TD, Tate P: *Anatomy and physiology,* St Louis, 1989, Times Mirror/Mosby College Publishing.)

FIG 8–15.
Right patella. **A,** Anterior view. **B,** Posterior view. (From Seeley RR, Stephens TD, Tate P: *Anatomy and physiology,* St Louis, 1989, Times Mirror/Mosby College Publishing.)

Intercondylar eminence
Lateral epicondyle
Head
Medial epicondyle
Tibial tuberosity
Tibia
Fibula
Lateral malleolus
Medial malleolus

FIG 8–16.
Right tibia and fibula, anterior view. (From Seeley RR, Stephens TD, Tate P: *Anatomy and physiology,* St Louis, 1989, Times Mirror/Mosby College Publishing.)

biceps femoris: outer hamstring
semimembranosus: inner hamstring
semitendinosus: inner hamstring.

pes anserinus: the distal tendon portion of the gracilis, sartorius, and semitendinosis muscles, which at their attachment on the proximal medial tibial side are similar to a goose's foot in appearance.

popliteus m.:   a muscle in the posterior superior tibia that has its tendon insertion into the posterior femur. It is important in lateral injuries of the knee in that the structure may be involved or

encountered on arthrographic examination or as a part of surgical procedure.

quadriceps m.:   the four divisions of muscles that are the bulk of the anterior thigh that become a tendon that surrounds the patella and ends on the tuberosity of the tibia. They function in extending the knee and, in the case of the rectus femoris, help to flex the hip. The quadriceps femoris group of muscles includes the **vastus lateralis, vastus medialis, vastus intermedius,** and **rectus femoris.**

Muscle Compartments
Muscles act in groups to bring about movements, primarily as agonists, antagonists, synergists, and prime movers. There are many muscle groups and compartments throughout the body. The most commonly referred to muscle groups are in the leg, because swelling within the compartments can lead to irreversible muscle change and loss of motor function. Therefore, the four compartments of the leg are defined here and the function and names given of the muscle groups of the lower extremity.

Achilles tendon: the tendinous heel cord that is the extension from the **triceps surae** group of muscles.

anterior c.:   contains the muscles responsible for dorsiflexion of the ankle and the large and lesser toes; included are the **tibialis anterior, extensor hallucis longus, extensor digitorum longus,** and **peroneus tertius.**

deep c.:   contains the flexors of the toes and ankle and are known as the **tibialis posterior, flexor digitorum longus,** and **flexor hallucis longus.**

gastrocsoleus muscle: refers to the combination of the two largest muscles contributing to the Achilles tendon.

lateral c.:   contains the muscles that evert or plantar flex the ankle; they are the **peroneus longus** and the **peroneus brevis.**

posterior c.:   contains the **triceps surae** muscles, which make up the bulk of the calf; included are the following:

gastrocnemius: the most posterior muscle of the calf, leading to the Achilles tendon, that flexes both the ankle and knee.

plantaris: the smaller ankle flexor that leads to the Achilles tendon over the medial side.

soleus: the larger deep ankle flexor of the calf leading to the Achilles tendon.

Ligaments

The knee is an encapsulated joint that has several layers of fascial tissue. The deeper layer is referred to as the **joint capsule,** but numerous ligaments and tendons make up this capsule (Fig. 8–17).

anterior and posterior cruciate l.: the two deep ligaments within the knee that are crossed.

infrapatellar l.: the infrapatellar tendon. Since this "tendon" bridges two bones and not a muscle to bone, it is more correctly referred to as the infrapatellar ligament. Its bursa is the infrapatellar bursa.

lateral collateral l.: strong fibrous ligament of the lateral knee joint with fibers from the femur to the tibia and fibula. This ligament is sometimes called the **tibial collateral,** but caution should be taken to distinguish this from the ankle ligaments.

ligaments of Henry and Wrisberg: small ligaments of attachment for the meniscus in the posterior knee.

ligamentum mucosa: not a true ligament but the thin, filmy membrane that sometimes divides the knee joint.

medial collateral l.: strong fibrous ligament on the medial side of the knee connecting the femur with the tibia. There is a **superficial** and a **deep ligament** in most knees. The posterior oblique ligament is composed of fibers that arise from the medial collateral ligament and attach more posteriorly in the joint.

proximal tibiofibular l.: ligament between the fibular neck and tibia.

tibiofibular l.: when used without distinction as to distal or proximal, refers to the ligaments just above the ankle; these ligaments are divided into the anterior, middle, and posterior tibiofibular ligaments.

Arteries and Veins (Fig. 8–18)

anterior tibial a.: main artery of the anterior leg supplying the extensors and peroneal muscles.

deep femoral a.: the largest branch of the femoral artery in the upper thigh that travels closely to the femur and gives off numerous circumferential branches around that bone; the branches are referred to as the **perforating arteries.**

femoral artery and vein: large artery and vein of the thigh that originate in the groin area; they penetrate posteriorly through fascia above the knee (Hunter canal) and become the popliteal artery and vein.

highest genicular a.: large branch from the femoral artery supplying the muscles and joints on the medial aspect of the knee. Branches above the knee may be referred to as medial and lateral superior genicular, medial and lateral inferior genicular, anterior and posterior tibial recurrent, and fibular arteries.

other arteries near the ankle: perforating, anterior and posterior medial malleolar, and anterior and posterior lateral malleolar arteries.

peroneal a.: travels along the posterior fibula supplying deep calf muscles and collateral circulation of the leg.

popliteal artery and vein: continuation of the femoral artery and vein as they emerge behind the knee, dividing distally to that joint and giving off the anterior tibial artery and posterior tibial artery.

posterior tibial a.: large artery of the posterior leg supplying most of the muscles of the calf and deep spaces; a major branch is the peroneal artery.

saphenous vein: large vein of the subcutaneous tissue in the medial thigh; continuous to the medial side of the ankle.

FIG 8–17.
Major joints in terms of disease and surgical sites. **A,** Hip. **B,** Knee. (From Hilt NE, Cogburn SB: *Manual of orthopedics,* St Louis, 1980, The CV Mosby Co.)

FIG 8–18.
Blood vessels of the pelvis and lower limb. **A,** Arteries of the pelvis and lower limb—the internal and external iliac arteries and their branches. The internal iliac artery supplies the pelvis and hip, and the external iliac artery supplies the lower limb through the femoral artery. **B,** Veins of the pelvis and lower limb—the right common iliac vein and its tributaries. (From Seeley RR, Stephens TD, Tate P: *Anatomy and physiology,* St Louis, 1989, Times Mirror/Mosby College Publishing.)

Other Structures

infrapatellar fat pad (retropatellar fat pad): a distinct mass of fat behind the patellar tendon extending into the anterior joint of the knee. Also called **Hoffa fat.**

medial and lateral menisci: referred to as the **semilunar cartilages,** which are fibrocartilaginous structures interfacing the medial and lateral rim of the femorotibial joint; serve to help distribute the weight load on the two cartilaginous surfaces by changing shape and position during motion.

interosseous membrane: a very strong fibrous membrane between the fibula and tibia, extending throughout most of the length of the bones.

plica: a fold, pleat, band, or shelf of synovial tissue; minor structures, but may be large enough to produce symptoms and demand surgical attention. Specific locations include the transverse suprapatellar, medial suprapatellar, mediopatellar (also called medial patellar shelf), and infrapatellar plica (also called ligamentum mucosa, which does not produce symptoms).

prepatellar bursa: a bursa in the fat in front of the kneecap.

suprapatellar pouch: the extension of the anterior knee joint to about 12 cm above the joint line.

Nerves of the Lower Limbs

common peroneal n.: a brief segment of nerve that divides into the superficial and deep peroneal nerve just distal to the fibular head.

deep peroneal n.: nerve that supplies voluntary function of the toe and ankle extension; the sensory branch is between the first and second toes.

posterior tibial n.: nerve of the posterior leg that supplies the outer and deep calf muscles and eventually the muscles of the foot and sensation on the sole of the foot.

saphenous n.: nerve branch from the femoral nerve; supplies only sensation to the medial leg.

sciatic n.: nerve of the posterior thigh, supplying muscles of the posterior thigh and dividing into the common peroneal and posterior tibial nerves.

superficial peroneal n.: nerve that supplies the voluntary muscle function which turns the ankle out; also supplies sensation on the dorsum of the foot.

sural n.: large sensory nerve of the calf deriving branches from both the peroneal and posterior tibial nerves.

Surgery of the Lower Limbs

The Femur and Tibia

Caldwell and Durham p.: for quadriceps rupture; a transfer of the biceps femoris tendon to quadriceps tendon.

D'Aubigne: for tumor of femoral condyle or tibial plateau; use of attached patella to act as graft for joint surface.

Enneking: for malignancy of distal femur or proximal tibia; resection of affected bone and use of graft taken from healthy bone and fixation with rod and patellar screws.

Gage p.: for spasticity of hamstring muscle; transfer of semitendinosus to rectus femoris.

Grant, Surrall, and Lehman p.: for spastic flexion contracture of knee; anterior closing wedge osteotomy of distal femur.

Lewis and Chekofsky p.: for malignant tumor of proximal femur; resection of proximal femur.

Moore p.: for malunion distal femur in child; excision wedge of bone, using fragments as a graft after correcting deformity.

Sage p.: for hamstring spasticity with dislocating patella and internal rotation deformity of hip; lengthening of rectus femoris.

Sutherland p.: for hamstring spasticity with weak quadriceps muscle; transfer of semitendinosus and semimembranosus to patellar extensor mechanism.

Tachdjian p.:   for hamstring spasticity in a child; lengthening of semitendinosus, semimembranosus, and biceps femoris.

Wagner p.:   for correction of leg length discrepancy (LLD); a method of shortening the femoral or tibial diaphysis, shortening the metaphysis of the femur or tibia, or lengthening the femur or tibia.

White p.:   for leg length discrepancy; a method of shortening the femur.

The Knee

Knee injuries account for a large percentage of the surgical procedures of the lower limbs because many muscles arising in the thigh and leg affect that joint. Often more than one procedure is indicated at the same time. Over the years, some of the combinations of procedures have acquired eponymic designations. To give a general purview of surgery of the knee, the single procedures and their modifications are listed first, and the combined procedures are listed last.

Knee Surgery for Internal Derangement

Andrews p.:   for anterior cruciate laxity; extracapsular tenodesis by using iliotibial band.

Campbell p.:   use of fascial strip from quadriceps tendon to replace anterior cruciate ligament.

Cho p.:   for anterior cruciate deficiency, intraarticular use of semitendinosus tendon.

Clancy: for anterior cruciate–deficient knee, use of midpatellar tendon with attached patellar and tibial bone. Also, for posterior cruciate laxity; use of mid patellar tendon graft.

Drez p.:   for anterior cruciate replacement; use of patellar tendon.

Ellison p.:   extraarticular repair to replace anterior cruciate function; rerouting iliotibial band under the lateral collateral ligament.

Engebretsen p.:   for anterior cruciate ligament deficiency; use of semitendinosus tendon with an LAD prosthetic graft as augmentation.

Ericksson p.:   for anterior cruciate instability; midportion of patellar tendon and portion of bone redirected through tibia and into posterior lateral femoral condyle.

five-in-one repair: five procedures for severe ligamentous injuries to the knee; includes a medial meniscectomy, medial collateral ligament repair, vastus medialis advancement, semitendinosus advancement, and a pes anserinus transfer. Also called **Nicholas procedure.**

Fox-Blazina p.:   extraarticular repair to replace anterior cruciate function by rerouting the iliotibial band under the lateral collateral ligament and placing it distal to original attachment.

Hey-Groves p.:   a reconstruction of the anterior cruciate ligament using tensor fasciae latae graft.

Hughston and Degenhardt: for posterior cruciate–deficient knee; use of medial head of gastrocnemius.

Hughston and Jacobson: for posterolateral instability; advancement of bony attachment of fibular collateral ligament and popliteus tendon to a superior and anterior direction.

Insall p.:   for anterior cruciate laxity; use of iliotibial band and bone block as replacement.

Insall and Hood p.:   for posterior cruciate ligament laxity; use of medial gastrocnemius and bone block as replacement.

Jones p.:   repair of the anterior cruciate ligament using a portion of the patella and patellar ligament. A **Lam modification** of this procedure is also used.

LAD (ligamentous anterior dislocation) composite graft: a synthetic anterior cruciate replacement designed to be used with tissue graft.

Leeds-Keio: a prosthetic Dacron mesh replacement for the anterior cruciate ligament.

ligamentous advancement: implies a soft-tissue procedure only. The ligament is detached and then pulled up or down and reattached to bone. This is done for the medial and lateral collateral ligaments.

Lindeman p.: for anterior cruciate ligament rupture; gracilis tendon transfer as a replacement.

Loose p.: for anterior cruciate instability with pivot shift; portion of iliotibial band is redirected through lateral femoral condyle and around lateral joint.

MacIntosh p.: using infrapatellar and quadriceps tendon for transfer over posterior lateral femoral condyle for anterior cruciate ligament replacement. Also, iliotibial band used in reconstruction to provide anterior cruciate stability.

Marshall p.: for anterior cruciate ligament laxity; portion of patellar tendon and fascia is directed through notch and over lateral femoral condyle.

Mauck p.: detachment of a segment of the tibia containing the medial collateral ligament and replacement of that block of bone in a position that tightens the ligament.

meniscectomy: excision of the medial or lateral meniscus. There are other menisci in the body, but meniscectomies are usually done on the knee. A **partial meniscectomy** is the removal of the torn portion only or a definite attempt to leave meniscal margins of an even width.

Muller p.: for posterolateral instability; reinforcement with iliotibial band graft.

over-the-top p.: for anterior cruciate deficiency; any procedure that places the transferred ligament over the lateral femoral condyle rather than through the condyle.

Pagddu p.: for anterior cruciate–deficient knee; intraarticular use of gracilis and semitendinosus tendons.

Paulos p.: for anterior cruciate–deficient knee; use of medial patellar tendon and retinaculum through tibial grove.

reverse Mauck p.: detachment of a segment of the femur containing the medial collateral ligament and insertion of this block of bone into a position that tightens the ligament.

Slocum p.: a pes anserinus transfer (pes transfer). This is commonly done in association with other procedures and involves a change in the direction of pull of tendons inserting just below the medial knee joint; designed to help replace dynamic stability in ligamentous laxity.

triad knee repair (O'Donoghue p.): a repair involving the anterior cruciate ligament, medial collateral ligament, and a medial meniscectomy.

vastus medialis advancement: a procedure done rarely by itself but more commonly in association with procedures for ligamentous laxity of the knee and/or chronic subluxing patella. It is a tightening of the vastus medialis muscle.

Wirth Jager p.: for posterior cruciate ligament deficiency; use of proximally based semitendinosus and gracilis tendon for replacement.

Yount p.: for severe contracture of posterior knee; division of iliotibial band and biceps tendon.

Zaricznyj p.: for anterior cruciate–deficient knee; use of double strand semitendinosus for replacement.

Zarins and Rowe: for anterior cruciate–deficient knee; simultaneous "over the top" of semitendinosus and iliotibial band with posteromedial and posterolateral capsular reefing.

Knee Surgery for Chronic Subluxation of the Patella

Campbell p.: fascial tissue transfer and vastus medialis reefing.

Emslie-Trillat p.: medial displacement of anterior tibial tuberosity on a bone pedicle for subluxing patella.

Galeazzi p.: for chronic lateral subluxing patella; use of fold of medial strip of parapatellar capsule, strip is brought across inferior to superior patella and back again.

Hauser p.: inferomedial displacement of a block of bone with the infrapatellar tendon attached.

Hughston p.: lateral release with quadricepsplasty and patellar tendon transfer as needed.

Insall p.: lateral retinacular release and lateral advancement of vastus medialis.

Maddigan, Wissinger, and Donaldson p.: for chronic lateral subluxing patella; wide lateral advancement of vastus medialis.

Maquet p.: anterior tibial tuberosity displacement on bone pedicle for patella alta.

Roux-Goldthwait p.: medial displacement of the lateral portion of the infrapatellar tendon.

Sargent p.: lateral release and advancement of vastus medialis over patella with attachment to exposed, bleeding patellar surface.

Silfverskiöld p.: for knee flexion contracture (in cerebral palsy); transection of medial and lateral head of gastrocnemius muscle and motor branch to medial gastrocnemius.

Southwick slide p.: medial displacement of bony attachment of the patellar tendon, replacing the lateral defect with bone from the medial side.

Stanisavljevic p.: for congenital dislocating patella; massive patellar tendon and quadriceps refashioning.

West and Soto-Hall p.: patellectomy and medial advancement of the quadriceps mechanism for patellar osteoarthritis.

Patellar Surgery

Cave and Rowe p.: for osteoarthritis of the patella; partial patellectomy with fold of infrapatellar fat sewn onto the posterior patella.

Codivilla p.: for neglected quadriceps tendon rupture; direct repair and advancement of fold from superior quadriceps mechanism.

Houston and Akroyd p.: for sleeve fracture of patella; tension band wire fixation with two Kirschner wires.

Magnuson p.: for unstable fracture of the patella; arthroplasty of the knee (fascia) in an attempt to remodel, and use of encircling metal wire.

Martin p.: for patellar fracture; fixation with a wire loop.

McLaughlin p.: for quadriceps or patellar tendon rupture; a reinforcing encircling wire is attached to patella or tibia, respectively.

Miyakawa p.: patellectomy with fabrication of a fold taken from the thick tissue well superior to the patella and reinforcing the patellar area to provide better mechanical force.

patellar or femoral condylar shaving (skiving) direct removal of diseased cartilage from the patella and femoral cartilage, usually done in combination with treatment of other chronic knee injury problems.

patellectomy: removal of the kneecap.

patellectomy (partial): this procedure has two different meanings: (1) total removal of cartilage from the patella, and (2) removal of a portion of the bone following a fracture.

Scudari p.: for fresh quadriceps rupture; repair with reinforcing flap from superior quadriceps mechanism.

Total Knee Arthroplasty

Total knee arthroplasty (TKA) is the replacement of both sides of the knee joint by metal or plastic components. See Internal Prostheses in this chapter for various types of prostheses.

Quadricepsplasty

Any repair or reapproximation of the quadriceps mechanism is called a quadricepsplasty.

Judet quadricepsplasty: for knee fibrosis; parapatellar and intraarticular adhesion release with intraoperative manipulation.

Thompson quadricepsplasty: for knee fibrosis; isolation of vastus lateralis and medialis from rectus femoris and capsular incision.

Tendon Transfers

Surgical releases for muscle imbalance or knee contractures are referred to as tendon transfers.

Baker p.: patellar tendon advancement; semitendinosus transfer for knock-kneed gait caused by internal rotation deformity of the hip.

Bickel and Moe p.: translocation of the peroneus tendon.

Caldwell and Durham p.:   for quadriceps paralysis; transfer of biceps femoris to quadriceps mechanism.

Chandler p.:   patellar tendon advancement.

Ecker, Lotke, and Glazer p.:   for neglected infrapatellar tendon rupture; transfer of gracilis and semitendinosus for reinforcement.

Eggers p.:   transfer of the biceps femoris tendon associated with capsular releases and soleus neurectomy.

Galleazzi p.:   for chronic subluxation of the patella; transfer of the semitendinosus.

Hughston p.:   for chronic subluxation of the patella; patellar tendon transfer fixed by staple and redirection of vastus medialis.

Kelikian p.:   for old patellar tendon rupture; transfer of the gracilis tendon.

Sutherland p.:   for internal rotation deformity in hip affected by cerebral palsy; lateral transfer of medial hamstring.

Tachdjian p.:   for hamstring tightness in cerebral palsy; plastic lengthening of hamstring sheaths and tendons.

Genu Recurvatum Procedures

Brett and Campbell: tibial osteotomies.

Heyman p.:   reinforcement of posterior capsule using multiple tendon transfers; soft tissue release and transfers.

Perry p.:   posterior capsular repair with multiple tendon transfers.

Knee Arthrodeses
Brittain
Charnley
Key
Lucas and Murray
Putti

The ankle arthrodeses are listed under foot and ankle procedures in Chapter 11.

Tibial Osteotomies
Campbell
Cotton
Coventry
Ferguson-Thompson-King
Brett
Pott
Lucas and Cottrell

Lower Limb (Below Knee) Surgery

Anderson p.:   for unequal leg lengths; tibial lengthening using an external skeletal fixator.

Anderson and Hutchins p.:   for unstable tibial fractures; a method of skeletal pins and casting for fixation.

beefburger p.:   for failed total knee arthroplasty; debridement with interposition of acrylic cement between leveled edges of femur and tibia, followed by brace immobilization.

Bosworth p.:   for anterior tibial epiphysitis; insertion of bone pegs into the tibial tubercle.

Brett p.:   for malunited proximal tibial fractures with knee recurvatum; bone graft applied to opened anterior tibial plateau hinged posteriorly.

Brown p.:   for congenital absence of tibia; transfer fibula to femoral intercondylar notch.

Carroll p.:   bone graft replacement of the distal end of the fibula for tumors.

d'Aubigne p.:   for tumors; a method of excision of femoral condyle or tibial plateau.

Fahey and O'Brien p.:   for excision of tumor; technique of excision of a portion of the shaft of a bone.

Forbes p.:   for nonunion tibial fracture; iliac bone graft to tibia.

Gilbert p.; Tamai p.:   technique of obtaining vascular fibular graft by using lateral approach.

Gill p.:   for long-bone nonunion; a half diameter slide graft of a 10- to 15-cm portion of bone.

Gruca p.:   for congenital absence of the fibula; construction of an ankle mortise by splitting of the fibula.

Hsu and Hsu p.: for ankle flexion contracture in muscular dystrophy; percutaneous tendocalcaneus lengthening.

Irwin p.: for paralytic genu recurvatum; a closing wedge osteotomy of the proximal tibia.

Langenskiold p.: for partial absence of fibula; fusion of distal tibia and fibula.

Lee p.: for depressed tibial plateau fracture; anterosuperior iliac spine used to replace joint surface.

Malawer p.: for malignancy of proximal fibula; resection of proximal fibula.

Nicoll p.: for tibial or other long-bone nonunion; dual onlay bone graft with cancellous bone in the middle.

Russell p.: for central depression lateral plateau; proximal portion of fibular head is used to support depression of joint surface.

Taylor p.: technique of obtaining vascular pedicle fibular graft through posterior approach.

Van Ness p.: for proximal focal femoral deficiency; a derotation osteotomy of the tibia to fit the limb more readily with a prosthesis.

Wagner p.: for leg-length disparity; shortening of proximal tibia or distal femur.

Weber p.: for persisting acute valgus deformity tibial shaft fracture in children; open reduction and removal of tissue.

Weiland p.: technique of obtaining vascular fibular graft by using lateral approach.

Wilson and Jacobs p.: for comminuted tibial plateau fractures; replacement technique for the lateral side using iliac crest graft.

The ankle and foot procedures are covered in The Foot and Ankle, Chapter 11.

SKIN GRAFTS

Skin grafts are of three major categories; split-thickness skin graft (STSG), full-thickness skin graft (FTSG), and pedicle and rotational flaps.

Split-Thickness Skin Graft

A split-thickness skin graft is 0.015 inch or 0.4 mm thick. Taking a graft this way leaves viable skin from the donor site and living cells in the graft. However, both donor site and the graft will appear different from normal surrounding skin. Names associated with skin grafts are **Blair-Brown, Douglas (mesh), Dragstedt,** and **Ollier-Thiersch.**

Full-Thickness Skin Graft

A full-thickness skin graft is a procedure that, throughout the entire surface of the graft, includes all the epidermis and, therefore, all the smooth skin coverage. This leaves behind a **donor site** that will need some form of closure or a split-thickness skin graft; for example, if a small necrosed area on a finger needs full skin coverage, a small ellipse of skin could be removed from the forearm; this is called a **pinch graft,** and the wound edges are closed.

Names associated with full-thickness skin grafts are **Braun, Davis, Esser (Stint), Krause-Wolfe, Reverdin,** and **Wolfe.**

Pedicle Grafts and Rotational Flaps

A pedicle graft is a layer of fat, dermis, and epidermis raised from a portion of the body having a sufficient blood supply to keep it alive. Pedicles are often used to cover large tissue defects, areas of exposed tendons, or areas where there will be considerable wear on the skin. The intended purpose of a pedicle is to eventually transfer this loose piece of skin and fat to cover another portion of the body. A flap is another name for pedicle, although the term connotes a local use in some cases; for example, a **rotational flap** is a rearrangement of the skin and fat in one area to cover a local defect. Pedicles may include muscle or bone.

A **delayed flap** is used for stimulation of the blood supply. An incision in the skin and fat with reapproximation of the wound margins into their original position is carried out. In a second or third procedure the flap is raised on a pedicle that is still attached, but now the distal part of that flap can be laid on another portion of the body. For example, a U-shaped incision is made in the leg and closed; 3 weeks later that skin is raised through the same incision and the flap that develops is laid on an open area of the opposite leg. This is called a **cross-leg pedicle graft.**

Other terms referring to pedicle grafts and flaps are bilobed, compound, compound lined, double pedicle, Verdan, jump, marsupial, tumbler, Tait, and island pedicle.

SURGICAL BLOCKS

The term **local anesthesia** is sometimes used to indicate a regional anesthesia. In precise parlance, **local anesthesia** indicates the injection of anesthetic agents at the site of the procedure. **Regional anesthesia** is infiltration of anatomic structure(s) proximal to the location of the procedure. Those used for orthopaedics are the following.

axillary b.:   injection of anesthetic agent into the nerves immediately around axillary artery, approached from the axilla; used for elbow, forearm, and hand procedures.

epidural b.:   infiltration of anesthetic agent into spinal canal but outside of the dura; can be used for so-called continuous drip anesthesia, where a catheter is left in place during procedure so that if more anesthesia is required it can be administered without repositioning the patient.

intravenous b.:   application of double tourniquet and the infiltration of anesthetic agents directly into vein to produce anesthesia in the limb below the tourniquet. Also called **Bier block.**

scalene b.:   injection of anesthetic agent into brachial plexus at the point of scalene muscles; used for shoulder and other upper limb procedures.

spinal b.:   infiltration of anesthetic agent into the spinal canal within the dura in the lumbar region. The proper positioning of patient during anesthetic infiltration is important in ensuring correct and sufficient anesthesia for procedures on the pelvis and lower limbs.

SURGICAL APPROACHES

A surgical approach implies the type of incision made by the surgeon to do a particular procedure. Many surgical approaches have been described by various surgeons whose names are applied to those approaches. However, those approaches are not all original and have been modified and improved over the years. Anatomically, the direction of the incision may be modified by another surgeon, whose name then becomes attached to that incision, although in fact it is designed for accessing the same area of the body. In many instances, an experienced surgeon may decide to plan an individualized approach in a given situation.

This prior consideration to surgical intervention may be described by the anatomic location and direction of the incision, for example, anterolateral or posterolateral approaches. More frequently, the anatomic terms are favored in describing where an incision is to be made, even though the eponyms are also used for a particular anatomic area described.

Approaches are listed by anatomic location, eponyms, and common uses for the incision. Those interested in the technique of an incision will use other references. At the end of this section is a list of common incision shapes.

Shoulder Approaches

anterior axillary a.:   usually used for repair of anterior dislocations; **Roberts.**

anteromedial a.:   used for repair of shoulder and acromioclavicular joint injuries; **Cubbins, Callahan and Scuderi, Roberts, Thompson and Henry, saber-cut.**

deltoid splitting a.:   used to approach the rotator cuff and subacromial bursa.

posterior a.:   used for repair of a posterior dislocation of the shoulder and lateral scapula. **Abbott**

and Lucas, Bennett, Harmon, Kocher, McWhorter, Rowe, Yee.

transacromial a.: used to approach the rotator cuff and bursa; **Codman, Darrach-McLaughlin, saber-cut.**

Humerus Approaches

anterolateral a.: an approach to the bone and radial nerve; **Thompson** and **Henry.**

anteromedial a.: an approach to the median and ulnar nerves.

posterior a.: an approach used to visualize the humerus, triceps, and radial nerve; **Henry.**

Elbow Approaches

anterior and anteromedial a.: for exploration of the median nerve, brachial artery, and other soft tissues; often associated with fractures.

anterolateral a.: for exploration of the radial nerve; **Henry.**

medial a.: for exploration of the ulnar nerve and medial epicondyle; **Campbell, Molesworth,** and **Campbell.**

posterior: for fractures of the distal humerus; **Bryan** and **Morrey.**

posterolateral a.: for elbow dislocations, radial head and distal humeral fractures, and arthroplasties; **Kocher.**

Forearm Approaches

posterior a.: in the proximal forearm used for fixation of proximal ulnar fractures and an approach to radial fractures; **Thompson.**

posterolateral a.: approach used for radial head fractures, some ulner fractures, and exploration of the deep radial nerve; **Boyd.**

anterior a.: used for visualization of most of the forearm muscles that flex the fingers and for internal fixation of fractures of the radius; **Henry.**

posterolateral (distal) a.: used for some distal forearm fractures, tendon transfers, and excision of the distal ulna; **Gordon.**

Pelvis Approaches

Avila a.: anterior approach along the iliac crest to reach the anterior sacroiliac crest.

Radley, Liebig, and Brown a.: to the ischium.

Hip Approaches

anterolateral a.: for open reduction and internal fixation of the femoral neck, prosthetic replacement, and some congenital dysplasia surgery; **Smith-Petersen, Van Gorder, Wilson, Cave, Callahan, Fahey.**

Hardinger a.: splitting gluteus medius and resection anterior portion of that muscle with part of vastus lateralis.

lateral a.: for internal fixation of hip fractures and prosthetic replacement; **Callahan, Charnley-Müller, Fahey, Harris, Hay, McLaughlan, Murphy, Ollier, Watson-Jones.**

medial a.: for congenital dysplastic hip surgery and other iliopsoas tendon approaches; **Ludloff, Young.**

posterior a.: for prosthetic replacement and repair of some pelvic fractures; **Abbot, Gibson, Guleke-Stookey, McFarland** and **Osborne, Moore, Osborne.**

Senegas (modified Ollier): for acetabular fractures; an extensive exposure of the involving detachment of the greater trochanter.

Femur Approaches

anterolateral a.: used for rod or plate fixation fractures; **Thompson.**

lateral a.: used for fracture fixation; **Eycle-Shymer** and **Shoemaker.**

posterior a.: used for some muscle surgery and fixation of fractures; **Bosworth.**

posterolateral a.: used for muscle procedures, fracture fixation, and nerve explorations; **Eycle-Shymer** and **Shoemaker, Henry.**

Knee Approaches

All approaches to the knee are for ligamentous and bony reconstruction, meniscectomies, and vascular explorations. The posterior approaches are more specifically devoted to neurovascular surgery but may also be used in ligamentous and bony reconstructive procedures.

anterior a.: Coonse and Adams, Bosworth, Putti, Jones and Brackett, Insall.

anterolateral a.: Kocher, Henderson.

anteromedial a.: Abbott and Carpenter, Langenbeck.

lateral a.: Bruser lateral, Aufranc, Henry, Hoppenfield, deBoer, Pogruna and Brown.

medial a.: Aufranc, Cave, Henry, Bosworth.

posterolateral a.: Henderson.

posterior a.: Abbott, Osgood, Bracket and Osgood, Putti and Abbott.

posteromedial a.: Banks and Laufman, Henderson.

transverse a.: Cave, Charnley, Cozen, Sir Henry Platt, McConnell.

trivector retaining a.: for extensive knee surgery such as a total joint replacement; an incision that is medial to the standard parapatellar incision, cutting into a portion of the vastus medialis muscle.

Lower Limb Approaches

anterior a.: for internal fixation of fractures; this is an exploration of the anterior deep spaces.

posterior a.: approach to the superomedial region of the tibia and gastrocnemius muscle; **Banks** and **Laufman.**

posterolateral a.: for peroneal nerve and muscle surgery and for some bone grafts; **Harmon, Henry, Huntington.**

posteromedial a.: for neurovascular exploration and internal fixation of fractures; **Phemister.**

Surgical Incisions Described by Appearance

J shaped	curvilinear
L curved	double
S-flap	linear
T shaped	longitudinal
T-tube	saber-cut
U shaped	split
Y incision	transverse
Z-plasty	

REPLANTATION MICROSURGERY

Microsurgery, the use of a binocular microscope to perform surgery, is a challenge for the skilled orthopaedic surgeon. It has been used extensively within other specialties but more recently adapted to a variety of orthopaedic conditions. Microtechniques are applied to nerve repair, vascular repair, replantation, free tissue transfers, and knee and spine surgery.

The integration of this technique provides the surgeon with a three-dimensional telescopic view of the operating field at magnifications of structures 2½ to 25 times the size. Nylon sutures of high tensile strength, finer than human hair, are used to reattach small blood vessels and nerves. To keep vessels open and carefully avoid constriction are the goals of this procedure. Use of the technique requires extreme patience and perseverance on the part of the microsurgical team.

Replantation of traumatically severed extremities has become a common practice in orthopaedic surgery and in musculoskeletal trauma management. The reintegration of tissues by way of microsurgical techniques has successfully restored functional use and eliminated the need for amputation in many cases. Hand and knee surgery have benefited greatly from microsurgery.

Replantation is truly a team effort, involving many hours of work with no room for compromise. The surgeon must spend many hours practicing and developing the skill, applying extreme patience and good judgment during application. The team approach is used to allow replacements during the long procedures.

Although other tissues heal in a short time, the regeneration of nerves may take from 1 to 2 years. Other technologic developments, such as the **laser scalpel,** are also useful in surgical procedures.

TREATMENT OF TUMORS

The prognosis for musculoskeletal tumors has improved with the addition of various chemotherapies and other interventions. Some of these therapies are used in conjunction with amputation and wide excisions.

adjuvant therapy: a method of treatment (i.e., radiation or chemotherapy) combined with another treatment (surgery) to improve therapeutic success.

chemotherapy: the use of drugs to treat tumors.

intralesional resection: surgical removal of tumor from within the surrounding capsule.

marginal resection: surgical removal of tumor through the capsule.

radiation therapy: the use of ionizing radiation to treat tumors.

radical resection: removal of an entire anatomical compartment, which includes tumor, tumor capsule and all muscle, bone, nerve and artery found within that compartment.

wide resection: surgical removal of tumor capsule and surrounding margin of surrounding tissue.

AMPUTATIONS

The least desirable procedure for any surgeon is an amputation of a part; however, sometimes it be-

comes necessary. An **amputation** is the removal of a part through bone, and a **disarticulation** is the removal of a part through a joint space. Both of these terms are interpreted by most as the same procedure, but there is a distinction.

Most amputations take place in the lower limbs and may be indicated by traumatic injury, burns, infection, loss of blood supply, or malignancy. Amputation may also be indicated when a nonfunctioning limb could be replaced by a functional prosthetic device or when a congenital defect could be improved cosmetically or functionally by the removal of a part.

The level of amputation is often based on preservation of as much of the residual limb as would heal well with the vascular and peripheral circulation intact. The most common levels fall into the following categories: above elbow (AE), above knee (AK), below elbow (BE), and below knee (BK).

In the present nomenclature, the description for limb absences can be reversed, that is, a leg, complete, is a complete leg amputation; if there is a partial amputation, it can be stated as to the level, for example, partial arm (upper one-third). Any amputation through an epiphysis or closer to a joint is considered a complete amputation; an amputation of the distal third to the distal growth plate (growth plate scar in an adult) is considered a complete leg amputation (Tables 8–2 and 8–3).

Following such a procedure the patient is often fitted right away with an artificial limb for the remaining residuum. The after treatment of the residual limb is most important in the adjustment and rehabilitation of the amputee, as are the psychologic aspects.

Before and after a prosthesis (artificial limb) is prescribed for an amputee, the physical medicine and rehabilitation team is an important link in teaching the patient prosthetic training. Prostheses have come a long way in appearance, fit, and functional use, and often it is not evident that a person is using a prosthesis. Chapter 7 discusses the many types of prostheses available. The following list of general terms applies to amputations.

TABLE 8–2.

Amputation Levels, Upper Limb

New Terms (with Abbreviations)	Current Terms	Eponyms
Shoulder (Sh), complete	Forequarter	Littlewood
Arm (Arm), complete	Shoulder disarticulation	Larrey, Dupuytren, Lisfranc
Arm (Arm), partial (upper ⅓)	Short (upper-third) AE	
Arm (Arm), partial (middle ⅓)	Medium (mid-third) AE	
Arm (Arm), partial (lower ⅓)	Long (lower-third) AE	
Forearm (Fo), complete	Elbow disarticulation	
Forearm (Fo), partial (upper ⅓)	Short (upper-third) BE	
Forearm (Fo), partial (middle ⅓)	Medium (mid-third) BE	
Forearm (Fo), partial (lower ⅓)	Long (lower-third) BE	
Carpal (Ca), complete	Wrist disarticulation	
Carpal (Ca), partial	WD, with some carpals still present	
Metacarpal (MC), complete		
Metacarpal (MC), partial	Partial hand amputations, usually	
Phalangeal (Ph), complete	without precise differentiation	Kutler
Phalangeal (Ph), partial		

Note: An amputation at the MCP joints of the ring and little fingers would be designated as Ph, 4,5, complete; an amputation of the same two fingers at the PIP joints would be Ph, 4,5, partial.

From Kay HW: A nomenclature for limb prosthetics, *Orthot Prosthet J* 28(4):37–47, 1974.

TABLE 8–3.

Amputation Levels, Lower Limbs

New Terms (with Abbreviations)	Current Terms	Eponyms
Pelvic (Pel), complete	Hemicorporectomy	
Hip (Hip), complete	Hemipelvectomy	King and Steelquist, Jaboulay, Gordon-Taylor, Sorondo-Ferré
Thigh (Th), complete	Hip disarticulation	Béclard, Boyd, Pack
Thigh (Th), partial (upper ⅓)	Short (upper-third) AK	Alouette
Thigh (Th), partial (middle ⅓)	Medium (mid-third) AK	
Thigh (Th), partial (lower ⅓)	Long (lower-third) AK	Kirk
Leg (Leg), complete	Knee disarticulation	Gritti-Stokes, Morestin, Callander, Pollock, Carden, Batch, Spittler and McFaddin
Leg (Leg), partial (upper ⅓)	Short (upper-third) BK	
Leg (Leg), partial (middle ⅓)	Medium (mid-third) BK	
Leg (Leg), partial (lower ⅓)	Long (lower-third) BK	Came
Tarsal (Ta), complete	Ankle disarticulation	Syme, Pirogoff, Guyon, Hancock, MacKenzie
Tarsal (Ta), partial		Chopart, Le Fort, Malgaigne, Vladimiroff-Mikulicz, Tripier
Metatarsal (MT), complete	Known collectively as partial	Lisfranc, Hey
Metatarsal (MT), partial	foot amputations	
Phalangeal (Ph), complete		
Phalangeal (Ph), partial		

From Kay HW: A nomenclature for limb prosthetics, *Orthot Prosthet J* 28(4): 37–47, 1974.

General Amputations

cineplastic (kineplastic) a.: amputation that includes a skin flap built into a muscle (the biceps being the most common); a portion of the prosthetic mechanism is activated by the muscle.

circular a.: one in which a perfect circular incision is made with single flaps.

closed a.: any amputation in which the wound is closed at the time of initial or secondary surgery.

disarticulation: any amputation in which the limb is severed through a joint.

guillotine (chop) a.: amputation making a straight cut through the limb.

open a.: any amputation in which the wound is left open for drainage, as opposed to a closed amputation.

stump revision: any surgery designed to revise the shape or scar of a residual limb.

Syme a.: The term is used to describe a special method of incision and closure for amputations at other locations, but describes a below-ankle amputation (removal of foot).

ASSOCIATED SURGICAL TERMS

ablate: to completely excise or amputate; the surgical removal of a part is referred to as **ablative surgery,** for example, the excision of a large tumorous mass and the surrounding soft tissue.

advancement: surgical or traumatic detachment of muscle, tendon, or ligamentous structure followed by reattachment at a more advanced point.

anastomosis: restoration of continuity of any vessel or organ; usually refers to the suturing of a tubular structure such as a blood vessel creating the passage between two distinct parts, such as end-to-end anastomosis.

anesthesia: loss of sensation with or without loss of consciousness as a direct result of the administration of a systemic drug agent. The term also describes the local or systemic loss of sensation caused by trauma or other injury.

approximate: to bring together or into apposition; this term is commonly used to refer to suturing of tissues or the repositioning of fractures.

aseptic: free from bacteria; aseptic technique is any technique designed to prevent contamination by bacteria.

aspiration: withdrawal of fluid from any open or closed space.

attenuate: to make thin, small, or fine; reduce in size.

autopsy: a postmortem and pathologic examination of the body by dissection; **necropsy.**

biopsy: the excision of a section of living tissue for microscopic examination and diagnosis. This may be performed on any tissue; for example, a bone marrow biopsy is performed by closed method (use of a needle or trochar); the terms **needle biopsy** and **closed biopsy** are often used. In the same sense, an **open biopsy** is one in which the tissue is examined before excision, and all or a sample of that tissue is sent for microscopic inspection.

The purpose of a biopsy is to determine the etiology and test for systemic, neoplastic, or reactive conditions. A biopsy is not made on normal anatomic tissue or where there is trauma or inflammation.

brisement (brēz-maw): the forcible breaking up of joint capsule, usually for conditions of partial fibrous ankylosis such as frozen shoulders.

broaching: the act of widening a bone medullary canal in such a fashion that it will accept the stem of a specific implant. The instrument used to do this is a **broach.**

callotasis: for limb length disparity, a transverse section of the bone of the short limb is stabilized with an external skeletal fixator and then the limb is gradually lengthened over a period of weeks.

catheterization: insertion of a tube into a cavity or blood vessel for drainage.

cauterization: the use of an electric current to stop local bleeding. This term also denotes the use of caustic materials such as silver nitrate to reduce local tissue granulation, as seen in open wounds.

cautery: an instrument designed to stop bleeding by destroying tissue through heat, electricity, or corrosive chemicals.

chamfer: applied to the act of smoothing off soft edges or rounding the end of a bone by making small cuts.

costoplasty: correction of rib deformity by osteotomies of rib, often used for correction of scoliosis deformities.

curettage: procedure in which a sharp, scraping instrument is used to remove abnormal tissue, growths, or obtain diagnostic specimens.

curette: sharp, scraping, spoon-shaped instrument used in curettage.

débridement (debreed-maw): cleansing a wound of devitalized, contaminated, or foreign material.

decompression: surgical relief of pressure to any structure.

dehiscence: a separation or splitting of the edges of a surgical wound, where the expectation was for the wound to remain closed.

delayed primary closure (secondary closure): the closure of an open wound by intention after the initial surgery or injury; this is often done when the risk of infection is very high.

diaplasis: the reduction of a fracture or dislocation by surgical means.

dismemberment: amputation of a limb.

dissection: separation of tissue for any reason. **Sharp dissection** is the use of a sharp instrument to facilitate dissection. **Blunt dissection** refers to the separation of tissues along natural lines of cleavage by the use of the fingers or other blunt instruments.

drainage: removal of fluid from a cavity. This term is often used to refer to material arising from open surgical wounds. **Dependent drainage** is an active effort to position a patient so that gravity will carry fluid away from the wound via catheterization.

ebonation: stripping of one tissue from another. In orthopaedics, this refers to a surgical or pathologic removal of hard, bony loose cartilage from the surface of bone.

electrocautery: surgical instrument used to control bleeding of a surgical wound. The use of this instrument is called **electrocauterization.**

enucleate: to remove whole and clean in its entirety an organ, tumor, or cyst by shelling out.

evacuate: to empty a cavity.

excise: to cut out.

exploration: the examination by direct surgical visualization; surgery done for the express purpose of examining tissue is called exploratory surgery.

extirpation: the removal in its entirety of diseased tissue, a structure, or mass; **excision.**

extraction: process of removal by pulling out.

extubation: the removal of a tube; used to refer to the tube inserted into the windpipe during anesthesia.

fixation: as applied to orthopaedics, implies the use of internal or external fixation, which is the use of metallic devices inserted into or through bone to hold a fracture in a set position and alignment while it heals.

fulguration: the use of high frequency electrocautery to destroy tissue during surgical procedures.

fusion: the uniting of two bony segments, whether a fracture or a vertebral joint.

granulation: the proliferation of numerous small blood vessels at a wound site to give the general appearance of a raw, red tissue. This is a normal healing process in that this rich vascular bed can modulate into normal tissue or act as a base for skin grafts or primary closure. **Granuloma** is a pathologic reaction to a foreign body or organism and should not be confused with granulation.

imbrication: the overlapping of tissue structures in closure of a wound and in repair of defects to improve the tightness of a structure.

implant: any substance inserted into the tissue for an indefinite period; this includes all internal prostheses, internal fixation devices, and other materials not absorbed by the body.

incision and drainage (I&D):   surgical incision into a cavity, usually for purpose of removing purulent (infected) material; most common example is the lancing of an abscess.

infiltration: usually refers to local injection of anesthetic solutions or fluids that then permeate soft tissue; may be a result of failure of intravenous fluids to go into the vein correctly.

infusion: introduction of any solution such as saline into a blood vessel or cavity.

injection: introduction of material, nutrients or medicine into tissues of the body by the use of a syringe and needle.

in situ: in orthopaedics, the fixation of a fracture in the position that it presents at the time of injury, usually a nondisplaced fracture; also used to describe a lesion that is highly localized.

in toto: in total; removal of an organ, cyst, or tumor in its entirety.

intubation: insertion of a tube into the trachea for entrance of air during surgical procedure; for example, endotracheal entubation.

in vitro: cells or tissue maintained in an artificial environment such that they can survive outside the living body usually for experimental purposes. (This term is sometimes italicized in the literature.)

in vivo: within the living organism, such as an experimental drug being used on an animal or human subject. (This term is sometimes italicized in the literature.)

irrigation: washing out of a wound or cavity with a solution. **Closed suction irrigation** is a specific system by which irrigating tubes are surgically implanted in a wound and used continuously after the time of surgery.

laser (light amplification by stimulated emission of radiation):   a device used in surgical procedures consisting of a resonant optical cavity in which a substance is stimulated to emit light radiation and a mirror that reflects the rays back and forth so molecules will emit more radiation. Finely directed laser light sources can be used to cut tissue, coagulate vessels, or cause the adhesion of one tissue surface to another.

lavage: the copious washing out or irrigation of a wound or cavity.

ligamentotaxis: use of strength of ligaments to bring about reduction of fracture fragments by using external skeletal fixation.

ligation: tying off; used particularly in reference to the tying of blood vessels at a surgical wound.

ligatures: sutures used to tie off blood vessels.

manipulation: the planned and carefully managed manual movement of a joint or fracture to produce increased joint motion or better position and alignment of the fracture. This term is sometimes used to denote a precise sequence of movements of a joint to determine the presence of disease or to reduce a dislocation.

marsupialization: incision into a cystic lesion with incorporation of the walls of the cyst to the exterior edges of the skin to produce constant drainage.

matte finish: a fine-ground-glass-appearing finish, designed for better cement to metallic surface fixation of internal prosthetics.

morcellation: breaking up of tissue for easier removal; also, to leave in place but in a refashioned shape such as bone graft material.

palliative: surgical procedure or use of medications to treat the symptoms without curing the disease process; used relative to the treatment of terminal conditions seen in cancer.

paracentesis: needle puncture into a cavity to aspirate fluid; usually done in the abdominal and thoracic cavities.

parenteral: the introduction (injection) of substances into the body by way of intravenous, intramuscular, subcutaneous, or intramedullary route, other than through the alimentary canal.

per primam: the healing of a surgical or traumatic wound by first intention, after closure. This means that the closure of the wound is successful and that there is no reopening of the wound due to failure of healing.

-pexy (suffix): fixation by solid tissue attachment. In orthopaedics, the most common term using this root is **scapulopexy,** a procedure whereby the scapula is fixed directly to the ribs.

phantom pain: the sensation of pain following amputation that seems to be in the part that has been removed. Eventually, the patient is able to localize the pain to the stump and loses the sense of the presence of the amputated part.

plication: taking tucks in a structure to shorten it; folds. **Fundiplication** is a combination of shortening and being part of the anatomy.

polyacetyl rod: synthetic polyester rod used for fracture fixation. The rod is bioabsorbable.

portal: small stab incision used for introduction of arthroscope or instrument into a joint.

primary closure: the closure of the wound edges at the time of trauma or surgery.

prosthesis: this term has a very broad meaning and includes all artificial limbs as well as materials implanted in the body to replace the structure, function, or appearance of the missing structure.

reefing: a folding in or overlapping of soft tissue by surgical suture designed to make that structure tighter.

reflect: in the surgical sense, to fold back tissue such as a muscle belly to expose deeper structures.

regimen: a system of therapy regulated to achieve certain results (e.g., diet, exercise following surgery).

release: incision into any soft tissue to produce relaxation of that tissue, for example, tendon release.

resection: partial excision of soft tissue or segment of bone; also, the removal of a portion of diseased nerve tissue, called a nerve resection.

retraction: a pulling back of tissue, whether done mechanically at the time of surgery or by scar formation after surgery; for example, a scar that is indented inward toward the body is considered a retracted scar.

revision: any surgical reconstruction of soft or hard tissue. A revision may be done at the time of initial trauma if damaged tissue is removed and normal structures are repositioned to compensate for that destruction. The term is more commonly used to describe a later surgical effort to reposition various tissues.

rongeur: to cut into bone with a sharp biting instrument called a rongeur, usually to remove bone that is diseased or obstructing visualization of deeper structures.

saucerization: creation of a saucer-like depression in bone in an effort to remove diseased bone. This is most commonly done for bone infections, and the wound is usually left open for drainage; it is also a saucer-like collapse of a crushed vertebrae on the horizontal surface.

scaffold: a support, usually of an absorbable fiber, for the ingrowth of tissue.

secondary closure: closure of a wound that had been left open after previous trauma or surgery. This is also called **delayed primary closure** and is done often when there was initially a high risk of infection.

sepsis: the presence of bacterial infection in blood or tissue from any source. This term is often used to describe the systemic condition resulting from an infection, for example, septicemia.

septic: contaminated with bacteria. A septic wound, otherwise known as a **dirty wound,** is one in which there is an existing infection with purulent material.

-stasis (suffix): to control flow or progression, for example, hemostasis.

stasis: condition arising from a static circumstance. For example, a stasis ulcer is one that is created in a patient kept in the same position for any length of time where blood or fluids stagnate.

stent: a support, flexible or rigid, usually biodegradable, designed to relieve excessive strain during graft or other tissue repair and remodeling.

subcutaneous: the fatty and fibrous tissues beneath the thick layers of skin.

subcuticular: the thick layer of skin below the epidermal layers. A subcuticular suture is used to close the skin by a continuous suture that pulls the deep layer of skin together, with the suture exiting at each end of the wound only.

sulcus: any normal groove or depression in bone or soft tissue.

suspension: usually refers to a soft tissue procedure designed to help hold some anatomic structure in a more functional position; tenodesis.

suture: any threadlike, pliable material that is used to close soft tissue; catgut, nylon.

tamponade: method to control bleeding by direct pressure.

-tome (suffix):   any instrument that cuts.

tourniquet: any instrument used to compress blood vessels to slow or stop circulation. If light pressure is applied by tourniquet, there will be congestion in the venous system. This is often used to help draw blood for laboratory testing. More secure tourniquet pressure, designed to stop all blood flow to a part, is used to prevent bleeding.

toxic: poisonous. This term is often used to describe the systemic condition of a patient with infection.

transect: to cut across the long axis of a tissue. For example, a tendon transection is often done to release the pull of that tendon at its point of insertion.

transfusion: term commonly used to describe the intravenous infusion of whole blood or blood components; however, any solution may be transfused.

transposition: the repositioning of an intact and attached tissue segment from one place to another. This term is often used in describing soft tissue and bone graft procedures.

-tripsy (suffix):   surgical crushing, for example, an osteotripsy is a procedure done in the foot to relieve a corn or callus caused by prominence of bone under the skin.

vest-over-pants closure: closure of fascia, particularly near joints, where one layer is closed on top of another to produce tightening or pull on the joint capsule.

viable: alive or capable of living; used to describe healthy tissue that appears to be intact.

Chapter 9

The Spine

The spine consists of three basic elements: bones, joints, and neural tissue. Together these components allow the spinal column to perform a variety of functions in the human body. The weight of the body is transferred through the vertebrae and disks, motion occurs through the intervertebral joints and disks, and the brainstem, spinal cord, and spinal nerves that travel in and around these bones and joints that are allowed to function in a protected environment.

The body has three main neural components: the central nervous system, the peripheral nervous system, and the autonomic nervous system. The **central nervous system** consists of the brain, brainstem, and the spinal cord. Protecting the spinal cord and spinal nerves are the meninges, composed of the dura mater, pia mater, and arachnoid. These protective layers help protect and isolate the central nervous system from the outside world. The brainstem and spinal cord travel within a tunnel-like structure called the spinal canal. The spinal cord gives rise to 31 pairs of spinal nerves or nerve roots that branch off along the length of the spinal cord and exit from the spinal canal through a tunnel called the foramen. After these nerve roots exit from the spine, they join other nerves to become **peripheral nerves.** Peripheral nerves contain the sensory fibers, voluntary muscle fibers, and fibers of the autonomic nervous system. The **autonomic nervous system** is composed of small nerve branches arising from the central nervous system and supplying **ganglia,** which are clusters of cells near but outside the bony limits of the vertebrae. The **sympathetic** and **parasympathetic nervous systems** are subdivisions of the autonomic nervous system, which is involved in the control of visceral organs and blood vessels. Most spinal nerves and peripheral nerves contain a mixture of sensory and motor fibers that supply specific muscles and provide sensation in particular locations in the body. By treating the anatomy of the spinal cord and its peripheral branches like a road map, a physician can often determine the cause of numbness, tingling, or weakness found on a sensory and motor examination.

The spine is made of bony segments known as **vertebrae.** These are separated by intervertebral disks and facet joints that permit motion. A complex arrangement of ligaments and muscles provide stability and motion of the spinal column. Neural elements exit and enter the spinal column through openings called foramina.

Each component of the spinal column depends on the others to function normally. If one part of the spine changes in character, such as in a fracture or a disk herniation, other structures can be affected, leading to arthritis, muscle fatigue, nerve or spinal cord damage, or irritation resulting in pain, numbness, weakness, or even paralysis in severe cases.

GENERAL ANATOMY OF THE SPINE

The 32 vertebrae composing the spinal segments are divided into five regions, with the segments numbered from top to bottom. They are the cervical, thoracic, lumbar, sacral, and coccygeal regions of the spine (Fig. 9–1).

It is very important to understand the designation of vertebrae, intervertebral disks, and nerves when making reference in writing. The proper description is as follows:

Vertebrae	Intervertebral disks	Dermatomes and nerve roots
C-1, L-5	C-2–3, L-4–5	C-2, L-5
T-4, S-2	T-3–4, S-1–2	T-3, S-2

These specific designations may be abbreviated without first being written out in tables and clinical or technical data, but it should be clear as to what part of the spinal anatomy reference is being made.

cervical spine: seven spinal segments (C-1 to C-7) and eight cervical nerve roots (C-1 to C-8) between the base of the skull (occiput) and the thoracic spine. The cervical spine differs from the rest of the vertebrae in one major aspect: the numbered nerve root exits the spinal canal above the correspondingly numbered vertebra's pedicle instead of below it.

thoracic (dorsal) spine: 12 spinal segments (T-1 to T-12) incorporating the 12 ribs of the thorax. Other than a slight increase in size from top to bottom, they are fairly uniform in appearance.

lumbar spine: five mobile segments of the lower back (L-1 to L-5). These are the largest of the vertebral segments.

sacral spine (sacrum): five fused segments of the lower spine that connect to the pelvis and have four foramina on each side.

coccygeal spine (coccyx): remaining three or four, somewhat fixed, fused segments at the end of the spine (tailbone) that articulate with sacrum above.

Except for the coccyx, sacrum, and the first cervical spine, there are anatomic parts that are common to all 32 spinal segments. Moving from anterior to posterior (front to back), the main vertebral parts are the following.

FIG 9–1.
Diagram showing the relation of the segments of the spinal cord and nerves to the segments of the vertebral column. (From Hamilton WJ, ed: *Textbook of human anatomy,* ed 2, London, England, 1976, The Macmillan Press, Ltd.)

facet joint (zygoapophyseal joint): small articular cartilage–surfaced joints connecting the posterior elements of one spine to the posterior elements of the neighboring spine.

foramen: an opening allowing for the egress of spinal nerve roots from between two vertebrae.

intramedullary: refers to medullaris, marrow; (1) within the medulla oblongata of the brain, (2) within the spinal cord, and (3) within the marrow cavity of bone.

lamina: the posterior part of the spinal ring that covers the spinal cord or nerves.

pars interarticularis: the posterior continuation of the spinal arch from the pedicle; the superior and inferior facets are connected to each other by the pars interarticularis.

pedicle: the first portion of the posterior spine arising from the vertebral body.

spinous process: the most posterior extension of the spine arising from the laminae.

transverse process: bony process arising from

midportion of the spinal ring just posterior to the pedicle and pars interarticularis.

vertebral body (Fig. 9–2): from a lateral view, it is the main rectangular portion; from an overhead view, oval.

CERVICAL SPINE ANATOMY

Bones and Landmarks

atlas: the first cervical vertebra (C-1), lying directly under the skull, through which the head articulates with the neck. The main connection to the vertebra below is a pivot around the odontoid process that is an upward projection of the body of the second cervical vertebra. The atlas is held to the odontoid by a ligament complex attaching it to the odontoid anteriorly and facet joints posteriorly, allowing rotation and flexion and extension between C-1 and C 2.

axis: the second cervical vertebra (C-2), about which the first cervical vertebra rotates, allowing

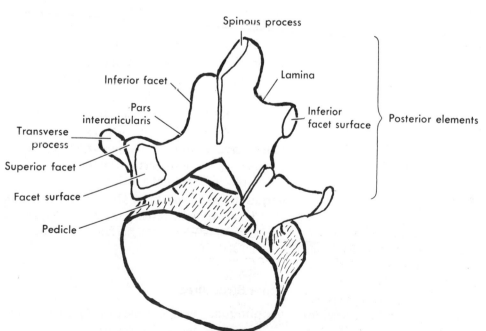

FIG 9–2.
Vertebral body and posterior elements.

head movement. It bears the **odontoid process,** the projecting part of the second cervical vertebra, which allows the first cervical vertebra (atlas) to rotate.

carotid tubercle: prominence of the transverse process of C-6 felt on the lateral side of neck.

cricoid ring: cartilage ring above the trachea and below the thyroid cartilage, the first cricoid ring is at the level of C-6.

hyoid bone: small, vertically oriented bones lateral to trachea, located at the level of C-3.

joints of Luschka (uncovertebral joints): unique to the cervical spine, these jointlike structures are formed by the apposition of posterolateral portions of adjacent vertebral bodies; forms the anterior portion of the canal where nerves pass through.

lateral mass: the lateral expansion of the spinal ring in the cervical spine, consisting of the facet joints and intervening bone as well as a tunnel through which the vertebral artery travels in the second through fifth cervical vertebra.

occiput: the base of the skull.

thyroid cartilage: widening expanses of cartilage above the trachea, the top marks the level of C-4, the bottom C-5.

Muscles

longissimus colli: long muscle immediately anterior to the cervical spine.

platysma: thin outermost muscle layer of the anterior neck.

posterior neck muscles: splenius, spinalis, and semispinalis.

scalenus: the deep lateral muscles of the anterior neck, including anterior scalene m. (scalenus anticus), middle scalene m. (scalenus medius), and posterior scalene m. (scalenus posticus).

sternocleidomastoid: large externally visible muscle of the anterior neck, enabling head to turn to either side.

strap muscles: a general term applied to the ribbon-like muscles in the anterior neck; they include omohyoid, sternohyoid, sternothyroid, and thyrohyoid.

Arteries and Veins

carotid artery: main artery to the head that divides into external and internal carotid arteries.

jugular vein: large obvious vein in the neck.

other arteries and veins: transcervical, facial, superior thyroid, and inferior thyroid.

vertebral artery: large artery that travels in the lateral masses of the cervical spine and eventually supplies the lower brainstem.

Nerves

cervical plexus: plexus of nerves that supply the neck muscles with branches named by muscles supplied, a portion of which is called the ansa cervicalis.

occipital nerve: nerve from the back of the neck that supplies motor function and sensation to the forehead; two parts—greater and lesser.

other nerves (twelfth cranial): transcervical, supraclavicular, posterior rami, facial, greater auricular, and hypoglossal.

phrenic nerve: nerve arising from three cervical nerve roots (C-3 to C-5); supplies the diaphragm.

spinal accessory nerve (eleventh cranial): the nerve from the brainstem that supplies the sternocleidomastoid muscles.

vagus nerve (tenth cranial): the long nerve in the anterior neck traveling with the carotid artery; responsible for many organ functions in the chest and abdomen.

Other Structures

esophagus: portion of the gut between the mouth and stomach in the anterior neck.

interspinous ligament: ligament between each of the spinal processes.

nuchal ligament: large posterior midline ligament in the neck from the base of the skull to the seventh cervical vertebra.

thyroid gland: near the "Adam's apple"; responsible for secretion of hormone that is involved in regulation of the rate of the metabolism.

trachea: the windpipe.

triangles: for surgical approaches and other considerations, the anterior half of the neck is divided into triangles—anterior, digastric, posterior, submental, and carotid.

THORACIC SPINE ANATOMY

thorax: the chest or rib cage; also refers to the space containing the lungs and heart. There are 12 vertebral segments and ribs; the lower two are called **floating ribs.**

costo-: combining form denoting relation to ribs.

costovertebral angle: juncture of tissue inferior and lateral to the twelfth rib and vertebral body.

costovertebral joint: junction of the rib with the thoracic spine.

costochondral junction: junction of the rib into cartilage in the anterior chest. NOTE: Most of the ribs have attachment to the cartilage rather than a direct junction with the breast bone.

sternum: the breast bone; further divided into three segments.
  manubrium: upper portion, proximal end.
  sternum: main portion.
  xiphoid: the dagger-like tip of the sternum, distal end.

diaphragm: the muscle between the abdomen and thorax; main muscle of normal breathing.

intercostals: the muscles between the ribs.

other thoracic spine and chest muscles: pectoralis, semispinalis, rotators, latissimus dorsi, and spinalis.

LUMBAR AND LOWER SPINE ANATOMY

Bones

lumbar spine: the five movable spinal segments of the lower back and largest of the spinal segments.

sacral spine (sacrum): the five segments fused together as a solid bone and below the last lumbar segment position.

coccyx: the three, and sometimes four, segments of bone just below the sacrum; referred to as the tailbone; the end of the spinal column.

sacroiliac joint: the junction between the sacrum and the ilium; resembles a large ear.

sacral ala: lateral portions of the sacral bone.

Disk and Spinal Canal

intervertebral (interspinal) disk: the structure that normally occupies the space between two moving vertebrae. It is more prominent in the cervical and lumbar spines. It is much like a radial tire. The centermost portion of the disk (**nucleus pulposus**) is normally composed of a gelatinous material that varies in consistency from a firm jelly material to a very thick and less pliable substance. This core is then surrounded by numerous layers of fibrous (fibrocartilaginous) material called the **annulus fibrosus.** That structure goes to the normal margins of the vertebral body, called the **anterior longitudinal ligament,** and to those on the spinal canal side posteriorly, the **posterior longitudinal ligament.**

ligamentum flavum: a band of yellow elastic tissue that runs between the laminae from the axis to the sacrum; it assists in maintaining or regaining erect position and serves to close in the spaces between the arches. It is important as a surgical structure in that a portion is usually removed during an exploration of the spinal canal.

spinal canal: the space between the vertebral body anteriorly and the lamina and spinal process posteriorly. The spinal cord extends to the level of the second lumbar segment in adults and the second sacral segment in infants. Below this level are numerous spinal nerves from the spinal cord. This lower portion resembles a horse's tail and is referred to as the **cauda equina** (horse's tail in Latin). The lower tip of the spinal cord is attached to the end of the spinal canal by a single filament called the **filum terminale.** The brain, spinal cord, and spinal nerves float in a water-like substance called the cerebral spinal fluid. This fluid is contained in a thin sac called the **meninges.** The thick, outer portion of that sac is called the **dura** or **dura mater.** The more flimsy inner coverings are the **arachnoid** (Latin for spider-like) and pia. The dura extends over the nerve roots out into the foramina. This saclike covering is called the **nerve root sleeve.** The dura also extends within the spinal canal down to the level of the second sacral segment. Any space within the dura from the first cervical to the second sacral level is considered **intradural.**

spinal cord: the part of the central nervous system below the level of the brainstem and above the cauda equina in the region of the cervical and thoracic and upper lumbar spine. Usually, the orthopaedist does not deal with the spinal cord—that is for the neurosurgeon. However, some affections of these parts may cause musculoskeletal problems.

long tracts: the nerve fibers that connect the spinal cord with the brain; main spinal nerve pathways.

pyramidal tract: carries the voluntary muscle messages from the brain.

dorsal column: the main, normal sensory tract to the brain.

spinal thalamic tract: the main tract of pain to the brain.

dorsal lateral column: the main tract of position and tone to the brain.

gray matter (anterior and posterior horns): the nerve cell bodies to muscle and sensory outflow and input, respectively.

Muscles

abdominal muscles: important for support of the spine, these muscles are the rectus abdominis, external oblique, internal oblique, and transversus.

artery of Adamkiewicz: an important source of blood supply to the lower portion of the spine, usually occurring at T-9 to T-11 level; however, not the only blood supply to the cord at that level.

iliopsoas muscle: large muscle starting at L-1 and becoming wider as it picks up segments from the lower lumbar spine; combines with the iliacus muscle before attaching to the lesser trochanter of the hip.

posterior spinal muscle segments: upper and lower posterior serratus m., spinalis m., semispinalis m., and rotators.

quadratus lumborum: a muscle lateral to the iliopsoas muscle of the spine running from the lower ribs to the ilium.

DISEASES AND STRUCTURAL ANOMALIES

Back and Neck Diseases

The spine is a complex organ that is a series of joints with attending bone, nerve tissues, muscles, and ligaments. In addition, there are two elements not common to other joints, namely, intervertebral disks and the spinal cord and nerves in the bony spinal canal. The nerves may be affected by either bone or disk disease; therefore, this section is divided into discussions of diseases affecting bone, nerves, spinal cord, vertebral disks, and congenital disorders.

Diseases of the spine may be treated by other medical specialties, particularly neurosurgery in the case of spinal cord and nerve lesions and injuries. However, the orthopaedist treats many diseases and conditions of the spine such as scoliosis, spina bifida, and degenerative disk disease. Treatment may last for years in the correction of some deformities.

General Bone Diseases of the Spine

The Latin word *vertebra* and the combining form *spondylo-* both denote the bony spinal segments. In some word combinations, the root word is assigned only to a specific part of the vertebra, such as spondylolysis in which the defect is always at the pars interarticularis. However, spondylo- in general means vertebra.

Spondylo- Root Diseases

spondylalgia: pain in vertebra(e).

spondylarthritis: arthritis of the spine.

spondylarthrocace: tuberculosis of the spine; **spondylocace.**

spondylexarthrosis: dislocation of a vertebra.

spondylitis: inflammatory disease involving the spine with inflammation of vertebrae, including types such as ankylosing, rheumatoid, traumatic, spondylitis deformans, Kümmell, and Marie-Strümpell d.

spondylizema: depression or downward displacement of a vertebra, with destruction or softening of one below it.

spondylodynia: pain in vertebra(e).

spondyloepiphyseal dysplasia: disorder of growth affecting both the spine and the ends of long bones.

spondylolisthesis: anterior displacement of one vertebra on the adjacent lower vertebra. A general term with multiple distinctions:

anterior displacement: forward movement of the superior segment on the inferior one.

lumbar lordosis: angle made by lines drawn from the superior surface of the first and fifth lumbar vertebra.

lumbosacral joint angle: angle between the inferior surface of the fifth lumbar vertebra and the top of the sacrum.

rounding of the cranial border: relationship of the height to the width of the rounded portion of the superior sacrum.

sacral inclination: relationship of the sagittal plane of the sacrum to the vertical plane.

sacrohorizontal angle: angle between the top of the sacrum and the horizontal line.

sagittal rotation: angular relationship between the body of the fifth lumbar vertebra and the sacrum; **sagittal roll, lumbosacral kyphosis, slip angle.**

wedging of olisthetic vertebra: measure obtained by dividing the height of the anterior border of the fifth vertebra by the height of its posterior border, multiplied by 100.

spondylolysis (Fig. 9–3): a fracture or defect in the pars interarticularis (a portion of bone between each of the joints of the back), allowing one vertebral body to slide forward on the next. May be referred to as **pars interarticularis defect.**

A classification system for spondylolysis and spondylolisthesis has evolved:

dysplastic: congenital abnormalities of the arch of the sacrum or the arch of L-5 that permit the slipping to occur.

isthmic: the lesion is in the pars interarticularis. Three types occur:

a. lytic, fatigue fracture of the pars interarticularis.

b. elongated but intact pars interarticularis.

c. acute fracture of the pars interarticularis.

degenerative: the lesion results from intersegmental instability of long duration.

traumatic: results from fracture in other areas of the bony hook than in pars interarticularis.

pathologic: generalized or localized bone disease is present.

spondylomalacia: softening of vertebrae; **Kümmell disease.**

spondylopathy: any vertebral disorder.

spondylopyosis: infection in vertebra(e).

spondyloschisis: congenital fissure (splitting) of vertebral arch.

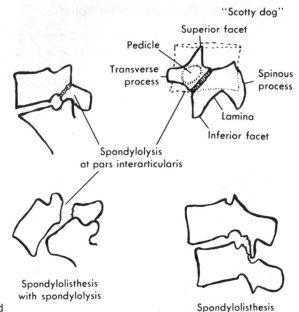

FIG 9–3.
Spondylolysis and spondylolisthesis seen in lateral view and oblique (Scotty dog) view.

spondylosis: bony replacement of ligaments around the disk spaces of the spine, associated with decreased mobility and eventual fusion; **marginal osteophyte.**

Rachio- Root Diseases

Rachio-, as relating to spine, is less frequently used than more specific combining forms.

rachialgia: pain in the vertebral column.

rachiocampsis: curvature of the spine.

rachiochysis: effusion of fluid within the vertebral canal.

rachiodynia: pain in the spinal column.

rachiokyphosis: humpbacked curvature of spine; kyphosis.

rachiomyelitis: inflammation of the spinal cord.

rachioparalysis: paralysis of the spinal muscles.

rachiopathy: any disease of the spine.

rachioplegia: spinal paralysis.

rachioscoliosis: lateral curvature of the spine.

rachisagra: pain or gout in the spine.

rachischisis: congenital fissure of the spinal cord.

Miscellaneous Spinal Disorders

alar dysgenesis: abnormality in development of the sacroiliac joint.

anisospondyly: different abnormal shapes of the vertebral bodies.

ankylosing spinal hyperostosis: arthritic disorder in which bridging osteophytyes located anteriorly and posteriorly on the vertebral body bind two or more vertebrae together; **Forestier disease.**

anterior spurring: ligament turning to bone on anterior side of vertebral body.

Baastrup d. (kissing spine): false joint formed by wide posterior spinous processes of the lumbar spine. This may become a source of pain.

camptocormia: severe forward flexion of upper torso, usually an excessive psychologic reaction to back pain.

cervical rib: riblike structure in the seventh cervical vertebra that may cause nerve root irritation.

coccyalgia: pain in the coccyx region; **coccygodynia, coccyodynia, coccydynia.**

crankshaft phenomenon: progressions of a spinal curve due to continued growth of the unfused anterior aspect of the spine following a posterior spine fusion for scoliosis in children. The deformity can be severe with increased lordosis and rotation despite little change in the curve as measured on an AP radiograph.

dysraphism: any failure of closure of the primary neural tube. This general category would include the disorder myelomeningocele. This definition includes the conditions in which there is an abnormal midline structure in the neural axis. Hence, diastematomyelia, in which the midline structure has fused but there is a bony spike from the anterior lying vertebral body is included within this term.

facet tropism: asymmetrical orientation of the facets comparing right to left side.

Grisel syndrome: subluxation of the atlantoaxial joint from inflammatory ligamentous laxity due to infection. Can result in neurologic complications.

interspinous pseudarthrosis: formation of a false joint between two spinous processes.

limbus annulare: a mass of bone situated at the anterosuperior margin of a vertebra. Arises from failure of fusion of the primary and secondary ossification centers.

lumbago: archaic term meaning back pain.

lumbarization: partial or complete formation of a free-moving first sacral segment so that it looks like a lumbar vertebra.

marginal osteophytes: excess bone formation at the margin of the vertebral body; **spondylosis.**

olisthy (Gr. *olisthanein,* to slip):   slipping of bone(s) from normal anatomic site; for example, a slipped disk.

paravertebral muscle spasm: spasm in the muscles on either side of the spinous processes (midline of the back); the term may be used to describe a physical finding or improperly used to define a disease process.

pseudoclaudication: increased pain and decreased strength in lower limbs associated with physical activity. Complaints are similar to those caused by an insufficient blood supply to the limb but are caused by diminished blood supply to the nerves in a narrowed spinal canal.

retrolisthesis: posterior displacement of the vertebra on the one below.

rudimentary ribs: nubbins of ribs seen below the level where the last rib normally occurs.

sacralgia: pain in the sacrum.

sacralization: fusion of L-5 to the first segment of the sacrum, so that the sacrum consists of six segments; with this abnormality, it is called **Bertolotti syndrome.**

sacralized transverse process: one or both of the lumbar spinous transverse processes abnormally joining with the sacrum; **sacralization.**

sacrodynia: pain perceived to be in the area of the sacrum but may originate elsewhere; **referred pain.**

sacroiliitis: inflammation of the sacroiliac joint. A very painful, often one-sided sacral area pain that follows delivery, is not due to sepsis, and will subside gradually and completely; **acute postpartum sacroiliitis.**

sciatica: pain radiating down the sciatic nerve into the posterior thigh and leg; can be caused by irritation of a nerve anywhere from the back to the thigh.

scoliorachitis: disease of the spine caused by rickets; abnormal bone mineralization.

Spinal Deformities

Spinal deformity is the abnormal angulation of the spinal column when a person is viewed from the back or the side. It can occur from a variety of causes and at any age. An **inclinometer** is a device used to measure the amount of trunk rotation on examination.

Structural Anomalies

Scoliosis is a general term that applies to any side-to-side curve in the back, that is, a lateral and rotational deviation of the spine from the midline. Such a curve may be termed **fixed curve,** which means that any attempt to eliminate the curve by motion is not successful. Curves may be C-shaped or S-shaped (Fig. 9–4).

A **compensatory curve** has a flexible segment above or below the fixed curve; this compensation will place the spine (above or below) into a vertical position with the head at the midline. The rotation of the spinous process is away from the apex of the curve. **Levorotatory scoliosis** means that this rotation of the most dorsal element of the spine is to the left if one is looking at the patient from behind. **Dextrorotoscoliosis** is the opposite condition. The apex of a curve is called the *convex side,* for example, a right lumbar scoliosis is a lateral deviation of the spine in the lumbar region, with the apex of that curve to the right; the *concave side* of the curve is the opposite side.

Scoliosis may be associated with vertebral anomalies (missing parts of the vertebrae) and with forward bending (round back); the latter is called **kyphoscoliosis.** Scoliosis may occur at birth (*congenital*), occur from known causes or diseases (*acquired*), or occur from unknown causes (*idiopathic*). An example will best illustrate the terminology. In a right thoracic, left lumbar, **uncompensated rotatory scoliosis,** viewed from behind, the upper back curves to the right and the lower back to the left; there is rotation of the spine, which may or may not be in both curves (unless so stated), and the center of the head is not in the midline when the patient is standing.

Other Spinal Deformities and Conditions

adolescent scoliosis: lateral curvature of the spine occurring during adolescence.

adult scoliosis: scoliosis occurring after skeletal maturity.

compensatory curve: a curve located above or below a rigid structural curve to maintain normal overall body alignment.

congenital scoliosis: scoliosis due to bony abnormalities present at birth involving either fail-

FIG 9–4.
Scoliosis. **A,** Normal. **B,** Right convex curve, uncentered. **C,** Right convex curve, centered. (From the American Orthopaedic Association: *Manual of orthopaedic surgery,* ed 5, Chicago, 1979, The Association.)

A   B   C ure of formation of a vertebra or separation of adjacent vertebrae.

double curve: two lateral curves in a single spine; **double major curve** is two lateral curves of equal magnitude, and **double thoracic curve** is two thoracic curves.

flattening of normal lumbar curve: condition in which the hollow of the back becomes shallow or even straight.

functional scoliosis: any scoliosis that is caused by leg length or other functional disorder and not by a primary curvature of the spine.

idiopathic scoliosis: structural lateral curvature of an unknown cause.

infantile scoliosis: lateral curvature of the spine that begins before age 3.

juvenile scoliosis: begins between the ages of 3 and 10 years of age.

kyphoscoliosis: lateral curvature of the spine associated with forward inclination of the spine.

kyphosis: round shoulder deformity, humpback, dorsal kyphotic curvature; may refer to any forward-bending area or deformity of the spine.

lordoscoliosis: lateral curvature of the spine associated with backward bending of the spine.

lumbar curve: curve with apex between the first and fourth lumbar vertebrae.

lumbar kyphosis: reverse of the normal curve of the low back.

lumbosacral curve: a lateral curve with its aspect at or below the fifth lumbar vertebra.

neuromuscular scoliosis: scoliosis caused by a muscle or central nervous system disorder.

reversal of cervical lordosis: change in the normal curvature of the cervical spine as seen on lateral radiograph. This is usually a straightening of the normal lordotic curve or an actual reversal and is most commonly caused by muscle spasm, indicating cervical disk abnormality.

structural curve: a fixed lateral curve of the spinal column.

thoracic curve: a spinal curvature with its apex between the second and eleventh thoracic vertebrae.

thoracolumbar curve: a spinal curve with its apex at the first lumbar or twelfth thoracic curve.

segmental instability: abnormal response to applied loads characterized by motion in the motor segment beyond normal constraints.

spinal stenosis: general term denoting narrowing of the spinal canal in the lumbar area leading to nerve root compromise; term often used for developmental abnormality that leaves a narrow, bony canal. There are four subgroups of this condition:

> **achondroplastic stenosis:** increased vertebral thickness, marked concavity of the vertebral body, and short pedicles.

> **constitutional stenosis:** normal-statured individuals with congenital variance in vertebral structure leading to a narrow canal.

> **degenerative stenosis:** gradual hypertrophy of the vertebral body margin, facet joints, and ligamentum flavum leading to stenosis.

> **combined stenosis:** for congenital or developmental reasons, the midsagittal diameter is decreased.

temporomandibular joint syndrome: complex of symptoms often seen in cervical sprain conditions. Symptoms include clicking in the jaw on opening and closing the mouth, soreness in the jaw, headaches, buzzing sounds, changes in hearing, stiffness in the neck and shoulders, dizziness, and swallowing disorders. It is believed that much of the reason for this symptom complex relates to change of the mandibular posture and the resultant change in cervical posture, or vice versa; **TMJ, craniomandibular cervical syndrome.**

thoracic outlet syndrome: mechanical problem related to the exit of arteries and nerves at the base of the neck leading down the arm, and can also involve the vein bringing blood back from the arm. Compression of these structures as they pass through a narrow foramen between the scalenus anterior muscle and first rib. Problem may be exacerbated by congenitally present additional cervical rib. An early sign is pain in the hand or shoulder. Arteries may be damaged in the process and cause an aneurysm in the area with possible breakoff of clot from the aneurysm.

traction spur: bony excrescence appearing on the anterolateral surface of the vertebral body near but not at the body margin that arises as a result of disk degeneration.

transitional vertebra: vertebra whose structure features some of the characteristics of the two adjacent vertebra. A common example is the fifth lumbar vertebra that has partial sacral components.

wedging: deformity of vertebral body, caused by trauma or gradual collapse, resulting in wedge-shaped vertebra; can also occur congenitally.

Eponymic Spinal Disorders

Marie-Strümpell d.:   inflammation of the spine, occurring as a rheumatoid-type disease in children.

Pott d.:   tuberculosis of the spine, usually in the lower thoracic segments.

Scheuermann d.:   inflammation of the anterior cartilage of the bodies of the lower thoracic and upper lumbar segments, causing pain in some older, growing children. There is more than 5 degrees of wedging of at least three adjacent vertebrae as seen on radiographs.

Schmorl nodes: developmental change resulting in inferior or superior extension of the intervertebral disk into the vertebral bodies.

Nerve Root Diseases of the Spine

The nerve roots in the spinal canal lie in close contact with the vertebrae and emerge through openings called foramina. In the neck, nerve root irritation may be localized at the place where it exits through the foramen, whereas in the lumbar spine, nerve root irritation usually occurs one level above the point of nerve exit.

Vertebrae and nerve roots of the spine are the same in number, except for the cervical spine—there are seven cervical vertebrae and eight cervical nerve roots (Fig. 9–1). This occurs because the first cervical nerve exits between the skull and the first cervical vertebra. Therefore, between C-7 and T-1 the eighth cervical nerve makes its exit. After this level, all nerves exit in conformance with the vertebra above the point of exit. When the examiner speaks of the *nerve roots* of the spine, it is recorded singularly as C-1 or C-2, whereas if the examiner is speaking of the *intervertebral disk* between the vertebrae, it is recorded in combination as C1–2 or C2–3. The vertebrae are recorded individually as C1 or L-4.

This section is concerned with the local spinal processes and the wide range of neurologic diseases seen by an orthopaedist and especially by a neurosurgeon.

cauda equina syndrome: sufficient pressure on the nerves in the low back to produce multiple nerve root irritation and commonly loss of bowel and bladder control.

compression of nerve root: mechanical process resulting from a tumor, fracture, or herniated disk; the resultant irritation is called **radiculitis** if there is actual inflammation around the nerve. Pain from this type of disorder is called **radicular pain.** A common lay term for pressure on the nerve is **pinched nerve,** as sometimes used by examiners. After surgery and a normal healing process, the patient may still have some irritation of the nerve, which is often referred to as **residual nerve root irritability. Sciatica** and **neuritis** may be used in describing these disorders, but the terms are not discrete in that the irritation of the nerve is not necessarily from within the spinal canal.

dermatome: refers to the distribution of sensory nerves near the skin that are responsible for pain, tingling, and other sensations (or lack of). The afferent nerve fibers (leading to the spinal cord) and cutaneous branches arise from a single posterior spinal nerve root and contain sensory fibers. Loss of sensation in a **dermatomal** distribution may indicate damage to a nerve root that is caused by a disk prolapse.

sclerotomal pain: more diffuse and ill-defined pain arising from voluntary muscles in spasm (**myotomic** distribution).

referred pain: sclerotomic in distribution and felt distant from its origin (e.g., bursitis in the shoulder produces pain in the lateral arm, and sciatic-like leg pain can be referred from the low-back area).

neurofibroma: fibrous tumor of a nerve, which may affect a nerve root and thus give the appearance of herniated disk disease.

radiculopathy: disease of the nerve roots in or near the spinal canal as a result of direct pressure from a disk, or inflammation of the nerve roots due to disk or spinal joint disease.

root sleeve fibrosis: scar tissue surrounding a nerve in the spinal canal or neural foramen; **epineural fibrosis.** If it is within the nerve, it is called **intraneural fibrosis.**

sacral cyst: abnormality in the spinal fluid sac in the sacrum.

Disk Diseases

A disk is described as having a soft or fluid-like center (nucleus pulposus) and is surrounded by radial, circular, and longitudinal fibers that are firm, like gristle in meat. These intervertebral disks (IV disks) are situated between the vertebrae and act as shock absorbers. Any portion of the disk may herniate or extrude into the spinal canal, causing irritation and pressure on a nerve (Fig. 9–5).

cartilage space narrowing: narrowing of any cartilage space; also called **disk space narrowing.**

degenerative disk disease: gradual or rapid deterioration of the chemical composition and physical properties of the disk space. This may involve a simple increase in the rigidity of the nuclear material to be more involved with cellular removal of abnormal tissue and an inflammatory response. If the ligaments around the disk space ossify, they are often referred to as bony "spurs." Because the disk changes in its physical properties, some clinicians will describe the condition as a disorganized disk; that is, the normal property of a soft center surrounded by more rigid, fibrous tissue is disrupted. The inflammation and muscle spasm that may result over a prolonged period are often referred to as a chronic cervical sprain, reflecting the abnormal stresses on the ligaments.

diskitis: inflammation or infection of the disk space.

disk space infection: infection in the space normally occupied by an intervertebral disk.

herniated intervertebral disk (HID): outpouching of a disk.

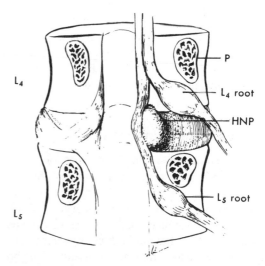

FIG 9–5.
Diagram of herniated nucleus pulposus (*HNP*) as seen from back with spinous processes and laminae removed from pedicles (*P*). Note that disk protrusion between fourth and fifth lumbar vertebrae impinges on fifth lumbar nerve root. (From Brashear RH and Raney BR: *Shand's handbook of orthopaedic surgery,* ed 9, St Louis, 1978, The CV Mosby Co.)

herniated nucleus pulposus (HNP): fibrous extrusion of semifluid nucleus pulposus through a ruptured intervertebral disk; damage results from pressure on the spinal cord or nerve roots, causing pain and disability; **HID, ruptured disk, slipped disk.** There are four recognized degrees of disk displacement:

intraspongy nuclear herniation: bulge of the disk within the annulus fibrosus.

protrusion: displaced nuclear material causes a discrete bulge in the annulus, but no material escapes through the annular fibers.

extrusion: displaced material reaches the spinal canal through disrupted fibers of the annulus, but remains connected to the central disk material.

sequestration: displaced material escapes as free fragment(s), which may migrate elsewhere.

intervertebral disk narrowing: narrowing of the space between any two vertebral bodies.

Naffziger syndrome: intervertebral disk disease, cervical rib, or some other disorder causes the scalene muscles to go into spasm, resulting in pressure on the major nerve plexus of the arm, causing pain in the neck, shoulder, arm, and hand; **scalenus anticus syndrome.**

Diseases of the Spinal Cord

Because *myelo-* is the Greek root for marrow, and because it was originally thought that the spinal cord was a part of the bone marrow, many words seem to denote bone diseases but actually refer to an affliction of the spinal cord. For that reason, the term *myelitis* is not used alone in this discussion; for example, it may be used to denote a disease of the bone marrow (osteomyelitis) or a disease of the spinal cord (poliomyelitis). This section contains a mixture of terms, some of which may not necessarily relate to the spine. Disorders that are most commonly congenital problems are discussed in a following section.

Myelo- Root Diseases, Acquired

myelalgia: pain in the spinal cord.

myelanalosis: wasting of spinal marrow; **tabes dorsalis.**

myelapoplexy: hemorrhage within the spinal cord.

myelasthenia: loss of nerve strength caused by some disorder of the spinal cord.

myelatrophy: atrophy (wasting away) of spinal cord because of lack of nutrition, causing it to diminish in size.

myelauxe: abnormal increase in size of spinal cord.

myeleterosis: abnormal alteration of the spinal cord.

myeloencephalitis: inflammation of spinal cord and brain; **myelencephalitis.**

myelomalacia: softening of the spinal cord.

myelomeningitis: inflammation of spinal cord and meninges (spinal membranes).

myeloneuritis: inflammation of spinal cord and peripheral nerves.

myeloparalysis: spinal paralysis.

myelopathy: functional disturbance and pathologic changes in the spinal cord. The myelopathies are defined as follows:

Nurick scale: classification scale for spinal cord compression due to spondylosis.

Grade 0: signs and symptoms of root involvement but without evidence of spinal cord disease.

Grade 1: signs of spinal cord disease but no difficulty in walking.

Grade 2: slight difficulty in walking but does not prevent full-time employment.

Grade 3: severe difficulty in walking that requires assistance and prevents full-time employment and avocation.

Grade 4: ability to walk only with assistance or with the aid of a frame.

Grade 5: chairbound or bedridden.

modified Frankel classification: scale for cord damage due to any cause.

Grade A: complete motor and sensory involvement.

Grade B: complete motor involvement, some sensory sparing including sacral sparing.

Grade C: functionally useless motor sparing.

Grade D: functional motor sparing.

Grade E: no neurologic involvement.

myelophthisis: wasting of the spinal cord; reduction of cell-forming function of bone marrow.

myeloplegia: spinal paralysis.

myeloradiculitis: inflammation of spinal cord and nerve roots.

myeloradiculopathy: disease of spinal cord and spinal nerve roots.

myelorrhagia: spinal hemorrhage.

myelosclerosis: hardening of the spinal cord.

myelosyphilis: syphilis of the spinal cord.

Other Spinal Diseases or Conditions, Acquired

central cord syndrome: most common of the incomplete traumatic spinal cord syndromes characterized by motor impairment that is proportionately greater in the upper limbs than in the lower, with bladder dysfunction and a variable degree of sensory loss below the level of the cord lesion.

ependymona: tumor of the spinal cord.

hematomyelia: effusion of blood (hemorrhage) into the substance of the spinal cord.

hematorrhachis: spinal apoplexy; hemorrhage into vertebral canal.

hyperlordosis: increase in the normal anterior concavity of the cervical or lumbar spine.

leptomeningitis: inflammation of the pia mater and arachnoid of the brain and spinal cord.

leptomeningopathy: disease of the arachnoid or pia mater of the brain and spinal cord.

lordosis: not a disease state, but the normal anterior concavity of the neck or low back.

meningioma: tumor arising from meninges, usually benign, does not recur if totally removed.

meningismus: apparent irritation of brain or spinal cord in which symptoms simulate meningitis but in which no actual inflammation of the membranes is present; **meningism.**

meningitis: inflammation of the meninges of the brain or spinal cord, caused by infectious agents such as bacteria, fungi, or viruses.

meningocele: local cystic protrusion of meninges through a cranial fissure; may be congenital or acquired.

meningoencephalomyelitis: inflammation of brain and spinal cord and their membranes.

meningomyelitis: inflammation of spinal cord, its enveloping arachnoid and pia mater, and sometimes the dura mater.

piriformis syndrome: a clinical diagnosis based on complaints of pain and abnormal sensations in the buttocks region with extension into the hips and posterior thigh as would be seen in sciatica. This is due to tightness of the piriformis muscle with pressure on the sciatic nerve.

syringomyelia: cavities filled with fluid in spinal cord, usually involving upper segments initially and involving the shoulder muscles.

Congenital Disorders of the Spine

Myelo- Root Diseases, Congenital

myelatelia: imperfect development of the spinal cord.

myelocele: herniation and protrusion of substance of spinal cord through defect in the bony spinal canal.

myelocystocele: cystic protrusion of substance of the spinal cord through a defect in the bony spinal canal.

myelocystomeningocele: cystic protrusion of

substance of the spinal cord, with meninges, through a defect in the spinal canal.

myelodiastasis: separation of the spinal cord.

myelodysplasia: defective development of any part of spinal cord.

myelomeningocele: herniation of cord and meninges through a defect in the vertebral column.

Other Spinal Disorders, Congenital

diastematomyelia: congenital defect associated with spina bifida in which the spinal cord is split in half by bony spicules or fibrous bands, each half being surrounded by a dural sac.

failure of segmentation: failure of a portion or all of two or more adjoining vertebrae to separate into normal units.

hemivertebra: incomplete development of one side of a vertebral body, resulting in a wedge shape. If two hemivertebrae are near each other, they may be **balanced,** that is, the two wedges point in opposite directions, and a lesser curve or no curve results. **Unbalanced** means that there is no opposing wedge for one or more hemivertebrae, and the net result is an abnormal curve.

interspinous pseudarthrosis (Baastrup d.): formation of a false joint between two lumbar spinous processes due to the congenitally large size of those processes.

segmental spinal dysgenesis: a rare set of distinct spinal anomalies including focal stenosis at the level of the dysgenesis with the spinal segments below that point being normal.

spina bifida: congenital defect common in the low back (lumbosacral region) of infants in which part of a vertebra does not fully develop (and in severe cases, nerve tissue) leaving a portion of spinal cord exposed. There are four forms of spina bifida:

spina bifida occulta (SBO): congenital defect consisting of the absence of a vertebral arch of the spinal column; normally, there are no symptoms.

myelocele (meningomyelocele): severe form.
meningocele: not as severe.
encephalocele: rare.

symmetric fusion: equal fusion throughout the vertebral body.

unsegmented bar: fusion on one side or the other of the vertebrae, which may involve the posterior elements or vertebral bodies; may occur at multiple levels and skip vertebral segments and may result in severe curves.

Eponymic Congenital Spinal Disorders

Arnold-Chiari syndrome: congenital combination of brain herniation and exposed spinal cord in the lower back. Two types are described:

Type I: cerebellum displaced caudally, brainstem normal, hydrocephalus occasionally present, onset of symptoms in adolescence.

Type II: commonly associated with myelomeningocele, caudal displacement of entire brainstem, cerebellar dysplasia, hydrocephalus in 90%, symptoms in infancy.

Jarcho-Levin syndrome: extensive defects of the spine with associated defects in the ribs leading to a small, stiff thorax and pulmonary compromise.

SURGERY OF THE SPINE

The two types of back surgery as applied to orthopaedics are the removal of disk fragments, bone, or ligaments causing pressure on neural elements from the spinal canal and fusion of two or more vertebral segments. The definitions of disk surgery are given to present some important distinctions between procedures of the cervical spine as compared with those of the lumbar spine and to clarify the misuse of terms related to spinal surgical procedures.

Before **invasive spine surgery** takes place, such as removal of a herniated disk, conservative measures are often initially taken in the form of medications, physical therapy, and activity modifications. When these measures do not relieve the patient's symptoms, tests to determine the cause of the symptoms are performed. These can include plain radiographs (x-rays), myelography followed by computer axial tomography (CAT), and magnetic resonance imaging (MRI).

For **myelography,** the patient is placed on a tilting table, and a needle is introduced into the subarachnoid space in the lower lumbar spine or upper cervical spine. Cerebrospinal fluid can be withdrawn for analysis and then one of several types of radiopaque contrast material injected. Currently, this material is water soluble. The contrast material infiltrates up and down the spinal canal to outline the nerve roots, nerve sleeves, dural sac, and, at higher levels, the spinal cord.

Multiple plain radiographs can be obtained at different angles and any given level to best outline the offending structure. A CAT scan is then taken to obtain better definition of the areas in question. MRI is often used as a substitute for myelography and CAT scanning because it does not require injection of contrast material into the spinal column.

The following spinal surgical procedures are performed by orthopaedic surgeons.

chemonucleolysis: a little used, but once common procedure for lumbar disk herniation. Under direct radiographic control, a chemical that denatures the protein or protein sugar complex in the disk space is injected. The injected disk tends to dissolve itself, and the remaining cartilage cells repopulate the disk and produce ground substance similar in composition to normal nucleus pulposus, or continued degeneration and scar formation takes place. This procedure is designed to speed up the process of relief of compression of the nerve root without surgery. The procedure carries a risk similar to standard diskectomy via laminectomy.

decompression: in relation to the spine this procedure is carried out to relieve pressure on the spinal cord or nerve roots. The pressure may result from fracture fragments, disk fragments, tumors, or infections. The approach may be anterior, lateral, or posterior.

decompressive laminectomy: a decompression done by removing the lamina and spinous process.

discectomy: the removal of intervertebral disk material placing pressure on neural elements. If the annulus of the disk is torn, the disk is protruded. If the fragment of the disk material is torn through a hole in the ligament, it is called an extruded fragment or extruded disk. If the fragment has migrated completely through the ligament, it is termed a sequestered disk or free fragment. The term **herniated nucleus pulposus (HNP)** is a catchall phrase for all of these conditions. In the neck, a fresh (soft) disk excision is sometimes done through a posterior approach (laminotomy). However, many cervical disk problems are approached anteriorly and include a spinal fusion.

foraminotomy: a procedure carried out alone or in conjunction with disk surgery. The foramina (tunnels or openings for the individual nerves to pass from the spine) may become narrowed because of disk impingement, intervertebral collapse, and spondylolisthesis. This surgical widening of the foramen is an attempt to relieve pressure on the nerve roots from a variety of causes.

laminectomy: removal of the lamina, the bony element covering the posterior portion of the spinal canal. This procedure removes the lamina on both sides of and including the spinous process. It may be performed at more than one level to approach the spinal cord and nerves for conditions including tumors and herniated disks. The spinal canal is approached from both sides of the spinous process, and the term is often inappropriately used in reference to the following two lesser procedures.

hemilaminectomy: the excision of only one side of the lamina (right or left) relative to the spinous process.

laminotomy (Fig. 9–5):   formation of a hole in the lamina without disrupting the continuity of the entire lamina to approach the intervertebral disk or neural structures. This is the most common approach to a herniated disk and is often mistakenly called a laminectomy.

laminoplasty: the lamina are hinged laterally, opened like a door, and secured in their new position with suture or bone to enlarge the spinal canal.

Spinal Fusions

A procedure where two or more adjacent vertebrae are induced to grow together as a single, solid bone by destroying the intervening joints and adding bone and/or bone substitutes and spinal hardware to induce bone growth between the adjacent vertebrae. The indications are spinal instability and arthritis. The excision of an intervertebral disk does not necessarily lead to symptomatic chronic degenerative arthritis or instability and is not in itself an indication for spinal fusion. However, it is often the case that disk surgery and spinal fusions are done concurrently for a variety of reasons. Fusions are sometimes done to restore adequate stability when it has been disturbed by a fracture, tumor, infection, or surgery. The lumbosacral region is the most common area for spinal fusions.

anterior spinal fusion: approaching the spine from the front, the intervertebral disk and/or vertebral body is removed and bone graft is inserted. Some variations of this procedure include the **Smith-Robinson, Cloward,** and **dowel procedures.**

cervical spinal fusion: spinal fusion involving the seven cervical segments. This may include the base of the skull, the occiput, and the first thoracic spine. The fusion may be anterior or posterior, with or without bone graft, and with or without fixation.

Aebi, Etter, and Cosica: anterior approach to inferior C-2 to fractured dens with screws.

Bohman: posterior triple spinous process wiring technique in the cervical spine to secure bone graft.

Brattstrom: use of acrylic cement for C-1 to C-2 fusion.

Brooks and Jenkins: loops of wire around lamina of C-1 and C-2 to hold bone graft between lamina.

Callahan: individual wire fixation of a strut bone graft to involved facets.

de Andrade and MacNab: anterior approach for cervical occipital fusion.

Gallie: wire around lamina of C-1 and spinous process of C-2.

Halifax: clamp across lamina of C-1 and C-2.

Mageri: wire looped around lamina of C-1 and C-2.

Magerl: transarticular facet screw fusion for posterior C-1 on C-2 with the use of bilateral screws directed from inferior posterior lateral mass to anterior superior C-1.

McAffee: anterior retropharyngeal approach to upper cervical spine; often used for fusion, allowing excision of tumor.

Meyer: for C-1 on C-2 instability, posterior fusion using vertical strut grafts and wires.

Newman: C-1 to C-2 posterior fusion without fixation.

Overton: a dowel graft that is applied across facet joints.

Robinson and Riley: an extensive anterior approach for fusion of C-1 to C-3 or lower.

Roy-Camille: for stabilization between the skull and C-2; posterior bone graft with wire and parallel vertical screw plate fixation from occiput to C-3.

Simmons: use of keystone-shaped graft in anterior fusion.

Spetzler: approach to anterior C-1 to C-3 by using a transoral approach for fusion following excision of tumor.

Wertheim Bohlman: for occipital cervical fusion; use of iliac crest graft and wire fixation from occiput to C-2.

Whitecloud and Larocca: anterior technique for cervical spine fusion using fibular graft.

Hibbs spinal f.: a lumbar spinal fusion that includes fusing the spinous process, lamina, and facet for stabilization.

posterior cervical spinal f.: spinal fusion done from the back, using the lamina, facets, and spinous processes of the neck.

   Southwick: a posterior fusion with wire attaching bone graft to the facet joints.

   Roger f.: posterior cervical fusion using iliac cortical and cancellous grafts.

posterior lumbar spinal f.: spinal fusion done from the back using the lamina, the facets, and spinous processes of the lower back.

   Albee: fusion of the spine using grafts across the spinous processes in spondylolisthesis.

   Bosworth: A fusion using an H-shaped bone graft in spondylolisthesis.

   Dwyer-Hartsill p.: for failed lumbar degenerative disk disease; pedicle screws wired to a rectangular frame along with posterolateral fusion.

   Gill: removal of the posterior spinal arch in spondylolisthesis.

   Gill, Manning, and White: a procedure sometimes combined with a posterolateral spinal fusion.

posterior spinal f.: a fusion of the cervical, thoracic, or lumbar regions primarily fusing the lamina and sometimes the facet joints, using iliac or other bone graft.

posterolateral interbody f. (PLIF): lumbar spine fusion that involves an interbony fusion accomplished through the posterior approach.

posterolateral f.: a fusion of both the lamina and transverse process, using the iliac bone for graft, usually in the lower lumbar and first sacral segments.

Spinal Instrumentation

Spinal instrumentation is comprised of metal devices that are secured to the vertebrae to hold them in a desired position and facilitate spinal fusion. They can be applied to the front, back, or side of the spine. Often these procedures cover a number of segments.

AO fixateur interne: a posteriorly placed spinal fixation device.

Banks-Dervin rod: for scoliosis fixation; a multiple level rod that is fixed with oblique spinous process to contralateral lamina screws.

Cotrel-Dubousset i.: posterior fixation device for spinal deformity, fracture, tumor, and degenerative conditions.

Dwyer i.: anteriorly placed screws and band device for correction of spinal deformities.

Edwards i.: a posterior rod and sleeve device used in stabilization of traumatic spinal conditions.

Harrington rod i.: an instrumentation and fusion using a straight, stiff rod for distraction or compression; associated with a posterior spinal fusion in the thoracic or thoracolumbar spine for scoliosis or trauma.

Isola i.: a posterior fixation device.

Jacobs locking hook i.: thick, threaded rods for fixation of various spinal deformities.

Kaneda: an anteriorly placed fixation device for spinal deformities.

Knodt distraction rod: for distraction stabilization of thoracic and lumbar spine.

Kostuick-Harrington i.: anteriorly placed device for spinal deformity correction.

Long Beach pedicle screw: posterolateral fusion screw and rod device.

Luque instrumentation: a posterior method of fixation.

Luque ISF: for posterolateral fusion fixation; a pedicle screw and plate device.

Rogozinski i.: a combined anteroposterior device used in correction of spinal deformities.

Roy-Camille: posterior pedicle screw and plate device for spinal stabilization.

Steffee plate: for posterolateral fusion fixation; plate and screw device.

Texas Scottish Rite Hospital: instrumentation used anteriorly and posteriorly.

Vermont (Krag): posteriorly placed internal fixation device.

Wiltse plate: screw plate device for posterior spinal stabilization.

Wisconsin (Drummond) interspinous segmental spinal i.: series of wires, rods, and buttons for multisegmental spine stabilization.

Zielke instrumentation: a method of fixation.

Miscellaneous Procedures on the Spine

Bradford p.: for kyphoscoliosis deformity; staged anterior and posterior approach for interbody fusion and correction of deformity.

Capner p.: draining of thoracic spinal abscess through an anterolateral approach.

coccygectomy: excision of the coccyx (tailbone).

coccygotomy: incision into the coccyx (tailbone).

commissural myelorrhapy: a longitudinal division of the spinal cord to sever crossing fibers.

cordotomy: transverse incision into the spinal cord.

corpectomy: excision of vertebral body usually combined with interposition of prosthesis or bone graft.

Dunn p.: for myelomeningocele spinal deformity; use of *contouring L-rod* for posterior stabilization.

eggshell p.: excavation of vertebral body for correction of deformity that is combined with spinal fusion.

facetectomy: excision of an articular facet of a vertebra.

Getty p.: for decompression of lumbar spinal stenosis; excision of lamina and portion of facet.

Goldstein p.: for scoliosis deformity graft incorporating posterior elements, including facet joints and ribs.

Hodgson p.: anterior approach to C-1 and C-2 area for drainage of tuberculous abscess.

kyphectomy: for kyphotic deformity in myelodysplasia; excision of kyphotic portion of lumbar spine combined with spinal fixation.

Leeds p.: for scoliosis, segmental wiring of a contoured square-ended Harrington rod.

Localio p.: for sacral tumor; a method of partial excision of the sacrum.

Loughheed and White p.: for drainage of lower abdominal abscess; coccygectomy and drainage from space anterior to sacrum.

MacCarthy procedure: for sacral tumor; a method of excision of the sacrum.

myelotomy: a procedure for severing tracts in the spinal cord.

rachicentesis: lumbar puncture for examination of the spinal fluid; rachiocentesis.

rachiotomy: incision into a vertebral canal for exploration.

rachitomy: surgical or anatomic opening of the vertebral canal.

radiculectomy: excision of a rootlet or resection of spinal nerve roots.

rhizotomy: division of the roots of the spinal nerves.

Risser p.: for scoliosis deformity; particular attention to fusion of facet joints and use of cast stabilization.

Roaf, Kirkaldy-Willis, and Cattero p.: drainage of thoracic spinal abscess through dorsolateral approach.

Schollner costoplasty: for rib deformity or scoliosis; multiple rib partial excisions.

Scott p.: use of cross-wire fixation transverse process to inferior pedicle in stabilization of spondylolysis fusion.

Seddon p.: drainage of thoracic spinal abscess through anterolateral approach with partial resection of rib.

Simmons p.: for cervical spinal kyphosis; a posterior osteotomy.

Smith Peterson p.: for correction of kyphotic deformity in ankylosing spondylitis; lumbar spine osteotomy.

Speed p. (Kellogg Speed): for spondylolisthesis spine fusion and anterior interbody fusion by using tibial cortical graft.

spondylosyndesis: surgical immobilization or ankylosis by fusion of the vertebral bodies with a short bone graft in cases of tuberculosis of the spine; **spondylodesis, Albee procedure.**

spondylotomy: incision into a vertebra or vertebral column; **rachiotomy.**

Tsuli p.: for severe cervical spondylosis; an expansive, multiple laminectomy.

Wiltse p.: a bilateral lateral spine fusion for spondylolisthesis.

Winter p.: for hemivertebra deformity; anterior and posterior approach with stabilization. Also a procedure for correction of congenital kyphosis, by using an anterior approach and strut bone grafts.

Spinal Approaches

anterior a.: when used to approach the cervical, cervicodorsal, dorsal, and lumbar spines, it is designed to provide sufficient surface for multiple segmental spinal fusions; **Hodgson, Roaf.**

anterior a.: for specific cervical spinal explorations and fusions; **Southwick** and **Robinson, Bailey** and **Badgley, Whitesides** and **Kelly, Henry** (to the vertebral artery).

anterolateral a.: an approach to the dorsal spine by rib resection to explore the spine anteriorly and in some cases to do spinal fusions and decompressions of the spinal cord.

dorsolateral a.: an approach to the dorsal spine by costotransversectomy, usually done for fractures and other affections of the spinal cord.

posterior a.: used for laminectomies and spinal fusions at any level; **Hibbs, Wagoner.**

Chapter 10

The Hand and Wrist

Where is there available a precision instrument that can either gently pick up eggs or lift 200 pounds; detect the weight of only four grains of sand, temperature differences of 1 degree, and the distance between two points less than 0.1 inch; be remote controlled, self-powered, and transportable to any part of the world? This priceless tool is available at no cost to almost all humankind—the hand.

A description of the intricate anatomic features of the hand and wrist is presented with illustrations. The sequence of definitions given here will help to define the basics of hand control, kinematics, and function. The chapter reflects changes in the anatomy format, with an explanation of zones, pulleys, and other miscellaneous names specific to the hand.

There are many abbreviations used in hand anatomy because of the lengthy Latin names, for example, flexor pollicis longus (FPL) tendon or metacarpophalangeal (MCP) joint. Usually the Latin name is spelled out initially and abbreviated subsequently. Appendix A (Orthopaedic Abbreviations) lists the many hand abbreviations used to simplify the terminology.

ANATOMY OF THE HAND AND WRIST

Bones (Fig. 10–1)

accessory bone: an extra bone that may develop in the carpus of the wrist as seen on radiographs; an anomaly.

carpal bones: the eight bones of the anatomic wrist, arranged in a proximal and distal row, and held firmly together by ligaments. The proximal row from lateral to medial include the **scaphoid (navicular), lunate (semilunar), triquetrum (triangular),** and **pisiform.** The distal row leading from the thumb side is composed of the **trapezium (greater multangular), trapezoid (lesser multangular), capitate,** and **hamate.**

carpus: the wrist; term applied to the structures of the wrist including the carpal bones.

DRUJ (*d*istal *r*adial *u*lnar *j*oint): acronym commonly used to describe that joint (pronounced "drudge").

fossae (fossa—*sing*): the scaphoid and lunate fossae are normal recesses in the articular surface of the distal radius that allow articulation of the scaphoid and lunate respectively.

metacarpals: the five long bones of the hand in the palm area. The bases of the metacarpal bones articulate proximally with the distal row of carpal bones.

phalanges: the bones of the thumb and fingers. Each phalanx has a body, proximal base, and distal head. There are two phalanges in the thumb (proximal and distal) and three phalanges in each of the four digits (proximal, medial, and distal).

sesamoids: small bones on the medial and lateral side of the base of the proximal phalanx of the thumb (metacarpophalangeal [MCP] joint). The sesamoids articulate with the head of the metacarpal bone to which muscles are attached. A sesamoid bone may also be found on the lateral

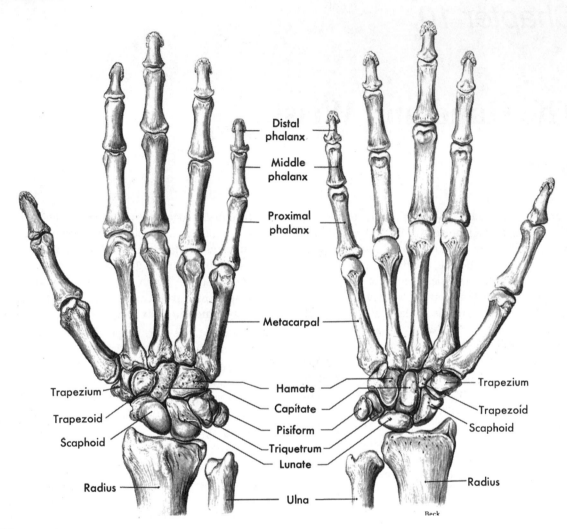

FIG 10–1.
Bones of the right hand and wrist, dorsal surface. (From Anthony C, Kolthoff N: *Textbook of anatomy and physiology,* ed 9, St Louis, 1975, The CV Mosby Co.)

side of the MCP joint of the index finger, and medial side of the MCP joint of the little finger.

sigmoid notch: the articular surface on the distal radius that accepts the ulna in the distal radio-ulnar joint.

styloids: bony protuberances off the radius and ulna that act as attachment sites for the radial and ulnar collateral ligaments, respectively. The ulna styloid is also an attachment for the triangular fibrocartilage complex.

tubercles: bony prominences that provide liga-mentous attachment. In the hand, these include the **scaphoid, trapezium, Lister tubercle,** and the **hook of the hamate.**

tuft: the terminal bony expansion of the distal phalanx.

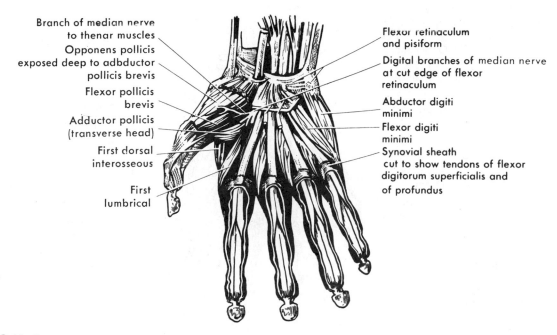

Branch of median nerve
to thenar muscles
Opponens pollicis
exposed deep to adbductor
pollicis brevis
Flexor pollicis
brevis
Adductor pollicis
(transverse head)
First dorsal
interosseous
First
lumbrical

Flexor retinaculum
and pisiform
Digital branches of median nerve
at cut edge of flexor
retinaculum
Abductor digiti
minimi
Flexor digiti
minimi
Synovial sheath
cut to show tendons of flexor
digitorum superficialis and
of profundus

FIG 10–2.
Muscles of the anterior aspect of the human hand; the palmar aponeurosis has been removed. (From DiDio LJA: *Synopsis of anatomy,* St Louis, 1970, The CV Mosby Co.)

Joints

The joints of the hand are remarkable for the variability of motion that supports the fingers and thumbs in many tasks (e.g., the carpometacarpal [CMC] joint of the thumb can move in all planes). The joints of the phalanges are the proximal, medial, and distal joints and are referred to as follows:

Carpometacarpal (CMC)
Distal interphalangeal (DIP)
Metacarpophalangeal (MCP)
Midcarpal (MC)
Proximal interphalangeal (PIP)
Radiocarpal (RC)

volar plate:　a thickening of the joint capsule of the volar aspect of the MP and IP joints that prevent hyperextension of these joints. Proximally, these begin with the "check-rein" ligaments.

Muscles

There are large muscles in the forearm that insert into the bones of the hand by means of their tendons (Figs. 10–2 and 10–3). These **extrinsic muscles** cause the hand and fingers to flex and extend (close and open). The **intrinsic muscles** are small and originate within the hand. These control positioning and to a large extent functional coordination of the fingers. In normal hand function all these groups work together in intricate unison.

Extrinsic Muscle Function

wrist flexors:　flexor carpi ulnaris (FCU), palmaris longus (PL), flexor carpi radialis (FCR); insert on the metacarpals, carpal bones, and ligaments; they cause strong wrist flexion.

wrist extensors:　extensor carpi radialis longus (ECRL), extensor carpi radialis brevis (ECRB), extensor carpi ulnaris (ECU); insert on the metacarpals.

Abductor pollicis brevis

Opponens pollicis

Flexor pollicis brevis

First palmar interosseous

Oblique head of adductor pollicis

Transverse head of adductor pollicis

Flexor pollicis longus

Deep transverse ligament

Split tendon of flexor digitorum superficialis reunited posteriorly to form a bed for profundus tendon

Profundus tendon

Vinculum longum for tendon of flexor digitorum superficialis

Flexor retinaculum (cut)

Pisiform

Hook of hamate

Abductor digiti minimi

Flexor digiti minimi brevis

Third and fourth dorsal interosseus

Third palmar interosseus

Tendon of flexor digitorum profundus

Tendon of flexor digitorum superficialis

Fourth lumbrical

FIG 10–3.
Muscles of the anterior aspect of the human hand. (From DiDio LJA: *Synopsis of anatomy,* St Louis, 1970, The CV Mosby Co.)

finger flexors: flexor digitorum profundus **(FDP)**, flexor digitorum sublimis or superficialis **(FDS)**, flexor pollicis longus **(FPL)** (thumb); insert on either the distal or the middle phalanges of the digits and cause powerful finger or thumb flexion.

finger extensors: extensor digiti quinti proprius **(EDQP)**, extensor digitorum communis **(EDC)**, extensor indicis proprius **(EIP)**; insert on the bones and extensor hoods of the fingers and cause extension of the digits.

thumb extensors: extensor pollicis longus **(EPL)** and brevis **(EPB)**.

thumb abductors: abductor pollicis longus **(APL)** and brevis **(APB)**.

thumb adductors: extensor pollicis longus **(EPL)** and adductor pollicis **(add poll)**.

Intrinsic Muscle Function

hypothenar muscles: opponens digiti quinti (or **minimi**) **(ODQ/ODM)**, flexor digiti quinti brevis **(FDQB)**, abductor digiti quinti (or **minimi**) **(ADQ/ADM)**; a less important group of intrinsic muscles that arise from the carpal bones and insert on the little finger, metacarpal, and proximal phalanx.

intrinsic muscles: lumbricals, dorsal interossei, volar interossei; arise from the metacarpals or from the flexor tendons and insert into the finger dorsal (extensor) mechanism and base of the proximal finger bone. They are responsible for spreading and bringing together the fingers and for firm coordination of motion at each finger joint.

thenar muscles: opponens pollicis **(OP)**, abductor pollicis brevis **(APB)**, flexor pollicis brevis (**FPB**) deep and superficial head, the deep head sometimes called first palmar interosseous (intrinsic muscles of the thumb); arise from the carpal bones and ligaments at the base of the palm and insert on the proximal phalanx or on the thumb metacarpal. They function to bring the thumb out and away from the palm and to oppose it to the other fingers. One intrinsic muscle arises from the metacarpals and crosses deep in the palm to the thumb. This adductor pollicis muscle pulls the thumb forcefully back in toward the palm (adduction).

Associated Forearm Muscles and Tendons
other muscles in the forearm: brachioradialis, pronator teres (PT), supinator, anconeus, and pronator quadratus (PQ); these do not extend to the hand but affect the position of the hand by actions such as rotation of the forearm (pronation and supination).

flexor wad of five: five muscles with a common origin in the medial elbow: pronator teres (PT), flexor digitorum profundus (FDP) and sublimis (FDS), palmaris longus (PL), and flexor carpi radialis (FCR).

flexor tendons of the wrist: flexor carpi radialis (**FCR**) is the radial wrist flexor that travels in its own tunnel and inserts at the base of the second metacarpal. The **flexor carpi ulnaris** (**FCU**) (the ulnar wrist flexor) is the more important and powerful. It has a primary insertion on the pisiform but will send fibers distally to intermesh with the hypothenar muscle fascia. These tendons, with a synovial lining, glide back and forth through the tunnel as the fingers and wrist are moved.

Zones
A surgical zone system has been established for the fingers, hand, wrist, and forearm. The anatomic zones are important in determining technical considerations for each zone, surgical approaches, and corrections for different disorders. The clinical impor-

tance of anatomic zones is that if an area is left unrepaired, specific deficits will occur in the extensor or flexor tendon zones.

zone I: from flexor digitorum profundus (FDP) insertion to flexor digitorum sublimis (FDS) insertion, anatomic structures found distal to the insertion of the sublimis tendon into the middle phalanx.

zone II: called "**no man's land,**" the anatomic structures found in the region just proximal to the A1 pulley up to zone I.

Camper chiasm: a bifurcation of the flexor digitorum sublimis (FDS) in zone II that allows passage of the flexor digitorum profundus (FDP) through it. This occurs just proximal to the insertion of the flexor digitorum sublimis (FDS) in the middle phalanx; **chiasma tendinum.**

zone III: anatomic structures at the origin of the lumbricals in the region of the arterial arch, from the carpal tunnel to zone II.

zone IV: the carpal tunnel.

zone V: anatomic area of the wrist proximal to the carpal tunnel.

Pulleys
Pulleys are thickened portions of flexor tendon sheaths that hold tendons in place. They are labeled as annular or cruciate, depending on the orientation of the fibers of the pulley. The most proximal pulley is located on the distal metacarpal and is labeled annular 1 (A1) and then annular 2 through 4. The cruciate pulleys are similarly labeled C1 through C3 (Fig. 10–4).

A1	zone II	C1	zone II
A2	zone II	C2	zone I
A3	zone II	C3	zone I
A4	zone I	A0	zone IV (palmar fascia)

Ligaments and Fascia

There are numerous ligaments named for the bones to which the ligaments are attached.

FIG 10–4.
This anatomic diagram of various parts of flexor sheath is helpful in understanding gliding of tendon. Maintenance of second annulus (A2) and fourth annulus (A4) is essential to retain appropriate angle of approach and prevent "bowstringing" of flexor tendons or tendon graft. (From Doyle JR, Blythe W: In American Academy of Orthopaedic Surgeons: *Symposium on tendon surgery in the hand,* St Louis, 1975, The CV Mosby Co.)

deep transverse metacarpal l.: specific distal ligaments between the second, third, fourth, and fifth metacarpophalangeal (MCP) volar plates.

juncturae tendinum: tendinous interconnection between extrinsic extensors over the dorsum of the hand. These allow synchronized digital extension; **connexus intertendineus.**

transverse carpal l.: the strong ligamentous band that lies across the arch of the carpal bones forming the roof of the carpal tunnel. It covers the median nerve and binds down the nine long flexor tendons of the thumb and fingers.

triangular l.: interconnecting fibers that join the two lateral bands dorsally and hold them in place. They are located over the proximal end of the middle phalanx just distal to the insertion of the central slip of the extensor tendon; **triangular fibrocartilage complex.**

vincula longa and breva: vascular and fibrous connections from the floor of the flexor tunnel to each of the two flexor tendons. The vincula breva lie close to the tendon insertions.

volar carpal l.: the ligament that spans and covers the median nerve and canal of Guyon, and runs from the transverse carpal ligament radially to the hypothenar fascia ulnarly. This ligament binds down the nine long flexor tendons of the thumb and fingers.

Extrinsic Wrist Ligaments

dorsal radiocarpal l.: (radiolunatotriquetrum).

volar l.: deep radioscaphocapite, long radioscapholunate, short radioscapholunate, and radiolunate and ulnar lunate.

Intrinsic Wrist Ligaments

arcuate (deltoid) l.: a major stabilizer of the midcarpal joint; ulnar arm (triquetrocapitate l.), radial arm (distal to scaphocapitate l.).

deep transverse intermetacarpal l.: fibrous interconnections between metacarpal heads II through V.

intermediate l.: lunatotriquetrum, scapholunate, and scaphotrapezium.

long l.: volar intercarpal ("U," deltoid arcuate).

short l.: interosseous.

space of Poirer: a weak area of the midcarpal joint, i.e., the arcuate ligament volar and distal to the lunate because the capitolunate l. is either absent or attenuated.

superficial transverse intermetacarpal l.: the expansion of the palmar fascia in the region of the distal metacarpals; **natatory l.**

Collateral Ligaments

The collateral ligaments of the elbow and wrist are supportive ligaments providing stability on the medial and lateral side of the wrist joint.

radial collateral l.: scaphocapitate l. (radial arm).

ulnar collateral l.: triquetrocapitate l. (ulnar arm).

Digital Collateral Ligaments

accessory l.: originates volar and deep to the main collateral ligaments and runs to the volar plate.

beak ligaments: volar ulnar ligaments that stabilize the carpometacarpal joint of the thumb; originates on the volar aspect of the triscaphe joint and inserts on the volar ulnar surface of the proximal thumb metacarpal.

dorsal extensor compartments: the six fascial compartments on the dorsum of the distal radius for the wrist extensors numbering from radial to ulnar; these are defined by extensor retinacular tunnels over the wrist.

I: abductor pollicis longus (APL) and extensor pollicis brevis (EPB).

II: extensor carpi radialis longus (ECRL) and brevis (ECRB).

III: extensor pollicis longus (EPL).

IV: extensor indicis proprius (EIP) and extensor digitorum communis (EDC) II–V.

V: extensor digiti minimi (EDM) or quinti (EDQ).

VI: extensor carpi ulnaris (ECU).

main l.: runs from the center of rotation of the metacarpal or phalangeal head to the proximal metaphyseal flair of the phalanx adjoining.

Palm

Palmar Fascial Compartments

flexor and extensor retinacula: special thickening of deep fascia where muscles of forearm become tendons and pass into the hand into a broad band of superficial fascia over the dorsum of the wrist; help to restrain the extensor tendons and prevent tendons from bowstringing away from wrist.

> *digital retinaculum:* the covering fascia of the finger flexors.

hypothenar eminence: prominence caused by intrinsic muscle mass on little finger side of the palm.

hypothenar space: deep space overlying the fifth metacarpal that may or may not be connected to the thenar space proximally.

Kanavel spaces: two fascial spaces of the palm, one thenar and one midpalmar, lying deep to the long flexor tendons and separated by a septum.

Landsmeer l.: fibrous tissue bands on the lateral side of the fingers that help to synchronize the motion of the two distal joints; **oblique retinacular ligaments.**

midpalmar space: a deep potential space that runs from the third to fifth ray.

natatory l.: another name for the superficial transverse intermetacarpal l.

palmar fascia: complex interwoven fascia in the palm of the hand that is a part of the expansion of the palmaris longus (PL) and protects the delicate structures in the hand.

palmar skin crease: the creases in the palm caused by natural folds in the skin. These are labeled as distal palmar crease (DPC), midpalmar crease (MPC), and thenar palmar crease (TPC), the "life line." The digital skin creases are labeled proximal, middle, and distal.

septa: two fibrous septa pass deeply from sides of palmar aponeurosis and separate muscles of the thenar and hypothenar deep spaces from midpalmar space.

thenar eminence: the prominence caused by intrinsic muscle mass on the thumb side of the palm.

thenar space: the potential space on the thumb side of the hand deep to the tendons and nerves.

web l.: expansion of the palmar fascia between the base of the fingers.

Bursa

All bursa are lined with synovial sheaths (tenosynovium). Following are the important ones in the hand.

intermediate bursa: occasionally seen anatomically as the bursa containing the index finger flexor tendon sheath.

radial bursa: sac containing the flexor pollicis longus (FPL) tendon sheath in the palm and thumb.

ulnar bursa: sac in the palm containing tendon sheaths of the index, long, ring, and little fingers and extending to the end of the little finger.

Miscellaneous

anatomic snuff box: the area of the lateral wrist formed between the extensor pollicis longus (EPL) tendon medially, and abductor pollicis longus (APL) and extensor pollicis brevis (EPB) tendons laterally. With the thumb abducted and extended, a triangular depression is made on the dorsum of the wrist at the radial border.

arcade of Froshe: tunnel through supinator muscle for the deep radial nerve; anatomic series of arches.

carpal tunnel: space in the wrist created by the volar carpal ligament. This space contains the flexor tendons of the fingers and thumb, as well as the median nerve.

Guyon canal: space between the hamate and pisiform bones at the wrist for the ulnar artery and nerve, covered by the ulnar side of the volar carpal ligament. Floor is the pisohamate ligament.

hook of hamate: bony prominence (tubercle) that provides ligamentous attachment.

Lister tubercle: bony prominence for ligamentous attachment.

slider crank mechanism: an engineering model of scaphoid motion in carpal kinematics.

The Fingers

central slip (tendon): the portion of the extensor tendon that inserts into the middle phalanx.

cutaneous l.: ligaments that restrain the skin during finger motion and include the following:
> *Cleland l.:* fibrous tissue bands on the lateral side of the fingers that stabilize the skin during finger movement, dorsal to Grayson l.
>
> *Grayson l.:* fibrous tissue bands of the finger extending from the volar distal interphalangeal (DIP) and proximal interphalangeal (PIP) joints to the lateral skin.

distal pulp: the mass of tissue of the volar distal finger. It is the soft cushion of the palmar surface of the distal phalanx.

dorsal expansion: the fibers spreading laterally at the base of the dorsal hood.

extensor hood: the fanlike expansion of the extensor communis tendon over the dorsum and sides of the *me*tacarpo*p*halangeal (MCP) joints. This complex structure brings together intrinsic and extrinsic tendons to control interphalangeal (IP) joint extension and metaphalangeal (MP) joint flexion or extension.

knuckle pad: the thick skin over the dorsum of the distal interphalangeal (DIP) and proximal interphalangeal (PIP) joints of the finger.

lateral bands: the portions of the intrinsic muscle tendons that run laterally across the proximal phalanx to the dorsum of the distal interphalangeal (DIP) and proximal interphalangeal (PIP) joints.

septa: fibrous tissue structures in the fingertips.

skin creases: indentations in the skin at the point of natural motion points of the finger. The digital skin creases are labeled proximal, medial, and distal.

web space: the skin web area between the base of the fingers.

The Nail

cuticle: the skin edge immediately covering the base of the fingernail.

eponychium: thin skin covering (epidermis) at the base of the nails on the dorsal surface; **cuticle.**

germinal matrix: the cells that generate the tissues that eventually form the nail from the base of the nail; primitive stage of development.

hyponychium: the thickened epidermis immediately under the distal portion of the nail; **subungual tissue.**

lunula: the white crescentic (half-moon shaped) area at the base of the nail.

nail matrix: the proximal portion of the nail bed from which growth mainly proceeds; also, the tissue upon which the deep aspect of the nail rests; **matrix unguis, nail bed.**

nail plate: the hard plate of the distal end of the dorsum of the fingers and thumbs. This rigid outer covering extends approximately 8 mm under the nail fold (parionychium) and arises from the nail bed (matrix unguis).

paronychium: a fold of skin (nail folds) that surround the nail at the base; the epidermis bordering the nail; **perionychium.**

subungual space: the potential space between the nail and nail bed; common site for a hematoma.

unguis: the horny cutaneous plate on the dorsal surface of the distal end of a finger; the **nail.**

Nerves and Arteries

antebrachial cutaneous nerve: medial/lateral and sensory to the thumb.

common digital arteries and nerves (Fig. 10–5):   the main branch of the various nerves or arteries in the palm; these then divide into the proper digital arteries and nerves.

dorsal digital artery and nerve: common and proper, the branches of artery and nerve in the dorsum of the finger.

lateral cutaneous nerve (of forearm):   sometimes provides sensation to the lateral side of the thumb metacarpal area.

Martin-Gruber connection: a connection between the median and ulnar nerve in the forearm where fibers that normally travel with the ulnar nerve from the brachial plexus distally, travel with median nerve until the midforearm and only enter the median nerve at that connection; **Martin-Gruber anastomosis.**

median nerve: the nerve that conducts sensations from the hand to the central nervous system and crosses under the small volar carpal ligament. Supplies some of the small muscles of the thumb including the opponens, the superficial head of the flexor pollicis brevis (FPB), and the abductor pollicis brevis (APB), but not the adductor and the deep head of the flexor pollicis brevis (FPB); provides sensation for most of the palm and volar thumb, long and index fingers, and thumb side of the ring finger. The

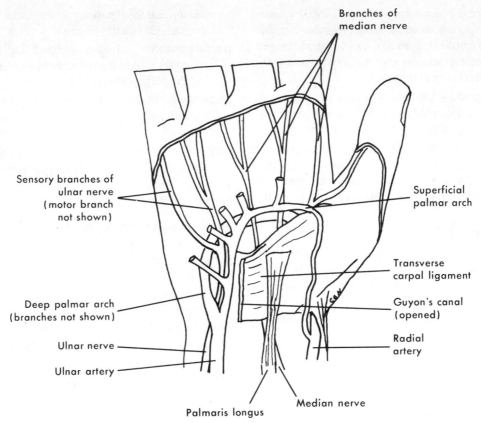

FIG 10–5.
Major arterial and nerve supply to the hand. Note the median nerve crossing under the carpal tunnel and the separate structure of the Guyon canal.

motor branch controls muscles surrounding the thumb.

Meissner's corpuscles: pressure receptors at nerve endings in the skin.

proper volar digital nerve and artery: the nerves and arteries after they have divided in the palm and travel along the two volar sides of the finger.

radial artery: major artery on the thumb side of the palm and wrist.

radial nerve, superficial branch: this nerve supplies sensation only; sensory distribution is over the dorsum of the thumb, index finger, long finger, and radial side of the ring finger.

Riche-Cannieu connection: the deep motor branch of the ulnar nerve may send a branch to join the motor branch of the median nerve. The relevance is that in injuries to the median nerve at the wrist, one may still retain motor function at the wrist.

superficial and deep palmar arterial arch: the superficial and deep connecting arcades of the radial and ulnar artery in the palm.

ulnar artery: artery on the little finger side of the palm and wrist.

ulnar nerve: the nerve crossing the wrist through the Guyon canal and supplying the adductor pollicis, deep head of the flexor pollicis brevis, and all small muscles of the hand, except the thumb and first two lumbricals. The sensation supplied is to the little finger and the little finger side of the ring finger.

Vater-Pacini corpuscle: pain pinpoint receptor.

vinculae: blood vessel bridges to the flexor tendons having a **vinculum brevum** and **vinculum longum.**

DISEASES AND STRUCTURAL ANOMALIES

Most of the diseases that affect the bones and joints of the hand are described in Chapter 2. The specific terminology for deformities caused by rheumatoid arthritis, nerve injuries, and congenital defects related to the hand is listed here. The terminology for diseases of the hand comprises many words not specific to other parts of the anatomy and is divided as follows.

Arthritic Deformities

arthritis (degenerative): commonly seen in the following joints: distal interphalangeal (DIP) (Heberden nodes), proximal interphalangeal (PIP; Bouchard nodes), metacarpophalangeal (MCP; posttraumatic or infection), carpometacarpal (CMC) digits (associated with CMC bossing), trapeziometacarpal (thumb), intercarpal (triscaphe, radiolunate, triquetrohamate, lunatotriquetral), radioscaphoid (seen in postscaphoid nonunions or with scapholunate advanced collapse [SLAC] wrist).

scapholunate advanced collapse (SLAC): after untreated scaphoid nonunion or untreated scapholunate dissociation, there is rotatory subluxation of the scaphoid. Typically will have radioscaphoid arthritis, sparing the radiolunate joint with proximal migration of the capitate.

arthritis (inflammatory): rheumatoid hand deformities that include the following: flexor or extensor tenosynovitis, tendon ruptures, caput ulnar syndrome (Vaughn-Jackson syndrome), intercarpal collapse or volar carpal subluxation, metaphalangeal volar collapse with ulnar deviation, thumb digits, boutonnière deformity, swanneck deformity, carpal tunnel syndrome, and intrinsic contractures.

attenuation (attrition) of tendons: erosion and eventual rupture of tendons by diseased synovium or bony spurs.

crystalline arthropathy (gout): with chronic hyperuricemia, there is recurrent joint inflammation, typically with fever and leukocytosis that affects fingers, wrists, and elbows; medical and surgical treatment indicated.

pseudogout: the deposition of calcium pyrophosphate crystals with episodic inflammation of wrist and metaphalangeal (MP) joints; chondrocalcinosis.

progressive systemic sclerosis (PSS): typically scleroderma, Reynaud subcutaneous calcinosis, resorption of the distal tufts. Diffuse hand involvement with skin thickening and fibrosis.

psoriatic arthritis (PA): typically of the distal interphalangeal (DIP), but any joint can be affected. Joint pain and stiffness can have similar clinical picture to rheumatoid arthritis.

pyogenic arthritis: bacterial infection of a joint.

systemic lupus erythematosus (SLE): deformity similar to rheumatoid arthritis with pain and swelling in the midproximal interphalangeal (PIP) joints and the wrists. Usually systemic, there is relative sparing of articular cartilage until late.

Arthritic Deformities (Specific)

boutonnière deformity: a fixed deformity of the finger consisting of flexion of the proximal interphalangeal joint and extension of the distal interphalangeal joint. A result of rheumatoid destruction of the extensor tendon mechanism at the proximal interphalangeal joint and also secondary to trauma without arthritis. Can be moderate to severe and indicates that a separate classification system exists.

diabetic cheirarthropathy: hand arthritis associated with diabetes; characterized by flexion contracture of the metacarpophalangeal and proximal interphalangeal joints of the fingers, with thickening, induration, and a waxy appearance of the skin.

mallet finger: drop of the distal phalanx due to traumatic or arthritic avulsion to the extensor tendon over the distal interphalangeal (DIP) joint, drop finger.

opera-glass hand: a rare, very advanced stage of arthritis in which the joints are destroyed and the bones become thin, fragile, and shortened.

radial drift: the position toward which the metacarpals tend to drift in rheumatoid arthritis—the alignment of the hand deviates toward the thumb; may apply to the thumb but usually specified.

swan-neck deformity: a static or dynamic position of the finger that exhibits distal interphalangeal (DIP) flexion and proximal interphalangeal (PIP) hyperextension. Seen in posttraumatic or rheumatoid patients. Anatomically, there is failure of the distal extensor mechanism, tightness of the central slip, and proximal interphalangeal (PIP) volar plate laxity. In rheumatoid arthritis, the classification system is as follows:
Type I: PIP joint flexible in all positions of MP joint.
Type II: PIP joint is limited in certain positions.
Type III: PIP joint is limited in all positions.
Type IV: stiff PIP with gross articular destruction.

tophus: accumulation of any crystalline material in the soft tissue; seen commonly in gout.

trapeziometacarpal arthritis: an arthritis at the base of the thumb; often occurs in the absence of systemic disease or previous trauma. Most common in women.

ulnar drift: the position of the fingers in rheumatoid arthritis; the fingers point away from the thumb and are often associated with radial drift at the wrist.

Neuropathies

reflex sympathetic dystrophy (RSD):   Usually posttraumatic (major or minor) pain dysfunction syndrome. Thought to be due to abnormal modulation of afferent pain signals with possible short-circuiting of somatic and autonomic nerve fibers. Attendant autonomic nervous system hyperactivity will produce abnormal peripheral small vessel response to cold and heat stimulus. Symptoms include hyperpathia (increased pain at rest), allodynia (painful response to a nonpainful stimulus), erythema (brawny edema), joint stiffness, and loss of skin elasticity. Osteoporosis and complete loss of dexterity result. Bone scan and tomography are diagnostic, and treatment includes physical therapy, oral medications, and a sympathetic ganglion blockade; also called **autonomic dystrophy, shoulder-hand syndrome, Sudeck atrophy, causalgia,** and **sympathetic maintained pain syndrome** (**SMPS**).

Sunderland classification (grades of nerve injury):
I neuropraxia: local conduction block, nerve in continuity, no wallerian degeneration, all have elements intact. No Tinel sign.
II axonotmesis: axonal damage; wallerian degeneration distally; endoneurium, perineurium, and epineurium intact; nerve sprouting; progress excellent.
III axonotmesis: axon and endothelium are disrupted, perineurium intact. Nerve mismatching with regeneration. Recovery is dependent on degree of neural matching, unpredictable; advancing Tinel sign and wallerian degeneration distally.
IV axonotmesis: axon, endoneurium, and perineurium violated. Nerve is grossly in continuity held by epineurium, advancing Tinel sign, regenerative units trapped in scar;

requires surgical intervention and traction (3-month wait before traction).

V neurotmesis: complete nerve transection requiring surgical intervention by repair graft or conduit.

VI neuroma in continuity: nerve grossly in continuity, but injured area is encased in nerve scar with varying degrees of nerve injury in each fascicle. The challenge is to identify the fascicles with a higher grade of injury and to repair these.

compressive neuropathy: loss of motor or sensory nerve function, acute or chronic, due to extrinsic compression. Entrapment can occur within tight fibroosseous tunnels or as a result of tumor, hemorrhage, or metabolic changes, causing swelling of soft tissues around the nerve.

Median Neuropathy

anterior interosseous nerve syndrome: anterior elbow and forearm pain and motor weakness of the flexor digitorum profundus (FDP) II, flexor pollicis longus (FPL), and pronator quadratus (PQ). Electromyography may be helpful. Conservative therapy may be tried for several months, and failing that, surgical decompression of the nerve is indicated.

carpal tunnel syndrome (CTS): a median nerve compression at the wrist caused by chronic synovitis surrounding the flexor tendons with repetitive finger motion or squeezing. Maximum pressure elevation occurs 3- to 4-cm distal to the volar wrist crease. Thenar motor loss may be included if untreated. Patient describes numbness, tingling, and dysesthesia in the hand at the median nerve distribution. Conservative therapy is indicated in chronic cases, and failing that, surgical decompression of the carpal tunnel is necessary. EMGs and nerve conduction studies are usually diagnostic.

pronator syndrome: entrapment of the median nerve in the elbow causes anterior elbow and forearm pain, with numbness, tingling, and paresthesias in the median nerve distribution. Elec-

trodiagnostics are occasionally helpful. Conventional therapy is tried for several months, and failing that, decompression of the median nerve is indicated.

Radial Neuropathy

posterior intraosseous nerve syndrome: compression of the motor branch of the radial nerve near the ***arcade of Froshe*** that causes weakness of the finger and wrist extensors. Electrodiagnosis and conservative treatment are not helpful. Surgical release of the radial nerve may improve function, but tendon transfers may be necessary.

radial sensory nerve entrapment (Wartenberg syndrome): the radial sensory nerve can become entrapped in the distal third of the forearm as it emerges between the brachioradialis and the extensor carpi radialis longus (ECRL). Patient experiences numbness and dysesthesia in the dorsoradial hand and wrist, provoked by hyperpronation of the forearm. Sensory nerve conduction studies are helpful, and surgical release is curative in most cases; **brachialgia statica paresthetica.**

radial tunnel syndrome: usually misdiagnosed as **resistant tennis elbow,** it is posterolateral elbow pain accentuated on resisted supination of the forearm or extension of the middle finger. Electromyography and nerve conduction studies are helpful. Treatment includes rest, splinting, and avoiding stressful activities.

wrist drop: a radial nerve palsy with loss of muscle control for wrist extension. This can be due to a variety of central and peripheral nerve conditions, but is most commonly associated with radial nerve palsy; **posterior intraosseous nerve syndrome.**

Ulnar Neuropathy

cubital tunnel syndrome: entrapment of the ulnar nerve at the elbow due to fibrous tissue in the fibroosseous arcade and the two heads of the flexor carpi ulnaris (FCU) as a result of prolonged elbow flexion. Early on, symptoms are sensory and involve the fourth and fifth digits; later, intrinsic motor weakness predominates. Surgical compression and/or ulnar nerve transposition is necessary.

Charcot-Marie-Tooth disease: In the hand, spontaneous deterioration of the neuromuscular complex will affect the ulnar nerve and cause severe intrinsic wasting with a characteristic clawhand deformity; **intrinsic minus deformity.**

double (multiple) crush syndrome: compression of a peripheral nerve (i.e., median or ulnar nerve) in two or more locations. There is cervical root compression at C-6 or C-7 and carpal tunnel syndrome. Three types exist: multiple anatomic regions along a peripheral nerve, multiple anatomic structure access to peripheral nerve with anatomic region superimposed on a neuropathy, or a combination of the above. These complex conditions require a multifactorial approach. Prognosis is guarded.

focal dystonia: a condition whereby muscles become imbalanced when some muscles are used more than others. This is due to repetitive motions of the hand, such as seen in musicians (pianists or string or brass instrumentalists). The brain does not send proper signals to the affected muscles, resulting in spasms and seizures of the hand. Sometimes the arm is affected. Treatment is in the form of electrical stimulation, ultrasound, exercise, or surgery.

intrinsic minus hand: in low ulnar nerve palsy, will cause intrinsic palsy with a characteristic metacarpophalangeal (MCP) hyperextension; proximal interphalangeal (PIP) and distal interphalangeal (DIP) sensory deformity. Results from any interruption of intrinsic function; intrinsic minus deformity, intrinsic plus deformity; **clawhand deformity.**

intrinsic plus hand: loss of extrinsic muscle function or intrinsic contracture will cause metaphalangeal flexion and interphalangeal extension.

monkey paw: an adduction and extension of the thumb where it cannot be opposed. It is unable to touch the tips of the fingers due to weakness of the opposing muscles of the thumb, as in a lesion of the median nerve.

peripheral neuropathy: intrinsic axonal or myelin pathologic condition usually due to an underlying metabolic malfunction or toxic state (i.e., diabetes, renal failure, alcoholic neuropathy).

Saturday night palsy: localized pressure palsy (e.g., in an alcoholic who falls asleep on a rested arm on a hard object); a first-degree neuropraxia occurs, which is worsened by an underlying alcoholic neuropathy.

tardy ulnar palsy: delayed chronic ulnar neuropathy secondary to chronic stretching of the nerve in the cubital tunnel due to cubitus valgus deformity at the elbow.

thoracic outlet syndrome: a constellation of signs and symptoms with multifactorial etiology. Common complaints include aching pain and heaviness in the neck, shoulder, and upper arm with numbness and tingling mainly to the fourth and fifth fingers. Symptoms worsen with arm elevation to include chest pain, tightness, and headaches. Thoracic outlet syndrome is believed due to compression of the brachial plexus over the cervical rib and between the scalenus anterior and scalenus medius muscles; in early adult life with shoulder sagging, brachial plexus traction can result. Initial treatment must include physiotherapy. Surgery may be indicated if symptoms persist for more than 1 year. Related conditions are *brachial plexus compression, scalenus anterior syndrome,* and *hyperabductor syndrome.*

ulnar tunnel syndrome: entrapment of the ulnar nerve at the wrist (Guyon canal). Could be acute or caused by repetitive trauma. Electrodiagnostics studies are helpful. Surgical release may be necessary.

vibration white finger syndrome: digital arterial or nerve injury in the hand from using tools with at least 2,000 to 3,000 cpm; characterized by Raynaud phenomenon: cold intolerance, numbness, tingling, and weakness with loss of dexterity.

Congenital Anomalies

Classification of Upper Limb Anomalies

The International Federation of Societies for Surgery of the Hand (IFSSH) has adopted a classification system for upper limb anomalies that affect hand function. An example is given for each group.

I. Failure of formation of parts.
   Transverse congenital amputations, constriction band syndrome (amniotic Streeter bands).
   Longitudinal (radial, ulnar) hemimelias, phocomelias, hypoplastic digits.
II. Failure of differentiation of parts (incomplete morphogenesis).
   Shoulder: Sprengel deformity.
   Arm and forearm synostosis: humeroradial, humeroulnar, radioulnar.
   Hand synostosis: syndactyly, camptodactyly, congenital trigger digit, clinodactyly.
III. Duplication.
   Polydactyly triphalangism, central polydactyly (polysyndactyly, mirror hand).
IV. Overgrowth (gigantism).
   Macrodactyly, lipofibromas, hamartoma of nerve, limb hypertrophy, hemihypertrophy.
V. Undergrowth.
   Brachydactyly.
VI. Constriction ring syndrome (amniotic Streeter bands).
VII. Generalized skeletal anomalies.
   Dwarfism, arthrogryposis, chromosomal anomalies (i.e., Madelung deformity); **Klippel-Feil syndrome.**

Agenesis

acheiria: absence of the hand.

acquired thumb flexion contracture: in children, a thumb flexion contracture that usually develops *after* birth, and, if present for more than a year, can be relieved by release of the A1 pulley at the volar base of the thumb. The thumb rarely catches or snaps. Hence, the term **congenital trigger thumb** is not appropriate for this condition.

acrosyndactyly: terminal interconnection of the syndactylyzed digits. These may or may not be connected proximally. The connection may be simple (skin) or complex (bone or other associated structures). These are commonly seen in Apert syndrome.

adactyly: absence of the digits.

amelia: total absence of the upper limb (congenital amputation).

amniotic bands: congenital circumferential crease rings that may be present at a fingertip or at upper arm level, or anywhere in between. This can be isolated or in conjunction with associated anomalies such as clubfoot or cleft palate. Neurovascular embarrassment depends on the depth of the crease and may be complete if the crease goes down to the bone. Four types are evident: (1) simple constriction rings; (2) rings associated with distal lymphedema or deformity; (3) rings associated with soft-tissue fusion of distal parts; and (4) intrauterine amputations. If there is any question of neurovascular compromise, Z-plasty releases are initiated in at least two stages; **constriction bands, Streeter bands, Streeter dysplasia.**

Apert syndrome: hand anomalies that include delta phalanx, metacarpal synostosis, complex syndactyly, and other anomalies including skull and facial. Digits are usually short, deformed, stiff, and at the tips "spoon hand."

aphalangia: absence of phalanges.

arachnodactyly: long spider-like fingers seen commonly in Marfan syndrome.

arthrofibrosis: joint capsular thickening and scarring with resistant stiffness seen in either posttraumatic situations, chronic spasticity, or an arthrogryposis.

arthrogryposis (arthrogryposis multiplex congenita): joint contractures present at birth; cause is not yet known. Muscle weakness with immobility leads to contractures. Absent skin lines give it a waxy appearance. There are three groups:

single localized deformity **(in upper extremity):** forearm pronation contracture, palm clutched thumb, selected loss of wrist and finger extensors, and intrinsic muscle contracture.

whole upper extremity involvement: no shoulder girdle musculature; thin, tubular arms and forearms; straight, stiff elbows; flexion and ulnar deviation of the wrist; and stiff fingers and adducted thumbs.

global rigidity with associated deformities: polydactyly or windblown deformity (intrinsic plus hand).

bifid thumb: a generic term for thumb duplication or preaxial polydactyly. Wassel classification is the most commonly used.

I: bifid distal phalanx (IP joint common).

II: duplicate distal phalanx (first proximal phalanx).

III: bifid proximal phalanx (MP joint common).

IV: duplicate proximal phalanx (first metacarpal most common).

V: bifid metacarpal (CMC joint common).

VI: duplicate metacarpal.

VII: triphalangeal thumb.

brachydactyly ("short fingers"): digital hypoplasia may result from an arrest of development and it may affect any or all component tissues in a digit. It can be isolated or in conjunction with other congenital anomalies.

camptodactyly ("bent finger"): congenital nontraumatic flexion contracture in the sagittal plane of the proximal interphalangeal joint of the little finger, usually accompanied by metacarpophalangeal joint hyperextension. This is usually associated with other anomalies, causes are multifactorial, treatment is difficult, and outcome is uncertain.

carpal coalition: a congenital fusion or synostosis between two carpal bones, most commonly lunate and triquetrum or capitohamate. These are usually asymptomatic.

cleft hand: a central ray deficiency (ectrodactyly, oligodactyly) secondary to failure of formation of parts. High association with extraskeletal (i.e., cardiac) defects that may be metacarpal and carpal anomalies or deficiencies. These present deep clefts that may extend down to the carpus. Despite the cosmetic appearance, function may be surprisingly good; **lobster-claw hand** (archaic).

clinodactyly ("bent finger"): radial or ulnar deviation of the digit tip in coronal plane. Usually this is expressed as radial deviation of the little finger at the distal interphalangeal joint and is associated with other anomalies.

congenital trigger thumb: a congenital locking or clicking of the thumb with flexion posture of the interphalangeal joint. Nodular formation on the flexor pollicis longus tendon or tendon sheath thickening is common. Tendon sheath release is curative.

delta phalanx: a triangular-shaped bone interposed in the digit between two normal phalanges. A C-shaped physis is common and will cause a sharp angular digital deformity.

Fanconi anemia: pancytopenia, hematophoretic anomalies associated with radial hemimelia (autosomal recessive).

flipper hand (phocomelia): congenital absence of the arms; the hands appear to arise directly from the shoulder.

floating thumb (pouce floutant): an unstable hypoplastic thumb that may be connected to the hand by skin and a simple neurovascular pedicle. These digits are generally useless and are best removed.

hemimelia: absence of the forearm and hand.

heart-hand syndrome (Holt-Oram syndrome): cardiac septal defects, autosomal and seen with radial ray deficiency.

hyperphalangism: an extra (fourth) phalanx interposed between the phalanges of a finger. There are no extra digits. The digits are usually short.

hypoplastic thumb: an incompletely developed thumb that can range from a short thumb to complete absence. This is usually seen in conjunction with many associated abnormalities. There are five types: short thumb, adducted thumb, abducted thumb, floating thumb, and absent thumb.

Kirner deformity: parrot-beak convexity of the nail bed due to volar bending of the distal phalanx. This may not be obvious until age 12.

macrodactyly: a disproportionately large digit apparent at birth or early childhood. In "true" case, all structural components may be enlarged including vessels and nerves. Commonly, there is a marked increase in subcutaneous fiber or fatty tissue.

Madelung deformity: congenital growth plate disorder of the volar ulnar physis of the distal radius. This will cause a severe volar and ulnar bowing of the radius, initially normal at birth, and the deformity becomes evident by 8 to 12 years of age.

mirror hand (ulnar dimelia): the forearm contains two ulnas and has no radius. Typically, the patient presents with eight digits. This is a rare spontaneous genetic mutation that, when present, can be passed down in an autosomal dominant fashion.

monodactyly: a single-digit hand that may also be seen as part of a spectrum of cleft hand disease.

Poland syndrome: thumb ray or finger deformity associated with absence of pectoral muscle head.

polydactyly: extra digits that may be complete or partially formed. These can be postaxial (ulnar side of the hand) or preaxial (on the thumb).

polysyndactyly (central polydactyly): polydactyly of the index and ring fingers, usually associated with complex syndactyly. These are usually bilateral.

radial clubbed hand: total or partial absence of radial structures of the hand and forearm (preaxial). There are four types: (1) short distal radius; (2) hypoplastic radius; (3) partial absence of the radius; (4) total absence of the radius. These may be accompanied by thumb, index, or long finger anomalies. Muscle or neurovascular anomalies can be isolated as part of a syndrome complex (i.e., VATER, Holt-Oram syndrome). Hand is radially deviated; **talipomanus.**

supernumerary digits: extra nubbins of fingers and thumb with no function.

symbrachidactyly: literally shortened, stiff digits. Seen commonly in the spectrum of cleft hand disease.

symphalangism: hereditary dysplasia and ankylosis of digital joints, most notably the proximal interphalangeal (PIP) joint. There may be partial or total bone bridging.

syndactyly: a congenital joining of two or more digits; the connection may be complete or incomplete, simple or complex. Simple-shared element of skin and subcutaneous tissue. Complex-shared element of skin, subcutaneous tissue, tendon, bone, and neurovascular structures.

synostosis: fusion between two adjacent parallel bones (i.e., metacarpals or radius and ulna). Term may also be used for humeral-radial fusion.

TAR syndrome: **t**hrombocytopenia, **a**bsent **r**adius; complete absence of the radius may be present (autosomal recessive).

trident hand: typical hand appearance of an achondroplastic dwarf.

triphalangeal thumb: interposition of an extra phalanx between two normal phalanges of the thumb; can at times be functionally normal or cause marked deformity or malfunction. The extra phalanx can be normal or be a delta phalanx. Often seen with congenital heart disease.

triplicate thumb: a variant form of preaxial polydactyly involving three thumbs; all are markedly diminished in size and may lack one or more tissue elements.

ulnar (postaxial) deficiency: this is usually isolated with severe limitation of elbow function; hypoplasia of ulna, partial aplasia of the ulna (absence of distal or middle third of the ulna), total aplasia of the ulna; **radiohumeral synostosis.**

ulnar variance: relative position of the distal ulnar joint referred to the level of the ulnar side of the distal radial joint, as determined on an anteroposterior radiograph that is obtained with neutral pronation and supination. A longer ulna is called a **positive variance,** and a shorter ulna is called a **negative variance,** measured in millimeters.

VATER syndrome: **v**ertebral anomalies, **a**nal atresia, **t**racheo**e**sophageal fistula, **r**enal and vascular anomalies, accompanied by a radial clubhand.

congenital ulnar drift: ulnar deviation of the digits at the metacarpophalangeal (MCP) joint with proximal interphalangeal (PIP) joint flexion deformity. Thumb webbing is also present. General muscular hypoplasia in the arm is present. Associated with craniofacial deformities and a markedly narrowed mouth; also called **windblown hand, whistling face syndrome, Freeman-Sheldon syndrome.**

Muscle and Tendon Disorders

trigger finger (acquired):   entrapment of finger flexor tendons usually under the proximal A1 pulleys; usually due to a disproportion between the flexor tendon and the flexor tendon sheath. Usually, the cause is obscure, with thickening of the pulley tissues and/or nodular formation about the tendon. This can be secondary (i.e., due to diabetes, rheumatoid arthritis, or gout). Conservative measures and steroid injections may help, but surgery is usually curative.

boutonnière deformity (posttraumatic):   usually due to a central slip rupture of the middle phalanx with an injury to the triangular ligaments. Volar subluxation of the lateral bands below the flexion axis of the proximal interphalangeal (PIP) joint will cause a fixed flexion attitude of the PIP joint.

carpal pedal spasm: an intrinsic plus position with wrist flexion usually seen in hypercalcemia.

de Quervain disease: stenosing tenosynovitis of the first dorsal extensor compartment, usually involving the extensor pollicis brevis (EPB) and abductor pollicis longus (APL).

intersection syndrome: pain and swelling over the place where the muscles of the first dorsal extensor compartment cross over the muscles of the second compartment. This is believed to be a tenosynovitis of the second dorsal compartment.

quadregia: in a setting where the profundus tendon to a digit is contracted or repaired too tightly, there will be a limitation of proximal excursion of the remaining flexor digitorum profundus (FDP), causing a weak grip (as all the FDP tendons usually share a common muscle belly).

tetraplegia: neurologic injury secondary to cervical spine trauma. Altered functional capacity of the hand, depending on the level of injury. This will also dictate operative and nonoperative intervention. A system has been devised:

Tetraplegia International Classification

Functional Group	Root Level Intact
Brachioradialis	C-5, C-6
Extensor carpi radialis longus	C-7 (possibly C-8)
Extensor carpi radialis brevis	C-7, C-8
Pronator teres	C-7, C-8
Flexor carpi radialis	C-8
Extensor digitorum communis	C-8
Extensor pollicis longus	T-1
Partial digital flexion	T-1
Lacks intrinsics only	T-1
Miscellaneous (i.e., Brown-Séquard syndrome or syringomyelia)	

Volkmann contracture: contracture affecting the volar forearm musculature as a result of scarring after an ischemic insult. This is the usual sequela of an untreated volar muscle compartment syndrome (seen in muscle crush injuries or forearm fracture). Circulation is usually impaired in the center of the forearm. The flexor digitorum profundus (FDP) and flexor pollicis longus (FPL) muscles are most severely affected. There is a mild, moderate, classic, or severe type.

"no man's land": usually refers to an injury to the digital flexor tendons at zone II (under the A1 and A2 pulleys). Until recently, injury to this area was fraught with technical difficulty and poor results.

Vascular Disorders

acrocyanosis: seen in Raynaud phenomenon. With exposure to cold, the fingers become deep blue and cold. This is usually due to peripheral vasospasm.

Buerger disease (thromboangiitis obliterans): an inflammatory thrombosis seen in smokers, usually in men. Digital arteries are affected. The disease is progressive, leading to digital loss and possibly loss of the whole hand.

hypothenar hammer syndrome: an ulnar artery aneurysm or thrombosis due to repetitive striking of the hypothenar eminence and the hook of hamate region against a hard blunt object; typically, localized pain, digital pallor, and cold sensibility are common symptoms.

Kienböck disease: a posttraumatic, vascularly mediated avascular necrosis of the lunate with subsequent collapse, dislocation, and arthrosis. MRI and bone scan have fine-tuned the classification; **isolated dislocation.**

Lichtman classification for Keinböck disease is as follows:
  Stage I: normal radiographic findings, positive bone scan, questionable linear fractures.
  Stage II: lunate sclerosis without collapse. MRI subclassification:

IIA: T2 focal signal intensity increase.
IIB: T2 focal signal intensity loss.
IIC: T2 generalized signal intensity increase.
IID: T2 generalized signal intensity loss.
Stage III: lunate sclerosis, fragmentation, and collapse.
Stage IV: stage III plus degenerative changes of the carpus.

Traumatic Disorders

factitious edema: history of minor trauma followed by persistent dorsal forearm pain, swelling, and tenderness due to repeated self-inflicted trauma; **secretan edema.**

Palmer classification: for triangular fibrocartilage injury.
  Class 1: traumatic.
    Type A: central perforation.
    Type B: medial avulsion (ulnar attachment), with or without distal ulnar fracture.
    Type C: distal avulsion (carpal attachment).
    Type D: lateral avulsion (radial attachment), with or without sigmoid-notch fracture.
  Class 2: degenerative (ulnocarpal impaction syndrome).
    Stage A: TFCC wear.
    Stage B: TFCC wear with lunate and or ulnar chondromalacia.
    Stage C: TFCC perforation with lunate and or ulnar chondromalacia.
    Stage D: TFCC perforation with lunate and/or ulnar chondromalacia and lunotriquetral-ligament perforation.
    Stage E: TFCC perforation with lunate and or ulnar chondromalacia and lunotriquetral-ligament perforation, and ulnar carpal arthritis.

peritendinous fibrosis: scarring around a tendon.

Stener lesion: in a complete tear of the ulnar collateral ligament of the metacarpophalangeal (MCP) joint of the thumb, the ligament may avulse distally and roll up proximally, causing an interposition of the adductor aponeurosis. Non-operative treatment will usually result in a chronically unstable thumb.

turret exostosis: a painful mass on the dorsal aspect of the middle phalanx seen on lateral x-ray as an exostosis (**bone spur**). This is believed to be traumatic in origin.

Specific Dislocations

Wrist Dislocations and Instability

In a distal radius dislocation, the radius is dislocated in reference to the ulna. However, the standard terminology describes the position of the ulna in relationship to the radius.

carpal instability dissociative (CID; Linsheid):   a carpal collapse pattern due to a ligamentous disruption in the proximal carpal row (i.e., scapholunate lunotriquetral pattern).

carpal instability nondissociative (CIND):   a carpal collapse pattern due to disruption of ligaments connecting the proximal and midcarpal row or due to other extrinsic factors (i.e., radial malunion; Dobyns).

Desault d.:   involves the radiocarpal joint with dorsal displacement of carpus and ulnar styloid process.

dorsal intercalated segment instability (DISI):   a zigzag collapse pattern seen best on the lateral views of the wrist. The lunate appears to send its distal face dorsally. This can occur as a result of displaced scaphoid fractures, scapholunate instability, a nondissociated carpal instability. Commonly, the lunate follows the triquetrum volarly without the scaphoid to contract its movement. The capitolunate angle is greater than 20 degrees and the scapholunate angle is greater than 70 degrees when the wrist is held in neutral posture.

lumbrical plus finger: posttraumatic contracture of the lumbrical will cause a paradoxical extension of the PIP and DIP joints each time an attempt is made to flex the digits.

lunate d.:   volar semilunar dislocation in the wrist; a type of dislocation often not recognized.

perilunate d.:   involves all carpals, which are shifted posteriorly, leaving the lunate in proper position; may be associated with a scaphoid fracture, in which case it is termed a **transscaphoid perilunate d.** Rarely do other carpi dislocate singularly or in association with fractures about the wrist. Wrist instabilities may be associated with fractures but specifically relate to ligamentous instabilities of the carpal bones. A devastating injury where all the connecting ligaments between the lunate and its surrounding carpal bones are severed. Commonly, the capitate sits dorsal to the lunate. The lunate may dislocate volarly as part of the spectrum.

transscaphoid perilunate dislocation: similar to the perilunate dislocation except that the stress lines extend through the body of the scaphoid itself rather than the scapholunate ligament. The radial styloid may be fractured as well.

volar flexed intercalated segment instability (VISI):   a zigzag collapse pattern with the lunate distal face turned volarly. This is seen best on lateral x-rays of the wrist. These can follow triquetral lunate instability or nondissociated instability patterns. An average reduced scapholunate angle of over 35 degrees.

Hand Dislocations

Dislocation can occur at all the small joints of the hand. Dislocations at the carpometacarpal (CMC) and metacarpophalangeal (MCP) joints generally occur in a dorsal direction. Dislocations at the MCP joints can sometimes be reduced without surgery. Dislocations in the hand are often associated with intraarticular fractures. Fracture-dislocations often require surgical reduction and fixation to realign joint surfaces.

Bennett d.:   lateral or dorsal displacement of the first CMC joint.

boutonnière deformity: flexion contracture of the proximal interphalangeal (PIP) joint that may progress to subluxation. Associated with hyperextension contracture of the distal interphalangeal (DIP) joint. Deformity begins with rupture of the extensor tendon insertion of the PIP joint and later becomes a fixed deformity.

carpal instability: partial or complete dislocations between individual wrist bones, causing a click-clunk with wrist movement. Most often occurs at the scapholunate joint but can occur at the triquetrolunate, midcarpal, and even the radiocarpal joint.

gamekeeper thumb: a hyperabduction injury with partial subluxation and instability of the thumb MCP joint due to traumatic rupture of the ulnar collateral ligament. Commonly due to a ski-pole strap injury; **skier's thumb.**

Nail and Skin Disorders

acanthosis nigricans: dull, gray, friable nails with leukonychia; can be an external marker of an internal malignancy.

beak deformity (hook nail):   with amputation of the tip of the distal phalanx, the nail may grow over the edge of the finger. It is unsightly and occasionally painful.

chromonychia: color changes in the nail unit.

clubbing: an increase in the unguophalangeal angle of greater than 180 degrees with fibrovascular hyperplasia of the nail unit.

Dupuytren contracture (palmar fibromatosis):   inflammatory process of the palmar fascia, occasionally extending into the fingers, in which severe contractures and nodular proliferation (skin dimples) may result. There are three phases: proliferative (nodular), involutional, and resolved. In the resolved state, the remaining constricting tissue is referred to as bands.

epidermoid cyst: benign cyst composed of epidermal fragments that have been pushed to the deeper layers by minor trauma.

leukonychia: whitening of the nail plate.

macronychia: an unusually large or wide nail.

micronychia: small, short, or narrow nail.

onychalgia: nail unit pain.

onychia: inflammation of the nail plate.

onychogryphosis: nail plate hypertrophy that is hornlike resulting from trauma; **onychogryposis.**

onycholysis: distal separation of the nail plate from the underlying nail bed.

onychomadesis: proximal separation of the nail plate from the nail matrix.

onychomycosis: fungal infection of the nail unit.

onychophagia: nail biting.

onychoptosis: loss of the nail plate.

onychorrhexis: spontaneous longitudinal splitting of the nail plate.

pitted nail: surface pits of nails less than 1 mm in diameter.

racket nail: thumbnail shorter than it is wide. Usually, the distal ends of the fingers are also short.

reedy nail: fingernail marked by longitudinal furrows.

scleroderma: an autoimmune disease that causes the skin of the hands to become thin, tense, and shiny; interphalangeal joint stiffness, distal ischemic ulceration, and autoamputation are common.

spoon nail: a central depression of the nail with raised sides.

subungual exostosis: a bone spur emanating from the distal phalanx dorsally under the nail bed, causing pressure pain, necrosis, and possible infection of the nail bed.

subungual hematoma: usually posttraumatic with nail bed laceration under an intact nail.

A collection of blood under the nail plate, under pressure, can destroy the nail bed unless decompressed by a hole drilled into the nail plate (i.e., a hot paper clip tip).

turtle-back nail: a distorted fingernail, being more convex than normal.

unguis incarnatus: ingrown nail.

watch crystal nail: a nail as broad as it is long and convexed lengthwise and crosswise; seen in pulmonary osteoarthropathy.

Other Specific Terms

Bouchard node: thick nodular swelling due to bone spurs in the proximal interphalangeal joints, not necessarily associated with systemic arthritis.

carpal bossing: prominence seen particularly at the dorsal index carpometacarpal (CMC) joint; may be painful but usually causes no symptoms.

flexor origin syndrome (reverse tennis elbow):   tendonitis of pronator teres and wrist and finger flexor muscle origin on medial epicondyle of elbow.

ganglion: a clear, viscid, fluid-filled sac found near the wrist joints or fingers, arising from capsuloligamentous structures; rarely associated with other diseases; most commonly found on dorsum of wrist.

glomus tumor: small vascular lesion that is usually very painful and associated with hypersensitivity to pressure or temperature; usually in fingertip.

hand-foot syndrome: swelling in hands and feet as seen in sickle cell disease.

Heberden node: a thick nodular swelling due to bone spurs in the distal interphalangeal joints; not necessarily associated with systemic arthritis.

inclusion cyst: a noninfectious process following healing of laceration or puncture wound; germinal matrix of dermal growth, causing mass comprised of desquamated dermal cells.

mucous cyst: a misnomer; this is a ganglion of the distal interphalangeal joint, which makes a cyst under the skin in the eponychial area.

Preiser disease: spontaneous loss of blood supply and collapse of scaphoid, usually seen in young adults.

stenosing tenosynovitis: a bulbous swelling of the tendon, causing the tendon to catch as it passes through the pulley (the thick fibrous tunnel that holds the tendon in place); sometimes caused by rheumatoid arthritis; **trigger fingers, snapping tendons.**

Infections

The hand has many structures that are vulnerable to infections. When edema and swelling place pressure on muscles, tendons, blood vessels, and nerves, function is disrupted and compartmental ischemia could result. Adhesions or fibrosis following infection may reduce hand function temporarily or permanently. Terms related to infections are the following.

collar-button abscess: a digital web space infection usually in the subdermal fatty layers. Drainage is usually required; **shirt-stud abscess.**

deep space infection (palmar space infection):   refers to infection of the thenar or midpalmar spaces.

epidermoid cyst: benign cyst composed of epidermal fragments that have been pushed to the deeper layers by minor trauma.

eponychia: a nail-fold infection involving the entire eponychial fold and lateral nail fold. These are relatively rare.

felon: a subcutaneous abscess involving the tissue of the distal fingertip. These may be under great pressure and require drainage, usually through a midlateral approach.

Hansen disease (leprosy):   commonly involves the hands; caused by *Mycobacterium leprae*. Peripheral neuropathy predominates with intrinsic atrophy and clawing. Later, soft-tissue necrosis can result in actual loss of digits.

herpetic whitlow: a fascicular outbreak with an erythematous rim seen usually in fingertips of health care workers. These are commonly misdiagnosed and mistakenly drained. Supportive treatment is the mainstay. These are usually self-limited.

horseshoe abscess: in those hands where thenar and hypothenar spaces are interconnected, an abscess may spread to both sides of the hand in the shape of a horseshoe. Palmar space infection usually results from a penetrating wound. The deep spaces of the hand may fill with purulent material. Drainage is the key.

Kanavel sign: for pyogenic flexor tenosynovitis; there is a flexed position of the finger, symmetrical enlargement of the finger, excessive tenderness over the course of the tendon sheath, and extreme pain on passive extension of the digit.

Meleney infection: life- or limb-threatening infection with anaerobic bacteria or microaerophilic streptococcus. Amputation is usually required to save the patient's life; **gas gangrene.**

paronychia: infection in the soft-tissue folds around the nail that usually results from injection of *Staphylococcus aureus* by a sliver of nail tissue, a manicure instrument, or a tooth. Drainage is mandatory.

pyogenic granuloma: an exophytic friable growth over the surface of the skin. These are usually caused by *Staphylococcus aureus* and will require complete excision to effect a cure.

subungual abscess: a collection of pus under the nail plate or over the nail bed.

tenosynovitis: inflammation of the tendon sheath. Causes are multifactorial and include overuse, rheumatoid arthritis, infection, and nonspecific onset.

verruca vulgaris: a viral wart involving the nail or skin tissue. A carbon dioxide laser is usually curative.

SURGERY OF THE HAND AND WRIST

Surgical procedures of the hand and wrist are more commonly described anatomically than by eponyms. All terms, including eponyms, are listed according to the goals of the surgical procedure.

Arthrodeses of the Fingers

chevron a.: a rigid stable construction for interphalangeal (IP) joint fusion; a precise, chevron-shaped fitting of the bone cuts of the joint to be fused with resection of the joint surface.

interphalangeal a.: cup and cone technique useful for metacarpophalangeal (MCP) or interphalangeal (IP) fusion, allows for fine adjustment of angles and rotatory alignment after joint surfaces have been prepared.

Moberg dowel graft: for an interphalangeal (IP) arthrodesis where there has been bone loss or nonunion. A finger joint fusion using a small squared bone peg.

Potenza a.: a finger joint fusion using bone peg taken from the adjacent phalanx or metacarpal.

trapeziometacarpal fusion: for advanced trapeziometacarpal disease in the thumb in young, active patients.

Arthrodeses of the Wrist

intercarpal a.: for wrist instability or collapse patterns, Kienböck disease, rheumatoid arthritis, localized degenerative changes in the carpus. These include triscaphe (scaphotrapeziotrapezoid), scaphocapitate, capitolunate, scapholunate, lunatotriquetral capitohamate (four-poster fusion). Moberg dowel grafts are useful in securing these fusions.

radiocarpal a.: commonly a total wrist fusion with or without autogenous graft. Useful for (1) a heavy laborer with posttraumatic arthritis, (2) failed radiocarpal arthroplasty, (3) rheumatoid arthritis, (4) tetraplegia with deformity of the wrist, (5) tendon transfer surgery to stabilize the wrist.

radioulnar fusion: for the creation of a one-bone forearm for advanced disease of the distal radio-ulnar joint.

SLAC procedure (scapho/unate advanced collapse):   for the common combination of radioscaphoid and midcarpal arthritis often seen in chronic nonunions of the scaphoid; a mid-carpal arthrodesis with excision of scaphoid.

total wrist a.:   fusion of the distal radius and prox-imal and distal carpal rows. Useful salvage pro-cedure for severe carpal arthritis.

triscaphe a.:   of the scaphotrapeziotrapezoid (SST) articulation. Useful in localized arthritis and for rotatory subluxation of the scaphoid.

Arthrodeses of the Wrist (Eponymns)

Abbott a.:   using only cortical bone grafts; **Abbott-Saunders-Bost a.**

Brockman-Nissen a.:   intraarticular wrist fusion.

Carroll a.:   rabbit ear–shaped bone graft fusion.

Gill-Stein a.:   extraarticular fusion using the dor-sal distal radius as the graft; **radiocarpal a.**

Haddad-Riordan a.:   intraarticular fusion using iliac crest bone graft.

Liebolt a.:   fusion using chips of bone graft.

Nalebuff a.:   fusion that includes use of a Stein-mann pin.

Seddon a.:   intraarticular fusion involving resec-tion of the distal ulna.

Smith-Petersen a.:   fusion that includes resec-tion of the distal ulna.

Wickstrom a.:   fusion of the wrist using bone graft inserted into both the radius and carpus.

Arthroplasties

An arthroplasty is the reconstruction of joints to restore motion and stability. It involves the meta-carpophalangeal (MCP), carpometacarpal (CMC), and proximal interphalangeal (PIP) joints of the fingers and wrist, often with implants. The hand spe-cialist frequently treats joint destruction commonly found in rheumatoid arthritis.

An implant arthroplasty involves a prosthetic re-placement of joints by metallic or silicone-rubber parts, usually for arthritic conditions or traumatic ankylosis. Swanson silicone-rubber arthroplasty is a popular choice. Other prosthetic devices for the hand and wrist are the AMC total wrist (**Volz, Steffe, Swanson**).

anchovy procedure (Carroll):   rolled palmaris longus (PL) graft placed into the space that re-mains after trapezium excision for pantrapezial arthritis.

Blatt capsulodesis: dynamic rotatory subluxa-tion of the scaphoid. A proximally based flap of dorsal wrist capsule is attached to the distal pole of the scaphoid; this will prevent downward movement of the distal pole during radial devia-tion of the wrist; **dorsal capsulodesis.**

capsulectomy: proximal interphalangeal (PIP) joint flexion contractures unresponsive to con-servative treatment; proximal release of the joint capsule (volar plate) will improve movement.

Carroll (Froimson) a.:   an interposition rolled tendon (palmaris longus [PL]) used as a spacer when the trapezium is removed for pantrapezial arthritis.

Darrach resection: resection of the distal 1 to 1.5 cm of distal ulna at the wrist. Once consid-ered as the standard procedure for the treatment of a myriad of distal radioulnar joint problems; now useful primarily in the elderly and for se-vere rheumatoid arthritis. (**Albright and Chase.**)

Eaton volar plate a: a chronic subluxation of the proximal interphalangeal (PIP) joint after a dis-placed large volar lip fracture of the proximal end of the middle phalanx, greater than 50% of the articular surface. If left untreated, a chronic subluxation results. The volar plate is then ad-vanced into the fracture site and tightened to pre-vent subluxation.

Fowler metacarpophalangeal (MCP) a.: for arthritis of the MCP joint. The metacarpal is cut in the form of a chevron at the base of the proximal phalanx and then cut into a V shape, with an interposition of extensor tendon fusion.

hemi-resection interposition arthroplasty (Bowers): for distal radioulnar joint arthritis, resection of the articular surface of the distal ulna and interposition of a rolled tendon graft.

matched ulnar resection: popularized by Watson; resection of the articular surface of the distal ulna to match the shape of the radial styloid notch. This is useful for the treatment of distal radioulnar joint instability and arthritis.

Neibauer prosthesis: silicone hinge joints with built-in ties; useful in metacarpophalangeal (MCP) joint arthroplasty.

perichondral autografts: use of osteocartilaginous grafts (from ribs) to resurface the injured articular surface of a small joint in the hand.

proximal row carpectomy: a salvage procedure whereby the scaphoid, lunate, and triquetrum are excised. This is useful in treating advanced arthritis involving the radiocarpal joint if wrist motion is still desired by the patient.

radial styloidectomy: excision of the tip of the radial styloid; useful in isolated radioscaphoid arthritis or as part of the SLAC wrist reconstruction.

Stefee thumb a.: a cemented metal polyethylene prosthesis useful in thumb metacarpophalangeal (MCP) arthroplasty.

Suave Kapanje (Lauenstein procedure): fusion of the articular surface of the distal radioulnar joint with proximal resection of a distal ulnar segment of approximately 1.5 cm to facilitate motion.

suspensionplasty (LRTI-Burton): for advanced trapeziometacarpal arthritis, removal of the trapezium, and placement of half of the flexor carpi radialis (FCR) as an anchor to the metacarpal and as a spacer. An improvement on the classic "anchovy" procedure.

Swanson a.: complete array of silicone implants for all digital articular joints, carpal bones, total wrist arthroplasty, distal ulna, and proximal radius. This is most useful in rheumatoid arthritis for the reconstruction of metacarpophalangeal (MCP) joints. Its use in the carpus had to be discontinued because of concerns regarding silicone synovitis.

Swanson prosthesis (silicone): most useful for metacarpophalangeal (MCP) and proximal interphalangeal (PIP) arthroplasty in rheumatoid arthritis. In selected situations, a total wrist arthroplasty is useful (i.e., in bilateral involvement). Carpal silicone arthroplasty is now falling out of favor because of silicone synovitis.

trapezial hemiarthroplasty: resection of the distal half of the trapezium, sparing the scaphotrapezial joint; useful for trapeziometacarpal arthritis.

Tupper a.: in metacarpophalangeal (MCP) joint arthritis, the volar plate may be used as an interpositional material after excision arthroplasty.

Vainio metaphalangeal (MP): MCP joint resectional arthroplasty with interposition of the extensor tendon and collateral ligaments.

Voltz a.: a metal-polyethylene cemented total wrist arthroplasty useful in selected cases of end-stage degenerative or rheumatoid arthritis.

Zancholli capsuloplasty: a volar plate advancement of the metacarpophalangeal (MCP) joint of the thumb to treat congenital hyperextension.

Zancholli-Lasso procedure: transfer of the flexor digitorum sublimus tendon (FDS) to the lateral band or the A2 pulley to prevent MP hyperextension and clawing; found in low ulnar nerve palsy.

Zancholli static-lock procedure: a volar plate advancement (plication) for the treatment of MP hyperextension; seen in claw deformities in low ulnar nerve palsy.

Neurologic Procedures

cable nerve grafts: a method of uniting strands of nerve graft and interposing them into a gap to repair a polyfascicular nerve discontinuity (of historic interest).

epineural repair: repair of lacerated nerve segments by repairing the epineurium. This is useful in digital nerves or in oligofascicular proximal nerves.

epineurotomy: the opening of the epineurium during a neurolysis procedure. This can be useful in certain cases of chronic nerve compression.

funiculectomy: for chronic end neuromas; peeling back the epineurium and resecting nerve fascicles, with reclosure and ligation of the epineurium. May aid in the treatment of end neuromas.

group fascicular repair: a perineural repair; useful in treating laceration of mixed motor and sensory nerves. Presumably, exact anatomic re-approximation will facilitate maximal functional return.

internal neurolysis: presumably, internal dissection of intraneural scarring will facilitate return of nerve function. Originally thought to be useful in the treatment of carpal tunnel syndrome but now found to be harmful in many cases. This technique, however, is useful in the removal of intraneural neurilemmoma.

medial epicondylectomy: one method to decompress the ulnar nerve in the cubital tunnel by removing its bony floor, the medial epicondyle of the distal humerus.

Moberg procedure (key pinch): for tetraplegia; to restore the ability of key pinch in group II or III level tetraplegia. This includes carpometacarpal (CMC) thumb arthrodesis, extensor pollicis longus (EPL) tenodesis, and flexor pollicis longus (FPL) tenodesis or transfer.

neurectomy: the resection of a portion of nerve of an end neuroma (and presumed buried in bone or muscle).

neurotization: in patients with a profound brachial plexus injury with a flare anesthetic arm, the use of a live intercostal nerve grafted to a distal neural segment of the brachial plexus has restored some upper extremity function in select patients.

Trauma Procedures

Bentzon procedure: attempt to convert a painful scaphoid nonunion to a painless pseudarthrosis by soft-tissue (capsular flap) interposition; of historic interest.

Bevin Aurglass technique: a digital web-deepening procedure for the correction of burn syndactyly.

distal finger amputation revision: procedure performed following traumatic amputation involving the distal phalanx (fingertip) by the following techniques:
  finger flaps: to preserve sensation.
    Atosoy: volar single V-Y advancement.
    cross-finger flap: a section of skin with its blood supply intact from a neighboring finger used to cover open area.
    Kutler: lateral double V-Y advancement.
    thenar flap: one raised from the thumb side of the base of the palm.
    Wolfe graft: free skin (pinch) graft; a section of full-thickness skin placed on the open area.

Fisk-Fernandez volar wedge: anterior cortical cancellous bone graft for the correction of scaphoid nonunion or malunion.

Herbert screw osteosynthesis: the use of a dumbbell-shaped bone screw with variable pitch to affect rigid compressive internal fixation of a scaphoid fracture or nonunion. This can be used with or without bone graft.

Kapandji fixation: for distal radius fracture; use of two K wires inserted at 90 degrees at fracture site lateral and posterior and then angled 45 degrees anteriorly.

metacarpal lengthening (Matev): useful for irretrievable thumb amputation at the metacarpophalangeal (MCP) joint level; metacarpal osteotomy, application of a distraction device, slow distraction, and later bone grafting will partially restore length of the thumb ray. Secondary first web deepening may be required.

Russe bone graft: for scaphoid nonunion fracture; cortical cancellous graft placed by a volar approach through a longitudinal trough in the volar surface of the scaphoid that will enhance bony union.

Microvascular Procedures

anastomosis: term used for the direct repair of nerves and blood vessels.

Chinese flap (radial forearm flap): a radial forearm rotation flap based on the radial artery to repair radial and hand defects.

lateral arm flap: a free flap based on the posterior radial collateral artery; useful for covering large, full-thickness defects in the dorsum of the hand.

toe-thumb transfer: complete transfer of a toe with its full complement of neurovascular, tendinous, and bone structures to the hand to add to a digit or thumb on a posttraumatic or congenitally deficient hand.

wrap-around procedure: the medial aspect of the great toe with its neurovascular bundles is removed from the toe and wrapped around a free bone graft at the tip of an amputation stump. This is then reattached using microvascular techniques. The donor site is secondarily grafted to close its defect.

Congenital Deformity Repairs

Barsky macrodactyly reduction: (1) filleting out of the distal phalanx, then placing all distal structures on to the end of the middle phalanx (this will shorten the macrodactylous digit); (2) hemiresection of the middle phalanx and primary distal interphalangeal (DIP) joint fusion.

Bilhaut-Cloquet procedure: for Wassel II thumb duplication (bifid thumb). The narrow half of each thumb tip is united with the other, discarding the central units and allowing the thumb to become one phalanx.

Bonola technique: a dorsally based closing wedge osteotomy of the distal phalanx to correct a Kirner deformity.

Carstan reverse wedge osteotomy: for the treatment of a delta phalanx; a central wedge is reversed and turned 180 degrees to straighten a digit.

Krukenberg procedure: in the congenital absence of a hand, the radius and ulna are surgically separated and covered with soft tissue so that the two bones will act as a claw.

radialization/centralization: an attempt to rebalance the hand and wrist on to the distal forearm in radial clubbed hand.

Skin, Nails, Fascia Procedures

advancement flaps (Kleinert-Atosoy): called V-Y flaps; flaps cut either from the volar pad or from the radial and ulnar pad of the distal fingertip for the reconstruction of fingertip injuries with skin and subcutaneous loss.

axial cutaneous flaps (scapular flap): free or island flap on a subscapular artery pedicle for medium-sized defect coverage in the hand.

axial flag flaps: a rotational skin flap based on a dorsal digital artery used for digital skin and subcutaneous defects.

axial pattern skin flap: a long skin flap possible because of an underlying vascular supply running along its long axis underneath.

cocked-half flap (Gillies): reconstruction of a thumb amputation at the metacarpophalangeal (MCP) joint level with a local skin graft, iliac crest graft, and skin graft.

composite nail bed flap: a full-thickness nail bed graft from a toe to cover a defect in a finger nail bed.

cross-finger flap: the dorsal skin of one digit is flapped over itself to create coverage for a volar skin defect of an adjacent digit.

escarotomy: in the management of deep thermal burns, burned and contracted skin is incised to decompress deeper tissues and prevent further necrosis.

fasciectomy: generic term used to describe excision of the palmar fascia, usually when involved in Dupuytren disease.

fasciotomy: (1) opening of muscle compartments and decompressing intrinsic muscle spaces in compartment syndrome; spaces to be decompressed are interosseus muscles (through dorsal incisions or volar thenar and hypothenar compartments); (2) incision into a Dupuytren central cord to release contracture; this is useful in elderly and debilitated patients, but contracture recurrence is common.

Macindo procedure: a form of palmar fasciectomy for Dupuytren contracture when the palmar skin is left open to granulate.

Moberg flap: useful in thumb tip reconstruction; the volar half of the thumb soft tissue is elevated with its neurovascular structures, and by flexing the interphalangeal (IP) joint of the thumb, the flap is then stretched over the thumb tip.

neurovascular island transfer: a method of transferring sensibility to an important part of the hand such as the thumb tip from a less important part of the hand, whereby a portion of skin is left connected to its neurovascular structures and passed subcutaneously to a different part of the hand.

onychectomy: removal of a fingernail.

onychotomy: the method of cutting into a nail, usually to remove a mass under the nail.

pedicle flap: a procedure that permits an island of skin and subcutaneous tissue to be transferred from one place to another on its own vascular supply, using multiple operative stages.

pedicle grafts: a term used for pedicle flaps but also includes *pedicle bone grafts. Island pedicle grafts and neurovascular pedicle grafts* are pedicle, skin, or subcutaneous tissue containing blood and nerve supply, thus providing sensation for the skin graft.

thenar flap (Smith-Albin):   for fingertip coverage, an H flap is raised on the thenar eminence and the digit tip is flexed down to it. By 10 to 14 days, the flap provides a good skin and soft-tissue coverage to the distal digit tip. However, digital stiffness is common.

Muscle and Tendon Surgery of the Hand

There are two types of tendon procedures: (1) restoration of tendon function by direct repair of a tendon, its advancement, or its transfer and (2) freeing of tendon from scar tissue, restrictive bands, or abnormal lining tissues. Because of these basic categories, tendon grafts and advancement procedures are listed here contextually and not in alphabetic order.

tendon advancement: done when the damage segment of a tendon is so near its insertion that a direct tendon-to-bone rather than tendon-to-tendon repair is necessary. One such technique is the **Wagner** advancement of the profundus tendon.

tenodesis: the fixation of a tendon onto two bony locations to keep a joint from flexing or extending beyond a selected range. This procedure lends itself to prevention of hyperextension of the metacarpophalangeal joints in ulnar claw deformity. Two commonly done are the Fowler and Riordan procedures.

tenorrhaphy: the repair of a lacerated tendon, either immediate or delayed.

tendolysis: often called tenolysis; a tendon release. It describes two different types of procedures: (1) one in which the tendon is freed from scar tissue or entrapment so that it may move properly and (2) tenosynovectomy, whereby all or part of the sheath of a functioning tendon is excised.

Tendon Repair Techniques

Numerous techniques and types of sutures are used in repairing tendons. A tendon repair is any reapproximation of a partially or completely severed tendon. The specific technique is directed at gaining maximal strength with minimal scarring.

Becker: multiple cross-stitching technique for approximation of fresh tendon edges.

Bunnell opponensplasty: the use of the flexor digitorum sublimis IV as a donor motor for thumb opposition using the pulley in the region of the flexor carpi ulnaris and the pisiform.

Kleinert: modification of Bunnell technique, burying suture knot at tendon edge.

modified Kessler suture: a direct end-to-end grafting suture for flexor tendon lacerations, especially in zone II. These are usually augmented with epitendinous sutures.

Pulver-Taft weave: the strongest method of reat taching two tendons where space is not at a premium. It involves weaving tendon ends in and out of each other.

Tsuge: multiple cross-stitching technique for tendon reapproximation.

Verdan: multiple cross-stitching technique for tendon reapproximation.

Other specific techniques include **Tajima, Halsted, Salvage,** and **Silverskiold procedures.**

Tendon Grafts and Transfers

A tendon transfer is the relocation of a tendon from one place to another. The tendon retains attachment to its muscle. By contrast, free tendon graft requires complete excision of a tendon and its repositioning in a new location. Tendon transfers may be static or dynamic.

central slip repair/reconstruction: procedure designed to repair the common extensor insertion into the proximal dorsal end of the middle phalanx, thus restoring active proximal interphalangeal (PIP) extension.

Clark pectoralis major transfer: transfer of the sternocostal portion of the pectoralis major muscle for the restoration of elbow flexion in brachial plexus injury.

crossed intrinsic transfer: in rheumatoid arthritis, with ulnar deviation of the digits at the metaphalangeal joint, a conjoined ulnar intrinsic tendon is released from one digit and placed into the radial conjoined intrinsic tendon of the adjacent digit on its ulnar side.

Green transfer: flexor carpi ulnaris (FCU) to extensor carpi radialis brevis (ECRB) transfer to correct a wrist flexion deformity in cerebral palsy. Overcorrection is common.

Jones transfer: in radial nerve palsy, tendon transfer designed to restore thumb, digital, and wrist extension.

flexor pronator slide: release of the flexor pronator muscle group origin allowing the muscle to slide distally. This helps correct wrist and digital flexion deformity and forearm pronation deformity in cerebral palsy.

flexor tenolysis: method used to free flexor tendon from its surrounding scars approximately 4 months after flexor tendon repair with secondary tendon adherence.

Fowler tenodesis: static tendon grafts originating in the extensor retinaculum, passing volarly to the deep transverse metacarpal ligament, and inserting it into the radial lateral bands. A procedure to prevent hyperextension of the metacarpophalangeal (MCP) joint as seen in the claw deformity of low ulnar nerve palsy.

tenovaginotomy: procedure designed to release stenosing tenosynovitis by incising a retinaculum or flexor pulley.

static tendon transfer: transfer of a free tendon graft that is attached to two or more bony locations such that the active movement of one joint will cause the passive movement of some other joint. For example, a tendon appropriately inserted proximal to the wrist and in the fingers will cause flexion of the fingers if the wrist is extended.

dynamic tendon transfer: one that brings about motion by direct action of muscle contraction.

Tendon transfers are commonly required to replace or assist voluntary muscle function that is lost because of nerve injury, nerve disease, or direct and indirect sequelae of trauma to the muscle. Substantial numbers of transfers are used in central nervous system paralyses such as those caused by strokes and polio. Transfers are listed by categories that define function.

Camitz procedure: the palmaris longus, with its distal attachment tubularized, is passed under the thenar eminence and attached to the radial aspect of the base of the proximal phalanx of the thumb to act as an opponensplasty. This is useful in chronic carpal tunnel syndrome.

finger extension: Boyes procedure.

finger flexion: for flexion of the metacarpophalangeal joint (intrinsic transfer); Boyes, Fowler, Bunnell, Stiles-Bunnell, Riordan, and Pulver-Taft procedures, and Brand I and Brand II procedures.

Huber transfer: a procedure designed to restore thumb opposition based on a transfer into the thenar eminence of the abductor digiti minimi, that is, a neurovascular pedicle.

opponensplasty: the use of any of the intrinsic or extrinsic muscle tendon units to restore thumb opposition (i.e., in median nerve palsy); **Brand, Burkhalter, Groves, Goldner, Riordan, Phalen-Miller, Littler, Huber, and Fowler procedures.**

Steindler flexorplasty: in brachial plexus injury causing paralysis of elbow flexion (biceps and brachialis) with sparing of distal forearm musculature, the flexor pronator mass with the medial epicondyle of the distal humerus is transferred anteriorly and proximally on the humerus to effect elbow flexion.

thumb abduction: pulling thumb away from the side of the hand; Boyes procedure.

thumb adduction: pulling the thumb to side of index finger; Boyes, Bunnell, Edgarton-Grand, and Royle-Thompson procedures.

wrist extension: Boyes procedure, using pronator teres to the extensor carpi radialis brevis muscle.

Tenosynovectomy

Tenosynovectomy refers to the excision of thickened tendon sheath and other tissue surrounding a tendon, commonly seen in infection, chemical irritation, and rheumatoid arthritis (synovectomy). It also refers to the following two procedures in hand surgery.

abductor pollicis longus release: a release of the fibrous canal surrounding the abductor pollicis longus at the wrist for symptoms of de Quervain syndrome (pain on abduction of the thumb). Also called **de Quervain release.**

trigger finger release: a release of fibrous covering of tendon (pulley) at the base of the finger to prevent a tendon with nodular changes from snapping with motion of the finger. Also called **snapping tendon release.**

Other Tendon Procedures

boutonnière reconstruction: a classic extensor tendon reconstruction for boutonnière deformity, designed to restore active extension of the proximal interphalangeal (PIP) joint and to prevent its flexion posturing. This procedure is fraught with difficulty, and prognosis is guarded; Littler, Matev, Fowler procedures.

Hunter rod (active tendon implant):   a silicone rubber tendon replacement that can function as a permanent tendon. This implant has a proximal loop that can be sewn into forearm motor muscles.

Kortzeborn procedure: this is a lengthening of the extensor tendons of the thumb and formation of a fascial attachment of the thumb to the ulnar side of the hand to relieve "ape hand" deformity.

passive tendon implant: a silicone-rubber tendon spacer or rod that is used to form a new synovium-filled channel. It is removed during a second-stage procedure, and a tendon graft that is threaded through. Useful as a two-stage procedure when the tendon bed is extremely scarred and a direct tendon graft is impossible.

swan-neck revision: surgery designed to eliminate a swan-neck deformity in the fingers by revision of tendons; **Swanson revision, Littler modified tendon revision.**

Other Hand and Wrist Procedures

capsular release (capsulectomy): an incision of a joint capsule done to regain lost motion caused by contractures.

capsulodesis: in hand surgery, the capsule, which may include the dorsal or volar plate, may be tightened to help hold an affected joint in a position that can no longer be held voluntarily. This is done often for nerve injuries and is commonly called the **Zancolli** procedure (for claw-hand deformity); **volar capsular reefing, Blatt dorsal capsulodesis.**

carpal tunnel release: a division of the strong ligamentous band (transverse carpal ligament) that covers the median nerve and flexor tendons of the finger and thumb. This is usually done to relieve pressure on the median nerve that may result from arthritis, trauma, or unknown causes. A *tenosynovectomy,* if necessary, may be done through the same incision.

carpectomy: the removal of the proximal row of carpal bones, usually indicated in some forms of arthritis or severe spastic contractures.

dermodesis: the removal of a segment of skin and then closure of the skin margins to shorten skin and restrict motion of a joint. It is frequently done in conjunction with a *Zancolli* capsulodesis for ulnar clawhand.

Dupuytren contracture release: named after a French surgeon, this surgical procedure is the excision of the contracted fibrotic bands of the palmar fascia. However, the skin is often adherent and recurrent deformity is a problem. Specific techniques for resection of these bands are:

Luck procedure: percutaneous transection of fibrotic bands without removal of tissue.

McCash procedure: transverse skin incision with transection of bands and then passive stretch dressing applied, leaving the wounds open.

ganglionectomy: the excision of a ganglion, which usually occurs on the dorsum of the wrist or the base of the fingers.

K-wire fixation: in a Kirschner wire (K-wire) fixation, small threaded or nonthreaded wires are used to transfix fractures or to produce traction with the use of an external appliance.

mallet finger revision: designed to regain active extension of the distal interphalangeal joints of the finger.

Fowler release: technique used at the proximal interphalangeal joint for a mallet finger.

palmar fasciectomy, fasciotomy: the release, with or without resection of tissues, of shortened, thickened, and contracted fasciae in the palm or finger in flexion deformities resulting from Dupuytren contracture.

phalangectomy: the excision of a part or all of a phalanx because of trauma or arthritis. Rarely performed in the hand, more commonly done in the foot.

pollicization: any operation replacing a congenitally or traumatically missing thumb by reconstruction of the index, long, ring, or little finger such that it acts or functions as a thumb; **Buck-Gramko, Riordan, Littler, Gillies,** and **Verdan procedures.**

ray amputation: a procedure to remove a metacarpal and all phalangeal segments of a finger distal to that metacarpal.

replantation: a microsurgical procedure that requires the reattachment of nerves, veins, and arteries to attempt restoration of function to a freshly severed part such as a finger.

revision polydactyly: polydactyly usually affects the thumb and little finger. Revision requires reattachment of specific tendons or ligaments; **Marks and Bayne.**

synovectomy: removal of synovium in joints. The procedure is done frequently for rheumatoid arthritis.

wafer procedure: for ulnar plus wrist; resection of the distal 2 mm to 3 mm of the ulnar head, leaving the styloid intact.

Approaches

Wrist

dorsal a.: on the back side of the wrist, this approach is used for tendon transfers, fusions, and ganglionectomies.

Henry approach: for volar forearm.

volar a.: approach from the palmar aspect of the wrist, used for carpal tunnel releases, tendon explorations, and some bony procedures.

medial a.: an approach to the ulnar side of the wrist used for some tendon transfers and for the Darrach procedure; **Smith-Petersen.**

lateral a.: used on the radial side of the wrist for tendon transfers, radial styloidectomy, and visualization of the navicular bone.

Hand

Surgical approaches are too numerous and complicated to describe here. Refer to Edmonson AS and Crenshaw AH, eds: *Campbell's operative orthopaedics,* ed 9, vol 1, St Louis, 1996, Mosby.

Chapter 11

The Foot and Ankle

The human foot is a marvelous anatomic structure that provides a stable base to support large amounts of weight and shift in any direction while structural support is still maintained. The bones of the foot are so arranged as to allow balance of full body weight and the ability to walk on varying types of terrain. The average person will walk an estimated 20,000 to 46,000 miles in a lifetime and, for that reason, will at some time seek the expertise of a foot and ankle specialist in orthopaedic surgery or a podiatrist for foot-related problems.

The **orthopaedic surgeon** treats many major problems related to the feet—repair of congenital deformities (clubfeet), tendon lengthenings, fusions, and other complicated surgical procedures necessary for foot and ankle correction. Problems of the feet are so numerous that treatment and care has become a subspecialty of orthopaedics. The Foot and Ankle Society of the AAOS has been directly responsible for establishing a subspecialty devoted to injuries, diseases, and surgery of the foot and ankle. This subspecialization is now a part of many residency training programs.

The **podiatrist,** a doctor of podiatric medicine, is a specialist who may be board certified in foot and ankle surgery or primary care podiatric medicine. His or her practice is devoted to the diagnosis and treatment of diseases and disorders in the human foot, offering instructions to patients in proper shoe fit and foot care. This may involve conservative management, surgery, biomechanics (prosthetic/orthotic corrections), or treatment of patients with systemic diseases (diabetes) that affect the foot.

The **pedorthist,** a board-certified specialist in special footwear modifications and orthoses, provides services such as footwear modifications and filling prescriptions for special lines of shoes, customized inserts, and numerous foot support orthotics in the treatment of a variety of conditions.

In larger institutions, the orthopaedist may work in association with a *podiatrist* and *pedorthist* in the care of patients with ankle- and foot-related problems. The current trend is toward a team approach with advantages being that all aspects of patient care can be addressed in one setting. This team includes the orthopaedist, podiatrist, pedorthist, orthotist, and physical therapist. These specialists work independently but may also make up the orthopaedic foot and ankle service team. For that reason, we have included many terms specific to podiatry along with the generally interchangeable terms of anatomy, diseases, and surgery of the foot and ankle.

ANATOMY

The human foot is composed of 26 bones and is divided into three functional units: the hindfoot (talus and calcaneus); midfoot (cuneiforms, cuboid, and navicular); and forefoot (metatarsals and phalanges). The calcaneus, talus, navicular, and cuboid joints permit most of the motion in turning the ankle inward (inversion) or outward (eversion).

The bones of the midfoot create longitudinal arches that allow for smooth distribution of weight and compensate for uneven terrain throughout the supporting structure. As weight is systematically shifted from the heel to the ball of the foot, forces increase to as much as two to four times the body weight. The tarsals, metatarsals, and ligaments form a springy arch that gives supporting strength, aided by the dynamic balance of coordinated muscular counterforces.

On weight bearing, force is transmitted across the heel, the lateral border of the foot, and the ball of the foot. The great toe joint supports the body's weight in the thrust of push-off, and the heel absorbs the impact of heel strike. All work together in supporting various gait patterns and weights and adjusting to different terrain, making the foot fascinating to study. Figs. 11–1 to 11–4 will assist in understanding these structures. Injuries around the ankle joint receive the most attention and are discussed in Chapter 1.

Bones of the Ankle and Foot

accessory navicular (os tibiale externum): an "extra" bone on the medial side of the navicula, actually a tertiary center of ossification. On motion, it may be a source of pain between the small ossicle and main navicular bone.

calcaneus: the heel bone; largest of the bones of the foot, joins with the talus and cuboid. The combining form is *calcaneo,* for example, calcaneotalus ligament, calcaneofibular or fibulocalcaneal ligament.

cuboid: cube-shaped bone on the lateral side of the foot, just anterior to the calcaneus and articulating with the base of the fourth and fifth metatarsals.

cuneiforms: three wedge-shaped bones lying just proximal to the first three metatarsals and articulating with the navicular bone. These are called the first, second, and third cuneiforms or medial, lateral, and middle cuneiforms.

forefoot: portion of foot containing metatarsals, phalanges, and sesamoids.

Phalanges:
3. Distal
2. Middle
1. Proximal

Metatarsals

Cuneiforms

Navicular

Talus

Cuboid

Calcaneus

FIG 11–1.
Bones of right foot viewed from above. Tarsal bones consist of cuneiforms, navicular, talus, cuboid, and calcaneus. (From Anthony C, Kolthoff N: *Textbook of anatomy and physiology,* ed 9, St Louis, 1975, The CV Mosby Co.)

FLEXOR DIGITORUM
LONGUS TENDONS

FLEXOR DIGITORUM
BREVIS TENDONS

ADDUCTOR HALLUCIS
MUSCLE (TRANSVERSE
HEAD)

FLEXOR HALLUCIS
LONGUS TENDON

LATERAL PLANTAR
NERVE (DEEP BRANCH)

DORSALIS PEDIS
ARTERY

PLANTAR ARCH

ABDUCTOR HALLUCIS
MUSCLE

ADDUCTOR HALLUCIS
MUSCLE (OBLIQUE HEAD)

FLEXOR HALLUCIS
BREVIS MUSCLE

PERONEUS LONGUS
TENDON

MEDIAL PLANTAR
ARTERY

FLEXOR DIGITORUM
LONGUS TENDON

FLEXOR DIGITORUM
ACCESSORIUS MUSCLE

MEDIAL PLANTAR
NERVE

LATERAL PLANTAR
NERVE

LATERAL PLANTAR
ARTERY

ABDUCTOR DIGITI
MINIMI MUSCLE

ABDUCTOR HALLUCIS
MUSCLE

FLEXOR DIGITORUM
BREVIS MUSCLE

CALCANEAL BRANCH

F. PRICE.

FIG 11–2.
The arteries and nerves of the plantar surface of
the foot (With permission from Hamilton WJ: *Textbook of human anatomy,* ed 2, 1976, Macmillan
Press, Ltd.)

FIG 11–3.
Muscles of sole. **A,** First layer. **B,** Second layer. **C,** Third and fourth layers. (With permission from Hamilton WJ: *Textbook of human anatomy,* ed 2, 1976, Macmillan Press, Ltd.)   *(Continued)*

hallux (*pl.* halluces):   the great toe.

hindfoot: calcaneal (heel bone) and talar (ankle bone) portion of the foot; **rear foot.**

malleolus: the prominence of bone on either side of the ankle. The medial and lateral malleoli

come from the tibia and fibula, respectively. The posterior malleolus is deep to the Achilles tendon and is a part of the tibia.

metatarsals: the five long bones of the foot between the tarsals and the phalanges.

FIRST DORSAL
INTEROSSEUS

TRANSVERSE HEAD
OF ADDUCTOR
HALLUCIS

SECOND PLANTAR
INTEROSSEUS

OBLIQUE HEAD
OF ADDUCTOR
HALLUCIS

FLEXOR HALLUCIS
BREVIS

MEDIAL CUNEIFORM
BONE

NAVICULAR BONE

PERONEUS LONGUS

HEAD OF TALUS

TIBIALIS POSTERIOR

TALUS

LONG PLANTAR
LIGAMENT

C

FIG 11–3, cont'd.

midfoot: portion of foot containing the navicula, three cuneiforms, and cuboid.

midtarsal joint: this joint comprises the talo-navicular and calcaneocuboid articulations and permits adduction-abduction and inversion-eversion motions of the forefoot.

navicular: tarsal bone on medial side of foot that articulates proximally with head of talus and distally with three cuneiforms. Formerly called the **scaphoid.**

os: bone; also used in conjunction with a whole bone such as the calcis (calcaneus). However, os usually refers to small ossicles (small bones) or anatomic variants:

os intercuneiforme: between the medial and intermediate cuneiform.

os intermetatarseum: between the proximal fourth and fifth metatarsal.

os peroneum: in the peroneal tendon at the proximal cuboid.

os sustentaculum: the medial junction between the talus and calcaneus.

os talocalcaneus: the large accessory bone bridging the lateral talus and calcaneus.

ossa tarsi: the seven proximal bones of the foot connecting the tibia and fibula to the five metatarsals. The combining form *tarso* is used often, for example, tarsometatarsal joints and ligaments; **tarsus, bony tarsus, tarsus osseus.**

os tibiale externum: medial navicular of foot; **accessory navicular.**

os trigonum: posterior to talus; can be easily confused with a fracture of the posterior lateral tubercle of the talus; **Bardeleben bone.**

os vesalianum: directly proximal to the fifth metatarsal.

phalanx: the toe; more specifically, the two distal bones of the great toe and three distal bones of the four small toes. The fifth toe is sometimes fused and has two phalanges only.

sesamoid: two seed-shaped bones in the flexor hallucis brevis tendon located beneath the first metatarsal head, helping to plantarflex the great toe.

subtalar joint: the main shock absorber for the foot; this joint comprises the talocalcaneus articulation and permits triplane movement of the hindfoot.

sustenaculum tali: a process of the medial calcaneus that supports the talus.

FIG 11–4.
A, Retinacular and synovial sheaths of ankle region, medial view. **B,** Retinacular and synovial sheaths of ankle region, lateral view. (With permission from Hamilton WJ: *Textbook of human anatomy,* ed 2, 1976, Macmillan Press, Ltd.)

talocalcaneal bar: denotes a bony or fibrocartilaginous bridge in a place where one is not usually present.

talus: large bone beneath tibia that helps make up one third of the ankle joint, permitting the foot to go up or down. The talocalcaneal (subtalar joint) below the ankle joint allows the heel to turn in and out. The talonavicular ligaments (spring ligaments) originate from the talus; **astragalus.**

Muscles, Tendons, Ligaments

abductor hallucis: short muscle on medial side that pulls the great toe away from other toes and supports medial longitudinal arch.

Achilles tendon (heel cord):   the long tendon of the calf composed of the gastrocnemius, soleus, and plantaris muscles and inserting into the calcaneus; **tendocalcaneus.**

adductor hallucis: short muscle that attaches to base of great toe, pulls it toward the second toe, and prevents splaying of metatarsal bones.

anterior tibial tendon (tibialis anterior):   long tendon of anterior leg inserting into the medial cuneiform and first metatarsal; helps to dorsiflex the foot.

extensor digitorum longus and brevis: long tendon from limb and short tendon from foot that pull the lesser toes up in dorsiflexion (extension) and stabilize the lesser metatarsophalangeal joints. There is no brevis tendon to the fifth toe.

extensor hallucis longus and brevis: long tendon from limb and short tendon from foot that pull the great toe up in dorsiflexion (extension) and stabilize the first metatarsophalangeal joint.

flexor digitorum longus and brevis: long tendinous insertion from the tibia and short muscle from the foot that insert into the distal and middle phalanges and plantarflex the toes and MP joints.

flexor hallucis longus and brevis: long tendons from fibula and short muscle (flexor digitorum longus) from foot to great toe that acts as flexor of great toe in walking; supports medial longitudinal arch of foot and is important in equilibrium.

interossei muscles: group of small muscles between the metatarsals that extends into the extensor hoods and flexors at the metatarsophalangeal (MTP) joints.

intrinsic and extrinsic muscles: similar to the hand, the intrinsic muscles arise from the bones of the foot and the extrinsic muscles from the bones of the leg. The intrinsic muscles are:

- abductor hallucis
- abductor digiti minimi
- adductor hallucis
- dorsal and plantar interosseous
- extensor digitorum brevis
- flexor digitorum brevis
- flexor digiti minimi
- lumbricals
- quadratus plantae

peroneal muscles (peroneus longus, brevis, and tertius):   the tendons arising from these muscles travel posterior to the lateral malleolus and insert into the dorsolateral and plantar aspects of the foot. After crossing the plantar aspect of the foot, the longus inserts into the base of the first metatarsal, the brevis inserts into the base of the fifth metatarsal, and tertius into the dorsum of the foot about the cuboid.

posterior tibial tendon (tibialis posterior):   long tendon from posterior leg passing along medial side of the foot, inserting diffusely into the plantar aspect of the midfoot.

quadratus plantae: muscle of the plantar arch associated with the flexor digitorum longus.

Ligaments

Ligaments are named for specific bony attachments including the following:

collateral l.:   of the phalangeal and metatarsophalangeal joints.

deep transverse metatarsal l.

dorsal and plantar cuneocuboid l.

dorsal and plantar cuneonavicular l.

dorsal and plantar intercuneiform l.

dorsal and plantar metatarsal l.

dorsal and plantar tarsometatarsal l.

talocalcaneal l.

talonavicular l.

bifurcated ligament: in the foot, this ligament arises from the upper anterior calcaneus and attaches to both the cuboid and navicula.

deltoid ligament: triangular ligament on the medial side of the ankle, running from the tibia to talus and calcaneus.

lateral collateral ligaments: three ligaments that give stability to the lateral aspect of the ankle joint; **anterior talofibular ligament, calcaneofibular ligament, and the posterior talofibular ligament.**

Lisfranc l.:   a ligament passing between the medial cuneiform bone and second metatarsal bone.

long plantar l.:   bridges the more proximal plantar aspect of the calcaneus to the cuboid, covering peroneal tendons.

short plantar l.:   shorter of two plantar ligaments bridging the calcaneus and cuboid.

spring l.:   very strong and key ligament of the arch; **plantar calcaneonavicular ligament.**

The Nail

eponychium (cuticle):   the epidermal layer covering the nail root.

hyponychium: the thickened epidermis underneath the free distal edge of the nail plate.

lunula: half-moon-shaped (lighter) area at the proximal base of the nail next to the root.

nail matrix: the proximal portion of nail bed from which growth chiefly proceeds; also, the tissue upon which the deep aspect of the nail rests; **matrix unguis, nail bed.**

nail plate (*unguis*):   hard portion of epidermis on dorsal side of hallux and phalanges from which the nails grow.

Miscellaneous Foot Terms

ankle mortise: a rectangular cavity formed by the tibia and fibula; a joint space to receive the talus.

fat pad: thick fibrous collection of fat on the plantar surface of the foot.

Feiss line: the line that travels from the medial malleolus to plantar aspect of the first metatarsophalangeal joint.

Haglund process: posterosuperior tuberosity of the calcaneus; **bursal projection.**

Meyer line: in a normal foot, a line that passes through the big toe to midpoint of heel.

plantar fascia: dense fascia of the plantar aspect of foot arising from calcaneus and inserting into base of proximal phalanges; **plantar aponeurosis.**

ray: complex of the metatarsals and phalanges that, on anteroposterior radiographs, appear as five rays.

sinus tarsi: small channel between the mid–anterior lateral calcaneus and talus; **tarsal sinus.**

web space: web of skin between and at the base of each toe.

Arteries, Veins, Nerves

calcaneal branch a. and n.:   supplies the heel (os calcis, calcaneus).

digital artery and nerves: terminal arteries and nerves that travel together on the sides of the toes.

dorsalis pedis a.:   branch from the anterior tibial artery, going into the dorsum of the foot.

malleolar a.:   anterior, medial, and lateral branches supply the medial and lateral malleolus.

plantar a. (deep branch):   supplies the plantar surface of the foot on medial and lateral side.

plantar arch: medial plantar artery that transverses the foot to anastomose with lateral plantar artery.

plantar nerve: terminal portion of posterior tibial nerve that divides into medial and lateral plantar nerves, giving off sensory branches to plantar side of foot and motor branches to intrinsic muscles of foot.

posterior tibial artery, nerve, and vein: travel through a fascial tunnel on the inner ankle (tarsal tunnel) and branch to supply the plantar aspect of the foot and toes.

DISEASES AND CONDITIONS OF THE FOOT AND ANKLE

The pathologic and neuromusculoskeletal changes that take place in the foot can be the result of multiple entities. For one, excessive weight, overuse, improper shoe fit, and similar causes can place stress and strain on the feet. Simple effects on the foot can relate to dermal abrasions, blisters, ulcers, fissures, bunions, corns, calluses, fungi, and other infections. The more severe problems involve peripheral vascular (ischemia) diseases, metabolic disorders (diabetes, gout), musculoskeletal changes (deformities), and trauma (fractures, dislocations). All of these may cause or contribute to disability and inability to function. Diseases and conditions of the foot are listed alphabetically for reference. Other diseases are listed in Chapter 2.

Achilles tendonitis: inflammation of Achilles tendon due to overstretching. The deeper sac becomes inflamed between the calcaneus and Achilles tendon.

ainhum: condition where there is spontaneous lysis, usually of the fourth or fifth toe but sometimes other toes.

anonychia: absence of toenail(s).

athlete's foot (tinea pedis): fungal infection of skin on the plantar surface of the feet and between the toes and nails caused by one of the dermatophyte species (*Trichophyton* or *Epidermophyton*); disease consists of scaling, fissures, maceration, and eroded areas between the toes; **dermatomycosis pedis.**

blue foot syndrome: bluish discoloration of the feet most commonly caused by vascular disturbances.

bunion: localized enlargement at the first metatarsal head area either because of malposition of the first metatarsal or because of overgrowth of bone at the first metatarsal head. This deformity may or may not affect the position of the great toe. If the great toe is affected, then one of the following designations would be appropriate: hallux abductus with bunion, hallux adductus with bunion, hallux abductovalgus with bunion.

bunion (dorsal): overgrowth of bone (exostosis) on the dorsal surface of the first metatarsal head or a dorsal malposition of the first metatarsal.

bunionette: similar to the bunion deformity but affecting the fifth metatarsal, causing the metatarsal head to be prominent laterally; often referred to as a "tailor's bunion."

bursitis: inflammation of a fluid-filled sac that is normally present around a bony prominence to cushion it.

calcaneal spur syndrome: spur-shaped calcium deposits at attachment points of tendinous fibrous tissues in the midfoot and hindfoot region, with excrescence on lower surface of calcaneus; causes tenderness and pain and is exacerbated with weight bearing.

callosity: hard, thickened skin on the bottom of the foot like a clavus; **tyloma, keratoma, callus** (pl. **calluses**).

clavus: any corn or hyperkeratotic tissue involving a toe; a reaction of skin to intermittent chronic pressure, producing extra layers of hard skin; caused by restrictive foot wear or by abnormal position or motion of the toes.

clavus (soft):   soft skin thickening between the toes, usually between the fourth and fifth toes; **heloma molle, soft corn, clavus mollis.**

clawtoes: hyperextension of the metatarsophalangeal joints associated with PIP and DIP joints, producing a clawlike appearance; **claw toe deformity.**

clubfoot: foot deformity resulting in the appearance of a golf club. The components include forefoot adduction with medial displacement of the talus, ankle equinus, and heel varus. The result is that the foot turns in with the heel pulled medially.

coalition: a bridge between two bones; may be fibrous (syndesmosis), cartilage (synchondrosis), or bone (synostosis), for example, a calcaneonavicular bar that is a bridge between the calcaneus and navicular bones; **tarsal bars.**

congenital bars: bridging of bone from one tarsal bone to another, with the most common being calcaneonavicular bars.

congenital rocker-bottom flatfoot: condition present at birth; abnormal equinus position of talus with valgus position of the heel, resulting in a foot that looks like a rocker and has a prominence below the medial ankle; **congenital vertical talus, congenital convex pes valgus.**

curly toe: a supinated and medially deviated toe.

dactylitis: infarcts in the small bones of the foot due to sickle cell disease.

dorsiflexed metatarsal: a metatarsal that is malpositioned so that its head is higher than the adjacent metatarsal heads, resulting in limitation of motion of the involved metatarsophalangeal joint.

dropfoot: paralysis of the dorsiflexor muscles of the foot causing foot and toes to drag when walking; **footdrop.**

Dupuytren contracture: a contracture of the plantar fascia of the foot; also, a flexion deformity of the toe caused by involvement of the plantar fascia.

Egyptian foot: a foot with a short first ray.

equinus: abnormal position of flexion and used in combining form with other words to denote anatomic, location; ankle equinus, forefoot equinus, metatarsus equinus.

exostosis: bony growth protruding from the surface of bone.

flail foot: a foot with poor neuromuscular function and control.

flatfoot: a foot with depressed arches. This term covers a wide range of conditions. In most cases, a flatfoot is due to minor imbalances of the muscles that control the arch and is referred to as **flexible flatfoot.** If the muscle changes occur during adult life or if there is an injury, the term **acquired flatfoot** might be used. Many individuals with flatfeet go through life with no functional interferences.

foot cramps: an involuntary action involving a muscle-tendon reflex contraction, stretching the tendon, which sends nerve messages to spinal cord, which in turn stimulates the muscle even more, producing a painful cramp. This can be related to abnormal levels of minerals (calcium, potassium, magnesium), a decrease in blood supply to the muscle, a pinched nerve, holding the foot in pronation for a length of time, or a problem with the muscle itself.

forefoot equinus: describes a high-arched foot characterized by excessive plantar flexion of forefoot in relation to hindfoot.

forefoot valgus: describes pronated position of forefoot with respect to the hindfoot.

forefoot varus: describes supinated position of forefoot with respect to hindfoot.

ganglion: soft-tissue mass filled with fluid usually coming from a joint or a tendon sheath in mid- or hindfoot.

gastrocnemius equinus: tightness of the gastrocnemius muscle that restricts ankle plantar flexion when the knee is fully extended.

gout: deposits of uric acid crystals usually in the great toe producing ankle pain and inflammation. Aspiration of joint fluid can help differentiate gout from an inflammatory condition due to bacteria. There is recurrent pain and tophi lumps.

Greek foot: a foot with a long first ray.

Haglund deformity: prominent posterosuperior aspect of the calcaneus; **retrocalcaneal exostosis** or a "pump bump."

Haglund syndrome: pain on the superior and lateral side of the heel usually associated with a callus of the skin, bony prominence, and bursitis. A variety of conditions and shoe types can contribute to this condition; **retrocalcaneal exostosis.**

hallux abductus: great toe pointing toward second toe (transverse plane deformity).

hallux adductus: great toe pointing toward midline of body (transverse plane deformity).

hallux dolorosa: flatfoot condition resulting in pain of the great toe.

hallux elevatus: fixed dorsiflexed position of entire first ray.

hallux extensus: fixed dorsiflexed position of the great toe.

hallux flexus: fixed flexion position of great toe.

hallux malleus: hammer toe deformity of the great toe; cock-up deformity of the distal interphalangeal joint.

hallux rigidus: painful, stiff metatarsophalangeal joint with limitation of motion and pain on dorsiflexion; caused by arthritic changes.

hallux valgus: great toe pointing toward second toe, often rotated in frontal plane so that the nail plate is facing away from second toe.

hallux valgus interphalanges: a hallux valgus deformity caused by deformity of the phalanx.

hallux varus: great toe pointing toward midline of body, often rotated in frontal plane so that the nail plate is facing second toe.

hammer toes: descriptive of a variety of deformities of the second to fifth toes; increased flexion of the distal toe, causing prominence of the bones of the dorsal aspect of the proximal interphalangeal joint. Term more properly reserved for hyperextension of MP joint with fixed flexion of the PIP only.

hard corn: a particularly hard, thickened area of skin over the dorsum of the toe; **heloma durum, clavus durum, hard clavus.**

heel spur: an overgrowth of bone at the plantar aspect of the calcaneus.

hindfoot equinus: characterized by the increase of calcaneal inclination angle (high-arched foot) in relation to the forefoot.

ingrown nail: condition of the nail growing into the skin distally; **unguis incarnatus, onychocryptosis.**

intractable plantar keratosis: well-defined callous tissue with a central core located beneath a metatarsal head and usually the result of abnormal pressure from the metatarsal.

lobster foot: congenital cleft between metatarsal producing a lobster claw appearance.

macrodactyly: enlargement of a toe or toes.

Madura foot: a severe fungal infection of the foot.

mallet toes: flexion of the distal joint of the second to fifth toes, such that the toenails are pointing into the ground when walking.

malum deformans: a deep foot ulcer commonly associated with diabetes mellitus.

metatarsal cuneiform exostosis: an overgrowth of bone usually involving the dorsal surface of the first metatarsal base and first cuneiform.

metatarsalgia: pain in the plantar aspect of the metatarsal area caused by a variety of disorders.

metatarsus abductus: turning out of the forefoot (metatarsals); **m. valgus.**

metatarsus adductocavus: forefoot turned inward in association with a high arch, usually seen in clubfoot deformity that includes heel varus (talipes equinovarus).

metatarsus adductus: turning in of the forefoot (metatarsals); **m. varus.**

metatarsus atavicus: abnormal shortness of the first metatarsal bone.

metatarsus equinus: see equinus.

metatarsus latus: broad foot; widened forefoot.

metatarsus primus varus: refers to wide splaying between first and second metatarsals and can be the cause of a bunion deformity.

Morton foot: short, hypermobile first metatarsal; **Morton syndrome.**

Morton neuroma: thickening of the plantar nerve just beyond the metatarsal head in the web spaces; usually found between the third and fourth toes, followed by the second and third toes.

myletoma: a fungal infection of the foot.

non–plantar grade foot: failure of part of the sole of the foot to contact the supporting surface.

onychauxis: thickening, fragmentation, and discoloration of a nail, most frequently the great toenail.

onychocryptosis: condition of nail growing into the skin distally; **ingrown nail, unguis incarnatus.**

onychomycosis: fungal infection of the nail plate.

osteochondrosis: disruption of the blood supply to a growth center of a bone. These have been given eponyms after the persons who first reported them:

Köhler disease: osteochondrosis of the navicular bone.

Freiberg infraction: osteochondrosis of the metatarsal head.

Sever disease: osteochondrosis of the calcaneus apophysis.

overlapping toe: a toe that overlaps an adjacent toe; commonly affecting the second toe, which overlaps the great toe.

pachyonychia: thickening of toenails, commonly caused by a fungus or trauma; **onychauxis.**

paronychia: an inflammation surrounding the nail plate.

peroneal spastic flatfoot: overall descriptive term applies to many flatfeet, including congenital bony bars (bridges).

Persian slipper foot: the clinical appearance of the paralytic form of vertical talus where the lateral column of the foot has an abducted plantar contour and the medial longitudinal column is elongated and convex. The lateral toes are elevated and clawed, which is the basis for the term.

pes: generally speaking, the term *pes* (foot) is used as a prefix to denote an acquired affection of the foot, for example, pes planus, better known as *flatfoot.* The terms *pes* and *talipes* are generally interchangeable.

pes cavus: high arches in midfoot with pain along the medial longitudinal arch (instep) after prolonged walking or standing.

pes planus: lowering of the longitudinal arch; flatfoot. There are two basic categories:

flexible pes planus: flatfoot with general laxity in which the foot appears normal when not bearing weight but flattens with weightbearing.

rigid pes planus: nonflexible flatfoot that is present whether bearing weight or not.

pigeon toe: term that is often applied to any intoeing gait.

plantar flexed metatarsal: a metatarsal that is malpositioned so that its head is lower than the adjacent metatarsal heads, resulting in abnormal pressure, which may produce a plantar callus.

plantar wart: a virus affecting the plantar surface of the foot; **verruca vulgaris.**

podagra: although literally means pain in the foot, this term is usually used for a painful attack of gout in the great toe.

polydactyly: congenital deformity, excess number of toes.

polysyndactyly: condition in which more than two toes are joined together.

prehallux (os tibiale externum): accessory navicular.

pronation: complex motion of the foot that produces *flattening* of the arch. This motion is normal during gait; however, excessive pronation can lead to pathologic changes of the foot.

pump bumps: a thickening of skin forming a callus in the back of the heel above the calcaneus as a result of tight-fitting shoes.

rocker-bottom foot: deformity of the foot such that the arch is disrupted and resembles a chair rocker bottom. This may be a complication of clubfoot treatment or myelomeningocele.

skew foot: skewed appearance caused by a series of deformities that include the base of the first metatarsal lying medial on the cuneiform, resulting in forefoot varus and concavity at the arch, pronation with inward rotation of the talar head and lateral displacement of the navicula and medial cuneiform, and heel valgus. Condition is difficult to treat by nonsurgical methods; **z-foot.**

splay foot: abnormally wide forefoot caused by abnormally wide metatarsal angles.

squatters: a dorsal articular facet on the talar neck in people who squat a lot of the time or are in jumping sports.

stiff ray: immobility of all joints of any toe or toes.

subungual exostosis: an extopic bone spur under a nail.

supination: complex motion of the foot that produces an *increase* in the arch. This motion is normal during gait; however, excessive supination can lead to pathologic changes of the foot.

syndactyly: congenital anomaly of the foot (or hand) marked by a complete webbing attachment between the toes or two or more toes; may contain bone or merely soft tissue.

tailor's bunion: painful prominence on lateral side of fifth metatarsal head. Term derived from historical cross-legged sitting behavior of tailors.

talipes: generally speaking, the term *talipes,* meaning ankle and foot, is used as a prefix to denote an affection of the foot, for example, talipes equinovarus (clubfoot).

talipes calcaneocavus: high-arched foot with fixed dorsiflexion; **pes c.**

talipes calcaneus: abnormally dorsiflexed hindfoot, with increased dorsiflexion of the calcaneus; **cavus foot, pes c.**

talipes calcanovalgus: abnormally dorsiflexed hindfoot with turning out of the heel; **pes c.**

talipes calcanovarus: abnormally dorsiflexed hindfoot with turning in of the heel; **pes c.**

talipes cavovalgus: high arch and turning out of the heel; **pes c.**

talipes cavovarus: high arch associated with turning in of the foot; **pes c.**

talipes equinovalgus: plantar flexion and turning out of the calcaneus; **pes e.**

talipes equinovarus: turning of the heel inward with increased plantar flexion. More precisely, a clubfoot often having the components of talipes equinovarus with metatarsus adductus. This condition can result from disease, causing paralysis, or from unknown causes; **clubfoot, pes e.**

talipes planovalgus: depression of the longitudinal arch associated with heel valgus; **pes planovalgus.**

talipes planus: depression of the longitudinal arch: no specified heel valgus is implied by this term; **pes planus, flatfoot.** A *flexible pes planus* is flatfoot with general laxity but no other specific disease process.

vertical talus: a spectrum of conditions where the talus is oriented in a plantar flexed and medially directed position resulting in a flatfoot with heel valgus. In the more severe congenital form, it is usually associated with the neurological disorder **congenital convex pes valgus.**

SURGERY

Procedures related to the foot and ankle are listed by abnormality. There are many types of procedures available for a single condition but not all are listed here; for example, of more than 50 operations for bunions, only a few are described. For easy reference, definitions of specific surgical terms are presented alphabetically.

Bunions

Akin
Austin
Bunionectomy
Chevron osteotomy
Closing abductory wedge osteotomy (CAWO)
Crescentic osteotomy
DuVries
Hauser
Juvara
Keller
Keller with prosthesis
Lapidus
Ludloff
Mann
Mayo
McBride
McKeever
Mitchell
Opening abductory wedge osteotomy (OAWO)
Reverdin-Green
Silver
Stone
Wilson

Clubfeet (Talipes Equinovarus)

Barr
Barr and Record
Brockman
Dunn-Brittain
Dunn-Brittain triple anthrodesis
Dwyer

Garceau
Garceau-Brahms
Gelman
Heyman
Lloyd-Roberts
McCauley
Ober
Phelps
Siffert-Foster-Nachamic
Tohen
Turco

Pes Planus (Flatfeet and Related Disorders)

Anderson-Fowler
Batchelor-Brown
Coleman
Durham
Evans
Grice
Grice-Green
Hammon
Hark
Harris-Beath
Herndon-Heyman
Hoke
Ingram
Kidner
Lowman
Miller
Osmond-Clarke
Pridie-Koutsogiannis
Subtalar arthroereisis
Vulpius-Compere
White
Young

Ankle Arthrodeses

Blair
Campbell
Charnley
Chuinard-Peterson
Horwitz-Adams

Lambrinudi
Sliding

Achilles Tendon Lengthenings

Baker
Bosworth
Bugg and Boyd
Hauser
Lindholm
Lynn
Ma-Griffith
Strayer
TAL
Vulpius-Compere
White slide
Z-plasty

Metatarsus Adductus (M. Varus)

Berman-Gartland
Fowler
Heyman-Herndon-Strong
Kendrick
Lange
Peabody

Ingrown Nails (Onychocryptosis)

Avulsion of nail plate
Bartlett
Bose
Cotting
Fowler
Frost
Heifetz
Jansen
Matricectomy
Phenolization
Quenu
Rose
Steindler
Suppan
Watson-Cheyne

Winograd
Zadic

Cavus Deformity

Cole
Gould
Hoke-Kite
Jahss
Samilson

Toe Abnormalities

Brahms
Clayton
Cone arthrodesis
Cracchiolo
Digital prosthesis
Farmer
Hibbs
Hoffman
Intermediate phalangectomy
Johnson-Spiegl
Jones
Kates-Kessel-Kay
Kessel and Bonney
Lipscomb
Larmon
Osteotripsy
Partial ostectomy
Syndactylization
V-Y plasty
Z-plasty

Small Toe Deformities

Cylindrical osteotomy
Dickson-Diveley
DIP fusion
Dorsal-V osteotomy
Dorsal Wedge osteotomy
DuVries plantar condylectomy
Giannestras
Girdlestone-Taylor

Kiehn-Earle-DesPrez
McElvenny
Metatarsal wedge resection with prosthesis
PIP fusion
Ruiz-Moro

Footdrop

Campbell
Gill

Forefoot Equinus (High-Arched Foot)

Elmslie-Cholmely
Japas
Steindler

Fractures

Essex-Lopresti
Gallis
McReynolds
Thomas
Warner-Farber

Muscle, Tendon, and Ligament Injuries

DuVries
Ellis Jones
Evans
Jones
Staples-Black-Brostrom

Paralytic and Spastic Conditions

Freid-Green
Hoffer
Kaufer
Liebolt
Majestro-Ruda-Frost

Miscellaneous

Lisfranc amputation
Pierrot-Murphy

Descriptions of Procedures

Akin: for bunion deformity or deformed great toe; an osteotomy of the proximal phalanx of the great toe.

Anderson p.:   for lateral ankle instability, use of plantaris tendon for lateral ligament reconstruction.

Anderson and Fowler p.:   for pes planus; an opening wedge osteotomy of the distal lateral calcaneus with tibial bone graft, closing wedge osteotomy of the medial cuneiform, and capsulotomy of the talonavicular joint.

arthroereisis: a general term for surgery of a joint. In the foot, it is a joint stabilization by implant (e.g., stabilization of subtalar joint in a pes planus deformity with expectation of removing the implant when the foot position has stabilized).

Austin: for bunion deformity; an osteotomy in the form of a chevron made in the distal aspect of the first metatarsal; **chevron procedure.**

avulsion of nail plate: a nonpermanent removal of the nail plate, either partial or complete, without disrupting the matrix cells that produce the nail plate.

Baker: for Achilles tendon tightness; relaxation of proximal tendon with a rectangular sliding slot incision.

Baker and Hill p.:   for dynamic foot varus deformity due to cerebral palsy, transposition of posterior tibial tendon anterior to medial malleolus.

Banks p.:   for nonunion medial malleolus; resection of nonunion, addition of locally obtained tibial cancellous bone and screw fixation.

Barr p.:   for paralytic clubfoot; transfer of the posterior tibial tendon to the third cuneiform or metatarsal.

Barr-Record p.:   for clubfeet; subcutaneous plantar fasciotomy and tendon Achilles lengthening (TAL) done as separate procedures, with tibiotalar fusion.

Bartlett p.:   for ingrown toenail; excision of wedge of skin with no excision of nail.

Batchelor-Brown p.:   for flatfeet; fusion of the subtalar joint with a fibular bone graft.

Berman and Gartland p.:   for metatarsus adductus; dome-shaped osteotomy of all five proximal metatarsals.

Bircher, Weber p.:   for malunion ankle fracture with diastasis; osteotomy and corrective fibular lengthening with screw and plate fixation.

Bose p.:   for ingrown toenail; excision of wedge of skin without excision of nail.

Bosworth p.:   for repair of old rupture of Achilles tendon; fashioning direct tendon graft from median raphe (central portion of tendon).

Boyd amputation: an amputation at the ankle with tibial calcaneal fusion.

Brahms p.:   for mallet toe; transfer of flexor digitorum profundus to dorsum of proximal phalanx.

Bridle p.:   for foot paralysis, posterior tibialis tendon transfer through interosseous membrane to dorsum of foot, and dual anastomosis to anterior tibialis and anteriorly transposed peroneus longus.

Brockman p.:   for clubfoot; a soft tissue release of the medial capsule of the foot as well as a release of the posterior tibial tendon.

Bugg-Boyd p.:   for repair of old Achilles tendon rupture; use of fascia lata graft.

bunionectomy: a general class of many different operations that are designed to correct bunion deformity.

Campbell p.:   For dropfoot or talipes equinus of certain origins; creates a posterior bone block to prevent plantar flexion.

cheilectomy: removal of an exostosis usually on the dorsal surface of the distal first metatarsal.

chevron osteotomy: for bunion deformity; an osteotomy in the form of a chevron made in the distal first metatarsal.

Chopart amputation: of the forefoot through the talonavicular and calcaneocuboid joint.

Chrisman-Snook p.:   repair of lateral collateral ligament of ankle using peroneus brevis tendon. Also called modified **Elmslie procedure.**

Cincinnati incision: an incision to correct clubfoot.

Clayton p.:   for deformity of toes in rheumatoid arthritis; resection of proximal phalanx and entire metatarsal heads of all toes.

closing abductory wedge osteotomy (CAWO):   for bunion deformity; proximal metatarsal osteotomy with closure of wedge to bring first metatarsal closer to second metatarsal.

Cole p.:   for cavus foot deformity; an anterior tarsal wedge osteotomy with fusion.

Coleman p.:   for talipes valgus; soft tissue and tendon release associated with a subtalar fusion.

condylectomy: for painful callus; removal of a condyle from a metatarsal or phalanx.

cone arthrodesis: for fusion of the first metatarsophalangeal joint; the metatarsal head is shaped into a cone, and a cone wedge is cut into the proximal phalanx at a proper angle to accept the metatarsal head for fusion; **Wilson p., Johnson and Barington p.**

cotting: for ingrown nail; excision of a nail.

Cracchiolo p.:   for deformity of toes in rheumatoid arthritis; silastic implant arthroplasty for MP joints all toes.

crescentic osteotomy: dome-shaped osteotomy at the base of the first metatarsal to correct a bunion deformity.

cylindrical osteotomy: to shorten long bones; removal of a cylinder of bone.

Dias and Giegerich p.:   for triplane fraction of ankle; open reduction with screw fixation when required.

Dickson-Diveley p.:   for clawing of big toe; the distal interphalangeal joint is fused, and the extensor hallucis longus is transferred to the long flexor.

digital prosthesis: excision of interphalangeal joint with insertion of prosthetic device in that space.

Dillwyn-Evans p.:   for severe resistant clubfoot deformity, Achilles and posterior tibial tendon

Z-plasty, talonavicular joint capsulectomy, resection, and fusion calcaneocuboid joint.

DIP fusion: for mallet toes; removal of the distal interphalangeal joint and then fusion.

dorsal-V osteotomy: for plantar callosity; an osteotomy at the neck of a lesser metatarsal to allow the metatarsal to assume a slightly higher position.

dorsal wedge osteotomy: for plantar callosity; an osteotomy at the base of a metatarsal to allow the metatarsal to move to a higher position.

Drennan p.:   for ankle flexion weakness; posterior transfer of anterior tibial tendon.

Dunn-Brittain: for paralytic clubfeet; a method of triple arthrodesis excising most of the head of the talus.

Dunn-Brittain triple arthrodesis: removal of entire navicular bone.

Durham p.:   for flatfoot; closing wedge osteotomy-fusion of cuneiform-navicular joint.

DuVries plantar condylectomy: for plantar callosities; resection of plantar condyles from the lesser metatarsals.

DuVries p.:   for chronic instability of deltoid ligament of ankle; cross-shaped imbrication of deltoid ligament. Also, a modified McBride bunion procedure with vertical medial capsular imbrication and suturing of lateral capsule to second metatarsal head.

Dwyer p.:   lateral closing wedge osteotomy of the calcaneus; associated with soft-tissue release for clubfeet and other disorders.

Ellis Jones p.:   for subluxing peroneal tendon; reconstruction of retinaculum using portion of Achilles tendon.

Elmslie p.:   for lateral ankle instability; peroneal tendon used in ligament reconstruction.

Elmslie-Cholmely p.:   double wedge osteotomy for certain high-arched feet.

Essex-Lopresti p.:   for fractured calcaneus; use of a Steinmann pin or other metal pin to help achieve and hold fracture reduction.

Evans p.:   for lateral collateral ligament instability of ankle; use of peroneus brevis tendon.

Evans p.:   for severe flatfoot deformity; distal lateral opening wedge osteotomy of the calcaneus.

exostectomy: removal of any excess prominences of bone.

Farmer p.:   for hallux varus; soft-tissue repair with the use of a skin flap.

Fowler p.:   for metatarsus varus with severe cavus deformity; plantar fascia and muscle release associated with an opening wedge osteotomy of the first cuneiform. Also, for deformity of toes in rheumatoid arthritis; resection of proximal phalanx and varying portions of metatarsal heads of all toes. Also, for ingrown toenail; excision of entire nail.

Freid-Green p.:   for paralysis of posterior tibial muscle; transfer of the peroneus longus, flexor digitorum longus, flexor hallucis longus, or extensor hallucis longus to posterior tibial tendon.

Frost p.:   for ingrown nail; a skin flap is made over the lateral nail bed, with removal of the nail and bed followed by closure of flap.

Fulford p.:   for spastic valgus deformity of foot; peroneus brevis elongation.

Gallie p.:   for malunion calcaneus; subtalar arthrodesis using a tibial bone graft.

Garceau p.:   for clubfeet; anterior tibial tendon transfer.

Garceau-Brahms p.:   for paralytic clubfeet; transection of the motor branches of the plantar nerve.

Gelman p.:   for clubfeet; identical to the McCauley procedure, except that the inferior calcaneonavicular ligament is not incised.

Giannestras p.:   for plantar callosity; proximal shortening of metatarsal.

Gill p.:   for dropfoot; wedge of bone taken from the superoposterior calcaneus with insertion of that block into the posterior tibiotalar joint.

Girdlestone p.:   for curled toes deformity; transfer of the long flexors of the involved toe(s) to the extensor hood mechanism (top of toe).

Gould p.: for pes cavus due to tight plantar fascia; a double plantar fasciotomy through a lateral heel approach proximally and a distal medial approach.

Grice p.: for congenital talipes valgus; a soft-tissue medial and lateral foot release procedure.

Grice-Green p.: for talipes valgus; tibial bone graft to subtalar joint. Also, for paralysis of gatrocsoleus; transfer of peroneus longus, peroneus brevis, and posterior tibial tendon.

Hammon p.: first metatarsal osteotomy and bone graft for a dorsal bunion.

Hark p.: for congenital talipes valgus; multiple extensor and flexor Z-tendon lengthenings with bony repositioning.

Harris-Beath p.: for flatfoot; talonavicular and subtalar arthrodesis.

Hauser p.: (1) for bunion deformity; excision of the medial exostosis and transfer of the adductor tendon from the proximal phalanx to the distal metatarsal; (2) for tight heel cord; division of proximal posterior and distal medial two-thirds of the Achilles tendon; (3) for Achilles tendon tightness; partial incision at two levels with passive stretching and casting

Heifetz p.: for ingrown nail; excision of affected ingrown side of nail and nail bed.

hemiphalangectomy: for shortening or straightening of a toe; resection of a portion of the phalanx.

Herndon-Heyman p.: for congenital talipes valgus; medial and lateral foot release with tendon lengthening.

Heyman p.: for clubfeet; soft-tissue release for clubfoot, including deltoid ligament.

Hibbs p.: for clawtoes and cavus feet; plantar fascia release with transfer of the extensor digitorum longus to the third cuneiform.

Hiroshima p.: for spastic equinus and equino-

varus deformity; anterior transfer of long toe flexors.

Hoffer p.: for spastic inversion of foot; transfer of anterior tibial tendon to cuboid.

Hoffman-Clayton p.: resection of metatarsal head; resection of metatarsal heads and bases of proximal phalanges for cock-up deformities of toes as seen in rheumatoid arthritis.

Hoke p.: (1) triple arthrodesis done with reshaping of the head of the talus; (2) for flatfeet; navicular bone and two medial cuneiforms are fused.

Hoke-Kite p.: for calcaneocavovarus deformity; excision and fusion with some shortening of talonavicular joint and a posteriorly closing wedge fusion of the talocalcaneal joint.

Hueter-Mayo p.: for simple bunion deformity; resection of prominent portion of first metatarsal.

Ingram p.: for congenital talipes valgus; Z-plasty lengthening of peroneus brevis tendon, medial release, reduction of navicular bone, and anterior tibial tendon transfer.

Intermediate phalangectomy: for hammer toe deformity; excision of the middle phalanx.

Jahss p.: for cavus foot with clawtoes; excision of metatarsotarsal joint with dorsal wedge closed to reduce cavus and with adequate bone excision to relax plantar fascia.

Jansey p.: for ingrown toenail; excision wedge of skin without excision of nail.

Japas p.: for high-arched feet; a combination of plantar fascia release and dorsal wedge osteotomy of the tarsal bones.

Johnson and Spiegl p.: for hallux varus; fusion of interphalangeal joint great toe and transfer of extensor hallicus longus to lateral proximal phalanx.

Jones p.: for cock-up deformity of great toe and other problems; transfer of the extensor hallucis longus to the distal first metatarsal; currently done with a distal interphalangeal joint fusion.

Jones p.: an ankle repair of the fibular collateral ligament using the peroneus brevis muscle.

Joplin p.:   for splay foot deformity; transfer of fifth toe flexor to first metatarsal.

Juvara p.:   for a bunion deformity; an oblique osteotomy at the proximal portion of the metatarsal to correct an abnormal transverse and/or sagittal plane deformity.

Karlsson p.:   for lateral ankle ligament instability, reconstruction using original ligament.

Kashiwagi p.:   for malunion calcaneus fracture; lateral subtalar and calcaneocuboid joint fusion.

Kates-Kessel-Kay p.:   for deformity of toes in rheumatoid arthritis; resection of metatarsal head only.

Kaufer p.:   for spastic inversion of foot; transfer of posterior tibial tendon to peroneus brevis.

Keller p.:   for hallux rigidus or bunion; resection of the proximal phalanx of the great toe.

Kendrick p.:   for metatarsus adductus; soft-tissue release for all tarsal metatarsal joints.

Kessel-Bonney p. (Moberg p.):   for lack of great toe extension; a closing wedged osteotomy of proximal phalanx.

Kidner p.:   for an accessory navicular bone; removal of the accessory navicular bone with or without transfer of the posterior tibial tendon under the navicular bone.

Kiehn-Earle-DesPrez p.:   for plantar ulcer; closure of ulcer and transfer of extensor digitorum longus to distal metatarsal shaft.

Lambrinudi p.:   a triple arthrodesis done by resection of the head and inferior portion of the talus.

Lange p.:   for metatarsus varus; simple oblique osteotomy of the second, third, and fourth metatarsals; lateral closing wedge osteotomy of the first metatarsal at the base.

Lapidus p.:   for bunion correction; a closing wedge and fusion at the junction of the first metatarsal and cuneiform bone and adductor release.

Larmon p.:   for rheumatoid foot deformity; arthroplasty by resection of medial metatarsal head and proximal phalanx of great toe and resection of plantar part of metatarsal head of lesser toes.

Liebolt: for paralytic equinus foot; a two-stage procedure involving a Hoke triple arthrodesis followed by an ankle fusion.

Lindholm p.:   for repair of ruptured Achilles tendon; fashioning of fascial flaps from superior tendon.

Lipscomb p.:   for deformity of toes in rheumatoid arthritis; resection of proximal phalanx and plantar metatarsal head of all toes.

Lisfranc amputation: amputation through the tarsometatarsal joint.

Lloyd-Roberts p.:   for clubfoot deformity in early childhood; soft-tissue release.

Lowman p.:   for flatfeet; transfer of the anterior tibialis with navicular cuneiform fusion.

Ludloff p.:   for hallux valgus; oblique osteotomy of the first metatarsal.

Lynn p.:   for repair of Achilles tendon rupture; use of fanned out portion of plantaris tendon to cover direct repair.

Ma-Griffith p.:   for Achilles tendon rupture; percutaneous technique of suture repair.

Majestro-Ruda-Frost: for spastic posterior tibial tendon; intramuscular lengthening.

malleolar osteotomy: a procedure or approach that provides access to the lateral side of the ankle joint in fracture reductions or in excising abnormal bone or cartilage.

Mann p.:   a modified McBride bunion procedure with vertical medial capsular imbrication and suturing of lateral capsule to second metatarsal head.

matricectomy: for toenail deformity or chronic disease; excision of all or a part of the nail plate (matrix) to eliminate growth of the nail.

Mayer p.:   for deformity caused by poliomyelitis; transfer of peroneal tendon.

Mayo p.:   for bunion exostosis of first metatarsal head without significant angular deformity; excision exostosis.

McBride p.: excision of the medial exostosis, medial capsular reefing, sesamoidectomy, and transfer of the adductor hallucis tendon into the distal first metatarsal.

McCauley p.: very extensive medial release of multiple joint capsules, tendon sheaths, and abductor hallucis, and, if needed, posterior capsulotomy later.

McElvenny p.: (1) excision of a plantar nerve neuroma; (2) for hallux varus; lateral capsular reefing procedure associated with use of the extensor hallucis brevis tendon for repair.

McKeever p.: for hallux valgus or rigidus; fusion of the first metatarsophalangeal joint.

McReynolds p.: for fractured calcaneus; open reduction and fixation with staples using a medial approach.

Meisenbach p.: for callosity on plantar aspect of foot; dorsal displacement of metatarsal head(s).

metaphyseal head resection with prosthesis: removal of the metatarsal head to create an artificial joint with a silastic implant.

metaphyseal osteotomy: through the neck of the metatarsal head.

Miller p.: for severe flatfoot deformity; navicular-cuneiform metatarsal fusion for hallux varus with repositioning of stump of adductor hallucis and transfer of abductor hallucis to lateral proximal phalanx.

Mitchell p.: a distal metatarsal osteotomy for bunion deformity; breaking and shifting of metatarsal with excision of exostosis and medial capsular reefing.

Naughton-Dunn p.: for severe foot deformity; a triple arthrodesis with wedge resection.

neurectomy: excision of a neuroma anywhere in the body; in the foot, excision of an interdigital neuroma between the second and third or third and fourth toes.

Ober p.: for paralytic clubfeet; a method of transfer of the posterior tibial tendon to the third cuneiform or metatarsal.

onychotomy: incision into the nail bed.

opening abductory wedge osteotomy (OAWO): for bunion deformity; osteotomy of the first metatarsal base with use of bone graft to open the wedge and bring the first metatarsal closer to the second.

opening wedge osteotomy: for bunion deformity; in orthopaedics, a variety of procedures with or without tendon transfers, with proximal cut in the metatarsal and reduction of the deformity.

Osmone-Clarke p.: for talipes valgus; soft-tissue release of the medial and lateral foot with peroneus brevis tendon transfer.

osteotripsy: for callosities; may be any percutaneous reduction of a bony prominence.

panmetatarsal head resection: usually for severe arthritic deformity; resection of all of the metatarsal heads.

pantalar fusion: for instability of the hindfoot; fusion of the tibiotalar, subtalar, calcaneocuboid, and talonavicular joints.

partial ostectomy: to relieve pressure on the skin; removal of bony prominence.

Peabody p.: (1) for metatarsus varus; resection of the proximal portion of the second, third, and fourth metatarsals, with osteotomy of the fifth and capsular release of the first metatarsals; (2) for paralysis of gastrocsoleus complex; transfer of anterior tibial tendon to the calcaneus.

Perry p.: for talipes equinovarus; split transfer of anterior tibialis to proximal third metatarsal, and flexor hallucis longus to dorsum of fourth metatarsal.

phenolization: for nail deformity in which a permanent elimination of a part or all of nail plate is desired. Phenol is applied to the nail matrix after the nail plate is removed to destroy any further nail growth.

Pierrot-Murphy p.: for dorsiflexion of the ankle weakness; transfer of Achilles tendon anteriorly on calcaneus.

PIP fusion: operation commonly done for claw-toes or hammer toes; removal of the proximal interphalangeal joint and then fusion.

Pridie-Koutsogiannis p.:   for flexible flatfoot with excessive heel valgus; medial displacing osteotomy of calcaneus.

Putti-Mayer p.:   for treatment of polio foot deformity; transfer of posterior tibial tendon.

Quenu p. (Fowler p., Zadik p.):   for ingrown toenail; excision of nail bed germinal matrix through skin flap incision, leaving distal nail intact.

Reverdin-Green p.:   for bunion deformity; a closing wedge osteotomy of the first metatarsal head.

Richardson p.:   for malunited calcaneal fracture; posterior subtalar fusion using iliac bone graft as necessary.

Rose p.:   for ingrown nail; removal of the ellipse of soft tissue to ingrown portion of nail.

Ruiz-Mora p.:   proximal phalangectomy of the fifth toe for cock-up (or curly toe) deformity.

Samilson p.:   for calcaneocavus foot; a crescentic osteotomy of the calcaneus.

Siffert-Foster-Nachamie p.:   for paralytic club-feet; triple arthrodesis.

Silver p.:   excision of medial first metatarsal exostosis with lateral capsular release and medial capsular imbrication.

Staples-Black-Brostrom p.:   for acute, severe ankle sprain; method of repair of lateral collateral ligaments.

Steindler matricectomy: for nail deformity; removal of a part of the nail matrix to eliminate one border of the nail plate.

Steindler p.:   plantar release of the proximal muscles and fascia of the foot for high-arched feet.

step down osteotomy: for abnormally long lesser metatarsal; an osteotomy to shorten the bone.

Stone p.:   for hallux rigidus; resection of the dorsal first metatarsal exostosis.

Strayer p.:   for tight heel cord; gastrocnemius lengthening leaving soleus intact.

subtalar arthrodesis: for arthritis and other conditions of the talocalcaneal joint; fusion of the talus to the calcaneus.

subtalar arthroereisis: for severe flatfoot with calcaneal valgus; insertion of an inert spacer into the subtalar joint.

Suppan p.:   for nail deformity; this is a name applied to a variety of procedures to eliminate all or a part of the nail matrix.

syndactylization: a soft-tissue procedure in which two adjacent toes are intentionally joined together. Syndactyly is the condition of an abnormal fusion of two or more digits.

TAL (tendon Achilles lengthening):   a variety of procedures used to lengthen a tight or spastic Achilles tendon.

talectomy: excision of the talus for severe soft tissue contractures.

Thomas p.:   for malunion calcaneus; subtalar arthrodesis using an iliac crest graft.

Tohen p.:   for spastic equinovarus deformity of foot; transfer of conjoined extensor hallucis longus and anterior tibial tendon to second or fifth metatarsal.

transmetatarsal amputation: an amputation through the midportion of the metatarsals.

triple arthrodesis: for flail hindfoot and other deformities caused by arthritis. Procedure involves fusion of the calcaneus to the cuboid, navicula to the talus, and talus to the calcaneus.

Turco p.:   for clubfeet; soft-tissue release of the posteromedial capsule as well as Achilles tendon lengthening.

Valpius-Compere p.:   for Achilles tendon tightness; proximal inverted V-shaped lengthening.

V-Y plasty: for clawtoes; transection of skin in V-shaped incision with closure in the shape of a Y.

Warner-Farber p.:   for trimalleolar fractures with large posterior fragment; detachment of the fibula from tibia to get screw fixation of posterior fragment.

Watson-Cheyne p.: for ingrown toenail; excision of vertical wedge avoiding bone; **Burghard p., O'Donoghue p., Mongensen p.**

Watson-Jones p.: for lateral ankle instability, use of peroneus brevis tendon in reconstruction of lateral ligament.

Westin p.: for paralytic talipes calcaneus, a tenodesis of the Achilles tendon to the fibula.

White slide p.: for Achilles tendon tightening in spastic hemiplegia, anterior fibers of the Achilles tendon are cut distally, and medial fibers are cut proximally. The foot is then dorsiflexed, producing the slide.

Whitman talectomy p.: talectomy for calcaneovalgus foot.

Whitman-Thompson p.: for talipes calcaneus or talipes calcaneovalgus; complete excision of the talus.

Wilson p.: for bunion deformity; an oblique osteotomy of the first metatarsal neck area.

Wilson and Jacob p.: for tibial plateau fracture; use of patella and its cartilage surface for joint replacement graft.

Winograd p.: for an ingrown nail; excision of an ingrown portion of toenail, with curettement of the nail bed.

Wolf p.: for plantar callosity; proximal shortening of the metatarsal.

Wu p.: for bunion deformity; a lateral and plantar displacement of the first metatarsal neck osteotomy with Herbert screw fixation. Also, for great toe fusion; a three Herbert screw fixation.

Young p.: anterior tibialis transfer for flatfoot.

Z-plasty: for tight heel cord; complete Z-shaped cut requiring suturing of Achilles tendon.

Zadik p.: for ingrown nail; excision of the entire nail.

Approaches

Ankle and Foot

anterior a.: for tendon repairs, transfers, and some ankle fusions; **Kochler, Ollier.**

lateral and posterolateral a.: for repair of fractures, ligamentous injuries, and some tendon transfers; **Kocher, Gatellier** and **Chastang.**

medial and posteromedial a.: for ankle fractures, tendon transfers, and correction of clubfeet; **Broomhead, Colonna** and **Ralston, Koenig** and **Schaefer, Garceau.**

Chapter 12

Physical Medicine and Rehabilitation: Physical Therapy and Occupational Therapy

PHYSICAL THERAPY

Physical medicine and rehabilitation (PM&R) is a medical specialty that is based on the fundamentals of neuromuscular physiology, exercise physiology, and functional anatomy.

The **physiatrist** is the physician specialist in PM&R certified by the American Board of Physical Medicine and Rehabilitation after completing a residency and other requirements. In some distinct centers for rehabilitation, a physiatrist is the medical director of the unit. However, some units are organized on a programmatic basis and have a group of other medical specialists overseeing individual programs: for example, a rheumatologist with the arthritis program, a neurologist with the neuromuscular disease program, and an orthopaedist with the musculoskeletal program.

The **physical therapist** is a health care professional who has completed an entry-level education program accredited by the Commission on Accreditation in Physical Therapy Education. Board-certified physical therapy specialty are in the following areas: cardiopulmonary, neurologic, clinical electrophysiologic, orthopaedic, pediatric, geriatric, and sports physical therapy.

In a hospital setting, the rehabilitation team may include the occupational therapist, speech therapist, rehabilitation nurse, social worker, and psychologist. Additional members might include a vocational counselor, special educator, prosthetist/orthotist, and numerous medical specialists depending on patient needs. The physical therapist assistant is a skilled technical health worker who, under the supervision of a physical therapist, assists in the patient's treatment program.

The goal of the rehabilitation team is to enhance each patient's physical capabilities by employing the team members' individual professional skills, expertise, and knowledge to evaluate, plan, and implement treatment interventions tailored to the needs of the patient. In this patient-centered approach, the patient and/or family participates in setting realistic goals to be achieved during the rehabilitation process.

In association with orthopaedic surgery, the rehabilitation team works closely with and is considered an integral part of the orthopaedic rehabilitation program. The physical therapist consults with the orthopaedist and other primary care physicians in the evaluation and treatment of patients and establishes the treatment plan.

Services are provided for preoperative and postoperative care of the surgical patient after restorative surgery, trauma, or correction of congenital anomalies. In addition, treatments include the prevention of pulmonary complications after surgery. Strengthening and range-of-motion exercises are designed for patients with ligamentous tears and fractures. Amputees fitted with prostheses are instructed in their use and maintenance. The patient with a spinal cord injury is taught activities of daily living (ADL), gait with braces, the use of assistive devices, and exercises to improve function. Large rehabilitation centers are designed to most effectively address these patients' needs.

Physical therapist services provide identification, prevention, remediation, and rehabilitation of patients with acute or prolonged physical dysfunction. Such intervention encompasses examination and analysis, therapeutic application of physical and chemical agents, exercises, and education to promote functional independence.

Physical therapy treatments may include the evaluation and treatment of abnormal gait patterns resulting from pathologic conditions, such as muscle weakness, paralysis, or biomechanical defects. Patients may also be referred for rehabilitative services for treatment of neuromuscular diseases (e.g., arthritis, stroke, or spinal cord injuries), temporomandibular joint (TMJ) syndrome, and chronic pain. The goal is to decrease pain, increase function, and prevent deformity.

Physical Therapy Services

Physical therapists practice in a variety of settings: acute care hospitals, rehabilitation centers, skilled nursing facilities, convalescent homes, home health, schools, industry, sports clinics, pediatric facilities, and private practice.

The following is a quick reference to typical services (though not inclusive) that are routinely provided by the physical therapist.

Evaluation (General)
Strength
Functional ability
Range of motion
Cognitive level
Coordination
Sensation
Ambulatory status

Evaluation (Specific)
Manual muscle testing
Cardiopulmonary function
Electroneurophysiologic
Neurodevelopmental
Isokinetic
Gait
Posture
Muscle tone
Wound
Neonatal
Thermography
Functional capacity evaluation

Treatment Techniques
Therapeutic exercise
  Passive
  Active-assistive
  Active
  Resistive (isometric, isotonic, concentric, eccentric, isokinetic)
  Work hardening
Specific techniques
  Proprioceptive neuromuscular facilitation (PNF)
  Bobath (neurodevelopmental)
  Rood
  Brunstrom
Muscle reeducation
  Brushing
  Icing
  Tapping
  Quick stretch
  Neurodevelopmental training
Mobility
  Bed (bedbound patient)
  Transfer techniques
  Wheelchair mobility and safety
  Ambulation—parallel bars, walker, crutches, cane, prosthetic, orthotic

Hydrotherapy
Cold/ice
Heat (moist)
Whirlpool (for increasing circulation, decreasing pain, debriding open wounds)
Therapy pool (for gravity-free exercise and ambulation)
Paraffin

Physical modalities
Electrical stimulation
Functional electrical stimulation (FES)
Diathermy
Transcutaneous electrical nerve stimulation (TENS)
Ultrasound
Infrared
Ultraviolet

Mobilization
Soft tissue
Joint

Cardiac care
Cardiac rehabilitation
Cardiac stress testing

Pulmonary
Bronchial drainage
Breathing exercises

Pediatric
Neurodevelopmental
Scoliosis care (education and exercise, pre- and postoperative care)
Musculoskeletal

Intermittent compression
Edema control

Traction
Cervical
Pelvic
Extremity

Patient education (an essential element of most treatment plans)

Consultation Services
Consultative services are available for patients with special or extraordinary needs that require the recommendations of a multidisciplinary group.

Physical Therapy Modalities

cervical traction: a means of separating the cervical vertebrae 1 to 2 mm to help relieve painful neck conditions or cervical radiculopathies; may be intermittent or continuous.

contrast baths: alternately exposing affected limb to warm and cool water for specified periods. This is a means of reducing swelling, diminishing pain, and improving joint range of motion.

diathermy: electromagnetic waves with a specific wavelength (shortwave diathermy, microwave diathermy) used as a means of producing heat deep inside tissues.

electrical stimulation:

alternating current: sinusoidal or faradic; stimulates normally innervated muscles to relieve pain and relax muscle spasm.

galvanic: direct current used to stimulate denervated muscles and for ion transfer (iontophoresis).

high-voltage pulsed galvanic: to relieve pain and relax muscle spasm. Stimulates normally innervated muscles.

iontophoresis: the use of direct current (D.C.) to drive water-soluble ions through the skin. Dexamethasone, xylocaine, and lidocaine are commonly used to treat acute and subacute localized inflammation and pain.

MENS (microamperage electrical nerve stimulation): microamperage current that is below patient's threshold; to relieve pain.

TENS (transcutaneous electrical nerve stimulation): Self-contained, modulated galvanic current (low voltage) that seems to block painful afferent nerve impulses. Helps to control pain so patient may exercise.

fluidotherapy: the use of forced warm air through a container holding fine cellulose particles to provide dry heat and exercise to upper and lower extremities. Both the temperature and the particle agitation can be controlled for edema and desensitization of hypersensitive area.

hot packs: silicone gel, clay, or other material in bags that can be heated to provide superficial heat for tissues.

hydrotherapy treatments: as commonly used today, immersion of affected limbs (sometimes including the trunk) in a tank of water at a specified temperature. The water may be moving (whirlpool), which is one means of debriding tissue. There are also tanks in which patients may sit (Lo-Boy) and in which they may be almost totally immersed (Hubbard tank). In a pool, the buoyancy of water can assist patients with partially paralyzed legs to walk.

interferential current: application of two medium-frequency alternating currents that interfere with each other. Used for pain control and muscle stimulation.

intermittent compression: a boot or sleeve that encloses the leg or arm and is alternately pressurized with air and then deflated. The inflate/deflate action provides a pumping effect that reduces disabling edema. It is often prescribed for breast cancer patients after a mastectomy and for lymphedema that may result.

paraffin bath: a combination of wax and mineral oil at 126° F used as a means of heating the hands or feet.

pelvic traction: application of pelvic belt with caudad pull, which may be continuous or use greater force intermittently.

phonophoresis: the use of ultrasound to drive molecules of medications through the skin to the underlying tissues.

RICE: an acronym for the initial treatment of an injury; **r**est, **i**ce, **c**ompression, and **e**levation.

ultrasound: ultrahigh-frequency sound waves that mechanically vibrate soft tissue. Secondary deep heat may develop according to method of application.

Physical Therapy Procedures

accupressure: sustained deep pressure over muscular trigger points.

aerobic exercises: exercises in which oxygen consumption is inhaled at a rate sufficient for a continuous process of energy production for muscle contraction; the goal is to increase endurance required for long-distance running or after cardiac complications.

anaerobic exercises: exercises in which the expenditure of energy is at a faster rate than that for which the cardiorespiratory mechanism can provide, the goal being to exert the maximal amount of force or energy in a short amount of time, as in a 40-yard dash.

aquatic exercise: exercise performed in a pool or large hydrotherapy tank that uses the buoyancy of water.

closed chain exercise (closed kinetic chain):   exercise that occurs when the distal segment of an extremity is fixed, such as performing a squat, in which the foot is in contact with the ground. Motion can take place in all planes.

Codman exercises: exercises for a stiff shoulder in which the patient is bent over at the waist (90 degrees) and the hand hangs like a pendulum toward the floor. A weight may be placed in the hand and the arm is then moved through various arcs to increase the ROM in that shoulder.

concentric contraction: muscle shortening; also called **positive work.**

cross-training: a complex training regimen in which two or more sports or activities are combined into either a solitary or a cyclical program to exercise different muscle groups, and to provide variety and protection from repetitive use syndromes.

DeLorme exercises: originally established on the basis of the 10 repetition maximum (RM), which is the maximal amount of resistance a muscle can lift through full ROM exercises

10 times; the term is frequently interchanged with progressive resistive exercises (PRE), which are designed to build strength and increase endurance through graduated resistance for a prescribed number of repetitions.

eccentric contraction: muscle lengthening, also called "negative work"; strengthening exercises in which the external force overcomes the actively contracting muscle, forcing the muscle to lengthen.

gait training: the use of parallel bars, crutches, walkers, and canes with specific instructions to the patient. Weight bearing may be described as non–weight bearing (NWB), partial weight bearing (PWB), or full weight bearing (FWB). Ambulation with crutches is often described as three-point gait, and with walker, four-point gait.

isokinetic exercises: constant velocity; strengthening exercises requiring special equipment in which there is an accommodating resistance, resulting in a maximal force against the contracting muscle throughout its full ROM. Can be used for the spine as well as the upper and lower extremities.

isometric exercises: muscle contraction without joint movement in which the resistance may be provided by a fixed object (wall, stabilized bar) or the antagonistic muscle group (flexors versus extensors); a muscle-strengthening exercise that does not impel muscle to work through its range of motion; **constant angle.**

isotonic exercises: muscle contraction with movement of the joint through a specified ROM against a fixed amount of resistance; **constant force.**

joint manipulation: any skilled manual technique applied to a joint that moves one particular surface in relation to another.

joint mobilization: skilled passive movements applied to joint surfaces to restore "joint play" and range of motion or to treat pain.

joint play (accessory movement): involuntary movements of joint surfaces allowed by

capsular elasticity that allow for normal, pain-free voluntary motion.

lumbar stabilization: exercise program to stabilize the torso by developing the "corset" muscles of the lumbar spine, particularly the abdominal muscles.

McConnell taping: the technique of specific taping to correct abnormal tilt, glide, and rotation of the patella in patients with patellofemoral disorders.

McKenzie (extension) exercises: exercises performed to decrease the compression on the intervertebral disk.

muscle energy technique: manual technique that uses active contraction of a patient's muscle to correct joint dysfunction.

myofascial release: manual therapy technique that applies prolonged stretching to release restrictions in the muscle-fascia system.

open chain exercises: exercise that occurs when the distal segment of an extremity is free, such as performing a seated knee extension exercise. Non–weight bearing and usually in one plane of motion; open kinetic chain.

pulley exercises: a rope on pulley system used to increase ROM of a joint or strengthen muscles; resistance can be applied by another limb or by weights.

range of motion (ROM) exercises: designed to maintain or increase the amount of movement in a joint. They may be one of the following:

   passive: force is applied to bring about motion in a joint or joints by either a therapist or the patient, without any muscle function in these joints.

   active-assistive: exercise performed by the patient but requiring assistance from a therapist, another extremity, or a mechanical device because of muscle weakness or pain.

   active: exercise performed by patient without assistance or resistance; the therapist is only an instructor-observer.

resistive exercise table: commonly used for lower extremity problems, such as after knee surgery; resistance can be applied by weights (NK™ table in some locales) or by a graded hydraulic system.

spray and stretch: use of a vapocoolant, such as Fluori-Methane or ice, for treatment of trigger points in muscles. The vapocoolant is sprayed over a stretched muscle to increase range of motion.

Swiss ball exercises: use of an inflatable gymnastic ball with various movements for mobility, strength, balance, coordination, and stabilization of the spine and the extremities.

therapeutic massage: soft tissue manipulation using techniques such as friction, stroking, and kneading to reduce muscle spasm and edema, stimulate circulation, and encourage relaxation. Also used to stretch scar tissue.

Williams (flexion) exercises: for patients with low back pain; exercises are performed to open the lumbar intervertebral foramina and decrease the compression on the facet joints by flexing the lumbosacral spine, thereby stretching the extensors of the back and strengthening the abdominal muscles.

Tests and Measurements*

Given that the circulation is intact, the major parameters in assessing the function of a limb are range of motion, sensation, and strength. These can be tested directly by the application of forces to the muscle and stimuli to the skin or can be assessed indirectly by electrodiagnostic modalities such as electromyography. In muscle testing, strength is graded by the following scale as assessed directly by the examiner. Range of motion (ROM) is measured with a goniometer, an instrument that measures joint motion in degrees.

*For more specific information on various tests and examinations, an excellent source is American Orthopaedic Association: *Manual of orthopaedic surgery,* ed 6; Chicago, 1985, The Association.

Key to manual muscle evaluation†

100%	5	N	Normal: Complete ROM against gravity with full resistance
75%	4	G	Good: Complete ROM against gravity with some resistance
50%	3	F	Fair: Complete ROM against gravity
25%	2	P	Poor: Complete ROM with gravity eliminated
10%	1	T	Trace: Evidence of contractility
0	0	0	Zero: No evidence of contractility
S		Spasm	If spasm or contracture exists,
C		Contracture	place S or C after the grade of a movement incomplete for this reason

dynamometer: an instrument to measure muscle strength and its effects from exercise, such as a handgrip d. that can be adjusted to test strength in different positions of grasp; or from a bicycle d. that measures muscular, respiratory, and metabolic effects of exercise, recording directly from a pressure gauge; **ergometer.**

computerized isokinetic dynamometer: an apparatus that can be used to test and record the maximal strength of a muscle as it acts on a joint through a full range of motion. The recording is used to evaluate the progress of a patient's condition during recovery or to confirm the existence and extent of injury.

Sensory Testing

heat and cold testing: (self-explanatory).

pinprick test: a gross test to check two variables: (1) the actual ability to feel a pinprick and (2) the ability to determine the difference between sharp and dull.

pressure testing: involves sensation produced by touch to a localized area using an instrument that indicates the pressure needed to produce sensation.

proprioceptive testing: tests the ability to sense the position of a body part with the eyes closed.

†From Daniels L, Worthingham C: *Muscle testing: techniques of manual examination by comparison,* ed 4, Philadelphia, 1980, WB Saunders.

tendon reflex examination: graded from 0 to 4 and varies widely in meaning from examiner to examiner; the test is performed by striking the tendon briskly and watching muscle reaction.

two-point discrimination: ability to perceive difference between one or two points of touch at the fingertips or elsewhere; this test of fine sensation is measured in centimeters or millimeters.

vibrator sense examination: tests the patient's ability to feel vibrations with use of a tuning fork.

Electrical Testing

electromyography (EMG):   an electrodiagnostic test conducted on a special machine that evaluates the capability of nerves and muscles to transmit and respond to normal or stimulated electric impulses. The muscle is evaluated by direct insertion of a small needle to which the muscle responds with characteristic contractile activity, which is referred to as "insertional activity." Once the muscle has acclimated to the presence of the needle, individual muscle fiber activity can be seen electrically on an **oscilloscope** and is described by the specific wave patterns. Disorders affecting the nerves, such as a herniated disk, will eventually cause changes in the wave pattern of the muscle. Other disorders commonly evaluated with this study include entrapment syndromes and other neuropathic and muscle disorders. **Conduction time** is the measurement of nerve stimulation applied through the skin, allowing the nerve to transmit impulses. The conduction time is increased in neurologic disorders, such as vitamin B_1 deficiency and carpal tunnel syndrome caused by local nerve pressure.

nerve conduction velocity (NCV):   a diagnostic test often performed with the EMG, this is a test of the integrity of peripheral nerve(s) that involves placing an electric stimulator over the nerve and measuring the time required for an impulse to travel over a segment of nerve; useful in the diagnosis of nerve entrapment syndrome and polyneuropathies.

OCCUPATIONAL THERAPY

Occupational therapy is the art and science of directing a patient's participation in selected tasks to restore, reinforce, and enhance performance, facilitate learning of those skills and functions essential for adaptation and productivity, diminish or correct abnormalities, and promote and maintain health. Its fundamental concerns are the capacity, throughout the life span, to perform with satisfaction to self and others those tasks and roles essential to productive living and the mastery of self and the environment.

The registered occupational therapist (OTR) is a professional who possesses unique skills and credentials, has been educated in a baccalaureate or master's curriculum accredited jointly by the Committee on Allied Health Education, American Medical Association, and the American Occupational Therapy Association (AOTA), and has passed the national certification examination of the American Occupational Therapy Certification Board (AOTCB) and holds current registration with that body. A certified occupational therapy assistant (COTA) has satisfactorily completed an occupational therapy assistant curriculum approved by AOTA, has passed a national certification examination, holds current certification with the AOTCB, and works under the supervision of an OTR. Graduate programs for OTRs prepare the therapist for the role of specialized practitioner, educator, or researcher. Most U.S. jurisdictions regulate Occupational Therapy, the majority through licensure laws.

Specific Occupational Therapist Services

Specific occupational therapist services include but are not limited to the following:

- Education and training in activities of daily living (ADL).
- Administering and interpreting such tests as manual muscle and range of motion.
- Design, fabrication, and application of slings and orthoses.

- Developing perceptual-motor skills and sensory integrative functioning.
- Restoration of hand functioning.
- Instruction in work simplification, energy conservation, and use of proper body mechanics during activity for work, leisure, and/or daily living.
- Guidance in the selection and use of adaptive equipment.
- Therapeutic activities to enhance functional performance.
- Prevocational evaluation and training and physical capacity evaluation.
- Consultation concerning adaptation to home or work environments.

Occupational Therapy Assessment

Services are provided to all age groups in a variety of settings, including hospitals, hand clinics, rehabilitation facilities, sheltered workshops, schools, extended care facilities, private homes, community agency clinics, and industrial settings.

Cases most frequently referred to occupational therapists by orthopaedists are amputation, arthritis, hand trauma, fractures (hip, femur, tibia, ankle, humerus, radius, ulna, wrist), total joint replacement, sports injury, osteoporosis, elbow and shoulder arthroplasty, spinal cord injury, and chronic pain. One-fourth of AOTA's more than 40,000 members work with orthopaedic patients.

Before treatment is given, each potential patient's case is *screened* to determine the need for occupational therapy. This is followed by assessment, which consists of obtaining and interpreting data necessary for treatment, including that needed to plan for and document the evaluation process and treatment results. The occupational therapy evaluation includes assessment of functional abilities and deficits as related to the patient's needs.

Specific Evaluations, Tests, and Devices

Specific evaluations, tests, and devices used in the assessment process include but are not limited to the following:

Baltimore therapeutic equipment work simulator (BTE):   a device used for evaluation and work hardening.

bulb dynamometer: a soft, cylindrical, rubber-filled squeeze bulb that measures gross isometric grasp and pinch, calibrated in pounds per square inch, measuring force in pounds by multiplying the reading by 4.

Crawford small parts dexterity test: of fine eye-hand coordination and manipulation of small hand tools.

functional capacities assessment: simple rating scale on living skills, indicating progress according to 10 functional levels.

Jamar dynamometer: measures gross isometric grasp in five positions and records in either pounds or kilograms.

Jebsen-Taylor hand function test: consisting of seven subtests to measure major aspects of hand function related to activities of daily living.

LIDO™ lift and workset: provides rehabilitation and evaluation of physical work-related activities.

Martin Vigorimeter: to test handgrip strength.

Minnesota rate of manipulation test: to measure dexterity from seventh grade to adult level.

O'Connor finger dexterity test: designed to measure fine motor ability.

Pennsylvania bimanual worksample: measures finger dexterity of both hands, gross movements of both arms, eye-hand coordination, ability to use both hands simultaneously.

pinch: three-point lateral and fingertip prehension tested with pinch gauge recorded in pounds or kilograms.

Purdue pegboard: measures gross movements of arm, hand, and fingers and fingertip dexterity.

Smith physical capacities evaluation (Smith PCE):   objective test to measure ability of individual to perform selected aspects of occupations.

two-point discrimination: measured with calibrated metric aesthesiometer.

Valpar component work sample series: consisting of 16 work samples designed to measure 17 work behaviors by task analysis; developed for workers with industrial injuries.

volumeter set: accurately measures hand and distal forearm edema for objective monitoring of edema-reducing treatment modalities.

VonFrey hair test (Semmes-Weinstein monofilament): a series of monofilaments with different ratings to determine amount of sensory loss.

WEST (work evaluation systems technology): evaluating work tolerance of upper extremities and/or total body, including ability to measure lifting capabilities and torque strength of hand.

Occupational Therapy Treatments

Occupational therapy treatment refers to the use of specific activities or methods to develop, improve, or restore the performance of necessary functions, compensate for dysfunction, or minimize debilitation. The therapist plans for and documents treatment performance. The following are categories of necessary functions treated in occupational therapy for orthopaedic problems*:

Activities of daily living/physical daily living skills (ADL/PDLS) are components of everyday activity, including self-care, work, and play/leisure activities. These may also be referred to as life skills or life tasks and consist of the following.

bathing: ability to obtain and use supplies and soap, rinse and dry all body parts, maintain bathing position, transfer to and from bathing position, use adapted bathing equipment such as bath mitt, tub bench, grab bars, scrub brush, etc.

dressing: ability to select appropriate clothing, obtain clothing from storage area, dress and undress in sequential fashion, fasten/unfasten clothes and shoes, and don and doff appliances, for example, glasses, prostheses, or orthoses.

*Definitions taken from *Occupational Therapy Product Output Reporting System and Uniform Terminology for Reporting Occupational Therapy,* ed 2; Rockville, MD, p 415.

feeding/eating: ability to set up food, use appropriate regular or adapted utensils and tableware, and bring food or drink from table to mouth.

functional communication: ability to use equipment or systems to enhance or provide communication, such as writing equipment, telephones, typewriters, communication boards, call lights, emergency systems, braille writers, augmentative communication systems, and computers.

functional mobility: ability to move from one position or one place to another as in bed mobility, wheelchair mobility, transfers (bed, chair, tub, toilet, car), and functional ambulation with or without adaptive aids, driving, or use of public transportation.

grooming: ability to obtain and use supplies to shave, apply and remove cosmetics, wash, comb, style and brush hair, care for nails, care for skin, and apply deodorant.

toilet hygiene: ability to obtain and use supplies, clean self, and transfer to and from and maintain toileting position on bedpan, toilet, and/or commode.

Work activities include home management tasks such as clothing care, cleaning, meal preparation and clean-up, household maintenance, care of others, and safety procedures. The latter is important in preventing falls in areas such as bathroom, kitchen, and stairs

Vocational activities consist of vocational exploration, job acquisition, and timely and effective job performance.

Play or leisure involves choosing and engaging in activities for amusement, relaxation, spontaneous enjoyment, or self-expression.

sensorimotor skills: consist of performance patterns of sensory and motor behavior prerequisite to self-care, work, and play and leisure performance, such as:
Range of motion (ROM)
Gross and fine coordination
Muscle control
Coordination
Dexterity

Strength and endurance
Sensory awareness, including
   tactile awareness
   stereognosis
Kinesthesia
Proprioceptive awareness

cognitive skills: necessary mental processes, including orientation, conceptualization/comprehension (concentration, attention span, memory), and cognitive integration (applying diverse knowledge to environmental situations, including ability to generalize and problem solve).

prevention and minimization of debilitation: refers to programs for persons with predisposition to disability, as well as for those who have already incurred a disability, and include the following:

   energy conservation: activity restriction, work simplification, time management, or organization of the environment to minimize energy output.

   joint protection: procedures to minimize stress on joints, including use of proper body mechanics, avoidance of static or deforming postures, and avoidance of excess weigh bearing.

   positioning: placement of body part in alignment to promote optimal functioning.

therapeutic adaptations: design or restructuring of the physical environment to assist self-care, work, and play and leisure performance through selecting, obtaining, fitting, and fabricating equipment, as well as instructing client, family, and staff in its proper use and care, including making minor repairs and modifications for correct fit, position, or use.

Some categories of therapeutic adaptation are:

orthotics, splints, or slings: to relieve pain, maintain joint alignment, protect joint integrity, improve function, or decrease deformity.

   dynamic splints: to allow for or provide motion by transfer of movement from other body parts or by use of outside forces such

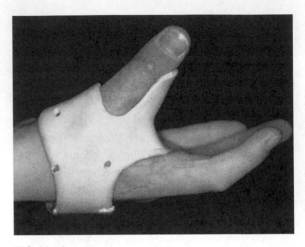

FIG 12–1.
Standard type C-bar web spacer for preventing contractures in burn patients. (Permissions: EC Jeter, OTR, National Naval Medical Center, Bethesda, Md.)

as springs, rubber bands, carbon dioxide, or electricity.

   functional fracture bracing (using thermoplastics): proximal or distal to fracture, in combination with hinge joint to provide motion and allowing weight bearing to enhance osteogenesis.

   static splints: with no moving parts, designed to maintain joint in desired position (Fig. 12–1).

prosthetics: artificial substitutes for missing body parts to augment functional performance, with occupational therapy especially involved in upper extremity prosthetic checkout and training.

assistive/adaptive equipment: additions or devices that assist in performance or in structural or positional changes, such as installing ramps and bars, changing furniture heights, adjusting traffic patterns, and modifying wheelchairs.

Some typical adaptive equipment examples for orthopaedics are reachers, sockdonners, elevated toilet seats, leg-lifter straps, and walker adaptations (platforms and walker bags).

Chapter 13

Musculoskeletal Research

Orthopaedic research involves the clinical and basic scientific investigation of the embryology, growth, development, and remodeling of the musculoskeletal system and its response to disease, trauma, and aging. Another major part of orthopaedic research is the evaluation of medical and surgical intervention in musculoskeletal diseases. Over the past 20 years, a much broader understanding of cellular response to chemical messages, and the chemical and physical stimuli for these messages, has developed. As a result, orthopaedic research often overlaps with other disciplines including biochemistry, biomechanics, genetics, immunology, and biomaterials.

A major area of investigation has been in fracture healing and the factors that positively and negatively affect that process. Better clinical management includes more precise fixation, less invasive procedures, better salvage of more severe injuries, and better maintenance of function during the repair process. Daily clinical decisions are based more on an understanding of the biology rather than the use of simple timing rules. Rehabilitation research has led to a speedier recovery after total knee replacement, hand surgery, and knee ligamentous reconstruction.

Another major advance has been in internal joint prosthetics. However, more investigation is needed into the methods of fixation, as well as the materials, products, and chemical reactions that follow. Techniques that allow for three-dimensional radiographic rapid motion pictures in high detail make it possible to analyze the rapid force accelerations important to prosthetic wear and brace effectiveness. The utility of these devices, as well as the field of sports medicine, will expand rapidly in the near future as a result of techniques that allow evaluation of multiple joint motions in three dimensions.

Approximately one-third of patients seen by primary care physicians in the United States have musculoskeletal problems. Arthroscopy has tremendously enhanced the surgeon's ability to improve the course of a disease process within joints. The economic savings from less hospitalization and decreased patient discomfort and morbidity have made musculoskeletal research one of the foremost achievements in orthopaedics.

Because research provides a scientific basis for most decisions made in orthopaedic surgery, there is an increasing need for high-caliber professionals in musculoskeletal research. This type of research requires the commitment and dedication of many different types of investigators. This team may consist of the principal investigator, assisted by junior investigators, orthopaedic surgeons, biochemists, physicists, engineers, physiologists, dentists, veterinarians, laboratory technicians, and many others from the medical and scientific areas. Research endeavors may take months or years, with the ultimate goal to improve the quality of care through the application of biologic and engineering principles to the musculoskeletal system. Interdisciplinary cooperation has been the hallmark of this field of endeavor.

A **research proposal** is an application for a research grant. This proposal is written up by the investigator(s), who submits a protocol outlining the proposed research plan, goals, and potential benefits. In addition, the investigator(s) must estimate time, personnel, laboratory space and equipment, and amount of funds required to accomplish the project. Once this information is gathered, the proposal goes before a grants committee reviewing board, which then decides whether it justifies funding. Sometimes a proposal is granted but funds not provided, or only part of a project is funded. Many worthwhile research proposals must await funding before proceeding.

A **research grant** is the name for funds provided to support a specific research project. This support may be given through a large health institution, such as the National Institutes of Health (NIH), corporation, pharmaceutical company, private endowment, or government agency. The Orthopaedic Research and Education Foundation (OREF), an independent organization, is currently a principal private supporting mechanism, offering fellowship programs in clinical and laboratory investigations. Another group, the Orthopaedic Research Society (ORS), meets yearly to present papers and exchange ideas with those performing research within the orthopaedic community. The American Academy of Orthopaedic Surgeons Research Advisory Committee (RAC) monitors and advises on administrative requirements for orthopaedic research.

Once research protocols have been investigated and experiments completed, investigators disseminate data on results and benefits obtained through various journals to all clinicians in the field. This chapter presents an overview of research terms.

GENERAL RESEARCH TERMINOLOGY

The following terms are likely to be found in many areas of research.

ANOVA: acronym for **an**alysis **of** **v**ariance; a statistical method for detecting significant differences between groups.

assay: assessment of the relative amount of a chemical in solution. Quantity is commonly expressed in terms of parts per million (PPM) or parts per billion (PPB).

cell components: of the many chemicals and parts of a cell, the most commonly described are the following:
centriole
endoplasmic reticulum
filaments
golgi apparatus
lysosome
microsome
microtubule
mitochondria
nucleolus
nucleus
plasma membrane (cell membrane)
polyribosomes
ribosome
vessicle

circadian: pertaining to a periodic biologic cycle, often a 24-hour period.

confidence interval: the chance that the average of a given set of data would fall within a set of numerical bounds if the experiment or survey were to be repeated. Typically, a confidence interval of 95% is selected when presenting clinical data.

ELISA (enzyme-linked immunosorbent assay): a competitive binding assay using an immunoglobulin attached to an enzyme-generated chromophoric substance that, when the complex attaches to a specific antigen (as seen on a macromolecule), will reveal and quantitate the amount of antigen by the generation of the chromophore.

hertz (Hz): a unit of frequency equal to one cycle per second.

HPLC (high-performance liquid chromatography, high-pressure liquid chromatography): means of making rapid separation of biochemical solutes with the use of a solid-support column under high pressure and based on ion-exchange, gel-permeation, or partition principles.

in vitro: analysis of reaction taking place outside the body but attempting to simulate a chemical reaction that takes place within the body. In the literature, the word is usually written in italics to read *in vitro.*

in vivo: an investigation carried out in tissue within a living body. In the literature, the word is usually written in italics to read *in vivo.*

lysosomal proteases: degradative enzymes found in lysosomes; generally active at acid pH; may be associated with extracellular matrix breakdown.

metalloproteinases (metalloproteases): protein-cleaving enzymes that have an association with zinc metal ion (Zn^{++}) to be active. There are now at least 15 metalloproteinases known. They have overlapping functions. Some of the major musculoskeletal metalloproteinases are:

collagenases (metalloproteinases I and XIII): cleaves specific collagens at specific points in the molecule.

gelatinase (metalloproteinase II): cleaves specific collagens, fibronectin, and proteoglycans.

stromelysin (metalloproteinase III, transin, proteoglycanase): cleaves core protein and, thereby, aggrecan from hyaluronic acid.

microsphere: a small sphere usually made of glass that is injected intravenously for studies of conditions such as blockage of small vessels and muscle injuries.

negative predictive value: the likelihood that a patient/sample for whom/which the test is negative actually does not have the index disease or status; determined by dividing the number of true positives by the sum of the true positives and false positives.

positive predictive value: the likelihood that a patient/sample for whom/which the test is positive actually has the index disease or status; determined by dividing the number of true nega-

tives by the sum of the true negatives and false negatives.

radioactive tracers: a variety of radioactive compounds commonly used to study the localization of specific elements or compounds. Those most commonly used in orthopaedics include the following:

^{45}Ca (calcium)

^{3}H (equal to tritiated, for example, tritiated thymidine)

^{51}Cr (chromium)

$^{35}SO_4$ (sulfate)

^{67}Ga (gallium)

^{99m}Tc (technetium)

^{85}Sr (strontium)

reagent: any substance with specific biologic or chemical action added to the solution of another substance to produce a chemical reaction.

scanning electron microscopy (SEM): to examine minute objects, a beam of electrons focused across a specimen produces an enlarged three-dimensional surface contour image of that specimen on a cathode ray tube. A photograph is then obtained.

sensitivity: the percentage of time that a given test is positive where the condition is known to exist (number of true positives divided by number of true positives plus false negatives).

specificity: the percentage of time that a test is negative for a condition where the condition does not exist (number of true negatives divided by number of true negatives plus the number of false positives).

superoxide radical: highly transient and chemically reactive species of oxygen atom that has an unpaired free electron. The presence of these or other radicals can lead to degradative biochemical pathways.

tissue inhibitor of metalloproteinase (TIMP): a specific protein that inhibits metalloproteinases.

transmission electron microscopy (TEM): to examine the internal structure of minute objects, a beam of electrons is transmitted through a specimen slice to produce an enlarged two-dimensional picture similar to that produced by a light microscope.

MEASUREMENTS

Most of the measurements used in the current orthopaedic literature are in the metric system, more specifically, the International System of Units. The basic units are the meter for length, kilogram for mass, second for time, and Centigrade for temperature. The basic measurements are listed in the box below.

Dalton (Da):   1/12th the mass of the C_{12} atom. This unit is used in expressing the weight of molecules, as opposed to molecular weight, where the value given is the mass of 6.23×10^{23} molecules of the material. The term dalton is essentially equivalent to the term molecular weight.

BONE HEALING AND METABOLISM

Research directed at chemical reactions in living tissue will often overlap with microscopic and elec-

tron microscopic techniques. After centuries of technologic refinement in the fields of biochemistry and histology (study of cells), the two fields have developed the ability to see or visually outline molecular structures and confirm by picture what is observed by the biochemist. Many terms listed in this and other sections are part of the investigatory vocabulary of the histologist, electron microscopist, and biochemist.

bone morphogenic protein: a family of proteins involved in the stimulation of bone formation.

bone salts: calcium (Ca), phosphate (PO_4), and hydroxyl (OH) ions are the main components of the bone crystal that is directly attached to the collagen molecule. The process by which this attachment occurs is very complicated. Associated terms include the following:

apatite ($Ca_{10}[PO_4]_6[OH]_2$)
alkaline phosphatase
acid phosphatase
brushite
calcium phosphate, dibasic (brushite, $CaHOP_4$ $2H_2O$)
amorphous calcium phosphate ($Ca_9[PO_4]_6$)
calcium pyrophosphate (CaPPi)
calcium phospholipid phosphate

Exponent of log base 10	Distance	Weight	Pressure	Force
10^{-15}	Femtometer	Femtogram = fg		
10^{-12}	Picometer	Picogram = pg	Picopascal	
10^{-9}	Nanometer	Nanogram = ng	Nanopascal	
10^{-6}	Micron	Microgram = μg	Micropascal	
10^{-3}	Millimeter	Milligram = mg	Millipascal	
10^{-2}	Centimeter			
10^{0}	Meter (39.37 inches)	Gram = g		
10^{3}	Kilometer	Kilogram = kg	Pascal (1 newton per 1 square meter) Kilopascal (KPa)	Newton (1 kg mass accelerated 1 m/sec^2)
10^{6}			Megapascal (MPa)	
10^{9}			Gigapascal (Gpa)	
10^{12}			Tetrapascal (TPa)	

phospholipid
proteolipid
phosphatidylserine
phosphatidylinositol
pyrophosphate (PPi, PYP)

calbinden (calcium binding protein): a 40 kDa protein involved in cytoplasmic transport of calcium.

calcitonin: a short-chain protein hormone that is involved in bone accretion. The activity of this hormone will reduce the level of serum calcium by its effect on new bone addition at the point where this is taking place.

cement line: the refractile boundary of an osteon, interstitial lamellar system, or border between cartilage and bone. This line marks the completion point of local development or remodeling of bone. Also called a **tide mark.**

Gla protein (γ-carboxyglutamic acid): amino acid seen particularly in osteocalcin (a protein involved in bone mineral formation).

insulin-like growth factor I (IGF-1, somato-medin C, Sm-C): protein growth factor that is produced in local or distant cells. Stimulates DNA production, cell differentiation, and production of specific cell products.

matrix vesicles: extracellular units that are involved in the initiation of calcium apatite crystal formation.

osteocalcin: vitamin K–dependent Gla protein involved in a number of bone formation processes, including the placement of calcium into mature apatite crystals; **bone Gla protein.**

parathyroid hormone (PTH): long-chain polypeptide involved in bone crystal removal and elevation of serum calcium; has multiple functions in that it affects the increase of calcium retention by the kidneys and has many other metabolic effects.

phosphoproteins: type of protein generated by bone cells. There are at least three different ones, and their function is unknown.

RGD: abbreviation for an amino acid sequence of arginine, glycine, and aspartine that is seen characteristically in adhesive proteins such as laminen.

transforming growth factor superfamily: a group of cytokines associated with cartilage and bone stimulation. This family includes the bone morphogenic proteins.

vitamin D: although a vitamin, it is metabolized by the body and functions as a hormone. Vitamin D is changed chemically by the liver and kidney, aiding in the absorption of calcium by the gut, retention of calcium by the kidney, and removal and replacement process in bone metabolism. Related terms are the following.

1,25-dihydroxycholecalciferol (equivalent of **1,25-dihydroxyvitamin D_3** and **1.25-DHCC**)

25-hydroxycholecalciferol (equivalent of **25-HCC) 24,25-dihydroxycholecalciferol**

Wolff's law: the clinical observation that states bone will form and remodel in the direction of forces acting on it.

ELECTROBIOLOGY

Over the past 20 years, the application of electrical or magnetic fields about fracture sites has been found to stimulate bone formation in the presence of fracture nonunion. The electrical stimulation is done by the direct insertion of electrodes into bone using a continuous current. Another method of treatment involves the external application of magnets with the field driven by an external electrical current. As a result of years of research, electrical or magnetic stimulation is now an approved form of treatment. Terms commonly used in reference to this work are the following:

anode: an electrical pole that has a positive charge and attracts negative ions.

capacitor (capacitive coupling): in orthopaedic bone stimulation application, not a true capacitor. Two plates are placed parallel to a resistor and applied to the skin on opposite sides of a nonunion. A high-frequency (60 kHz) current then produces small currents in the deep tissues.

cathode: an electrical pole that has a negative charge and attracts cations, which are positively charged ions. In the stimulation of bone formation this is the active pole around which the bone is formed.

magnetic field: the magnetic force field developed as a result of a fluctuating electrical current. The field has polarity that is described by north and south poles. In the stimulation of fracture healing, the magnetic polarity is directed so that the forces are perpendicular to the site of the fracture.

Clinically used electromagnetic pulses are of two general types. One is a short burst of rapid pulses with repetitions of 15 times per second. This pulse is used mostly in nonunion bone stimulation. The second is a single wider pulse at 72–75 Hz used to stimulate vascular ingrowth such as in avascular necrosis; **pulsed electromagnetic fields (PEMF).**

stress-generated potentials (SGP): any electrical potential produced by mechanical deformation of tissues, particularly bone cartilage and ligaments.

piezoelectric potentials: a charge that is developed on molecular surface of a material, such as bone collagen and apatite crystals due to bending of that material.

streaming potentials: potentials created near the charged molecular surface created by the passage of charged ions in fluids during the course of deformation.

zeta potential: the relative electrical potential produced at the point of the slip plane of passing fluid that contains electrically charged ions. This slip plane is usually 7 Å from the surface.

CARTILAGE AND JOINTS

The surface of bone at the joint is covered with a glistening white to blue-white tissue called hyaline cartilage. This cartilage is composed of living cells that slowly replace themselves, getting nourishment from the circulation in bone and fluid in the joint. For the most part, there is no vascular circulation in cartilage. The matrix, material between the cells, is composed of collagen and proteoglycan aggregates. Since much of the research on bone and soft tissues involves collagen, these terms are listed separately.

Proteoglycans are found in almost all tissues of the body. However, cartilage has a relative much higher concentration of proteoglycans. Proteoglycans come in many forms, depending on the anatomic location. The basic structure of proteoglycan aggregates is a number of proteoglycan subunits composed of specific glycosaminoglycans attached to the protein core. The subunits are then attached by link protein to hyaluronic-acid chain. The final structure is a molecule that may well have a molecular weight of well over a million. The glycosaminoglycans that make up the side chain of these subunits will vary from one area of the body to the next and will also vary in specific glycosaminoglycan disorders. The various subunits are described with specific chemical compounds.

aggrecan (proteoglycan subunit): large proteoglycan composed of a core protein with numerous GAG chains covalently attached; forms aggregates with hyaluronic acid and link protein.

biglycan (DPG-I): core protein with two GAG chains.

cathepsins: a variety of lysosomal enzymes that can degrade matrix components.

chondrocalcin: 35-kDa protein found in the epiphyseal (bone growth) plate. It is involved in the formation of calcium apatite crystals in the area of hypertrophied cartilage. This is also known as C propeptide (CPII) for its derivation from the cleavage of C propeptide from type II procollagen.

chondroitin sulfate: a sulfated sugar with 40 to 60 repeating units of glucuronic acid (glucuronate) and N-acetylgalactosamine; makes up part of aggrecan chondroitin sulfate C (dermatan sulfate).

core protein: the central protein of the proteoglycan subunit.

decorin (DPG-II): core protein associated with a single GAG.

glucosamine: glucose with a nitrogen-containing group. It is a hexosamine.

glycosaminoglycans (GAG, mucopolysaccharides): linear sugar polymers of repeating disaccharides, usually acid, and containing an amino sugar and sugar.

keratan sulfate: a GAG with 5 to 20 repeating units of galactose and N-acetylglucosamine; makes up part of aggrecan.

hyaluronic acid: GAG of glucuronic acid (glucuronate) and N-acetylglucosamine that makes up the core of the proteoglycan aggregate.

hyaluronidase: enzyme that breaks up hyaluronic acid.

link protein: specific 44,000 to 50,000 molecular weight protein that connects proteoglycan subunit to hyaluronic acid chain.

proteoglycan: protein chain associated with amine sugar side chains that may contain highly charged sulfate and carboxyl groups.

proteoglycan aggregate: complex structure of proteoglycan subunits attached by link protein to hyaluronic acid chains (Fig. 13–1).

stromelysin (metalloproteinase II): specific lysozyme for cleavage of aggrecans from hyaluronic acid; has other actions.

FIG 13–1.
Synthesis and degradation of type II collagen, one of a family of 17 or more collagens that are characterized by the triple helix. Antibodies developed in rabbit and mice can be used to detect minimal (ng/ml) quantities of these biochemical products. (Courtesy of A. Robin Poole, PhD, DSc, Director, Joint Diseases Laboratory.)

COLLAGEN

Collagen is a protein material found in all connective tissues of the body. It is the basic ingredient in gelatin. Collagen is produced by cells and acts as the supporting structure that lends cohesion to a variety of connective tissues. Bone is almost purely a combination of collagen and bone crystals. Some collagen is found in cartilage. The tendons and ligaments are composed mostly of collagen, but the mix of collagens is slightly different type than the collagen found in bone.

There are now at least 17 types of collagen known. All collagens are characterized by a portion of the molecule containing a triple helical region or regions where the three protein chains have a gly-x-y amino acid repeat. Bone is predominantly made up of a fibrillar collagen called type I collagen, composed of two $\alpha1$ chains and one $\alpha2$ chain. On the other hand, cartilage is composed mostly of type II collagen, which is composed of three identical $\alpha1$ chains. The following terms are related to collagen metabolism.

collagenase: enzyme that breaks down collagen molecules.

cross-linking: the chemical attachment of molecular chains to make fibrils and fibrils to make collagen fibers.

fiber: when applied to collagen, denotes the complete collagen fiber that is composed of many collagen fibrils.

fibril: mature collagen with intermolecular cross-links completed.

hydroxylysine: amino acid that is hydroxylated after incorporation into protocollagen.

hydroxylisinonorleucine: an amino acid important in cross-linking.

hydroxyproline: amino acid that is hydroxylated after incorporation into protocollagen.

hydroxypyridinoline: an amino acid important in cross-linking of collagen to stabilize collagen molecules in fibrils.

lysinonorleucine: an amino acid important in cross-linking of collagen to stabilize collagen molecules in fibrils.

procollagen: triple-helical collagen molecule that has C and N terminal nonhelical propeptides that are cleaved in the matrix after the procollagen molecule is incorporated into the fibril. (Fig. 13-2).

pyridinoline: an amino acid important in cross-linking of collagen to stabilize collagen molecules in fibrils.

BIOMECHANICS

The terms used in biomechanics come more from a physics textbook than from anything normally seen in orthopaedics. The "loads" on bones, muscles, and joints can be studied from the static and dynamic standpoints, looking at forces, work accomplished, and any deformation. The energy absorbed by the system is analyzed with an eye to the deformation and recovery or permanent deformity resulting from the deformation, as in fractures and ruptures. Because much of the tissue is complex, there are peculiarities in its responses that prompt study of elasticity is various structures under the heading of **viscoelasticity.**

The study of motion and the forces that produced the motion is known as **kinesiology.** In human research, the interest in the relationship of motion between two parts of the body, such as the leg and thigh, is known as **kinematics.** The gliding of joints is studied in terms of lubrication and viscoelasticity.

Another area of research in biomechanics is the field of design. The shape and material composition of implants are studied from the standpoints of stress, strain, deflection, fatigue, wear, and friction. The body's immunologic response to new implant materials of metals, alloys, ceramics, and plastics has enabled the musculoskeletal system to have thousands of "spare parts," available through use of engineering principles and research. With wider acceptance of

Type II collagen fibril
(contains type XI collagen)

Decorin core

HA   DS

G3

CS

CS

KS

G2

G1   Link

Type IX
collagen

CS

— 100 nm

A.R. Poole, 1991

FIG 13–2.
Complex relationchip of proteoglycan to collagen that results in the ability of cartilage to tolerate forces greater than 10 atmospheres a million times a year during adult life. (From Koopman WJ: *Arthritis and allied conditions,* ed 13, Williams & Wilkins, 1996.)

implants, the field of biomechanics is drawing an ever-increasing number of nonorthopaedic members to the team.

There is considerable overlap in biomechanical terminology; therefore, the frequently used terms are in alphabetic order.

acceleration: change in velocity per unit of time.

angular acceleration: rate of change of average angular velocity. The instant center is that point about which the rotation occurs (degrees/sec^2).

linear acceleration: rate of change of velocity in a straight line (m/sec^2).

allowable stress: a stress value that is higher than that of normal loads but is lower than the yield stress of the material. The unit of measure is newtons per square meters (pascals) or pounds per square inch.

angular displacement: change of angular position of a line measured in degrees.

anisotropic material: a material in which the mechanical properties vary depending on the spatial direction of forces.

average angular velocity: angular displacement divided by the time taken for that displacement (degrees/sec).

average velocity: displacement divided by the time taken for that displacement (cm/sec).

bending: deformation of a structure in response to a load applied to an unsupported portion of that structure.

bending moment: a quantity at a point in a structure equal to the product of the force applied and the shortest distance from the point to the line along which the force is acting. The unit of measure is newton meters or foot-pound force.

bending moment diagram: a diagram showing amount of bending moment at various sections of a long structure subjected to bending loads.

biomechanical adaptations: biologically mediated changes in the mechanical properties of tissues (material properties and/or structural changes) in association with the application of mechanical variables to those tissues.

brittle failure: failure by fracture before permanent deformation occurs, for example, breaking glass versus plastic failure seen in the bending of a willow stick.

centroid: center of gravity for an object; the points of balance for an area; if you hang an area by the centroid, it will not rotate under its own weight.

center of gravity (center of mass): point in a body where the body mass is centered.

coefficient of friction: the ratio of tangential force to the interbody compressive force required to initiate motion between the two bodies. No units of measure.

compliance: amount of deformation caused by one unit of load.

compression: the force that tends to push two objects together, the unit of measure is newtons or foot-pound force (negative number).

couple: a pair of equal and opposite parallel forces acting on a body and separated by a distance. The moment or torque of a couple is defined as a quantity equal to the product of one of the forces and the perpendicular distance between the forces. The unit of measure for the torque is newton meters or foot-pound force.

coupling: a phenomenon of consistent association of one motion (translation or rotation) about an axis with another motion about a second axis. One motion cannot be produced without the other.

creep: the viscoelastic deformation of a material with time when it is subjected to a constant, suddenly applied load. The deformation-time curve approaches a steady state asymptomatically.

degrees of freedom: the number of independent coordinates in a coordinate system required to completely define the position of an object in space.

displacement: change in the position of a particle; compared with a specific point of reference when studying deformation or other motion.

ductile failure: failure of a structure because of excessive plastic deformation, such as pulling on a wire, with stretching and eventual breakage.

ductility: the property of a material to absorb relatively large amounts of plastic deformation energy before deformation. The opposite is brittleness.

dynamic load: a load that varies with time.

elastic behavior: exhibited when deformation caused by a load returns to original position when the load is removed, as in a rubber band.

elastic modulus: an index of the force on an object per unit of deformation.

elongation: the amount of deformation caused by a tensile stress or load; a measure of ductility.

energy: the ability to do work; the amount of work done by a load on a body, measured in newton meters or foot-pound force.

equilibrium: the condition of a body that is not accelerating; the sum of all forces acting on an object is zero. To clarify, an object will remain still or move in the same direction or at the same angular velocity unless there is some external force applied to change it; **Newton's law.**

fatigue failure: failure by fatigue either with or without permanent deformation, caused by cyclic loading; for example, to bend a paper clip a number of times to point of breaking.

fatigue fracture: a fracture or break in a material caused by repeated applications of loads that are less than the yield strength but greater than the fatigue limit.

fatigue limit: the load a material can endure indefinitely without bending or breaking when subjected to cyclic loading.

fatigue strength (endurance limit): the maximum load a material can withstand indefinitely without fracture.

force: any action that tends to change the state of rest or of motion of a body to which it is applied; unit of measure is newtons or pound force.

free-body analysis: a technique for determining the stresses at a point in a structure subjected to external loads.

helical axis of motion: a unique axis in space that completely defines a three-dimensional motion between two rigid bodies, analogous to instantaneous axis of rotation for plane motion.

hysteresis: a phenomenon associated with energy loss exhibited by viscoelastic materials when they are subjected to loading and unloading cycles.

impulse: product of the force and the time interval of application; measured in newton seconds or pound force seconds.

inertia: the property of all materials bodies to resist change in the state of rest or motion under the actioin of applied loads.

instantaneous axis of rotation: when a body moves in a plane, there is a point in the body or some hypothetical extension of it that does not move. An axis perpendicular to the plane of motion and passing through that point is the instantaneous axis (center) of rotation.

isotropic: the properties of a material are the same for all directions.

joule: unit of energy (work), unit of measure; 1 newton times 1 meter (newton meter).

kilopond (Kp): a force equal to the gravitational force applied to 1 kilogram of mass at the earth's surface; term becoming obsolete.

kinematics: division of mechanics (dynamics) that deals with the geometry of the motion of bodies; displacement, acceleration, and velocity, without taking into account the forces that produce the motion.

kinetic energy: the value assigned to the energy of a moving object.

loading: any force applied to an object. In orthopaedics, the normal forces acting on bone, joints, tendons, or ligaments, are called **functional loads,** loads that distract are **tensile loads,** and those that compress are **compressive loads.**

lubrication: means by which contact friction is affected.

> **boundary lubrication:** load carried by asperity (uneven) contacts through thin surface layers.
>
> **film lubrication:** load carried by a fluid film that separates the surfaces.
>
> **lambda ratio (λ):** compares fluid film thickness to surface roughness.
>
> **mixed film:** load carried both by asperity (uneven) contacts and fluid film.

mass moment of inertia: the quantitative measure of inertia for change in angular velocity. The unit of measure is kilogram meter squared or pound foot squared.

modulus of elasticity: the ratio of normal stress to normal strain in a material. The unit of measure for the modulus of elasticity (E) is newtons per square meter or pound force per square foot.

moment: quantity necessary to angularly accelerate a mass.

moment of inertia of an area: a measure of the area of a material in a certain manner about its centroid. The distribution is proportional to the strength in bending. The unit of measure is meters (or feet) to the fourth power.

momentum: product of mass and velocity of a moving body, may be angular or linear. When linear, the unit of measure is kilogram meters per second or pound feet per second.

newton: amount of force required to give a 1 kilogram mass an acceleration of 1 meter per second.

normal strain: the quantity described by the quotient of the change of length of a line and its original length.

normal stress: the quantity described by the quotient of distributed force and area when the force is perpendicular to the area.

pascal: newton per square meter.

plastic behavior: exhibited when deformation caused by a load does not return to the original position when the load is removed; for example, stretching gum.

plasticity: the property of a material to permanently deform when it is loaded beyond its elastic range.

Poisson's ratio: the ratio of transverse to axial strain, generally noted by the Greek letter ν (nu), and no unit of measure.

polar moment of inertia: a property of a crosssection of a long structure that gives a measure of the distribution of the material about its axis, proportional to torsional strength and stiffness. The unit of measure is meter or foot to the fourth power.

potential energy: energy that may be stored within a structure as a result of deformation or displacement of that structure. The unit of measure is newton meters (joules) or foot pound force.

rigidity: the amount of load required to give a structure one unit of deformation; same as **elastic modulus.**

shear modulus: the ratio of shear stress to the shear strain in a material. The unit of measure is newtons per square meter (pascals) or pound force per square foot.

shear strain: the change in angle between two lines originally at right angles in a solid (measured in radians).

shear stress: the quantity described by the quotient of force and the area, when the force is applied parallel to the area.

SI units: system of international units such as meter, kilogram, second, and Centigrade degree.

statics: the branch of mechanics that deals with the equilibrium of bodies at rest or in motion with zero acceleration.

stiffness: a measure of resistance offered to external loads by a specimen or structure as it deforms.

stiffness coefficient: the property of a structure defined by the ratio of force applied to the deformation produced. It quantifies the resistance that a structure offers to deformation.

strain: the change in length per unit length or in an angle of a material subjected to a load.

strain energy: energy stored in a body by virtue of its being deformed under the application of a load; for example, a spring.

strength: the maximal load that a structure can withstand before functional failure occurs (load strength) or the maximal energy that a structure can withstand before functional failure occurs (energy strength).

stress: the force per unit area of a structure and a measurement of the intensity of the force. Stress may be compressive, forces directed into the material; tensile, forces away from or distracting the material; or shear, forces parallel to the surface. Units of measure are newtons per square meter or pound force per square foot.

stress-strain diagram: the plot of stress, usually on y axis, versus strain, usually on x axis. Also called **load deformation curve.**

tension: force pulling a body apart (positive number).

torque: the force acting about a pivot point described by force times distance from the pivot point.

torr: a measure of pressure; one torr equals 1 mmHg pressure. One standard atmospheric pressure is equivalent to 760 torr.

torsion: a type of load that is applied by a couple of forces that are parallel and directed opposite to each other about the long axis of a structure.

torsional rigidity: the torque per unit of angular deformation. The unit of measure is newton meters per radian or foot-pound force per degree.

toughness: the ability of a material to absorb energy by bending without breaking.

ultimate load: the largest load a structure can sustain without failure. The unit of measure is newtons or pound force if the load is a force and newton meters or foot-pound force if the load is a torque or moment.

vector: a quantity that has both magnitude and direction.

viscoelasticity: the property of a material to show sensitivity to the rate of loading or deformation

viscoelastic stability: the type of stability in which the critical load is a function of time as well as the geometric and material properties of the structure.

viscosity: the property of materials to resist loads that produce shear; the ratio of shearing stress to shearing strain rate; the ratio of shearing stress to velocity gradient. Commonly represented by η (eta) or μ (mu). The unit of measure is newton seconds per square meter, or pound force per square foot, and poise (1 poise = 0.1 newton seconds per square meter).

wear: progressive loss of surface material due to relative motion of interacting surfaces.

   abrasive wear: wear due to gouging of soft surface elements by hard surface elements.

   adhesive wear: wear due to localized bonding, which pulls the wear particles from the surface.

   fatigue wear: wear due to repetitive loading of localized regions causing surface and subsurface cracks to propagate, leading to material fracture.

weight: the force applied by gravitational pull.

work: the product of force multiplied by the displacement through which the force moves.

yield stress: that point of stress on the load deformation curve at which appreciable deformation takes place without any appreciable increase in load. The unit of measure is newtons per square meter or pound force per square foot.

BIOMATERIALS

Historically many different types of materials have been used in attempts to replace bone and joints artificially. Wood, ceramics, and unsophisticated metals were the first materials used, and later metal alloys, including Vitallium and stainless steel, were accepted as having the least wear problems associated with little reaction from the body.

Research into biomaterials is currently directed at long-term use of joint replacement materials. From a bioengineering standpoint, loosening, fatigue failure, and wear are the major problems being investigated. Porous materials that allow bony ingrowth are being researched for the potential development of devices that do not require the use of polymethylmethacrylate "cement" fixation. Biodegradable materials for fracture fixation are also being studied.

metal alloy: a combination of metallic elements with no chemical bonding, but where the combination renders sought-after characteristics of nonreactiveness, durability, and certain biomechanical characteristics. Some standard alloys and some being investigated are the following:
cobalt chrome
Elgiloy
HS25
MP35N
multiphase alloy
nitrided titanium 6-4
stainless steel 316L
titanium
titanium 6-4
Vitallium

bioceramics: ceramic materials composed of glass, glass metals, or metal combinations, resulting in smooth, form-holding products; used mostly in joint replacement. Types are the following:
Alumina
Low-surface reactive bioglass
Nearly inert bioceramics
Resorbable bioceramics

Plastics

Plastics have been available for nearly a century. Plastics similar to what is seen in plastic bags have been polymerized to produce very strong, compacted plastic, which although not perfect, can tolerate repeated high force for years. Plastics are also used to create absorbable temporary sutures or scaffolds for tissue transplantation. The following are some biomaterial plastics used in orthopaedics.

absorbable scaffold (scaffold): a number of synthetic polymer meshes, pads, and porous lattice have been developed for tissue ingrowth. These polymers include **polyglycolic acid, polylactic acid (PLA), poly-L-lactone, polybutalone,** and **polylactide/glycolide (DL-lactic-co-glycolic acid = PLGA).**

ultrahigh molecular-weight polyethylene (UHMWPE): general term for plastic material where particles are pressed, with and without graphite fiber reinforcement, under very high pressures. Brands include **Enduron** and **Hylamer-M.**

synthetic ligaments: There are two basic types of synthetic ligaments under investigation: those that have cells growing into the fabric, and those that rely entirely on their structure. Some of the materials used are the following:
Carbon fiber
Coated carbon fiber
Dacron tape
Gortex
Polypropylene
Proplast
Woven bovine collagen
Zenotech

Appendix A

Orthopaedic Abbreviations

Many abbreviations are used in orthopaedic terminology that are not used by the general medical profession. The Joint Commission on Accreditation of Health Organizations (JCAHO) has directed that each hospital establish a standard list that is used and known by all specialties. However, the orthopaedic physician uses many more to expediently fulfill his needs in a clinical situation. The "physician's shorthand" given here is a compendium for recognition as a reference only.

Care must be taken when using abbreviations. In some cases, a single abbreviation may serve for several words. For example, the abbreviation "quad" could refer to quadrilateral (hip), quadriceps (musculature), and quadriplegic (paralysis). Therefore, consider the context of the material being read to determine which word is used. References vary widely in the use of capitalization of abbreviations.

DISEASES, CONDITIONS, AND SYNDROMES

AIDS: acquired immunodeficiency syndrome

ALPSA: anterior labrum periosteum shoulder arthroscopic lesion

ALRI: anterolateral rotatory instability (knee)

ALS: amyotrophic lateral sclerosis; anterolateral sclerosis

APC: anteroposterior compression (fracture)

ARDS: adult respiratory distress syndrome

AS: arteriosclerosis; aortic stenosis

ASI: acromial spur index

AVF: arteriovenous fistula

AVM: arteriovenous malformation

BIL: biceps interval lesion

CA: carcinoma

CHF: congestive heart failure

CP: cerebral palsy

CPPD: calcium pyrophosphate deposition (disease)

CREST: *c*aleinosis, *R*aynaud, *e*sophageal, *s*clerodactyly, *t*elangiectasia

CVA: cerebrovascular accident (stroke)

DDH: developmental dysplasia of the hip

DISI: dorsiflexed intercalated segment instability

DisI: dislocation

DJD: degenerative joint disease

DOMS: delayed-onset muscle soreness

DVT: deep vein thrombosis

EBV: Epstein-Barr virus

EDS: Ehlers-Danlos syndrome

FA: false aneurysm

FB: foreign body

FFC: fixed flexion contracture

fract or fx: fracture

FUO: fever of undetermined origin

HIV: human immunodeficiency virus

HNP: herniated nucleus pulposus

IDK: internal derangement of the knee

INFH: ischemic necrosis of femoral head

ITT: internal tibial torsion

LAD: ligamentous anterior dislocation

LCP: Legg-Calvé-Perthes disease

LE: lupus erythematosus

LLD: leg length discrepancy

LOM: limitation of motion

MACS: MAST-associated compartment syndrome

MCI: midcarpal instability

MD: muscular dystrophy

MESS: mangled extremity severity score (fractures)

MI: myocardial infarction

MS: multiple sclerosis

OA: osteoarthritis

OCD: osteochondritis dissecans

PE: pulmonary embolism

PFC: pelvic flexion contracture

PFFD: proximal femoral focal deficiency

PID: pelvic inflammatory disease

PMD: progressive muscular dystrophy

polio: poliomyelitis

PVC: premature ventricular contraction

PVD: peripheral vascular disease

quad atrophy: quadriceps atrophy

RA: rheumatoid arthritis

RSD: reflex sympathetic dystrophy

SAPHO: synovitis-acne-pustulosis-hyperostosis-osteomyelitis syndrome

SCFE: slipped capital femoral epiphysis

SLAP: superior labrum anterior to posterior (shoulder lesion)

SLE: systemic lupus erythematosus

SMA: spinal muscular atrophy

SMPS: sympathetic maintained pain syndrome

staph: *Staphylococcus* or implies *Staphylococcus aureus* species

strep: *Streptococcus*

sympt or sx: symptoms

TB: tuberculosis

TIA: transient ischemic attack

THR: total hip replacement

TMJ(s):   temporomandibular joint (syndrome)

TSS: toxic shock syndrome

URI: upper respiratory (tract) infection

UTI: urinary tract infection

VATER: *v*ertebral, *a*nd *t*racheosophogeal, *e*sophogeal, *r*adical

VDDR: vitamin D–dependent rickets

VDRR: vitamin D–resistant rickets

VISI: volar flexed intercalated segment instability

VS: vertical shear (fractures)

GENERAL ANATOMY

abd: abdomen

ANS: autonomic nervous system

ant: anterior

AV: arteriovenous; atrioventricular

BB to MM: belly button to medial malleolus (examination)

CNS: central nervous system

collat: collateral (ligament)

CSF: cerebrospinal fluid

CV: cardiovascular

D/3, distal/3:   distal third

DP: dorsalis pedis (pulse)

GB: gallbladder

GI: gastrointestinal

GU: genitourinary

HEENT: head, ears, eyes, nose, throat (examination)

inf: inferior

lig: ligature; ligament

LLL: left lower limb

LLQ: left lower quadrant

LSK: liver, spleen, and kidneys

LUL: left upper limb

LUQ: left upper quadrant

M/3, middle/3:   middle third

med: medial

mm: muscles; mucous membrane; millimeter

NV: neurovascular

P/3, proximal/3:   proximal third

PERRLA: pupils equal, round, regular to light accommodation

PNS: peripheral nervous system

PVS: peripheral vascular system

post: posterior

px: pneumothorax

quad: quadriceps; quadrilateral; quadriplegic

RLL: right lower limb

RLQ: right lower quadrant

RUL: right upper limb

RUQ: right upper quadrant

sup: superior

SPECIFIC ANATOMY

AAL or ant ax line: anterior axillary line

AC: acromioclavicular (joint)

ASIS: anterosuperior iliac spine

C-1 to C-7:   cervical vertebrae

C-spine: cervical spine

cva: costovertebral angle

CVA: cerebrovascular accident

D-spine: dorsal spine*

GHL: glenohumeral ligament

ICS: intercostal space (ribs)

*When reference is made to the dorsal and thoracic spines, they are one and the same. T-spine or D-spine may be used in clinical notes.

IS: interspace

L-1 to L-5:   lumbar vertebrae

LS: lumbosacral (spine)

L-spine: lumbar spine

MAL: midaxillary line

MCL: midclavicular line

MSL: midsternal line

PAL: posterior axillary line

PSIS: posterosuperior iliac spine

S-1 to S-5:   sacral vertebrae

SC: sternoclavicular (joint)

SI: sacroiliac (joint)

T-1 to T-12:   thoracic vertebrae

T-spine: thoracic spine*

Hand (Anatomy)

ADQ/ADM: abductor digiti quinti (or minimi)

abd poll: abductor pollicis

add poll: adductor pollicis

ADQ/ADM: abductor digiti quinti (or minimi)

APB: abductor pollicis brevis

APL: abductor pollicis longus

CMC: carpometacarpal

DIP: distal interphalangeal (joint); DIPJ

DP: distal phalanx

DPC: distal palmar crease

DRUJ: distal radioulnar joint

ECRB: extensor carpi radialis brevis

ECRL: extensor carpi radialis longus

ECU: extensor carpi ulnaris

EDC: extensor digitorum communis

EDL: extensor digitorum longus

EDQ/EDM: extensor digiti quinti (or minimi)

EIP: extensor indicis proprius

EPB: extensor pollicis brevis

EPL: extensor pollicis longus

FCR: flexor carpi radialis

FCU: flexor carpi ulnaris

FDL: flexor digitorum longus

FDP: flexor digitorum profundus

FDQB: flexor digiti quinti brevis

FDS: flexor digitorum sublimis (or superficialis)

FPB: flexor pollicis brevis

FPL: flexor pollicis longus

IP: interphalangeal (joint)

MC: metacarpal; midcarpal

MCP: metacarpophalangeal (joint)

MP: middle phalanx (or metaphalangeal) joint

MPC: midpalmar crease

ODQ/ODM: opponens digiti quinti (or minimi)

OP: opponens pollicis

PB: peroneus brevis

phal: phalanx or phalanges

PIP: proximal interphalangeal (joint); PIPJ

PL: palmaris longus

PP: proximal phalanx

PQ: pronator quadratus

PT: pronator teres

RC: radiocarpal

TPC: thenar palmar crease

UN: ulnar nerve (finger spreader)

Fingers

1st digit: thumb

2nd digit: index

3rd digit: long

4th digit: ring

5th digit: little

Hand (Diseases, Conditions)

CID: carpal instability dissociative

CIND: carpal instability, nondissociative

CLIP: capitolunate instability pattern

CTS: carpal tunnel syndrome

DISI: dorsal intercalated segment instability

MCI: midcarpal instability (volar, palmar, extrinsic)

PA: psoriatic arthritis

PSS: progressive systemic sclerosis

RSD: reflex sympathetic dystrophy

SLAC: scapholunate advanced collapse

SLE: systemic lupus erythematosus

VISI: volar intercalated segment instability

VATER: vertebral anomalies, anal atresia, tracheo-esophageal fistula, renal and vascular anomalies

Hand (Surgery)

AA: advancement ulnar arm of arcuate ligament

DC: dorsal capsulodesis

FQF: four-quadrant fusion

THF: triquetrohamate fusion

TLR: triquetrohamate ligament reconstruction

NC: neuroma-in-continuity

VC: volar capsulodesis

Foot and Ankle

CAWA: closing abductory wedge osteotomy

DIP: distal interphalangeal (joint); DIPJ

DP: dorsalis pedis pulse

HA: hallux abductus

HD: heloma durum (hard corn)

HM: heloma molle (soft corn)

HT: hammer toe

HV: hallux valgus

IHW: inner heel wedge

IPJ: interphalangeal joint

IPK: intractable plantar keratosis

MHW: medial heel wedge

MPJ: metaphalangeal joint

MPV: metatarsus primus varus

MT bar: metatarsal bar

MTA: metatarsus adductus

MTJ: midtarsal joint

MTP: metatarsophalangeal (joint)

MTV: metatarsus varus

OAWO: opening abductory wedge esteotomy

PIP: proximal interphalangeal (joint); PIPJ

PTP: posterior tibial pulse

PW: plantar wart

STJ: subtalar joint

TEV: talipes equinovarus

TMT: tarsometatarsal

SURGICAL PROCEDURES AND RELATED TERMS

5 in 1: five procedures done during same surgery for ligamentous repair of the knee for rotatory instability.

ACS: acetabular cup system

AML: anatomic medullary locking

Anes: anesthesia

AO: Arbeitsgemeinschaft für Osteosynthcsafragen

Bx: biopsy

CCK: constrained condylar knee

CR: closed reduction

CTR: carpal tunnel release

DCP: dynamic compression plate

en bloc: in a lump; as a whole

ESIN: elastic stable intramedullary nailing

H: per hypodermic

I&D: incision and drainage

IM: intramuscular; intermuscular; intramedullary (rod)

IV: intravenous

KMFTR: Kotz modular femur and tibia resection (system)

lam: laminectomy

lami: laminotomy

LASER: light amplification by stimulated emission of radiation; lower case in context

lat men: lateral meniscectomy

LC/DCP: limited-contact dynamic-compression (plate)

LCS mb: low-contact stress meniscal bearing

LCS rp: low-contact stress rotating patella

LIFO: locked intramedullary fracture osteosynthesis

LP: lumbar puncture

MARS: modular acetabulum reconstruction system

med men: medial meniscectomy

MSD: microsurgical discectomy

OR: operating room; open reduction

ORIF: open reduction/internal fixation

OW: open wedge (osteotomy)

PCA: porous-coated anatomic

PLIF: posterolateral interbody fusion

PO, postop: postoperatively

preop: preoperatively

prog: prognosis

PTT: patellar tendon transfer

PVS: peripheral vascular surgery

QSAC: quadrant-sparing acetabular component

RR: recovery room

SDR: surgical dressing room

STSG: split-thickness skin graft

Sub-Q, SQ, SC: subcutaneous (under the skin)

surg: surgical; surgery

TAL: tendon Achilles lengthening

TC: total condylar

TG: tendon graft

THA: total hip arthroplasty

THR: total hip replacement

TJR: total joint replacement

TKA: total knee arthroplasty

TT: tendon transfer

IMAGING TECHNIQUES

AGE: angle of greatest extension

AGF: angle of greatest flexion

ASES: American Shoulder and Elbow Surgeons (scales and ratings)

AP: anteroposterior

BMP: bone marrow pressure

CAT (scan):   computed axial tomography

CPA: condylar-plateau angle

CRT: cathode-ray tube

CT: computed tomography

CXR: chest x-ray examination

DEXA: dual x-ray absorptiometry

DPA: dual photon absorptiometry

DPD: dual photon densitometry

DSA: digital subtraction angiography

FTA: femorotibial angle

Gd-DTPA: gadopentetate dimeglumine

ISIS: integrated shape imaging system

IVP: intravenous pyelogram

KUB: kidney, ureter, and bladder view of abdomen

lat: lateral

MRI: magnetic resonance imaging

obl: oblique

PA: posteroanterior

QCT: quantitative computed tomography

R: roentgen unit, x-ray examination

RA: radium

rad: radiation absorbed dose

rem: roentgen-equivalent-man

SPECT: single photon emission computed tomography

SPGR: spoiled grass (image)

STIR: short tau inversion recovery

tomo: tomogram

XIP: x-ray in plaster (examination)

XOP: x-ray out of plaster (examination)

CASTS, SPLINTS, DRESSINGS

DBS: Denis Browne splint

FWB: full weight bearing

HCTU: home cervical traction unit

ICT: intermittent cervical traction

LAC: long-arm cast

LANC: long-arm navicular cast

LAS: long-arm splint

LLC: long-leg cast

LLS: long-leg splint

LLWC: long-leg walking cast

MAST: medical antishock trousers

MESS: mangled extremity severity score

NWB: non–weight bearing

PTB: patellar tendon bearing (cast, orthosis, prosthesis)

PWB: partial weight bearing

SAC: short-arm cast

SANC: short-arm navicular cast

SAS: short-arm splint

SDD: sterile dry dressing

SLC: short-leg cast

SLS: short-leg splint

tx: traction

PROSTHETICS AND ORTHOTICS

Amputation and Prosthesis Sites

AE: above elbow

AK: above knee

BE: below elbow

BK: below knee

ED: elbow disarticulation

HD: hip disarticulation

SD: shoulder disarticulation

WD: wrist disarticulation

General Terms

AML: anatomic medullary locking (total hip replacement)

APRL: Army Prosthetics Research Lab

ATH: anthropometric total hip

BFO: balanced forearm orthosis

CAD-CAM: computer-assisted design–computer-assisted manufacturing

CASH: cruciform anterior spinal hyperextension orthosis

CAT-CAM: contour-adducted trochanteric–controlled alignment method

CO: certified orthotist

CP: certified prosthetist

CPO: certified prosthetist and orthotist

CROW: Charcot restraint orthotic walker

CTO: cervicothoracic orthosis

CTSO: cervical thoracolumbosacral orthosis

DANA: designed after natural anatomy (prosthesis)

GSH: Green-Seligson Henry (nail)

IPSF: immediate postsurgical fitting

KB: knee bearing

LSP: lumbrosacral orthosis

M/L: medial lateral (narrow M/L)

NSNA: normal shape, normal alignment

NYU: New York University (inserts)

OKC: Oklahoma City cable (system)

PCA: porous-coated anatomic (total hip replacement)

PPO: passive prehension orthosis

PTB: patella tendon bearing; pretibial bearing (socket type)

PTBO: patellar tendon bearing orthosis

PTBS: patellar tendon bearing suspension

PTB-SC: patellar tendon-bearing–supracondylar

PTB-SP: patellar tendon-bearing–suprapatellar

PTS: patellar tendon socket

RGO: reciprocating gait orthosis

SACH: solid ankle cushioned heel

SAFE: stationary ankle flexible endoskeletal (foot)

SC: supracondylar

SCOPE: Sacramento, California orthotic-prosthetic evaluation

SCSP: supracondylar-suprapatellar

SOMI: sternal-occiput-mandibular immobilization orthosis

SP: suprapatellar

SPC: suprapatellar cuff

STEN: stored energy

TLSO: thoracic lumbosacral orthosis

TTAP: threaded titanium acetabular prosthesis

UCB: University of California (Berkeley) orthosis (Additional abbreviations within the chapter)

PHYSICAL MEDICINE AND OCCUPATIONAL THERAPY (EXERCISES AND TESTS)

A(ROM): active range of motion

AA: active-assistive (range of motion)

ABD: abduction

ADL: activities of daily living

ADD: adduction

AG: antigravity

AGE: angle of greatest extension

AGF: angle of greatest flexion

BME: brief maximal effort

CMS: circulation, muscle sensation

DKB: deep knee bends

DTRs: deep tendon reflexes

ERE: external rotation in extension

ERF: external rotation in flexion

FABER: flexion in abduction and external rotation

FADIR: flexion in adduction and internal rotation

FES: functional electrical stimulation

FF: further flexion

FFC: fixed flexion contracture

IRE: internal rotation in extension

IRF: internal rotation in flexion

MENS: microamperage electrical nerve stimulation

MMT: manual muscle testing

MT: muscle testing

OT: occupational therapy

P: passive

PCE (Smith):   physical capacities evaluation

PEMF: pulsating electromagnetic fields

PFC: pelvic flexion contracture

PNF: proprioceptive neuromuscular facilitation

PR: pelvic rock

PREs: progressive resistive exercises

PT: physical therapy

RICE: rest, ice, compression, elevation

RM: repetition maximum

ROM: range of motion

SLR: straight leg raising

TENS: transcutaneous electrical nerve stimulation

TT: tilt table

WC: wheelchair

WEST: work evaluation systems technology

WFE or Wms flex ex: Williams flexion exercises

∥ bars: parallel bars

Reflex Tests

aJ: ankle jerks

bJ: biceps jerks

eJ: elbow jerks

kJ: knee jerks

tJ: triceps jerks

Physical Therapy Modalities

CB: contrast baths

EMG: electromyography

HP: hot packs

HT: Hubbard tank

IR: infrared (light)

MWD: microwave diathermy

NCV: nerve conduction velocity

PB: paraffin baths

SWD: shortwave diathermy

US: ultrasound

UV: ultraviolet (light)

WPB: whirlpool bath

RESEARCH

ANOVA   analysis of variance

ELISA: enzyme-linked immunosorbent assay

cpm: counts per minute

Da: Dalton

GAG: glycosaminoglycans

Gla: γ-carboxyglutamic acid

Gpa: gigapascal

HPLC: high-performance (pressure) liquid chromatography

Hz: hertz

Kp: Kilopond

PEMF: pulsed electromagnetic fields

PPM: parts per million

PTH: parathyroid hormone

SEM: scanning electron microscopy

SGP: stress-generated potentials

TEM: transmission electron microscopy

TIMP: tissue inhibitor of metalloproteinase

UHMWPE: ultrahigh molecular weight polyethylene

MISCELLANEOUS

abd: abdominal (pad)

adm: admission

ASAP: as soon as possible

ASES:

BP: blood pressure

c̄: with; cum

C: Centigrade

Cath: catheter

CC: chief complaint

c/o: complaint of

CPR: cardiopulmonary resuscitation

decub: decubitus position; lying down

DIE: died in emergency room

disch: discharge

DL: danger list

DNR: do not resuscitate

DOA: date of admission; dead on arrival

DOE: date of examination

Dx or diag: diagnosis

ECG, EKG: electrocardiograph(gram)

EDC: estimated date of confinement

EEG: electroencephalograph(gram)

EOM: extraocular movement

expir: expiration

F: Fahrenheit

FH: family history

H&P: history and physical (examination)

HPI: history of present illness

Hx: history

L&W: living and well

mx: management

NB: note well

OD: oculus dexter (right eye); overdose

OPD: outpatient department

OS: oculus sinister (left eye). Also abbreviated OL.

OU: both eyes

p̄: after

P&A: percussion and auscultation

PE, Px: physical examination

PH: past history

PI: present illness

PMHx: past medical history

PRN: whenever necessary

prog: prognosis

pt: patient

PTA: prior to admission

R/O: rule out

ROS, SR: review of systems

RR: relative risk

RRE: round, regular, and equal

RTC: return to clinic

RV: return visit

s̄: without

SH: social history

SL: serious list

SOS: if necessary

stat: immediately

TPR: temperature, pulse, respiration

TPN: total parenteral nutrition (IM, IV, subcutaneous, intramedullary)

tx: treatment

VSL: very serious list

WD, WN: well developed, well nourished

WNL: within normal limits

x̄: except

⊖ **or ō:** negative

+ **or** ⊕**:** positive

Δ: difference, deltoid muscle

↑: increase

↓: decrease

>: greater than

<: less than

♂**:** male

♀**:** female

1°: primary

2°: secondary

3°: tertiary

PRESCRIPTIONS (℞)

Forms

amp: ampule

aq, aqu: aqueous; water solution

ASA: aspirin

caps: capsules

cpd: compound

ETOH: alcohol

fl: fluid

med: medicine

prep: preparation

quant: quantity

℞ (Latin): to take; recipe

sol, soln: solution

tabs: tablets

Amounts

dr, ℨ: dram (4 ml)

g: gram (15 grain)

gr: grain (60 milligram)

gt: drop

gtt: drops (0.05 ml)

kg: kilogram (1,000 gram)

mg: milligram (1/60 grain)

oz, ℥: ounce (8 dram, 30 ml)

qt: quart (32 oz, 0.946 liter)

s̈s̈: ½ (e.g., gt s̈s̈ = ½ drop)

wt: weight

Directions

Sig: let it be labeled; directions

When:

ac: before meals

ad lib: as desired

ASAP: as soon as possible

c̄c: with meals

dc, D/C: discontinue

hs: at bedtime

p̄: after

pc: after meals

pp: after meals (postprandial)

sos: repeat once if need exists

stat: immediately

sum: take

ut dict: as directed

How often:

bid: twice a day (ii)

prn, PRN: as often as necessary; ad lib

q: every

qam: every morning

qd: every day

qh: every hour

q3h: every 3 hours

qid: four times a day (iiii)

qn: every night

qod: every other day

qpm: every afternoon or evening

qs or QS: as much as suffices; quantity sufficient

quotid: daily

tid: three times a day (iii)

Where:

IM: intramuscular (injection)

IV: intravenous (injection)

NPO: nihil per os (nothing per mouth)

po: per os

pr: per rectum

Sub-Q: subcutaneous

NOTE: More specific laboratory abbreviations remain within that chapter.

Appendix B

Anatomic Positions and Directions

In orthopaedics, anatomic positions and directions are frequently used to provide an accurate description of specific anatomic locations. These basic directions may be compared to looking at a map to determine the longitude and latitude of an area. Humans are three-dimensional subjects with points of reference made in the orthograde (upright) position. The surface locations and anatomic planes are described as follows.

SURFACE LOCATION

The location of a structure is described in reference to a standing person facing the examiner with outstretched hands in a palms-up position. The basic directional terms are:

anterior (ventral): forward or front surface.

posterior (dorsal): back surface.

lateral: sides, away from midline.

medial: middle, toward the midline.

superior: upper area, above, toward the head.

inferior: lower area, below, toward the tail end.

These reference points may be combined to give a more precise location to a specific region on a surface or in structures deep within the body, for example, the exposed hip in a surgical procedure. When these terms are compounded and hyphen omitted, the combining forms may be:

Anteromedial
Anterosuperior
Posteromedial
Anterolateral
Dorsolateral
Posterosuperior
Anteroposterior
Posterolateral
Superolateral

ANATOMIC PLANES

The term *plane* comes from the Latin word, planus, meaning a flat, level surface. There are three directions of planes, all in reference to a standing person facing the examiner: vertical anterior to posterior (sagittal), vertical side to side (coronal or longitudinal), and horizontal (transverse).

anteroposterior planes

median (midsagittal) plane: vertical plane directly through the midline of the body, transecting the nose, navel, and spine, and dividing body into left and right halves.

median or sagittal plane: any of the anteroposterior planes through the midaxis, dividing body in half; the term sometimes implies the median plane only. If the word sagittal is used to denote the median plane, then other sagittal planes are called parasagittal planes.

vertical side to side planes:

coronal (frontal plane): a plane parallel with long axis of body at right angles to me-

Cranial or superior

Transverse plane

Coronal plane

Sagittal plane

Proximal end of lower leg

Medial surface of leg

Lateral surface of leg

Distal end of lower leg

(dorsal)

Posterior

Lateral

Medial

Anterior (ventral)

Lateral

Caudal or inferior

FIG B–1.
Anterior view of human figure demonstrating meaning of terms used in describing the body. (From Anthony CP, Kolthoff N: *Textbook of anatomy and physiology,* ed 9, St Louis, 1975, The CV Mosby Co.)

dian sagittal plane going through coronal sutures of the skull (approximately center of body) and dividing body into front and back parts.

longitudinal: lengthwise and parallel with long axis of body or part; any of the vertical side to side planes. Coronal and longitudi-

nal planes have been used interchangeably to describe each other. In this case, the context of the sentence will indicate the reference point of the plane.

horizontal (transverse) plane: any of the horizontal planes across the body at right angles to coronal and sagittal planes parallel to baseline.

SPECIFIC LOCATIONS

When describing limb anatomy, the nomenclature is very specific. The four appendages are correctly referred to as the upper and lower limbs, two forelimbs, and two hindlimbs. The **thigh** indicates that portion above the knee and the **shank** the portion between the knee and ankle. The **calf** is the posterior aspect and the **shin** the anterior aspect of the leg. The sole (bottom) of the foot is called the **plantar surface,** and the top is the **dorsal surface.** The **brachium** refers to that portion of the arm above the elbow and below the shoulder. The **antebrachium** refers to the portion of the arm below the elbow but above the wrist. The **ventral side** of the hand is the palm or **volar surface,** with the opposite side being the **dorsum** or **dorsal surface.** The forearm is similarly divided into volar and dorsal aspects.

JOINT MOTIONS*

Ranges of joint motion refer to the extent of movement within a given joint. Joint motion may be active, passive, or active assistive. The major joint areas involve the shoulder (glenoid), elbow (cubitus), hip (coxa), and knee (genu).

All the hinge joints have motion described in terms of **flexion** and **extension.** Except for the ankle, the 0-degree position occurs when the limb is held out straight, and the degree of flexion is then stated in terms of degrees from the 0-degree extended position. The knee and elbow will occasionally extend beyond the 0-degree limit, and this motion is expressed in degrees of **hyperextension.** The wrist has approximately 90 degrees of extention and 90 degrees of flexion (dorsiflexion and palmar flexion). Other measured motions include:

*Further information about the assessment and recording of joint motions is obtainable from American Academy of Orthopaedic Surgeons: *Joint motion—method of measuring and recording.* Chicago, 1985. The Academy.

circumduction: a maneuver or movement of a ball-and-socket joint in a circular motion; for example, the shoulder can circumduct 180 degrees with six movements possible.

flexion: to bend from the joint as in flexion movements of the spine at the waist (anterior or lateral). In the foot or hand is expressed as:

dorsiflexion: the toe-up motion of the ankle expressed in degrees from the 0-degree position of the foot at rest on the ground in standing position.

plantar flexion: the toe-down motion of the foot at the ankle expressed in degrees from 0-degree position of the foot at rest on the ground in standing position.

palmar flexion: of the wrist with palm up in flexion.

extension: extending distally away from body as in the limbs, or bending back posteriorly as in the spine.

pronation: palm-down position of hand with elbow at a 90-degree angle, brought about by the motion of the radius around the ulna (posterior rotation). In the foot, the plantar surface is turned down.

supinate, supination: palm-up position of the hand with elbow flexed at a 90-degree angle, brought about by motion of the radius around the ulna (anterior rotation). In the foot, the plantar surface is turned inward.

ulnar deviation: of the hand at the wrist such that the hand is directed in an ulnar direction; measured in degrees from 0 with hand in midline.

radial deviation: of the hand at the wrist such that the hand is directed radially; measured in degrees from 0 with hand in midline.

abduction: movement away from midline of body in frontal plane; applied to hip, shoulder, fingers, thumb, and foot. The midline reference point is a central line in the body for proximal joints and the central part of a limb for distal joints.

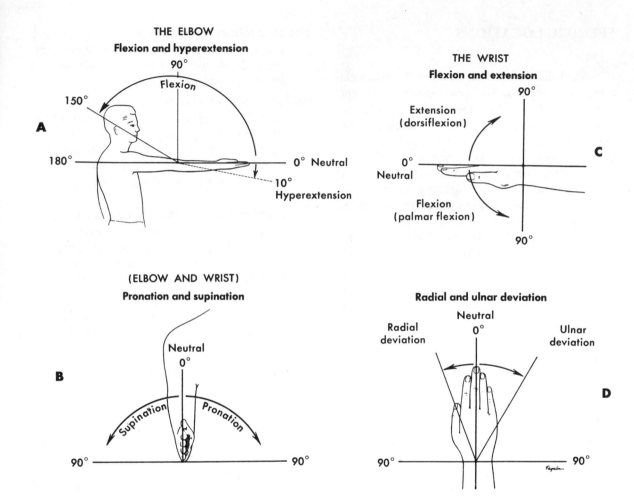

FIG B–2.
A, Elbow. *Flexion:* 0 to 150 degrees. *Extension:* 150 degrees to 0 (from angle of greatest flexion to 0 position). *Hyperextension:* measured in degrees beyond the 0 starting point. This motion is not present in all individuals; when it is, it may vary from 5 to 15 degrees. **B,** Elbow and wrist, *Pronation:* 0 to 80 or 90 degrees. *Supination:* 0 to 80 or 90 degrees. *Total forearm motion:* 160 to 180 degrees. **C,** Wrist. *Flexion* (palmar flexion): 0 to about 80 degrees. *Extension* (dorsiflexion): 0 to about 70 degrees, **D,** Wrist. *Radial deviation:* 0 to 20 degrees. *Ulnar deviation:* 0 to 30 degrees. (From American Academy of Orthopaedic Surgeons: *Joint motion—method of measuring and recording,* Chicago, 1985, The Academy.)

adduction: movement toward the midline in frontal plane as in abduction. On verbal transcription in clinical notes the person dictating will sometimes say "a-b-duction" or "a-d-duction" to clarify distinction between *abd*uction and *add*uction.

anteversion: in reference to the neck of humerus or femur, an anterior rotation.

eversion: turning outward, when applied to the heel, describes the degree of motion of the heel pushed outward with ankle in neutral position; when applied to the foot, describes the com-

THE HIP

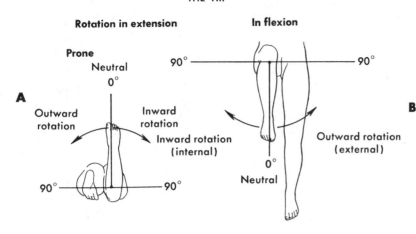

A

Rotation in extension

Prone
Neutral
0°

Outward rotation

Inward rotation

90°   90°

Inward rotation
(internal)

In flexion

90° ——————— 90°

Outward rotation
(external)

Inward rotation

0°
Neutral

B

C

Abduction

90° ————— 90°

0°
Neutral

Adduction

90° ————— 90°

0°
Neutral

FIG B–3.
The hip. **A,** *Inward rotation:* measured by rotating leg outward. *Outward rotation:* measured by rotating leg inward. **B,** *Inward rotation (internal):* measured by rotating leg away from midline of trunk with thigh as the axis of rotation, thus producing inward rotation of the hip. *Outward rotation (external):* measured by rotating leg toward midline of trunk with thigh as the axis of rotation, thus producing outward rotation of the hip. **C,** *Abduction:* outward motion of the extremity is measured in degrees from 0 starting position. *Adduction:* to measure, examiner should elevate opposite extremity a few degrees to allow leg to pass under it. (From American Academy of Orthopaedic Surgeons: *Joint motion— method of measuring and recording,* Chicago, 1985, The Academy.)

bined motions of dorsiflexion, pronation, and abduction.

inversion: when applied to the heel, describes the degree of motion of the heel pushed inward with ankle in neutral position; when applied to the foot, describes the combined motions of plantar flexion, supination, and adduction.

retroflexion: bending backwards

retroversion: turned toward the back; in reference to the neck of femur or humerus, a posterior rotation.

apposition: contact of two adjacent parts; bring-

ing together as in a finger movement, the thumb to index finger.

opposition: applied mostly to the thumb but also to little finger; describes the motion required to bring about opposition, or the setting opposite, of thumb against little finger (pulp surfaces). For the thumb, opposition is the combined action of abduction, rotation, and flexion.

external rotation: in frontal plane is away from midline.

internal rotation: in a frontal plane is toward the midline.

FIG B–4.
A, Hindpart of the foot. *Inversion:* heel is grasped firmly in cup of examiner's hand. Passive motion is estimated in degrees, or percentages of motion, by turning heel inward. *Eversion:* motion is estimated by turning heel outward. **B,** Forepart of the foot. *Active inversion:* foot is directed medial. This motion includes supination, adduction, and some degree of plantar flexion; can be estimated in degrees or expressed in percentages as compared with the opposite foot. *Active eversion:* sole of foot is turned to face laterally. This motion includes pronation, abduction, and dorsiflexion. (From American Academy of Orthopaedic Surgeons: *Joint motion—method of measuring and recording,* Chicago, 1985, The Academy.)

valgus: turned outward; the distal part is bent away from the midline; for example, genu valgus (bow-legged).

varus: turned inward; the distal part is toward the midline; for example, genu varus (knock-kneed).

ANATOMIC ASSOCIATED TERMS

The following are other associated terms referring to directions of anatomy or physical signs.

a, an: no, not, against.

ab: away from (a*b*duct).

ad: toward (a*d*duct).

AGE: angle of greatest extension.

AGF: angle of greatest flexion.

alignment: linear position of one part of an extremity compared with another; to bring into a straight line.

ambi: on both sides.

ambidextrous: using both right and left hands effectively.

amph-, amphi-: both ways, all around, both sides.

an-: not, against, without.

angulation: sharp bend of a structure to form an angle.

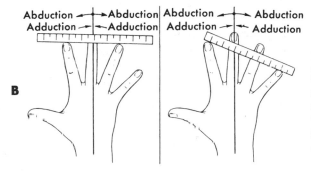

FIG B–5.
A, Nomenclature of fingers. To avoid mistakes, fingers and thumb are referred to by name rather than by number. **B,** Finger spread in abduction and adduction can be measured in centimeters or inches from the tip of index finger to tip of little finger. Individual fingers spread from tip to tip of indicated fingers (From American Academy of Orthopaedic Surgeons: *Joint motion—method of measuring and recording,* Chicago, 1985, The Academy.)

aniso: unequal, asymmetrical, dissimilar.

ante-: forward, before.

antecedent: to precede, or go before.

anteflexion: to bend forward.

anterior: front view, ventral side, face surface, superior.

antero-: before, in front of.

anteversion: tipping forward.

anticus: foremost, in the front.

antimere: the right or left half of the body; a segment of an animal body formed by planes, cutting the axis of the body at right angles.

apex: top, tip, point of activity, summit, vertex (refers to C-2).

apical: pertaining to apex; situated near point of reference.

apo-: away from.

asymmetric: lacking symmetry; uneven, as one limb to another.

axis: line of symmetry, rotation, or revolution; pivot dividing line; also second vertebra.

basal, basilar: base of a part.

bilateral: both sides.

cata-: prefix meaning down, against, or according to.

caudal, caudad: tail, inferior to or bottom point of reference, away from head.

centri-: center.

cephalic: head end, cranial end, uppermost point of reference.

circumference: around, outer circular boundary.

circumflex: describes an arc of a circle; winding around.

co-, com-, con-: together, with.

concave: rounded, depressed surface.

contralateral: opposite side.

convex: rounded, elevated surface.

coronal: a plane dividing the body with front and

THE THUMB

Zero starting position

Abduction   Rotation

Flexion

or

Flexion to tip of   Flexion to base of
little finger   little finger

FIG B–6.
Thumb opposition. The motion is a composite of three elements: abduction, rotation, and flexion. This motion is considered complete when tip, or pulp, of thumb touches tip of fifth finger or, according to some surgeons, when tip of thumb touches base of the fifth finger. (From American Academy of Orthopaedic Surgeons: *Joint motion—method of measuring and recording,* Chicago, 1985, The Academy.)

back portions. In the direction of the coronal suture; a longitudinal plane passing through the body at right angles to the median plane.

craniad: toward the head.

curvilinear: curved away from straight line.

de-:   away, from, down.

deep: depth from surface.

delta: triangle (deltoid).

dexter: right.

dia-:   between, through, across, apart.

diffuse: widely distributed.

dis-:   apart from.

distal: away from, furthest point of reference.

dorsal: back or posterior aspect.

ec-:   out, out from.

ectopic: located away from normal position; out of place.

em-, en-:   in, within.

endo-:   within, in.

epi-:   on, above, over.

eso-:   in, inward, inside.

ex-, exo-:   out, outside.

external: outside, describing walls, cavities, or hollow viscera.

extra-:   beyond, outside, without.

facet: flat surface.

flexure: curved or bent.

fore: in front of, before.

hyper-:   over, above, excessive.

hypo-:   under, below, deficient.

in-, ino-:   into, within.

inferior: below point of reference, underneath.

infra: below or under.

in situ: in its natural place or position.

inter-:   between.

intercalary: middle.

internal: inside; describing walls, cavities, or hollow viscera.

interstitial: spaces within a structure.

intra-:   within.

intro-:   into, beginning.

ipsilateral: same side.

iso-:   equal, symmetrical.

juxta: close to.

juxtaposition: apposition, near to, side by side.

lat, latero-, lateral: sides, right and left; away from median plane, outer surface.

latus: broad.

levo: left.

linea aspera: linea (line) and aspera (rough).

linear: elongated, straight line.

longitudinal: lengthwise, parallel to the long axis of the body or an organ (coronal or frontal planes).

medi-, medial: middle or median plane, toward midline, inner surface, link making halves.

megalo-: large.

meso-: middle intermediate.

met-, meta-: beyond, from one place to another, point of change.

multiangular: many angles.

oblique: slanted, inclined.

oblongata: oblong

palmar: side of hand surface, face up.

para-, par-: beyond, beside.

parallel: equal in lines or surface; in the same direction.

pars: a division or part; a particular part of a greater structure (e.g., pars interarticularis).

patent: open, unobstructed, apparent, evident.

peri-, peripheral: immediately around, sphere.

perpendicular: exactly upright; being at right angles to a given line or plane.

pivot: to turn as in a circular motion.

plantar: sole, bottom of the foot.

posterior, postero-, post-: after, behind, tail end, back, inferior to surface.

prone: face down (lying face down).

protract: pull forward.

proximal: close to nearest point of reference.

quadratus: four-sided.

re-: back, again.

recurvatum: bending backward; a flexure or hyperextension.

residual: left behind.

retract: pull back.

retrad: backward, toward back part.

retro-, retrograde, retroflex: bending backward, behind.

rotation: turning in a circular motion.

sinister: left.

striate: having transverse lines (muscles).

sub-: under.

summit: top.

super-, supra-: above, beyond, upon, over.

superficial: near the surface.

superior, supero-: uppermost side, above point of reference, toward head (cephalic).

supine: lying on back, face up.

sym-, syn-: together.

symmetric: exhibiting symmetry, even, alike.

terminal: end.

trans-, transverse: through, across, horizontal.

ultra: beyond.

unilateral: one side.

ventral: belly side (abdomen), anterior, front, face up.

vertex: top, summit, apex.

vertical: perpendicular to the plane of the horizon (vertex).

volar: underneath surface, palm or sole side up.

Appendix C

Etymology of Orthopaedics

The word "etymology" comes from the Latin *etymon,* meaning genuine or true, plus *logos,* word. Etymology is the study of the origin of words (*origo,* beginning).

In ancient times, the classic language was Greek and Latin in origin and nonmedical in use. Scientific language was attributed to early physicians and writers such as Hypocrates, Aristotle, and Galen. Latin terms were introduced by Galen (a Greek physician who moved to Rome), as well as by the Flemish anatomist, Versalius; Celsus, Aretaeus, and Chaucer also contributed to the scientific vocabulary.

Centuries later, scholars preferred the languages of Latin and Greek in science over other languages for a number of reasons, mainly, because of the ease in which words could be used interchangeably in combining forms based on roots, prefixes, and suffixes. Anglo-Saxon English has a limited capacity for compounding words and often requires numerous words to make a point. Therefore, Latin and Greek were retained as the main structure of scientific language as we know it today. Scholars for generations have studied word origins and discovered full histories for most words, found mostly in the authoritative Oxford English Dictionary.

Anatomy is a very descriptive science. Many words that are of nonmedical origin describe sizes and shapes (deltoid, lamboid, piriformus) or plants (sesamoid, sesame seed; nucleus, little nut; pisiform, pea-shaped), or are taken from living creatures (lupus, wolf; musculus, little mouse; cauda, horse's tail; lumbrical, worm.) Often, the Greek and Latin words that have the same meaning are very different; for example, clavicle (L, dim. of clavis, a key) and cleido (Gr, a fastener or key, used in combining form [sternocleidomastoid]).

Anglo-Saxon English favors monosyllabic words such as hand, foot, back, leg, arm, etc., and is augmented by many words from other languages such as Latin (L), Greek, (Gr), French (Fr), Italian (It), Spanish (Sp), Middle English (ME), German (Ger), and other non-classical origins.

A knowledge of word derivation is the best way to accurately use words in their proper form. A brief description of the origin of orthopaedic terminology is given here to aid in the understanding of this specialty.

a, an: (G) negative prefix before a word that signifies the thing named is deprived of its quality (e.g., anaerobic, anorexic); not, without.

abdomen: (L) belly. Area between the chest and pelvis.

accident: (L) from accidens, a happening; accidere, to happen; (G) cado, to fall. An unexpected happening.

acetabulum: (L) ace, vinegar cup + bulum, utensil, dim. of abrum, a holder or receptacle. Cup-shaped depression of the ilium (true hip) for holding head of femur.

acromion: (G) akron or akros, summit, peak + -omos, shoulder. Outermost tip of scapula.

acute: (L) acutus, sharp, from acuere, to sharpen (cf. acus, needle).

adhesion: (L) ad, to bring in + haerere, to stick; adhaesio, stuck to.

adipose: (L) adeps, adipis, fat. Term used to describe animal fat.

adventitia: (L) adventicius. Ad, to + veniere, to come. An adventitious bursa is one formed from surrounding tissues in an unusual situation (e.g., tailor's bursa, student's elbow). A tunica adventitia is applied to the outer covering of a structure or organ (artery).

etiology: (G) aeti, a cause + ology, a discourse. A study of causes.

agonist: (G) agonistes, a rival or combatant, a prime mover; a muscle concerned with carrying out a movement (contraction) as compared with antagonist.

ala, alar: (L) winglike structure; alar ligament of first cervical vertebra, and sacral ala, the lateral portion.

allograft: (G) allos, other + (L) graphium, grafting knife. To transplant tissue from same species.

amphlarthrosis: (G) amphi, on both sides + arthron, a joint. Limited mobility with movement in all directions. Diarthrosis and synarthrosis refer to incomplete joints (intervertebral disks).

analgesia: (G) an, not + algos, pain. Absence of pain.

ancone: (G) ankon, anconeus, elbow.

amputation: (L) amputare, to cut around and amputatio, a pruning. Hippocrates recommended this operation at the joint.

anesthcsia: (G) an, against + aisthesis, sensation + ia, condition. Absence of sensation.

anapophysis: (G) ana, back + apophysis, an offshoot. An accessory spinal process of a vertebra.

anastomosis: (G) an opening. Created by a natural, pathologic, or surgical communication between two normally distinct spaces or organs.

anatomy: (G) ana, apart + tome, a cutting; anatome, dissection. Hippocrates (420 BC) used word for a branch of medical education. The oldest treatise known on anatomy is an Egyptian papyrus (1600 BC) on dissecting bodies for medical purposes.

anconeus: (G) ancon, a bend, especially the elbow (cf. angle).

ankle: (A-S) from (L) angulus, an angle, corner, or bend; (G) bend.

ankylosis: (G) ankyl, stiff + osis, condition. Ancient term for stiffening of joints, loss of mobility.

annulus: (L) ring-shaped structure; annular fibrosis of intervertebral disks.

anomaly: (G) anomalia - an, against + omaly, ordinary. Abnormality or deviation from normal.

antagonist: (G) anti- or an, against, opposite + tagon, a struggle; agonistes, a rival. A muscle that opposes the action of another muscle (agonist).

anterior: (L) ante- before, more in front; from anterus, positive form of anterior. Antero- used in combining form.

apex: (L) tip.

aplasia: (G) a, against + plasia, to mold or form. A failure in tissue formation.

aponeurosls: (G) apo, away from + neuron, tendon. Before Aristotle (c. 350 BC) introduced the word neura for nerves, everything of a fibrous nature was called a neuron. Galen (c. 180 AD) was first to use the word aponeurosis to refer to the insertion of a muscle that was not by flesh fibers, but terminated in the white sheath.

appendages: (L) appendere, to hang to; appendicular, appendix, an extremity.

apophysis: (G) apo, from + physis, growth; offshoot. Outcropping, but not end of bone, but rather the outgrowth of bone without an independent center of ossification. A place for tendinous attachment.

arachnoid: (L) spider-like, resembling a web; cerebrum and cord covering.

arcuate: (L) arcualis, arch-shaped, bowed. Refers to arcuate line of rectus sheath.

arthritis: (G) arthro, joint + -itis, inflammation.

arthrodesis: (G) arthro, joint + desis, binding; fusion of a joint.

arthrology: (G) arthro, joint + -ology, treatise or discourse. Galen recorded two main orders of joints: diarthrosis (articulation with movement) and synarthrosis (articulation without movement). He then divided the diarthroses into enarthroses, arthrodies, and ginglymus. Synarthroses were divided into suture, symphysis, and gomphosis.

articulatio: (L) articulus, little joint, dim. of artus, fitted close. Artus was used for limbs, thus, articulatus, jointed. Galen, Pliny, and Celsus preferred the Latin "articulus" to the Greek "arthro"; however, both continue to be used.

artery: (G) aer, air + terso, to carry. Arteries were believed to be air carriers in vessels. Later, term included arteries carrying blood.

aspera: (L) asper, rough. Linea aspera is a roughened ridge on the femur associated with insertion of the adductor group of muscles.

asthenia: (G) asthenis, without strength; loss of strength, myasthenia—loss of muscle strength.

atlas: (G) from atlao, endure or sustain. Galen (c. 180 AD) called the atlas, protos spondylos, first cervical vertebra, and second vertebra epistropheus, to rotate upon. The term was later changed to refer to the axis.

atrophy: (G) atrophia, a wasting; a, lacking + trophia, nourishment. A decrease in size of an organ or tissue.

autogenous: (G) autos, self + genous, to produce; self-produced or originating within the body.

avulsion: (L) avulsio, to separate by force. From (G) ab, away from + (L) vellere, to pull.

axilla: (L) armpit. Uncertain origin, but thought to be a compound word from axis alae, meaning axle of a wing, where arm revolves at this point.

axis: (L) a line, real or imaginary, that runs through center of a body; or a pivot, about which a part revolves.

bacterium (pl. bacteria):   (G) bakterion, rod; rod-shaped one-celled organism.

biceps: (L) bi, two + ceps, head; caput; bicipital, having two heads. Refers to the biceps brachii and biceps femora muscle groups.

biopsy: (G) bio, life + op, vision. Excision of living tissue for microscopic examination.

blasts: (G) suffix meaning germ; used in reference to cells that make other cells, such as the osteoblasts, bone-making cells.

bone: (A-S) from (L) os and (G) osteon.

boss: (Fr) boce, a swelling; a rounded eminence, e.g., carpal bossing. Bosselated refers to having many small prominences.

brachium: (L) arm, from (G) brakhion, shorter; brachy, short.

brevis: (L) short. Refers to short flexor of fingers (flexor digitorum brevis).

brisement: (Fr) crushing as in breaking by force; pronounced breez-mon.

bruise: (Fr) bruiser, to break. Broken vessel.

bruit: (Fr) noise; pronounced broo-ee.

bunion: (G) bunion, bugnone, a lump; bouvos, a hill or eminence.

bursa: (G) bursula, a pouch or sac, a purse; (L) pouch, wine skin. A sac between tendons, tendon and bone, muscle and bone that acts as a gliding surface at pressure points where friction can occur. Named in association with their anatomic location.

cadaver (pl. cadavera):   (L) cadere, to fall, die.

calcar: (L) a spur, calcarine, spur-shaped; small spiny projection of bone.

calcaneus: (L) calx, a heel; os calcis, heel bone.

calcification: (L) calx, lime + facere, to make.

calcium: (L) calx, lime.

calisthenics: (G) kalos, beautiful + sthenos, strength.

callus: (G) kalon, callositas, dry wood; (L) callum, hard skin; (A-S) callus, new bone formation at site of fracture; callous, hard thickened skin.

canal: (L) canalis, channel. Conduit for vessels, nerves.

cancellous: (L) cancelli, lattice work. A resemblance of cancellous tissue in bone to lattice work.

capitellum: (L) capitella, small head. Knob-like protrusion of lateral condyle of the distal humerus.

capsule: (L) dim. of capsa, capsula, a little box; from capio, I receive.

caput: (L) a head; (G) capitulum, a little head. Modified to -ceps, as in biceps and triceps.

carpus: (L) carpus, wrist; (G) karpos, wrist.

cartilage: (L) cartilago, gristle; (G) chondro.

cauda: (L) a tail, from cadere, to fall. Hence, cauda equina, termination of the spinal cord, was believed to resemble a plaited horse's tail.

cell: (L) cella, a chamber.

cervical: (L) cervico, cervicalis, pertaining to the neck.

cheiro: (G) chiro, hand; (L) manus, to grasp.

chirurgery: (G) hand + work; one who works with his hands, a chirurgeon.

chondral: (G) from chondros, cartilage or gristle; (L) cartilago, gristle.

chronic: (G) chronos, time; of long duration.

circulation: (L) circulatio, movement in a circular course.

claudication: (L) claudicare, to limp or be lame. Disturbance of circulation.

clavicle: (L) claviculum, dim. of clavis, a key. Was probably related to claudere, to shut or close; (G) **cleido-** as in sternocleidomastoid. Both Latin and Greek use meant a key, bolt, fastener. The collar bone was likened to a key because it locks the shoulder girdle to the breast bone and because of its shape.

clinic: (G) klinikos, to recline, a bed.

clonus: (G) klonos, turmoil; convulsing movements of epileptics. Now refers to spasm in which rigidity and relaxation alternate.

coccyx: (G) cuckoo's beak, from kokkyx, a cuckoo. Coccyx, tip of spine.

collagen: (G) kolla, glue + gennan, to produce; a glue-like substance that holds connective tissues together. **Colloid,** kollodes, glutinous.

collateral: (L) con, together + lateralis, latus, side. Secondary, accessory.

comitans: (L) companion. Comes (sing.), cometes (pl.). A blood vessel that accompanies a nerve trunk.

comminuted: (L) com, together + minuere, to crumble. To break into pieces.

concussion: (L) concussus, a shaking, from concutio, shake violently. An old term for thunder.

condyle: (G) kondylos, knuckle, knob; projections at the end of bones.

conjoined: (Fr) to meet, touch, overlap; refers to the aponeurotic tendon.

contusion: (L) contusio, a bruise; from contundere: con, together + tundere, to break.

coracoid: (G) korax, a crow + oeides, shape; (L) corvus. Anything hooked or pointed like a raven's beak. Variant of coronoid.

corpus: (L) corporis, body; (G) is somatos, soma.

cortex: (L) corticis, rind; outer hard layer of compact bone.

costo: (L) costa, from costarum, of the ribs. Refers to costovertebral cartilage.

coxa: (L) kaksha, the hip bone.

crepitus: (G) krepis, a little noise, creaking; from crepitare, to crackle.

cribriform: (L) cribrum, a sieve + forma, form, sieve-like; anything perforated with holes (e.g., cribriform plate of ethmoid bone).

cricoid: (G) krikos, a ring + oeides, shape. Refers to cricoid cartilage shaped like a signet ring.

cruciate: (L) crux, shaped like a cross; refers to the two intraarticular ligaments of the knee joint that cross and give strong support to the knee.

cubitus: (L) elbow, from cubo, lying down (cf. decubitus). Cuboid is cube-shaped; (G) kyboides, cube.

cuneiform: (L) cuneus, a wedge + forma, shape. Anything wedge-shaped.

curettage: (Fr) curette, a cleanser; scraping out a cavity. Also called debridement.

dactylos: (G) a digit, of the fingers or toes.

debridement: (Fr) de + bridle; thus, unbridling. Originally, to cut away as restricting bands, and later to include tissue.

decubitus: (L) lying down; position of lying down, decubitus ulcer may occur.

dehiscence: (L) dehiscere, to gape; to burst open as in a wound.

deltoid: (G) delta (fourth letter of Greek alphabet); triangular-shaped.

dermas: (L) skin; cutis vera, true skin; corium, integumentary.

dermatome: (G) derma, skin + tome, incision. Refers to dermatome distribution of spinal cord segments and nerve distribution.

desmoid: (G) from desmos, band, a ligament.

diagnosis: (G) dia, through + gnosis, knowledge; to discern.

diaphragm: (G) dia, through + phragm, a partition, wall. Any partition of the body; more specifically, the abdominal diaphragm.

diaphysis: (G) dia, through + physis, growth. To grow through, produce. Refers to center of ossification for shaft of long bones situated between growing regions at end of bone (epiphysis, metaphysis).

diarthrosis: (G) a joint, a movable articulation; freely movable hinge joint.

diastase: (G) dia, through + stase, to stand. A standing apart, separation. Now refers to complete separation of bone.

diathermy: (G) dia, through + therme, heat.

digitorum: (L) digitus, fingers or toes.

diplegia: (G) di, two + plegia, stroke; paralysis affecting one side only.

disk: (L) discus, plate; flat, round, plate-like structure (intervertebral d.).

disease: (Fr) desaise; des, from + aise, depart from normal.

dislocation: (L) dis, apart + locus or locare, to place; dislocatio. Refers to separation of bone at joint area; formerly called a subluxation.

doctor: (L) from docere, to teach.

dorsum: (L) the back of a part.

dysfunction: (G) dys, difficult, painful + functio (L), a performance. Abnormal, impaired function.

dysplasia: (G) dys, bad + plasien, to form. Abnormal growth process.

dura: (L) hard. Refers to dura mater, the outermost and toughest of three membranes enclosing the spinal cord and brain. Syn. pia mater, soft.

dystrophy: (G) dys, bad, defective + troph, nourishment. Deficient by way of nutrition or metabolism; shortening of a muscle.

ebonation: (L) e, out + (A-S) ban, bone. Removal of bony fragments from a wound.

eburnate: (L) eburnus, ivory; refers to changes in bone density to an ivory-like structure in a process called eburnation.

ecchymosis: (G) ek, out + chymos, juice + osis, condition; ecchy, extravasation + mosis, to pour, shed. Extravasation of blood into tissue.

edema: (G) oedema, a swelling. Hippocrates referred to fluid buildup in tissue as oedematous, and the term continues to this day.

elbow: (A-S) from elboga; eln, forearm + boga, bend. From ell, a measure of length used in early times from shoulder to fingers; boga was a bending or bow.

embolus: (G) plug.

enarthrosis: (G) en, in + arthron, joint; a ball-and-socket joint.

enchondroma: (G) en, within + chondro, cartilage + oma, tumor; tumor within cartilage.

endoskeleton: (G) endo, within + (A-S) skeleton; the bony and cartilaginous parts of the skeleton that develop from mesoderm and not ectoderm and that are buried within the soft parts.

ensiform: (L) ensis, sword + forma, shape. Part of breastbone (xiphoid).

epicondyle: (G) epi, upon + kondylos, a knuckle, knob. Prominence on bone above or upon a condyle.

epidermis: (L) epi, upon + dermis, skin. Outer layer of skin.

epilepsy: (G) epi, upon + lepsy, falling sickness. Ancient term referring to infliction, seizures. The French terms are petit mal (short) and grand mal (large).

epimysium: (G) epi, upon + mys, muscle. The fibrous sheath enclosing a muscle.

epiphysis: (G) epi, upon + physis, outgrowth. Center of ossification where a part of the process ossifies separately before making an osseous union with the main portion of bone.

epithelium: (G) epi, upon + thele, nipple. Areas with nipple-like papillae. Together with the cognate word "endothelium" and the more recent "mesothelium," applies to surfaces of all kinds.

erythema: (G) erythros, red + ema, condition. To redden, to blush.

ethmoid: (G) ethmos, a sieve + oeides, form, shape, resembles. Cribriform, sieve-like. Perforations of the ethmoid plate.

etiology: (G) aetiology; refers to studying causes of disease.

eversion: (L) out + ventere, to turn the foot out at the ankle between the talus and calcaneus.

exacerbate: (L) ex, out + acerbus, harsh, bitter; from exacerbare and exasperate, an increase in symptoms, a flareup, to make worse.

exostosis: (G) ex, out + os, bone + osis, condition. A bony outgrowth.

extrinsic: (L) extrinsecus, coming from; extra, outside + secus, otherwise.

fabella: (L) dim. of faba, a bean; a bean-shaped sesamoid fibrocartilage that may develop in the lateral head of the gastrocnemius muscle behind the knee joint.

facet: (Fr) facette, little face; refers to the small, smooth articular surface of bone as in facet joints of the spine.

falx: (L) sickle-shaped structure; denotes a ligamentous opening, e.g. conjoined tendon.

fascia: (L) a band, bandage. Anatomic fasciae denote sheath-like fibrous connective tissue that supports, separates, and covers muscles, joints, and other tissues of the body.

femur: (L) dim. of ferendum, bearing; bearing weight as thigh bone.

fenestra: (L) a window; to open or make a window, fenestrate.

fiber: (L) fibra, thread-like; (G) fibrin, fibroid.

fibula: (L) a small clasp, or needle-like point, a broach, buckle; (G) anything pointed or piercing. Long, thin bone of lower limb behind the tibia.

fissure: (L) fissura, a cleft or groove; any groove in bone or fascia.

flap: (Dutch) flappens, to strike; named for a pedicle graft covering bone after resection.

flexor: (L) flectere, to bend; any muscle that flexes or bends a joint.

foramen: (L) forare, foro, to pierce; a natural opening or passageway in bone or fascia or vessels or nerves to pass through (e.g., obturator foramen).

fossa: (L) fovea, pit or hollow; (Fr) fodere, to dig. Any hollow depression in bone.

fracture: (L) fractura, a break; (Fr) frangere, to break.

ganglion: (G) ganglia, a knot, mass, tumor swelling.

gastrocnemius: (G) gaster, belly + kneme, leg. Refers to the large superficial calf muscle of the posterior lower limb.

genu: (L) to bend. Geniculum referred to a knot or node. (G) gony, gonu, knee; genu recurvatum, valgus, and varus.

gladiolus: (L) dim. of gladius, a sword; main part of sternum.

glenoid: (G) glene, shallow socket + oeides, shape. Cup-shaped depression of scapula of shoulder.

glia: (G) glue; supporting tissue of spinal cord.

gluteal: (G) gloutos, a rump, buttock; any rounded eminence.

gout: (L) gutta, a drop, meaning poison falling drop by drop into a joint as a cause of pain and disease. Hippocrates described gout in the foot as podagra.

gracilis: (L) thin, lean, slender; a muscle of the thigh.

hallux: (G) hallus, allomai, to leap; (L) great toe.

hamate: (L) hamatus, hamatum, hook-like process; hamate bone of wrist.

hamstring: (A-S) ham, back of thigh; flexor tendons behind knee that stand out like cords.

hang nail: (A-S) angnaegl, from ange, troublesome + naeagl, nail.

hemiplegia: (G) hemi-, half + plege, a stroke. Paralysis affecting one side of body.

histology: (G) histos, woven web + logos, a treatise; histo refers to any woven material, a web, and in Homer, the sail of a ship. The tissue structure of an organism or part.

humerus (L) ossa humeri that involved the scapula, clavicle, and humerus. Later changed to mean only upper arm bone.

hyaline: (G) hyalos, glass; hyaloid, glass-like that denotes clear matrix (e.g., hyaline cartilage of joint surfaces).

hyoid: (G) U-shaped; from Greek letter upsilon.

idiopathic: (G) idios, own, peculiar to oneself + pathos, disease. Refers to a condition or disease state without known cause.

index: (L) from dico, to point out, a pointer; hence, the forefinger.

ilium: (L) flank, from ilia, soft parts, because the iliac bone supports the gut. It is the wide portion of bone of the pelvis.

infection: (L) infectum, from inficere, to taint or tinge; to alter by invasion of a pathogenic agent, to infect.

inflammation: (L) inflammatic, from inflammare, to burn, or flame within. In the 18th century, Sauvages introduced suffix "-itis" to refer to inflammation.

innervation: (L) in, into + nervus, a nerve. Reciprocal innervation refers to muscles moving a joint.

innominate: (L) innominatus, from in, without + nomen, name. Given to three bones of the pelvis where compound bone was not named.

intramedullary: (L) within + medullaris, marrow. Within marrow cavity of bone.

intrinsic: (L) intrinsecus, situated inside; thus, intrinsic muscles have their origin and insertion entirely within a structure and thereby are limited to it.

insertion: (L) in, into + serere, to plant. Place of attachment of a muscle into a bone which it moves.

inversion: (L) ventere, to turn; to turn foot inward at the ankle.

ischemic: (G) isch, to keep back + aemia, blood. Deficiency of blood to a part.

ischium: (G) ischion, hip, meaning strength; lowermost bone of innominate bones forming the bony pelvis, seat bone. (L) coxa.

joint: (L) junctura, junctio, from jungere, to join; the point of articulation between two bones.

juxtaposition: (L) near, close proximity + positio, place. Adjacent to or side by side.

kinematics: (G) kinematos, movement; relates to biomechanics and muscle movements.

kyphosis: (G) kypho, hump + -osis, condition. Convex prominence of spine.

lacuna: (L) a pit, hollow space; refers to microscopic resorption areas in bone, cartilage, or cementum. Lacunula, small or minute lacuna.

lamella: (L) a little plate, dim. of lamina; layer of bone or ground substance of osseous tissue situated in places within bone.

lamina: (L) flat plate; refers to flattened part of either side of the vertebral arch when used alone.

latissimus: (L) latus, broad; refers to latissimus dorsi back sheath muscle.

levator: (L) levo, to lift, a lifter; refers to levator musculi.

ligamentum: (L) ligare, to tie, bind + mentum, a bandage. Fibrous band of tissue connecting articular ends of bone serving to bind them together to facilitate or limit motion.

limbus: (L) edge, fibrocartilagenous rim of a joint; refers to glenoid (shoulder) and acetabulum (hip).

linea aspera: (L) linea, line + aspera, rough. Roughened ridge on femur for insertion of adductus group of muscles.

lipos: (G) lipos, fat; lipoid, resembling fat.

lordosis: (G) lordo, curved, to bend; an exaggeration of the normal forward convexity in the lumbar region of the spine.

lumbar: (L) lumbus, loin; refers to lumbar region.

lumbrical: (L) lumbricus, worm; refers to the four small wormlike muscles of the palm of the hand and foot.

lunate: (L) luna, moon; crescent-shaped bone in wrist.

lunula: (L) dim. of luna; refers to half moon–shaped white area at base of nail.

lupus: (L) wolf; named for gradual skin disease, lupus erythematosus.

luxation: (G) luxatio, dislocation, from luxo, to dislocate; subluxate is a partial dislocation.

lymph: (L) lympha, water; clear, transparent fluid found in lymphatic vessels.

malacia: (G) malakia, softening; as of abnormal tissue softening.

malaise: (Fr) discomfort; indisposed, not well.

malleolus: (L) malleus, small hammer; refers to bony eminences on either side of the ankle.

manubrium: (L) a handle, from manus, hand + hibrium or habeo, to hold. Named for uppermost part of sternum (manubrium sterni) that is similar to the handle of a sword.

manus: (L) the hand; (G) cheir.

marrow: (A-S) mearh, unknown origin; (L) medulla. The spinal cord was formerly called the spinal marrow (14th c.). Now, any soft central part of bone.

matrix: (L) mater, mother tissue; refers to intercellular substance of tissue, the formative portion of a structure.

mediastinum: (L) medius, middle + stare, to stand; taken from "per medium tensum," that which is tight down the middle. (The term is applied to partitions and in no way is connected to the word mediastinus of Latin origin.)

medicine: (L) medicina, the art of healing; medicor meant to heal or cure. From 13th century, medicus applied to anyone associated with the art of healing in the care and treatment of patients.

medullary: (L) medullaris, marrow, from medius, middle (medio ossis); refers to the medullary cavity, medulla.

meninges: (G) meninx, a membrane; refers to membranes investing the spinal cord and brain.

melia: (G) melos, limb; refers to absence of a limb, e.g., hemimelia.

meniscus: (G) meniskos, crescent-shaped, dim. of mene, moon; the medial and lateral crescent-shaped intraarticular fibrocartilage in the knee.

metabolic: (G) metaballein, to change; refers to metabolism.

metacarpus: (G) meta, beyond + karpus, wrist. Five bony rays distal to the wrist.

metaphysis: (G) meta, beyond + physis, growth. The line of junction of the epiphysis and the diaphysis.

metaplasia: (G) meta, beyond + plasia, to form. Virchow described connective tissue group changes into another tissue of the same group, such as cartilage into bone.

metatarsal: (G) meta, beyond + tarsos, ankle. Five bony rays distal to the tarsal bones of the foot.

mnemonic: (G) memory; a very old system for remembering dating back to 477 BC.

mucous: (L) muco, slimy exudate from membrane.

muscle: (L) little mouse, dim. of mus, mouse and (G) myo; probably derived from the way muscles move under the skin. Galen gave first account of musculi by describing over 300. In 1543 BC, Versalius abandoned the system of naming muscles and accurately numbered them. In the 16th century, Jaque Dubois renamed muscles after parts to which they were attached (e.g., tibialis, peroneus), and others were named by shape (rhomboid), size (longus, brevis), or substance (membranous), or from number of heads (biceps, triceps). Borelli added to names the action of muscles (pulley, lever, wheel). In the 18th century, Winslow, Albinus, Cowper, Douglas, and Riolan named muscles as we know them today. Leonardo da Vinci lettered his illustrations and occasionally gave a muscle a special name.

myelos: (G) marrow, the pith of plants; refers to the marrow cavity of the spinal cord.

navicular: (L) navicula, little ship, dim. of navis, a ship; boat-shaped structure hollowed out in form. Both navicular and scaphoid are used for the boat-shaped carpal and tarsal bones. The BNA Conference adopted navicular as the correct term.

necrosis: (G) nekrosis, state of death; sequestrum of bone, sloughing of soft tissue. Insufficient blood supply to a part resulting in death of tissue.

nerve: (L) nervus, sinew and (G) neuron, sinew; refers to the nerve cells.

neurolemma: (G) neuro, nerve + lemma, sheath, husk. A thin membranous sheath covering a nerve fiber.

nodule: (L) nodulus, a knot; refers to a small node or collection of cells.

nucleus: (L) nux, nut, a little nut; the central part of a cell.

obturator: (L) obturare/obturo, to stop up, obstruct, or occlude; a membrane that covers an opening (e.g., obturator foramen).

occult: (L) from occulere, to hide or cover over; occultus, hidden, concealed.

odontoid: (G) ondon, tooth + oid, resembles; toothlike process of second cervical vertebra.

olecranon: (G) olenes kranon, olekranon, point of the elbow; elbow process at the proximal end of the ulna.

omohyoid: (G) omos, shoulder + hyoeides, U-shaped. Shoulder muscle formerly called because the muscle was attached to the scapula at one end and the hyoid bone at the other.

onychia: (G) onychos, onyx, nail; (L) unguis. Inflammation of nail bed.

organ: (G) organon, (L) organum, viscus, vicera.

orifice: (L) orificium, a natural opening.

orthopaedic: (G) orthos, straight + paes, a child. Literally means straightening of children. First introduced in 1741 by Nicholas Andry, French physician, who published the first book on orthopaedics. He proposed to prevent and correct deformities in children by exercise, diet, and mechanical means. His was the first work specifically devoted to the subject.

os: (L) os, ossis, bone; ossicle, ossiculum, small bone. (G) oste, allows for use in combining form.

ossification: (L) os, bone + facere, to make. Process of bone formation.

osteoblast: (G) osteo, bone + blast, a germ or sprout. A bone-producing cell.

osteoclast: (G) osteo, bone + klasis, to break up. Concerned with absorption and removal of unwanted tissue.

osteogenesis: (G) osteo, bone + genesis, origin. Bone production.

pain: (L) poena, a fine, a penalty.

palmaris: (L) palm, hand; palmaris longus and brevis muscles of hand.

palpate: (L) palpare, palpabilis, to touch; perceptible by feel, touch.

palsy: (Fr) paralysie, (ME) parlesie; term palsy appeared in 1300.

paralysis: (G) para, besides + lysis, to loosen, paralyein, to disable. Disabling limb condition.

paraplegia: (G) para, besides + plegia, a stroke. Formerly meant stricken on one side, and now refers to paralysis of both limbs and maybe the trunk.

paresis: (G) parienai, to let fall or pass; referred to muscle weakening and now includes partial paralysis.

pars: (L) a part of a larger structure; the pars interarticularis bridges the spine between articular facets.

paronychia: (G) para, besides + nychia, a nail. Refers to infection of marginal area of nail.

patella: (L) a saucer, small pan, dim. of patera, a round plate, and patere, to lie open or exposed; the kneecap.

patency: (L) patens, open, evident.

pathology: (G) pathema, disease + logos, word, reason. Study of the nature and cause of disease.

pectineus: (L) pecten, comb; muscle that flexes and adducts the thigh.

pectoralis: (L) from pectus, the breast; ancient term for an ornamental breast plate that was later included in medicine to mean the pectoralis major and minor muscles of the chest.

pedicle: (L) pes, pedis, foot, and pediculus, a little foot, stem; referred to stalks of plants originally, and later to structures of anatomy.

pelvis: (L) a basin, (G) tub or wooden bowl; any basin-shaped structure or cavity. Named for the large three innominate bones.

periosteum: (G) peri, around + osteon, bone. Hard protective fibrous membrane covering bone.

peritoneum: (G) peri, around + teinein, to stretch. Serous membrane that supports the abdominal cavity.

peroneal: (G) perone, pin, sewing needle, anything pointed for piercing; (L) fibula, brooch. Peroneal relates to the fibula; peroneus, perone, relates to one of three muscles of the leg causing motion of the foot.

pes: (L) pedis, a foot or foot-like projection; applied to different structures such as pes cavus (hollow), pes planus (flat), pes anserinus (goose foot).

phalanges: (G) phalanx, a band of soldiers; (L) internodia, because joints of fingers and toes were called nodes in close knit row. Refers to the distal, medial, and proximal phalanges of the hands and feet.

phlebo: (G) phleps, phlebos, vein; combining form for vein.

physician: (Fr) physicien; one who has successfully completed a prescribed course of studies in medicine.

pinna: a static wing-like projection.

pisiform: (L) pisum, pea + forma, shape. Pea-shaped bone of wrist and smallest of carpal bones, proximal row, ulnar side.

plantar: (L) planta, sole of foot, and (G) platus, planus, flat; from (L) plantaris, a sprout, twig, plant.

plaster: (G) emplastron, to form, mould. Hippocrates and Galen wrote extensively on the subject. Pliny described it in making casts. Originally, bandages were made of starch and paste, lime and eggwhite. The gypsum variety was made in Paris, thus plaster of Paris.

pleura: (G) a rib. Now applied to serous membrane lining the chest wall.

plexus: (L) a braid, plait, entanglement; a complex, especially of blood and lymphatic vessels, and nerves (e.g., brachial plexus).

pollex: (L) thumb, from polleo, strong; pl. pollices.

popliteal: (L) poples, the ham; ancient term from plicare, to fold. Refers to the popliteus muscle behind the knee between the hamstrings that flexes the leg and aids in rotation.

profundus: (L) deep seated; refers to source located deeper than indicated reference point (e.g., profundus tendon). Opposite of sublimis.

pronator: (L) pronatus, prone (face down), from pronare, to bend forward and pronus, turned, inclined; pronator muscle that allows pronation. Versalius used pronum and supinum to refer to muscles.

proprioceptive: (L) proprius, one's own, special + capere, to take, seize. A perception of sensations that creates awareness of what's going on within the body.

prosthesis: (G) prosthesis, an addition.

proximal: (L) nearest point of reference.

pulse: (L) pulsus, beating; pulsate, pulsare, throb.

quadriceps: (L) quadri, four + caput, head. Four-headed as a quadriceps muscle.

rachio: (G) rhachis, spinal column; used in combining form.

radius: (L) a staff, rod, spoke of a wheel; (G) radix, a ray. Refers to forearm bone shaped like a wheel spoke.

ramus: (L) rami, branch; a branch of any given artery or nerve of the spine.

ray: (L) radius; in orthopaedics, refers to the five rays of bones in the hands and feet.

rectus: (L) straight; refers to rectus abdominus muscle of the abdomen.

reflex: (L) reflexus, to bend back and (G) reflectere, to turn back; used to describe muscle movements of the body.

resection: (L) resectio, a cutting off; partial excision of a bone.

retinaculum: (L) halter, a tether, from retinere, to restrain; restraining fibers of fascia that hold a part in place (e.g., the patellar retinaculum, fibers that surround the knee cap and knee).

retroversion: (L) retro, back + versio, a turning.

rheumatoid: (G) rheuma, discharge + oid, resembling. Resembling rheumatism.

rhomboids (G) rhombus, kite-shaped; a four-sided figure with all sides equal. Refers to the rhomboid muscles, greater and lesser.

sacrum: (L) sacer, sacred, holy. In ancient times, the sacrum was used in sacrificial rites because it was the last bone to decay, and it was believed that the body would reform around it. Largest of vertebral bones, it protects and supports the lower organs.

sagittal: (L) sagitta, an arrow; the sagittal suture resembles an arrow. The sagittal plane is the medial vertical plane in line with the suture (i.e., the median plane of the body).

sarcolemma: (G) sarx, flesh + lemma, sheath. The delicate membranous sheath surrounding each individual muscle fiber.

sartorius: (L) sartor, a tailor; refers to a muscle whose action is to bring the leg into a flexed, adducted and laterally rotated cross-legged sitting position habitually adopted by tailors.

scalenus: (G) scalenos, uneven; refers to a triangle with unequal sides, and named for the neck muscle group of unequal length composed of the medius, minimus, and anterior m.

scaphoid: (G) skaphe, a small boat, and (L) scapha, skiff; scooped out, hence, boat-shaped bones in the hands and feet.

scapula: (L) scapulae, resembling a trough or digging tool and (G) spathula, broad implement, resembling a spade; the large, flat, triangular bone of the shoulder that articulates with the clavicle and humerus.

sciatic: (L) sciaticus, and (G) ischion, a hip joint; refers to pain in the loins and hip, and is associated with the large sciatic nerve.

sclerosis: German in origin; meant degeneration of tissue. Later, referred to a hardening process.

scoliosis: (G) a curvature. In early times, meant anything bent or curved. Now refers specifically to a lateral curvature of the spine.

semilunar: (L) semi, half + luna, moon. The crescent-shaped lunate bone of carpus, lunate bone.

septum: (L) saeptum, a partition.

sequestrum: (L) sequestrare, to separate, set aside; fragment of necrosed bone that has detached from surrounding tissue.

serratus: (L) serra, a saw, serrated, having a sawtooth edge; serratus anterior muscles, anterior (chest) and posterior (back).

sesamoid: (G) sesamon, sesame seed + -oid, resembling. Seed-shaped bones or fibrocartilage situated in tendons that move over a bony surface.

skeleton: (G) a dried up body; the framework of the body consisting of 206 bones.

soleus: (L) solea, a flat fish; the flat, triangular-shaped muscle that inserts into the tendocalcaneus of the lower limbs.

spasm: (G) spasmos, convulsion, to draw out or pluck; refers to tonic or clonic muscle spasms.

spina: (L) a thorn, (G) spondylos. In anatomy, thornlike projections were called spines dating back to the 14th century; the vertebral column with its spinous processes.

splay foot: (ME) splayen, to spread out + (A-S) foot. Flatfoot, pes planus.

sprain: (L) exprimere, to press, squeeze, strain; (Fr) espraindre, to wring.

stenosis: (G) stenos, narrow, a stricture; narrowing of a passageway.

sternum: (G) sternon, breast, chest + steros, hard, solid, and palpable. Thus, the breastbone composed of the manubrium (top portion), gladiolus (body), and ensiform or xiphoid process (lower portion).

stethoscope: (G) stethos, chest + skopein, to examine. Instrument used to mediate the sounds produced within the body.

styloid: (G) stylos, pillar and (L) stilus, any long, pointed instrument; the ulnar styloid is the large prominence of bone at the back of the wrist.

sublimis: (L) uplifted, up in the air; applied to physical position, such as sublimus tendon near the surface.

subclavian: (L) sub, under, below + clavis, key. Refers to muscle, artery, or vein under the clavicle (collar bone).

subscription: (L) subscriptus, written under.

supination: (L) supinatio, turning face upward; supinator muscle of forearm, or that of leg, turning leg or foot outward.

supraspinatus: (L) supra, above + spinatus, spines or thorn-shaped. Refers to the supraspinatus muscle above the spine of the scapula.

sural: (L) sura, calf; refers to calf muscle group, triceps surae (gastrocnemius, plantaris, and soleus muscles).

surgeon: (G) from chirurgeon, meaning the hand + to work. One who works with the hands.

surgery: (L) chirurgia, from (G) cheir, hand + ergon, work.

symphysis: (G) syn, together + phyein, to grow, growing together; a natural union. Refers to the symphysis pubis, two articular bones joined by fibrocartilage.

symptom: (G) symptoma, occurrence.

synarthrosis: (G) syn, together + arthrosis, a joint. An immovable joint.

syndesmosis: (G) syn, together + desmos, a band. A joint in which two bones are held together by ligaments.

syndrome: (G) concurrence, running together; clinical picture of a disease made by the presence of several typical signs and symptoms.

synergists: (G) syn, together + ergon, work. Refers to the smooth coordinated way in which muscles work together in the execution of movement, such as the synergist muscle group.

synostosis: (G) syn, together + osteon, bone. The union of two bones by osseous tissue such as the diaphysis and epiphysis of a long bone at the end of the growth period.

synovium: (G) syn, together + oon, egg, (L) ovum, egg white. Refers to the egg white appearance of fluid present in movable joints.

tabatiere anatomique: (Fr) anatomic snuff box; refers to space at the base of the thumb. Now called snuff box.

talipes: (L) talipedare, to be weak on the feet, to totter. Hence, talipes, club foot.

talus: (L) from Cicero, "ludere talis," to play at dice and taxillus, dice; bone resembling dice (talus, ankle bone). Formerly called astragalus.

tarsus: (G) from tarsomai, to become dry, tarsos; referred to anything flat or spread out. Thus it applied to the flat part of the feet.

tendon: (L) tendere, to stretch out; (Gr) tenon, a tightly stretched band; the elongated end of a muscle. Syn. sinew.

tensor: (L) tendere, tensum, to stretch; named for muscle that tenses or stretches and does not alter the direction of a part (e.g., tensor fascia).

teres: (L) from terere, to rub or grind smooth, well turned or rounded off; refers to the ligamentum teres, round ligament of the hip.

thecal: (G) sheath, capsule; relates to a tendon sheath, theca.

thenar: (G) from theino, to strike; referred to flat part of hand used to strike. Now refers to muscles of the palm divided into groups called thenar (major group) and hypothenar (lesser group).

thoraco: (G) thorax, chest, breast plate, stethos. In classical Greek, the thorax was armor (breastplate) to protect the chest and abdomen.

therapy: (G) therapeia, treatment, remedy, cure. First referred to the noun, therapeutae, healers, and later included treatment.

tibialis: (L) a pipe or flute, shin bone, varient of tubia, tube. In ancient times, musical instruments were made from shin bones of animals and objects of tubular form. Tibia, the larger anterior bone of the lower limb.

tourniquet: (Fr) tournier, to turn. Originally applied to a stick that turned to tighten a bandage or apply pressure over a large artery to stop blood flow.

trabecula: (L) little beam, dim. of trabs, trapes, timber; any large wooden beam, such as the rib of a boat or strands of supporting fibers. Refers to beamlike pattern or arrangement of bony lamellae in cancellous bone and muscle bundles raised up beneath ventricular endocardium of heart.

trapezius: (L) trapezion, an irregular, four-sided figure; referred to a four-sided geometrical figure with two sides parallel to two sides divergent. Named for a carpal wrist bone (os magnum), and for the trapezius muscle. The muscle was also called musculus cucullaris, because together with its fellow of the opposite side, it resembled a monk's cowl or hood.

trauma: (G) tro, to wound or hurt + ma, results of action. Any wound or injury to the body by exterior forces inflicted or by physical agent.

triceps: (G) tri, three + (L) tres, three + ceps, head; a three-headed muscle with a single insertion (e.g., triceps brachii in the arm and triceps surae of the lower limb that combines the gastrocnemius and soleus muscles).

triquetrum: (L) triquetrus, having three corners; refers to the wedge-shaped cuneiform bone of the wrist.

trochanter: (G) trochos, a wheel or runner; two bony processes below the neck of the femur for muscle attachment. Galen applied term to greater and lesser trochanters and bony protuberance because of the way it moved in the act of running.

trochlea: (L) trochilsa, a pulley and (G) trochos, a wheel; refers to trochlea of humerus, an articular cylinder around which the ulna moves, similar to a pulley, but cylinder does not turn. A structure having the function of a pulley, a ring through which a tendon or muscle projects.

tuberosity: (L) tuberosities, to roughen; any roughened areas of bone for muscle attachment (e.g., greater tuberosity of the humerus).

ulna: (L) from ell, a measure of length; (Gr) olene, the elbow. In earlier times, the word denoted the whole arm, and now refers to the inner and larger bone of the forearm and elbow opposite the thumb side.

unguis: (L) claw, talon, nail; the toe or fingernails under the nail bed.

uniceps: (L) unus, one + ceps, head. Having a single head or origin.

unilateral: (L) unus, one + latus, side; occurring on one side.

valgus: (L) bent outward, bow-legged; also, talipes valgus; hallux valgus.

varus: (L) bent, turned inward; talipes varus (foot), genu varum (knock-kneed).

vascular: (L) vas, a vessel or dish; hence, a vascular organ is one with a profuse blood supply.

vastus: (L) vast, wide and great; refers to the three large muscle groups of the thigh (v. lateralis, v. medialis, v. intermedius).

vena: (L) vein, vessel; refers to the vena cava, the large vein leading to the heart with an upper and lower distribution.

vertebra: (L) joint, from vertere, to turn and vertebratus, jointed or articulated. Refers to the 33 bony segments of the spinal column.

viability: (L) vita, life + habilis, fit. The ability to live, grow, and develop.

vinculum: (L) a band, cord, or anything that binds, from vincio, I bind; ringlike ligaments of the wrists and ankles.

viscera: (L) vis, strength, casing, cavity; internal organs enclosed in the abdominal cavity and thorax.

volar: (L) vola, palm of hand or sole, from vola manus, hollow of hand; (Gr) is ballo, to hurl. Palma referred to outstretched open hand.

vulnerable: (L) vulnerare, to wound; easily wounded.

whitlow: (ME) whitflawe, white flow; suppurative inflammation at the end of a finger or toe, deep-seated or superficial. Paronychia, felon.

wound: (A-S) wund; trauma to tissue.

xiphoid: (Gr) xiphos, a sword + oeides, shape, sword-shaped; sword-shaped bone of the inferior tip of the sternum to which ribs attach, ensiformus.

Appendix D

ICD Codes for Eponymic Musculoskeletal Disease Terms

The following is intended for quick reference to International Classification of Diseases (ICD) codes that may be hard to find because of the use of eponymic terminology. It is recommended that the specific number be cross-checked with the coding system you are using, as a second decimal digit is sometimes required by insurance companies. In the preparation of the assignment of codes to these eponymic terms we used as a supplemental resource *The 3-In-1 Code Book for Orthopaedics and Neurosurgery,* St. Anthony Publishing, 1993, Alexandria, Virginia.

Fractures are coded primarily for closed (skin not broken) fractures. Closed fractures usually have a .0 and then a fifth digit if required. Open fractures are usually .1 with a fifth digit for location if required.

Many conditions affect joints. The fifth digit (second to the right of the decimal) assigns the portion of bone involved. In general, the shoulder is 1, elbow 2, wrist 4, hip 5, knee 6, and ankle and foot 7.

Some insurers insist on a fifth digit, which is usually served by adding a zero if the given code is only four digits.

The code for open fractures is given to the right of the closed fracture code.

Addison's keloid 701.0
Ainhum 136.0
Albes-Schönberg disease 756.52
Albert achillodynia 729.5
Albright-McCune-Sternberg syndrome 756.59
Allman clavicle fractures classification 810.02 or .03 (open 810.12 or .13)
Anderson and d'Alonzo classification 805.02 (open 805.12)

Apert disease 755.55
Arnold-Chiari 741.0
Ashurst classification 824.3
aviator's astragalus 825.21 (.31 for open f.)
Baastrup syndrome 721.5
Babinski-Frohlich syndrome 253.8
backfire fracture 813.42 (open f.: 813.52)
backpack palsy 955.7
Badelon classification 812.42 (open f.: 812.52)
Bado 813.03 (open f.: 813.13)
Baker cyst 727.51
Bamberger-Marie disease 731.2
Bankart lesion 718.31
Barton fracture 813.42 (open f.: 813.52)
baseball elbow 726.31
baseball finger 816.02 (open f.: 816.12)
Bechterew's disease 720.0
Behçet syndrome 136.1
Bell palsy 351.0
Bennett dislocation 834.01 (open d.: 834.11)
Bennett fracture 815.01 (open f.: 815.11)
black dot heel 924.20
black heel syndrome 924.20
Blount disease 732.4
blue toe syndrome   Varies with source of embolism
Boeck sarcoid 135
boutonnière deformity finger 736.21
boot top fracture 823.2 (open f.: 823.32)
Bosworth fracture 824.2 (open f.: 824.3)
Bouchard node 715.14
boutonnière deformity 736.21
bowler's thumb 727.05
boxer's elbow 813.01 (open f.: 813.11)

boxer's fracture 815.04 (open f.: 815.14)
Boyd and Griffin 820s depending on location
Brailisford's disease 732.3
breaststroker's knee 717.7
Brendt and Harty fracture classification 825.21
    (open f.: 825.31)
Brodie abscess 730.1
Brown-Sequlard syndrome 344.89
Buchanan disease 732.1
Bucholtz fracture classification 808s
bucket handle meniscus tear
    medial 717.0
    lateral 717.41
Buerger disease 443.1
bump, runners 726.71
bumper fracture   Depends on bone involved
Burns disease 732.3
butterfly fracture   Depends on bone involved
Caffey disease 756.59
caisson disease 993.3
cartilage hair hypoplasia 756.9
cartwheel fracture 821.22 (open f.: 821.32)
cast syndrome 557.1
cauda equipna syndrome 344.6
Chadwick and Bentley fracture 823.8 (open f.:
    823.9)
chalk bone 756.52
Chance fracture 805.4
Chandler disease 732.7
Charcot disease 356.1
Charcot joint 713.5
Charcot-Marie Tooth disease 356.1
charley horse
    quadriceps or hamstring 843.8
    calf 844.8
chauffeur fracture 813.42 (open f.: 813.52)
chisel fracture 813.05 (open f.: 815.15)
Chopart amputation 897.0
Chopart dislocation 838.02 (open d.: 838.12)
clawfoot 754.71
    acquired 736.74
clawhand 755.59
    acquired 736.06
clawtoes 754.71
    acquired 735.5

clay shoveler's fracture 812.44 (open f.: 812.54)
Codman tumor M9230/0
collar button abscess 682.4
Colles fracture 813.41 (open f.: 813.51)
reverse 813.41 (open f.: 813.51)
Colonna fracture classification 820s depending
    on location
Colton fracture classification 813.01 (open f.:
    813.11)
Cotton fracture 824.8 (open f.: 824.9)
CREST (CRST) 710.1
Cushing disease 255.0
Danis-Weber classification 824s
Darrock-Hughston-Milch fracture 813.42 (open
    f.: 813.52)
dashboard fracture 808.0 (open 808.1)
Delbet fracture classification 820s depending
    on location
de Quervain disease 727.04
de Quervain fracture 814.01 (open f.: 814.11)
de Quervain syndrome 727.04
Desault dislocation 833.02 (open 833.12)
Diaz disease 732.5
Diaz fracture classification 824s
direct fracture   By region
DISH 721.6
DISI 842.01
diver disease 993.3
Down syndrome 758.0
Duchenne muscular dystrophy 359.1
Dupuytren contracture 728.6
Dupuytren fracture
    ankle 824.4 (open f.: 824.5)
    radius 813.42 (open f.: 813.52)
Duverney fracture 808.41 (open 808.51)
Ehlers-Danlos syndrome 756.83
Ellis-van Creveld 756.55
Engelmann disease 756.59
Epstein dislocation classification system 808s
    and 820s
Epstein fracture classification system 808s and
    820s
Erb disease 359.1
Erb-Goldflam disease 358.0
Erb paralysis 767.6

Essex-Lopresti fracture 813.05 (open f.: 813.15) or 833.01 (open f.: 833.12)

Essex-Lopresti (os calcis fractures)

Evans femur fracture classification 820s based on location

Ewing tumor M9260/3

Fairbanks changes in x-ray 719s

Fairbanks dysostosis 756.50

Fanconi anemia 284.0

Fanconi syndrome 270.0

Felix disease 732.1

Felty syndrome 714.1

Ferkel-Cheng classification talus OCD and fracture 825.21 (open f.: 825.31) or 732.5

Ferkel-Sgaglione classification of OCD and talus fracture 825.21 (open f.: 825.31) or 732.5

Fielding fracture classification system 820.22 (open f.: 820.32)

Freiberg disease 732.5

Frieberg infarction 732.5

Friedrich ataxia 334.0

Frohlich adiposogenital dystrophy 253.8

frozen shoulder 726.0

Frykman fracture classification system 813.4/.5 (fifth digit by specific type)

Galeazzi fracture 813.42 f.: (open 813.52)

gamekeeper thumb 842.12

Garden fracture classification system 820.0 (fifth digit by region)

gargoylism 277.5

Garré, chronic sclerosing osteomyelitis 730.1

Garrod disease 728.79

Gartland fracture classification 812.41 (open f.: 812.51)

Gaucher disease 272.7

golfer elbow 726.31

Gosselin fracture 824.8 (open f.: 824.9)

Gower muscular dystrophy 359.1

greenstick fracture   By region

Guillain-Barré syndrome 357.0

Gustillo (open) fracture   Depends on location

Haglund deformity
    congenital 755.67
    acquired 732.72

Haglund disease 732.5

Hand-Schuller-Christian disease 277.8

handlebar palsy 354.2

hangman fracture 805.02

Hass disease 732.3

hatchet head deformity 718.31

Hawkins fracture classification system 825.21/.31

Haygarth node 714.04

Heberden node 715.04

Henderson-Jones chondromatosis 727.82

Herbert and Fisher fracture classification system 814.02 (open f.: 814.11)

Hermodsson fracture 718.31

herpetic Whitlow 054.6

Hill-Sachs lesion 718.31

Hill-Sachs fracture 718.31

hip pointer 843.0

Hodgkin tumor M9650/3 (varies by cell type)

Hohl fracture classification system 823.0 (open f.: 823.1)

horseshoe abscess 682.4

hot cross bun skull 268.1 (rickets)

housemaid's knee 726.65

hump, dowager   General term

Hunter syndrome 277.5

Hurler syndrome 277.5

Ideberg fracture classification 811.03 (open f.: 811.13)

Iselin disease 732.5

Jaccoud's syndrome 714.4

Jacksonian epilepsy 345.5

Jaffe disease
    hereditary multiple exostosis 756.4
    osteoid osteoma M9191/0

javelin thrower elbow 726.31

Jefferson fracture 805.02

Jensen fracture classification 820.21 (open f.: 821.31)

Johansson classification system 820s, 821s

joint mice 727.82

Jones fracture 825.25 (open f.: 825.35)

jumper knee 726.69

Kaschin-Beck disease 716.0 (fifth digit by region)

Kawasaki disease 446.1

keloid, Addison 701.0

keratoma 701.1

Key and Conwell fracture classification 808s

Kidner lesion 755.69

Kienböck disease 732.3

Kienböck dislocation 833.03 (open d.: 833.13)

Kilfoyle fracture classification 812.43 (open f.: 812.53)

kissing spine 721.5

Klippel disease 723.8

Klippel-Feil disease 756.16

Kohler disease 732.5

Konig disease 732.7

Kocher fracture 812.44 (open f.: 812.54)

Kummel disease 721.7

Kyle fracture classification system 820.21 (open f.: 820.31)

kyphoscoliosis 737.30

Landouzy-Dejerine disease 359.1

Lange-Hansen classification fracture 824s

Le Fort fracture 824.2 (open f.: 824.3)

leadpipe fracture   By bone involved

Legg-Calvé-Perthes disease 732.1

Legg-Calvé-Waldenstrom disease 732.1

Legg-Perthes disease 732.1

Letterer-Siwe disease M9722/3

Letts Vincent Gouw classification fracture 821s, 822s

Letournel and Judet fracture classification 808s

Levine fracture classification 805.02 (open f.: 805.12)

linebacker arm 728.12

Lisfranc amputation 897.0

Lisfranc dislocation 838.3

Lisfranc fracture 825.25 (open f.: 825.35)

little leaguer's elbow 718.82

little leaguer's shoulder 718.81

lobster-claw deformity 755.58

loose bodies 717.6

lorry driver fracture 813.42 (open f.: 813.52)

Lou Gehrig's disease 335.20

Madelung deformity 755.54

Maffucci syndrome 756.4

Maisonneuve fracture 823.01 (open f.: 823.11) 837.0 (open f.: 837.1)

Malgaigne fracture 808.43 (open f.: 808.53)

mallet finger (if tendon only) 736.1

mallet fracture 816.02 (open f.: 816.12)

mallet toes 736.79

Mallory fracture classification E878.1

marathoner toe 703.8

marble bones 756.52

march fracture 825.25

Marfan syndrome 759.8

Marie-Bamberger disease 731.2

Marie-Charcot-Tooth disease 356.1

Marie-Strumpell disease 720.0

Maroteaux-Lamy syndrome 277.5

Mason fracture classification system 813.05 (open f.: 813.15)

Mast, Spiegel, and Pappas classification 823.8 of 823.9

Mauclaire disease 732.3

Mayo 813.01 (open f.: 813.11)

McCune-Albright syndrome 756.59

Meyers and McKeever 823.0 (open f.: 823.1)

milk-alkali disease/syndrome 999.1

milkmaid's dislocation 832.09

milkmaid's elbow 832.09

milkman syndrome 268.2

Milroy's disease 757.0

Monckeberg sclerosis 440.2

mongolism 758.0

Monteggia dislocation 835.03 (open d.: 835.13)

Monteggia fracture-dislocation 813.22 (open f.-d.: 813.32)

Montercaux fracture 823.01 (open f.: 823.11) 837.0 (open f.: 837.1)

Moore fracture 813.41 (open f.: 813.51)

Morel syndrome 733.3

Morquio syndrome 277.5

Morton neuroma 355.6

Morton toe 726.7

Mouchet's disease 732.5

Naffziger syndrome 353.0

nail-patella syndrome 756.81

Namaqualand hip dysplasia 732.1

Neer fracture classification 812.0s (open f.: 812.1s)

nightstick fracture 813.22 (open 813.32)

Ogden fracture classification system   By bone involved

Ogden fracture classification 823.0 (open f.: 823.1)

Ollier disease 756.4

opera glass hand 715.14

Osgood-Schlatter disease 732.4

Otto pelvis 715.35

Paget disease 731.0

Panner disease 732.3

paratrooper fracture 824.8 (open f.: 824.9)

parrot-beak meniscus tear 717.1–717.4 (depends on location)

Parsonage-Aldren-Turner syndrome 353.5

Parsonage-Turner syndrome 353.5

Pauwels 820's

Pellegrini-Steida disease 726.62

Perthes disease 732.1

Piedmont fracture 813.21 (open f.: 813.31)

Pierson disease 732.1

Pipkin fracture classification system 820.09 (open f.: 820.19)

pitcher elbow 718.82

Poland fracture classification system   By bone

Pott disease 730.88 and/or 015.0

Pott fracture 824.4 (open f.: 824.5)

Preiser disease 733.09

"pump bump"
   congenital 755.67
   acquired 732.72

Quénu and Küss modified fractures-dislocations classification 825s, 838s

Raynaud disease 443.0

Raynaud phenomenon 443.0

Reiter syndrome 099.3

reverse Colles fracture 813.41 (open f.: 813.51)

reverse tennis elbow 726.31

ring fracture 808s

ring man shoulder 733.99

Riseborough and Radin fracture classification system 812.4 (open f.: 812.5; fifth digit by region)

rocker-bottom foot 754.61

Rockwood classification 840.0

Rolando fracture 815.01 (open f.: 815.11)

Rowe and Lowell classification system for fracture-dislocations 808.0 (open f.-d.: 808.1)

Rüedi and Allgöwer 823.8 (open f.: 823.9)

rugger jersey (spine) 268.2

runner bump   Depends on location

runner knee   Depends on cause

Russel-Taylor classification 820s

Salter-Harris fractures (involving the physis in children)   Code number varies by fracture location

Samilson classification 715.11

Sanfilipo syndrome 277.5

Schatzker 823's

Scheie syndrome 277.5

Scheuermann disease 732.0

Schmorl node 722.30
   thoracic 722.31
   lumbar 722.32

Schwann tumor M9560/0, malignant/3

Segond fracture 823.00 (open f.: 823.10)

Seinsheimer fracture classification system 820.22 (open f.: 822.32)

Sever disease 732.5

Shepard fracture 825.21 (open f.: 825.31)

shepherd crook deformity 756.54

shoulder pointer 840.8

silver-fork deformity 813.41 (open d.: 813.51)

Sinding-Larsen-Johansson disease 732.4

skeletal amyloidosis 277.3

skier injury 823.22 (open f.: 823.32)

Skillern's fracture 813.44 (open f.: 813.54)

Smith dislocation 838.03 (open d.: 838.13)

Smith fracture 813.41 (open f.: 813.51)

snapping hip 719.65

Stieda fracture 821.21 (open f.: 821.31)

Stewart-Morel syndrome 733.3

Stickler syndrome 756.4

stiff man syndrome 333.91

Streeter bands 762.9

Stewart and Milford 820.09 (open f.: 820.19)

Sudeck atrophy not specified 337.20
   of upper limb 337.21

of lower limb 337.22
of other specified site 337.29
swan-neck deformity   General term
tackler arm 728.12
TAR syndrome 284.0 (thrombocytopenic component), 754.8
teardrop fracture 805–806
tennis elbow 726.32
reverse 726.31
tennis leg 844.8
tennis toe 703.8
Thiemann disease 732.5
Thompson and Epstein fracture classification
system 808s 820s, 835s
thrower elbow 726.31
thumb
bowler 727.05
gamekeeper 842.12
TIA 435.9
Tietze syndrome 733.6
Tile classification 808s
Tillaux Kleiger fracture 824.8 (open f.: 824.9)
TMJ syndrome 524.6
toe
mallet 736.79
marathoner 703.8
tennis 703.8
Torode and Zieg 808s
trigger finger 727.03 (congenital: 756.89)
triplane fracture 824.8 (open f.: 824.9)

Tronzo fracture classification system 820.21
(open f.: 820.31)
Trunkey fracture classification system 808s
Tscherne classification 823s
Turner syndrome 758.6
van Necks disease 731.1
VATER association 759.8
VDDR 275.3
VDRR 275.3
VISI 842.10
Volkmann contracture 958.6
Volkmann deformity 755.37
Volkmann fracture 824.8 (open f.: 824.9)
Voorhoeve disease 756.4
wagon wheel fracture 821.22 (open f.: 821.32)
Wagstaff fracture 824.2 (open f.: 824.3)
Waldenström disease 732.3
Watson-Jones 823.0 (open f.: 823.1)
weaver bottom 726.5
Weber [Danis-Weber] classification 824s
whiplash (assuming neck) 847.0
Whitlow, herpetic 054.6
willow fracture   By bone
Winquist-Hansen 820.3
wrist and fore arms, fractures of 813s and 814s
wryneck (wry neck) 754.1 (congenital)
Y fracture   By bone
Young fracture classification 808s
Zickle fracture classification system 820.22
(open f.: 820.32)

Bibliography

General

American Academy of Orthopaedic Surgeons, Heck CV, editor: *Fifty years of progress (1922–1983),* Chicago, 1983, The Academy.

American Medical Association: *International Classification of Diseases 9th Revision Clinical Modification,* Dover, Delaware, American Medical Association, 1997.

American Medical Association: *Manual of style,* ed 8, Baltimore, 1989, Williams & Wilkins.

American Orthopaedic Association: History of orthopaedics. In *Manual of orthopaedic surgery,* Chicago, 1985, pp 1–8, AAOS.

Brashear RH, Raney RB: *Handbook of orthopaedic surgery,* ed 10, St Louis, 1986, The CV Mosby Co.

Cozen L: *Office orthopaedics,* ed 4, Springfield, Ill, 1975, Charles C Thomas, Publishers.

Cyriax J: *Textbook of orthopaedic medicine: diagnosis of soft tissue lesions,* ed 8, vol 1, Philadelphia, 1984, Bailliere Tindall.

Dorland's illustrated medical dictionary, ed 27, Philadelphia, 1988, WB Saunders Co.

Glanz WD et al: *Mosby's medical and nursing dictionary,* ed 2, St Louis, 1986, The CV Mosby Co.

Hilt NE, Cogburn SB: *Manual of orthopaedics,* St Louis, 1977, The CV Mosby Co.

Simpson JA, Weiner ESC, eds: *The Oxford English dictionary,* ed 2, Oxford, New York, 1989, Clarendon Press/Oxford University Press.

Stedman's medical dictionary, illustrated, ed 25, Baltimore, 1990, Williams & Wilkins.

Thomas CL: *Taber's cyclopedic medical dictionary,* ed 16, Philadelphia, 1989, FA Davis Co.

Turek SL: *Orthopaedics: principles and their applications,* ed 4, vol 1, 2, Philadelphia, 1984, JB Lippincott Co.

Webster's II New Riverside Univesity dictionary, Boston, 1988, Houghton Mifflin Co.

Fractures

Allman FL: Fractures and ligamentous injuries of the clavicle and its articulation. *J Bone Joint Surg* 49A(4): 774–784, 1967.

Anderson IF: Osteochondral fractures of the dome of the talus. *J Bone Joint Surg* 71A:1143–1152, 1989.

Anderson LD, D'Alonzo RT: Fractures of the odontoid process of the axis. *J Bone Joint Surg* 56A(8):1663–1674, 1974.

Ashurst APC: Classification and mechanism of fractures of the leg bones involving the ankle: based on a study of three hundred cases from the Episcopal Hospital. *Arch Surg* 4:51–129, 1922.

Badelon O, Bensahel H, et al: Lateral humeral condylar fractures in children: a report of 47 cases. *J Pediatr Orthop* 8(1):31–34, 1988.

Bado JL: The Monteggia lesion. *Clin Orthop Rel Res* 50: 71–86, 1967.

Boyd HB, Griffin LL: Classification and treatment of trochanteric fractures. *Arch Surg* 58:853–866, 1949.

Buckholtz RW: Pathomechanics of pelvic ring disruptions. *Adv Orthop Surg* 10:167, 1987.

Cabenela ME, Morrey BF: Fractures of the proximal ulna and olecranon. In Morrey BF, (ed): *The elbow and its disorders,* Philadelphia, 1993, WB Saunders Co.

Canale ST, Kelley FB: Fractures of the neck of the talus. *J Bone Joint Surg* 60A(2):143–156, 1978.

Chadwick CJ, Bentley G: The classification and prognosis of epiphyseal injuries. *Injury* 18:157–168, 1987.

Colonna PC: Fracture of the neck of the femur in children. *Am J Surg* 6:793–797, 1929.

Colton, CL: Fractures of the olecranon in adults: classification and management. *Injury* 5:121–129, 1973.

Crenshaw AH: Fractures of shoulder girdle, arm and forearm. In Crenshaw AH, ed: *Campbell's operative orthopaedics,* ed 8, St Louis, 1991, Mosby–Year Book.

DePalma AF: In Connelly JF, ed: *The management of fractures and dislocations: an atlas,* ed 3, vols 1–2, Philadelphia, 1981, WB Saunders Co.

Dias LS, Tachdjian MO: Physeal injuries of the ankle in children. *Clin Orthop Rel Res* 136:230–233, 1978.

Essex-Lopresti P: The mechanism, reduction technique, and results in fractures of the os calcis. *Br J Surg* 39: 395–419, 1952.

Evans EM, Wales SS: Trochanteric fractures. *J Bone Joint Surg* 33B(2):192–204, 1951.

Ferkel RD, Cheng MS, Applegate GR: A new method of arthroscopic staging of osteochondral lesions of the talus. Presented at the American Academy of Orthopaedic Surgeons, Orlando, Fla, February 17, 1995.

Ferkel RD, Sgaglione NA, Del Pizzo W, et al: Arthroscopic treatment of osteochondral lesions of the talus: technique and results. *Othop Trans* 14:172–173, 1990.

Fielding JW, Magliato HJ: Subtrochanteric fractures. *Surg Gyn Obs* 122:555–560, 1966.

Frykman G: Fracture of the distal radius including sequelae-shoulder-hand-finger syndrome, disturbance in the distal radio-ulnar joint and impairment of nerve function: a clinical and experimental study. *Acta Orthop Scand* 108(suppl):1, 1967.

Garden RS: Malreduction and avascular necrosis in subcapital fractures of the femur. *J Bone Joint Surg* 53B(2): 183–197, 1971.

Gartland JJ: Management of supracondylar fractures of the humerus in children. *Surg Gynecol Obstet* 109:145–154, 1959.

Gustilo RB: *The fracture classification manual,* St Louis, 1991, Mosby–Year Book, Inc.

Gustilo RB, Mendoza RM, et al: Problems in the management of type III (severe) open fractures. *J Trauma* 24:742, 1986.

Gustilo RB, Merkow RI, Templeman D: The management of open fractures. *J Bone Joint Surg* 72A:299–304, 1990.

Hardcastle PH, Reschauer R, et al: Injuries to the tarsometatarsal joint: incidence, classification, and treatment. *J Bone Joint Surg* 64B(3):349–356; 1982.

Hawkins LG: Fracture of the neck of the talus. *J Bone Joint Surg* 52A(5):991–1002, 1970.

Helfet DL, Howey T, et al: Limb salvage versus amputation. *Clin Orthop Rel Res* 256:80–86, 1990.

Herbert TJ, Fisher WE: Management of the scaphoid fracture using a new bone screw. *J Bone Joint Surg* 66B:114–123, 1984.

Hohl M, Moore TM: Articular fractures of the proximal tibia. In Evarts M (ed): *Surgery of the musculoskeletal system,* ed 2, New York, 1990, Churchill Livingstone.

Ideberg R: Fractures of the scapula involving the glenoid fossa. In: *Surgery of the shoulder, Toronto,* 1984, BC Decker, pp 63–66.

Jensen JS: Classification of trochanteric fractures. *Acta Orthop Scand* 51:803–810, 1980.

Johansson JE, McBroom R, et al: Fracture of the ipsilateral femur in patients with total hip replacement. *J Bone Joint Surg* 63A:1435–1442, 1981.

Judet R, Judet J, et al: Fractures of the acetabulum: classification and surgical approaches for open reduction: preliminary report. *J Bone Joint Surg* 46A(8):1615–1646, 1675, 1964.

Judet and Letournal acetabular fracture classification. *J Bone Joint Surg* 73A:639–645, 1991.

Key JA, Conwell HE: *Management of fractures, dislocations and sprains,* St Louis, 1951, CV Mosby.

Kilfoyle RM: Fractures of the medial condyle and epicondyle in children. *Clin Orthop Rel Res* 41:43–50, 1965.

Klafs CE, Arnheim DD: *Modern principles of athletic training,* ed 5, St Louis, 1981, The CV Mosby Co.

Kulund DN: *The injured athlete,* Philadelphia, 1982, JB Lippincott Co.

Kyle RF, Gustilo RB, et al: Analysis of six hundred and twenty-two intertrochanteric hip fractures. *J Bone Joint Surg* 61A(2):216–221, 1979.

Lauge-Hansen N: Fractures of the ankle. II. Combined experimental-surgical and experimental-roentgenologic investigations. *Arch Surg* 60:957–985, 1950.

Letts M, Vincent N, et al: The "floating knee" in children. *J Bone Joint Surg* 68B:442–446, 1986.

Levine AM, Edwards CC: The management of traumatic spondylolisthesis of the axis. *J Bone Joint Surg* 67A(2): 217–226, 1985.

Mallory TH, Kraus TJ, et al: Intraoperative femoral fractures associated with cementless total hip anthroplasty. *Orthopaedics* 12(2):231–239, 1989.

Mason ML: Some observations on fractures of the head of the radius with a review of one hundred cases. *Br J Surg* 42:123–132, 1954.

Mast JW, Spiegel PG, et al: Fractures of the tibial pilon. *Clin Orthop Rel Res* 230:68–82, 1988.

Meyers MH, McKeever FM: Followup notes: fracture of the intercondylar eminence of the tibia. *J Bone Joint Surg* 52A(8):1677–1684, 1970.

Milch H: Fractures and fracture dislocations of the humeral condyles. *J Trauma* 4:592–607, 1964.

Müller ME, Allgöwer M, Schnieder R: *Manual of internal fixation,* ed 3, Berlin, 1991, Springer-Verlag, pp 152–157.

Müller ME, Nazarian S, et al: *The comprehensive classification of fractures of long bones.* Berlin, 1990, Springer-Verlag.

Neer, CSI: Displaced proximal humeral fractures. Part I: Classification and evaluation. *J Bone Joint Surg* 52A(6):1077–1089, 1970.

Neer CS, Howrowitz BS: Fractures of the proximal humeral epiphyseal plate. *Clin Orthop Rel Res* 41:24–31, 1965.

Oestern HH, Tscherne H: Pathophysiology and classification of soft tissue injuries associated with fractures. In Tscherne H, Gotzen L (eds): *Fractures with soft tissue injuries,* Berlin, 1984, Springer-Verlag, pp 1–8.

Ogden JA: Skeletal growth mechanism injury patterns. *J Pediatr Orthop* 2:371–377, 1982.

Ogden JA, Tross RB, et al: Fractures of the tibial tuberosity in adolescents. *J Bone Joint Surg* 62A(2):205–215, 1980.

Owen R, Goodfellow J, Bullough P: *Scientific foundations of orthopaedics and traumatology,* London, 1980. William Heinemann Medical Books, Ltd.

Pauwels F: *Der Schenkenholsbruck, em mechanisches Problem Grundlagen des Heilungsvorganges Prognose und kausale Therapie,* Stuttgart, 1935, Beilageheft zur Zeitschrift fur Orthopaedische Chirurgie, Ferdinand Enke.

Peterson L: *Sports injuries.* Chicago, 1986, Year Book Medical Publishing.

Pipkin G: Treatment of grade IV fracture-dislocation of the hip. *J Bone Joint Surg* 39A(5):1027–1042, 1957.

Poland J: *Traumatic separation of the epiphysis,* London, 1898, Smith, Elder and Company.

Riseborough EJ, Radin EL: Intercondylar T fracture of the humerus in the adult: a comparison of operative and non-operative treatment in twenty-nine cases. *J Bone Joint Surg* 51A(1):130–141, 1898.

Rockwood CA: Subluxations and dislocations about the shoulder. In: *Fractures in adults,* Philadelphia, 1984, JB Lippincott, pp 1192–1198.

Rockwood CA, Green D, Buckholtz: *Fractures in adults,* 3rd ed, vol 1–2, Philadelphia, 1984, JB Lippincott Co.

Rockwood CA, Wilkins KE, King RE: *Fractures in children,* vol 3, Philadelphia, 1984, JB Lippincott Co.

Rowe CR, Lowell JD: Prognosis of fractures of the acetabulum. *J Bone Joint Surg* 43A:30–59, 1962.

Rüedi T, Allgöwer M: Fractures of the lower end of the tibia into the ankle joint. *Injury* 1:92, 1969.

Russell TA: Fractures of the hip and pelvis. In Crenshaw AH, ed: *Campbell's operative orthopaedics,* ed 8, St Louis, 1991, Mosby–Year Book.

Salter RB, Harris WR: Injuries involving the epiphyseal plate. *J Bone Joint Surg* 45A:587–622, 1963.

Samilson RL, Preito V: Dislocation arthropathy of the shoulder. *J Bone Joint Surg* 65A(4):456–460, 1983.

Schatzker J, McBroom R, et al: The tibial plateau fracture. *Clin Orthop Rel Res* 138:94–104, 1979.

Schultz RJ: *The language of fractures,* Huntington, NY, 1976, RE Krieger Publishing Co.

Seinsheimer FI: Subtrochanteric fractures of the femur. *J Bone Joint Surg* 60A(3):300–306, 1978.

Seligson D, Pope M: *Concepts in external fixation,* New York, 1982, Grune & Stratton.

Stewart MJ, Milford LW: Fracture-dislocation of the hip: an end result study. *J Bone Joint Surg* 36A:315–342, 1954.

Thompson VP, Epstein HC: Traumatic dislocation of the hip: a survey of 204 cases covering a period of twenty-one years. *J Bone Joint Surg* 33A(3):746–778, 1951.

Tile M: Pelvic ring fractures, should they be fixed. *J Bone Joint Surg* 70B:1–12, 1988.

Torode I, Zieg S: Pelvic fractures in children. *J Pediatr Orthop* 5:76, 1985.

Tronzo RG: Special considerations in management. *Orthop Clin North Am* 5(3):571–583, 1974.

Watson-Jones: *Fractures and joint injuries,* Edinburgh, 1955, E and S Livingston.

Weber BG: Die Verletzungen des oberen Spurnggelenkes. In Bern: *Aktuelle Probleme in der Chirurgie,* 1966, Verlag Han Huber.

Winquist RA, Hansen ST: Comminuted fractures of the femoral shaft treated by intramedullary nailing. *Orthop Clin North Am* 11(3):633–647, 1980.

Young JWR, Burgess AR, et al: Pelvic fractures: value of plain radiography in early assessment and management. *Radiology* 160:445–451, 1986.

Zickle RE: An intramedullary fixation device for the proximal part of the femur: nine years experience. *J Bone Joint Surg* 58A:866–872, 1976.

Diseases

Aegerter E, Kirkpatrick JA: *Orthopaedic diseases: physiology, pathology, radiology,* ed 4, Philadelphia, 1975, WB Saunders Co.

Albright JA, Brand RA: *Scientific basis of orthopaedics,* New York, 1979, Appleton-Century-Crofts.

American Academy of Orthopaedic Surgeons and the International Society for the Study of the Lumbar Spine: *Glossary on spinal terminology,* document 675–680, Chicago, 1980, The Academy.

Bogumill GP, Schwamm HA: *Orthopaedic pathology: a synopsis with clinical and radiographic correlation,* Philadelphia, 1984, WB Saunders Co.

Dietz FR, Matthews KD: Update on genetic bases of disorders with orthopaedic manifestations. *J Bone Joint Surg* 78A:1583–1598, 1996.

Enneking WF: A system of staging musculoskeletal neoplasms. *Clin Orthop* 204:9–24, 1986.

Enzinger FM, Weiss SW: *Soft tissue tumors,* ed 2, St Louis, 1988, CV Mosby Co.

Fitzgerald RH, et al: *Orthopedic knowledge update,* 1987, American Academy of Orthopedic Surgeons.

Frassica FJ, Thompson RC: Evaluation, diagnosis and classification of benign soft-tissue tumors. *J Bone Joint Surg* 78A:126–140, 1996.

Gartland JJ: *Fundamentals of orthopaedics,* ed 5, Philadelphia, 1991, WB Saunders Co.

Mercier LR: *Practical orthopaedics,* ed 3, St Louis, 1991, Mosby–Year Book, Inc.

The Merck manual of diagnosis and therapy, ed 16, Rahway, NJ, 1992, Merck Research Laboratories.

Mirra JM: *Bone tumors: clinical, radiographic, and pathologic correlations,* ed 2, Philadelphia, 1989, WB Saunders Co.

Mourad LA: *Orthopaedic disorders,* St Louis, 1991, Mosby–Year Book, Inc.

Salter RB: *Textbook of disorders and injuries of the musculoskeletal system,* ed 2, Baltimore, 1984, Williams & Wilkins.

Schajowicz F, Ackerman IV, Sissons HA: Histological typing of bone tumors. In: *International Classification of Tumors,* vol 6, Geneva, 1972, World Health Organization.

Steinberg ME, Hayken GD, Steinberg DR: A quantitative system for staging avascular necrosis. *J Bone Joint Surg* 77B:34–41, 1995.

X-Ray Imaging

Ewald FC: Knee Society total knee arthroplasty roentgenographic evaluation and scoring system. *Clin Orthop* 248:9–13, 1989.

Greulich WW, Pyle SI: *Atlas of the development of the hand and wrist,* ed 2, Stanford, Calif, 1959, Stanford University Press.

Tanner JM, et al: *Assessment of skeletal maturity and prediction of adult height (TW2) method,* ed 2, London, 1983, Academic Press.

Todd, TW: *Atlas of skeletal maturity,* St Louis, 1937, The CV Mosby Co.

Test, Signs, & Maneuvers

American Academy of Orthopaedic Surgeons: *Joint motion: method of measuring and recording,* ed 6, Chicago, 1985, The Academy.

Gerhardt JJ: *Measuring and recording of joint motion: instrumentation and techniques,* ed 2, Toronto/Lewiston, NY, 1990, Hogrefe & Huber.

Hoppenfeld S: *Physical examination of the spine and extremities,* New York, 1976, Appleton-Century-Crofts.

Lliang MH, Katz JN, Phillips C, ed al: The American Academy of Orthopaedic Surgeons Task Force on Outcome Studies: the total hip arthoplasty evaluation form of the American Academy of Orthopaedic Surgeons. *J Bone Joint Surg* 73B:816, 1991.

Polly HF, Hunder GG: *Physical examination of the joints,* ed 2, Philadelphia, 1978, WB Saunders Co.

Trumbly CM: *Physical disabilities,* ed 2, Baltimore, 1983, Williams & Wilkins.

Laboratory

Henry JB, ed: *Clinical diagnostic management by laboratory methods,* ed 18, Philadelphia, 1991, WB Saunders Co.

Kjeldsberg CR, Knight JA: *Body fluids,* ed 2, 1987, American Society of Clinical Pathologists.

Casts, Splints, and Dressings

American Academy of Orthopaedic Surgeons: *Emergency care and transportation of the sick and injured,* ed 6, Chicago, 1997, The Academy.

Schmeisser GA: *A clinical manual of orthopedic traction techniques,* Philadelphia, 1963, WB Saunders Co.

Schneider RF: *Handbook for the orthopaedic assistant,* ed 2, St Louis, 1976, The CV Mosby Co.

Simon RR, Koenigsknecht SJ: *Emergency orthopaedics: the extremities,* ed 2, Norwalk, Conn, 1987, Appleton & Lange.

Prosthetics and Orthotics

American Academy of Orthopaedic Surgeons: *Atlas of orthotics,* ed 2, St Louis, 1985, CV Mosby Co.

American Academy of Orthopaedic Surgeons: *Atlas of limb prosthetics: surgical, prosthetic, and rehabilitation principles,* ed 2, St Louis, 1992 Mosby–Year Book, Inc.

Bunch WH, Keagy RD: *Principles of orthotic treatment,* St Louis, 1976, The CV Mosby Co.

Redford JB: *Orthotics etcetera,* ed 3, Baltimore, 1986, Williams & Wilkins.

Anatomy and Surgery

American Orthopaedic Association: *Manual of orthopaedic surgery,* Chicago, 1985, The Association.

Burchardt H: The biology of bone graft repair, *Clin Orthop* 174:28, 1983.

Casscells SW: *Arthroscopy: diagnostic and surgical practice,* Philadelphia, 1984, Lea & Febiger.

Crenshaw AH, editor: *Campbell's operative orthopaedics,* vols 1–5, ed 8, St Louis, 1992, Mosby–Year Book, Inc.

Epps CH Jr: *Complications in orthopaedic surgery,* ed 3, vols I and II, Philadelphia, 1994. JB Lippincott.

Friedlaender G: *Allografting.* St Louis, 1992, Mosby–Year Book, Inc.

Friedlaender GE: Immune responses to osteochondral allografts: current knowledge and future directions. *Clin Orthop* 174:58, 1983.

Haimovici H: *Vascular surgery: principles and techniques,* New York, 1984, Appleton-Century-Crofts.

Moore KL: *Clinically oriented anatomy,* ed 2, Baltimore, 1985, Williams & Wilkins.

Reckling F, Reckling JA, Mohn M: *Orthopaedic anatomy and surgical approaches,* St Louis, 1990, Mosby–Year Book, Inc.

Robertson PA: Prediction of amputation after severe lower limb trauma. *J Bone Joint Surg* 73A:639–645, 1991.

Rutherford RB, ed: *Vascular surgery,* ed 2, Philadelphia, 1984, WB Saunders Co.

Shahriaree H, ed: *O'Connors textbook of arthroscopic surgery,* ed 2, Philadelphia, 1992, JB Lippincott.

Tomford WW, Friedlaender GE: Bone banking procedures. *Clin Orthop* 174:15, 1983.

Weiland AJ: Current concepts review: vascularized free bone transplants. *J Bone Joint Surg* 63A:166, 1981.

Hand and Wrist

Green DP, ed: *Operative hand surgery,* ed 2, New York, 1988, Churchill-Livingstone.

Lichtman DM: *The wrist and its disorders,* Philadelphia, 1988, WB Saunders Co.

Mackinnon SE, Dellon AL: *Surgery of the peripheral nerve,* New York, 1988, Thieme Medical Publishers.

Scher RK, Daniel CR III, eds: *Nails: therapy, diagnosis, surgery,* Philadelphia, 1990, WB Saunders Co.

Tsuge K; In Steichen JB, ed: *Comprehensive atlas of hand surgery.* Chicago, 1989, Year Book Medical Publishers.

Foot and Ankle

Jahss MH: *Disorders of the foot,* vols I and II, Philadelphia, 1982, WB Saunders Co.

Mann RA: *Surgery of the foot,* ed 5, St Louis, 1986, The CV Mosby Co.

Occupational Therapy and Physical Therapy

American Occupational Therapy Association Commission on Practice Uniform Reporting System Task Force: *Uniform terminology system for reporting occupational therapy services,* Rockville, Md., The Association.

Kamenetz HL: *Dictionary of rehabilitation medicine,* New York, 1983, Springer Publishing Company.

Magee DJ: *Orthopaedic physical assessment,* ed 3, Philadelphia, 1997, WB Saunders Co.

Research

Brighton CT, Black J, Pollack S: *Electrical properties of bone and cartilage,* New York, 1979, Grune & Stratton.

Poole AR: Cartilage in health and disease. In McCarthy D, Koopman W, eds: *Arthritis and allied conditions. A textbook in rheumatology,* ed 12, Philadelphia, 1992, Lea & Febiger, pp 279–333.

Frankel V: Orthopedic biomechanics, Philadelphia, 1970, Lea & Febiger.

SUGGESTED READINGS

Journals and Tapes

AAOS Instructional Course Lectures (Park Ridge, Ill)

ACTA Chirurgiae Orthopaedicae et Traumatologiae Cechoslovaca (Praha)

ACTA Orthopaedica Scandinavica

Aktuelle Probleme in Chirurgie und Orthopadie (Bern)

Advances in Ortho Surg 1985 (Baltimore)

American Journal of Emergency Medicine (Philadelphia)

American Journal of Knee Surgery (Thorofare, NJ)

American Journal of Sports Medicine (Waltham, Mass)

Archives of Orthopaedic and Traumatic Surgery (Berlin)

Archives of Physical Medicine and Rehabilitation (Chicago)

Archivio Putti di Chirurgia Degli Organi di Movimento (Firenze)

Arthritis and Rheumatism (Philadelphia)

Arthroscopy (New York)

Audio Digest Foundation (AAOS Ortho Tapes) (Chicago)

Beitrage zur Orthopadie und Traumatologie (Berlin)

Bone (New York)

Bone Marrow Transplant (United Kingdom)

Bone and Mineral (Amsterdam)

Bulletin of the Hospital for Joint Diseases Orthopaedic Institute (New York)

Chirurgia Narzadow Ruchu I Ortopedia Polska (Warszara)

Chirurgia Degli Organi di Movimento (Bologna)

Clinical Orthopaedics and Related Research (Philadelphia)

Clinics in Sports Medicine (Philadelphia)

Continuing Education in Ortho Surg (Recert) (AAOS) (Chicago)

Foot and Ankle (Baltimore)

Hand Clinics (Philadelphia)

Hip (Philadelphia)

Instructional Course Lectures; AAOS (Chicago)

International Orthopaedics (NY)

Italian Journal of Orthopaedics and Traumatology (Bologna)

JAMA (Chicago)

Journal of Arthroplasty (New Brunswick, NJ)

Journal of Bone and Joint Surgery, American Volume (Boston)

Journal of Bone and Joint Surgery, British Volume (London)

Journal of Bone and Mineral Research (New York)

Journal of Foot Surgery (Baltimore)

Journal of Hand Surgery (St Louis)

Journal of Hand Therapy (Philadelphia)

Journal of Orthopaedic Research (New York)

Journal of Orthopaedic and Sports Physical Therapy (Baltimore)

Journal of Orthopaedic Trauma (New York)

Journal of Pediatric Orthopaedics (New York)

Journal of Prosthetics and Orthotics (Alexandria, Va)

Magyar Traumatologia, Orthopaedia es Helyreallito Sebeszet (Budapest)

Journal of Rheumatology (Buffalo, NY)

Journal of Sports Medicine and Physical Fitness (Torino, Italy)

Journal of the American Medical Association (Chicago)

Journal of the American Podiatric Medical Association (Bethesda, Md)

J Trauma (Baltimore)

New England Journal of Medicine (Boston)

Nippon Seikeigeka Gakkai Zasshi. Journal of the Japanese Orthopaedic Association (Tokyo)

Orthopaedic Audio-synopsis (AAOS) (Chicago)

Orthopaedic Clinical Update Monograph (AAOS) (Chicago)

Orthopade (Berlin)

Orthopedic Clinics of North America (Philadelphia)

Orthopaedic Nursing (Pitman, NJ) (NAON)

Orthopaedic Review (Lawrenceville, NJ)

Orthopaedic Survey (Chicago)

Orthopaedics (Thorofare, NJ)

Ortopediia Travmatologiia I Protezirovanie (Kharkov)

Pediatric Clinics of North America (Philadelphia)

Physical Therapy Journal (Alexandria)

Revue de Chirugie Orthopedique et Reparatrice de l'Appareil Moteur (Paris)

Skeletal Radiology (Berlin)

Spine (Hagerstown, Md)

Sports Medicine

Yearbook of Orthopaedic Trauma & Surgery (Chicago)

Yearbook of Orthopaedic and Traumatic Surgery (St Louis)

Yearbook of Orthopaedics (abstracts) (St Louis)

Yearbook of Sports Medicine (Chicago)

Yearbook of Sports Medicine (St Louis)

Zeitschrift fur Orthopadie und ihre Grenzgebiete (Stuttgart)

Osteopathic Medicine

Journal of the American Osteopathic Association (Chicago)

Index

A

A-, 386
AAA bone, 197
Ab-, 386
Abbott and Gill osteotomy, 194
Abbott and Lucas approach, 259–260
Abbott method, 123
Abbott-Fisher-Lucas arthrodesis, 215
Abbott-Saunders-Bost arthrodesis,
    314
Abbreviations
  anatomy, 372–375
  casts, splints, dressings, 376
  diseases, conditions, and syn-
     dromes, 371–372
  imaging techniques, 376
  miscellaneous, 378–379
  physical medicine and occupational
    therapy, 377–378
  prescriptions, 380
  prosthetics and orthotics, 376–377
  research, 378
  surgical procedures and related
    terms, 375
Abdominal muscles, 274
Abduction, 383
  fracture from, 14
Abduction bar, 159
Abduction orthosis, 179
Abduction sign, 125
Abductor hallucis, 329
Abductor lurch, 139
Abductor pollicis longus release, 320
Ablate, 264
Ablative surgery, 264
Abott arthrodesis, 314
Above-elbow amputation, 170
Abrasion, 88
Abrasive wear, 369
Abscess, 88
Absorbable scaffold, 370
A/C harness, 162
A/C joint separation, 31

Acanthosis nigricans, 311
Acceleration, 365
Accessory bone, 291
Accessory ligament, 221, 297
Accessory movement, 351
Accessory navicular, 324, 327
Accupressure, 350
Ace bandage, 162
Acetabular angle, 103
Acetabular deficiencies, 83–84
Acetabular fracture, 21, 28
Acetabular fracture-dislocation, 26
Acetabular head quotient, 107
Acetabular index angle, 103
Acetabular line, 107
Acetabular notch, 242
Acetabular prostheses, 207–208
Acetabular rim syndrome, 82
Acetabuloplasty, 245
Acetabulum, 242
Acheiria, 87, 305
Acheiropodia, 87
Achilles bulge sign, 135
Achilles reflex, 138
Achilles squeeze test, 132
Achilles tendon, 221, 249, 329
Achilles tendonitis, 331
Achillobursitis, 66
Achillodynia, 66
Achondroplasia, 61
Achondroplastic dwarfism, 61
Achondroplastic stenosis, 279
Acid phosphatase, 143
Acid-fast bacillus, 147
Aconeus, 235
AcP, 143
Acquired thumb flexion contracture,
  305
Acrocephalosyndactylism, 55
Acrocyanosis, 74, 309
Acromial angle, 103
Acromial profile, 110
Acromioclavicular joint, 227

Acromioclavicular ligament, 229
Acromioclavicular separation, 26
Acromioclavicular sprain, 33
Acromion, 82
Acromion process, 227
Acromionectomy, 231
Acromioplasty, 231
Acroosteolysis, 49
Acrosclerosis, 72
Acrosyndactyly, 305
Activated partial thromboplastin time,
  145
Active tendon implant, 320
Acute, 88
Acute calcific retropharyngeal ten-
  donitis, 66
Acute calcific tendonitis, 66
Acute osteomyelitis, 45
Acute postpartum sacroiliitis, 277
Ad-, 386
Adactylia, 87
Adactyly, 305
Adamantinoma, 49
Adaptic dressing, 162
Adaptive equipment, 356
Addis test, 132
Addison's keloid, 73
Adduction, 384
  fracture from, 15
Adduction sign, 125
Adduction test, forced, 126
Adductor brevis, 242
Adductor hallucis, 329
Adductor longus, 242
Adductor magnus, 242
Adductor muscle, of hip, 247
Adductor tubercle, 247
Adductor tuberosity, 247
Adductors of hip, 242
Adenopathy, 88
Adhesions, 88
Adhesive capsulitis, 69
Adhesive tape, 162

Adhesive wear, 369
Adipose tissue, 218
Adolescent scoliosis, 278
Adson maneuver, 123
Adult scoliosis, 278
Advancement, 264
Advancement flaps, 317
Adventitia, 223
Adventitious, 88
AE amputation, 170
Aebi, Etter, and Cosica fusion, 286
Aerobic exercises, 350
AFB, 147, 224
Afebrile, 88
AFO, 177
A-frame orthosis, 179
AGE, 386
AGF, 386
Aggravated, 88–89
Aggrecan, 362
Aggressive fibromatosis, 65
Agonists, 218
-agra, 89
Ahlback changes, 110
Ainhum, 331
Air pressure splints, 167
Air splint, 167
Airplane cast, 158
Airplane splint, 160, 182
Akin procedure, 338
Ala of the ilium, 240
Alanine aminotransferase, 142
Alar dysgenesis, 276
Albee fusion, 287
Albee procedure, 289
Albers-Schonberg disease, 43
Albert achillodynia, 66
Albright and Chase resection, 314
Albright syndrome, 55, 64
Albright-McCune-Sternberg syndrome, 55
Albumin, 142
Alexander view, 100
-algia, 89
Algodystrophy, 75
Algodystrophy syndrome, 49
Alignment, 386
Alk PO4 tase, 143
Alkaline phosphatase, 143
Allen maneuver, 123
Allen test, 127
Allergy, 89
Allis maneuver, 130

Allis sign, 130
Allman fracture classification system, 14
Alloantibodies, 150
Allogeneic, 197
Allograft, 197
Allowable stress, 365
ALP, 142, 143
ALPSA lesion, 34
ALS, 75
ALT, 142
Aluminum foam splint, 160
Alvers-Schönberg disease, 55
Ambi-, 386
Ambidextrous, 386
Amelia, 87, 305
American Shoulder and Elbow Surgeons system, 139
Aminoterminal propeptide, 146
Amniotic band syndrome, 87
Amniotic bands, 305
Amoss sign, 123
Amph-, 386
Amphi-, 386
Amputation neuroma, 77
Amputations, 262–264
    above-elbow, 170
    associated terminology, 264–268
    below-elbow, 170
    below-knee, 173
    Chopart, 173
    Lisfranc, 173
    partial hand, 170
    Syme, 173
    transfemoral, 174
    transtibial, 173
Amspacher and Messenbaugh osteotomy, 194
Amspacher and Messenbaugh procedure, 238
Amstutz and Wilson osteotomy, 194
Amyloidosis, skeletal, 54
Amyoplasia congenita, 59
Amyosthenia, 57
Amyotonia congenita, 59
Amyotrophic lateral sclerosis, 75
An-, 386
ANA, 143
Anaerobic culture, 147
Anaerobic exercises, 350
Analgesia, 89
Analgia, 89
Anastomosis, 89, 264

Anatomic femorotibial angle, 103
Anatomic neck, 227
Anatomic neck fracture, 6
Anatomic planes, 381–383
Anatomic position and directions, 381–389
    anatomic planes, 381–383
    surface location, 381
Anatomic snuff box, 298
Anatomy
    etymology of, 390–403
    in orthopaedic surgery, 189–268
    positions and directions, 381–389
Anchovy procedure, 314
Anderson and d'Alonzo fracture classification system, 14
Anderson and Fowler procedure, 338
Anderson and Hutchins procedure, 257
Anderson procedure, 257, 338
André Thomas sign, 127
Andrews procedure, 254
Anesthesia, 89, 259
    amputations and, 264
    surgical blocks, 259
Aneurysm, 70
Aneurysmal bone cyst, 49
Aneurysmorrhaphy, 224
Anghelescu sign, 123
Angiography, 117
Angioplasty, 117
Angiosarcoma, 74
Angles, radiographic, 103–107
Angular acceleration, 365
Angular displacement, 365
Angulation, 386
Angulation of fracture, 6
Aniso-, 387
Anisospondyly, 276
Anisotropic material, 365
Ankle
    abbreviations, 374–375
    anatomy of, 323–331
    arteries/veins/nerves of, 330–331
    bones of, 324–329
    clonus test, 135–136
    diseases/conditions of, 331–335
    dislocations, 32
    fracture-dislocation, 32
    fractures, 10–12, 14, 17, 21, 29
    joint, 180
    mortise, 330
    mortise diastasis, 10

muscles/tendons/ligaments of, 329–330
orthoses, 178
prosthesis for, 213
prosthetic components, 174–175
radiographic views, 102
sprains, 14, 33–34
surgery for, 336–345
surgical approaches, 345
tests, signs, and maneuvers for, 135
Ankle-arm index, 117
Ankle-brachial index, 117
Ankle-foot orthoses, 178
Ankylo-, 66, 69
Ankylodactylia, 69
Ankylosing spinal hyperostosis, 276
Ankylosing spondylitis, 73
Ankylosis, 69
Anode, 361
Anomaly, 89
Anonychia, 331
ANOVA, 358
Anserine bursa, 217
Antalgic gait, 139
Ante-, 387
Anteater nose sign, 109
Antebrachial cutaneous nerve, 237, 299
Antecedent, 387
Antecedent sign, 138
Antefemoral cyst, 68
Anteflexion, 89, 387
Anterior axillary approach, 259
Anterior compartment, 249
Anterior compartment syndrome, 71
Anterior control orthosis, 184
Anterior cruciate instability test, 132–133
Anterior cruciate ligament, 250
Anterior cruciate sprain, 33
Anterior dislocation, 32
Anterior drawer sign, 133, 135
Anterior hiatal sign, 109
Anterior iliofemoral ligament, 243
Anterior inferior iliac spine, 240
Anterior interosseous nerve, 237
Anterior interosseous nerve syndrome, 303
Anterior sacroiliac ligament, 241
Anterior shoulder dislocation, 31
Anterior spinal fusion, 286
Anterior spurring, 276
Anterior superior iliac spine, 240

Anterior talofibular sprain, 33
Anterior thoracic nerve, 229
Anterior tibial artery, 250
Anterior tibial sign, 132
Anterior tibial spine, 247
Anterior tibial tendon, 329
Anterior tibial tubercle, 247
Antero-, 387
Anteroinferior glenohumeral ligament, 229
Anterolateral rotatory instability, 85
Anteromedial approach, 259
Anteromedial cyst, 68
Anteromedial glenohumeral ligament, 229
Anteroposterior and mediolateral control orthosis, 185
Anteroposterior control orthosis, 185
Anteroposterior planes, 381
Anterosuperior glenohumeral ligament, 229
Anteversion, 89, 384, 387
Anticus, 387
Anticus reflex, 137
Anticus sign, 137
Anti-double-stranded DNA, 143
Anti-HBC, 150
Anti-HIV, 150
Anti-human immunodeficiency virus antibodies, 150
Antimere, 387
Antinuclear antibody, 143
Antistreptolysin O titer, 144
Anvil test, 123, 130
AO, 200
AO Classification System, 13
AO fixateur interne, 287
AO-Morscher plate, 203
Aortofemoral bypass, 224
Aortoiliac bypass, 224
AP view, 100
Apert disease, 55
Apert syndrome, 305
Apex, 387
Aphalangia, 87, 305
Aphasia, 89
Apical, 387
Apical lordotic view, 100
Apical view, 100
Apley sign, 133
Apley test, 133
Apo-, 387
Apodia, 87

Aponeurectomy, 218
Aponeurorrhaphy, 218, 222
Aponeuroses, 218
Aponeurotomy, 218
Apophyseal fracture, 4
Apophysis, 189
Apophysitis, 49
Apoplexy, 75
Apposition, 385
Apposition of fracture, 6
Apprehension test, 125
Approximate, 264
Apraxia, 75
APTT, 145
Aquatic exercise, 350
Arachnodactyly, 87, 305
Arachnoiditis, 75
Arbeitsgemeinschaft für Osteosynthesefragen, 200
Arcade of Frohse, 298
Arcade of Struthers, 235, 238
Arch support, 187
Archer's shoulder, 34
Arcuate ligament, 240, 297
Arizona universal leg support, 163
Arm (see also Upper extremities)
    anatomy of, 233–238
    blood vessels of, 236–237
    cylinder cast, 157
    muscles of, 235
    nerves of, 237–238
    surgery of, 238–240
Armstrong procedure, 231
Arnold brace, 185
Arnold-Chiari syndrome, 284
Aronson and Prager procedure, 238
Arrhythmia, 74
Arterial disorders, 70–72
Arterial insufficiency, 70
Arterial occlusive disease, 70
Arteriogram, 99
Arteriography, 117
    femoral, 98, 99
Arterioles, 223
Arteriosclerosis, 70
Arteriovenous fistula, 70
Arteriovenous malformation, 71
Arteritis, 73
Artery, 222, 223
Artery of Adamkiewicz, 274
Arthralgia, 67
Arthrectomy, 214
Arthrectomy catheter, 225

Arthrempyesis, 67
Arthritis, 67
  degenerative, 301
  gouty, 82
  hypertrophic, 67
  inflammatory, 301
  psoriatic, 301
  pyogenic, 301
  suppurative, 68
  trapeziometacarpal, 302
Arthro-, 67, 213
Arthrocace, 67
Arthrocele, 67
Arthrocentesis, 214
Arthrochalasis, 67
Arthrochondritis, 67
Arthroclasis, 214
Arthrodesis, 214, 215–216
  of elbow, 238
  of knee, 257
Arthrodial cartilage, 216
Arthrodynia, 67
Arthrodysplasia, 67
Arthroempyesis, 67
Arthroendoscopy, 214
Arthroereisis, 214, 338
Arthrofibrosis, 305
Arthrogram, 99, 214
Arthrography, 99
Arthrogryposis, 67, 306
Arthrokatadysis, 67, 82
Arthrokleisis, 67, 214
Arthrolith, 67
Arthrolysis, 214
Arthromeningitis, 67
Arthrometer test, 133
Arthroncus, 67
Arthroneuralgia, 67
Arthronosos, 67
Arthropathy, 67
Arthrophyma, 67
Arthrophyte, 67
Arthroplasty, 214, 314–315
  total knee, 256
Arthropyosis, 67
Arthrorheumatism, 67
Arthrosclerosis, 67
Arthroscopy, 214
Arthrosis, 40, 67
  cystic, 67
Arthrosteitis, 67
Arthrosynovitis, 67
Arthroxerosis, 67

Articular cartilage, 189, 216
Articular fracture, 4
Artifact, 138
Aseptic, 89, 264
Aseptic necrosis, 50
Ashhurst sign, 109
Ashurst fracture classification system,
  14–15
ASIF, 200
Asnis procedure, 245
Asnis screw, 200
ASO titer, 144
Aspartate aminotransferase, 142
Asphyxia, 89
Aspiration, 89, 264
Assay, 358
Assistive equipment, 356
Assmann disease, 50, 55
Association for the Study of Internal
  Fixation, 200
AST, 142
Asthenia, 89
Astragalus, aviator's, 10
ASVG, 225
Asymmetric, 387
Asymmetry, 89
Asymptomatic, 89
Asynergia, 89
Atavistic epiphysis, 192
Ataxia, 75, 89
Ataxic cerebral palsy, 76
Atheroma, 70
Atherosclerosis, 70
Athetoid cerebral palsy, 76
Athetosis, 89
Athlete's foot, 331
Atlanta brace, 179
Atlas, 271
Atonia, 75, 89
Atrophy, 74, 89
Attenuate, 264
Attenuation of tendons, 301
Atypical, 89
Austin procedure, 338
Autochthonous, 197
Autogenous, 197
Autogenous saphenous vein graft, 225
Autograft, 197
Autologous blood, 150
Autonomic nervous system, 269
Autopsy, 264
Autosomal, 92
AV fistula, 70

Avascular, 89
Avascular necrosis, 41, 50
Average angular velocity, 365
Average velocity, 366
AVF, 70
Aviator's astragalus, 10
Avila approach, 260
AVM, 71
Avulsion, 89
Avulsion fracture, 4
Avulsion of nail plate, 338
AxFem, 225
Axial cutaneous flaps, 317
Axial flag flaps, 317
Axial pattern skin flap, 317
Axilla, 227
Axillary artery, 229
Axillary block, 259
Axillary lateral view, 100
Axillary nerve, 229
Axillary vein, 229
Axillofemoral bypass, 225
Axis, 271, 387
Axis fracture, 22
Axonotmesis, 75

B

Baastrup disease, 276, 284
Babinski reflex, 136, 137
Babinski sign, 136
Babinski-Fröhlich syndrome, 55
Baciu and Filibiu arthrodesis, 215
Back
  diseases of, 274–277
  tests, signs, and maneuvers for,
    123–125
Backfire fracture, 8
Backpack palsy, 34
Bacterial species reports, 147–148
Bacteriologic studies, 147–148
Badelon fracture classification
  system, 15
Badgley arthrodesis, 215
Badgley nail, 200
Bado fracture classification system,
  15
Bail knee lock, 180
Bailey and Dubow osteotomy, 194
Bailey-Dubow nail, 200
Baker and Hill osteotomy, 194
Baker and Hill procedure, 338
Baker cyst, 85

Baker procedure, 256, 338
Balanced suspension, 163
Balkan frame, 166
Ball-and-socket joint, 214
Ball-and-socket osteotomy, 194
Balloon angioplasty, 225
Ballotment test, 127
Baltimore therapeutic equipment
    work simulator, 354
Bamboo spine, 109
Bandage, 156
Bandage adhesive, 162
Bankart fracture, 6
Bankart procedure, 231
Bankhart lesion, 31
    reverse, 31
Banks procedure, 338
Banks-Dervin rod, 287
BAP, 146
Bardeleben bone, 327
Barlow splint, 179
Barlow test, 130
Barr procedure, 338
Barre-Lieou syndrome, 75
Barr-Record procedure, 338
Barsky macrodactyly reduction, 317
Bartlett procedure, 338
Barton fracture, 8
    reverse, 9
Barton tongs, 164
Basal, 387
Basal neck fracture, 9
Baseball elbow, 34
Baseball finger, 9, 34
Baseball splint, 160
Baseline radiograph, 98
Basic hand splint, 181
Basilar, 387
Basile screw, 200
Basilic vein, 236
Basketball foot, 34
Batchelor plaster, 158
Batchelor-Brown procedure, 339
Bateman procedure, 231
Bathing, 355
Baumann angle, 103
Baumgard and Schwartz procedure,
    238
Baxter and D'Astous procedure, 245
Bayonet position, 6
Bayonet sign, 133
BE amputation, 170, 173–174
Beak deformity, 311

Beak ligaments, 297
Beaufort seating orthosis, 186
Bechtol prosthesis, 206
Becker muscular dystrophy, 59
Becker technique, 319
Beefburger procedure, 257
Beevor sign, 136
Behçet syndrome, 68
Bekhterev test, 123
Bell palsy, 78
Bell-Dally dislocation, 31
Bellemore and Barrett osteotomy, 194
Below-elbow amputation, 170
Below-knee amputation, 173–174
Below-knee suspension, 175
Bench test, 123–124
Bending, 366
Bending moment, 366
Bending moment diagram, 366
Benediction attitude, 127
Benediction sign, 127
Benign, 89
Bennett approach, 259–260
Bennett dislocation, 311
Bennett fracture, 9
Bennett orthosis, 184
Benoit-Gerrard, 200
Bent finger, 306
Bentzon procedure, 316
Berman and Gartland procedure, 339
Bertol method, 110
Bertolotti syndrome, 277
Betadine dressing, 162
Beta$_2$-microglobulin amyloidosis, 81
Bevin Aurglass technique, 316
BGP, 146
Biceps femoris, 249
Biceps groove, 227
Biceps muscle, 235
Biceps reflex, 138
Biceps tuberosity, 234
Bicipital groove, 227
Bicipital tendonitis, 65
Bickel and Moe procedure, 256
Bicompartmental knee replacement,
    212
Bier block, 259
Bifid thumb, 306
Bifurcated ligament, 330
Bifurcation, 89
Bigelow ligament, 243
Bigelow maneuver, reverse, 131–132
Biglycan, 362

BIL lesion, 34
Bilateral, 387
Bilhaut-Cloquet procedure, 317
Bilirubin, total, 142
Billet, 175
Bimalleolar fracture, 4
Bioceramics, 370
Biodegradable fixation, 200
Biomaterials, 369–370
Biomechanical adaptations, 366
Biomechanics, 364–369
Biometric prosthesis, 206
Biopsy, 264
Bipartite, 89
Bipartite patella, 85
Bipolar total hip replacement, 208
Bircher procedure, 339
Bivalve cast, 159
Black heel syndrome, 34
Blackburne ratio, 107
Black-dot heel, 34
Bladder, radiography, 99
Blade plate, 200
Blair arthrodesis, 215
Blatt capsulodesis, 314
Bleck procedure, 245
Blood and serum tests, general, 143–
    145
Blood bank
    procedures, 149–151
    products, 151
Blood components, abbreviations,
    151–152
Blood gases, 144
Blood urea nitrogen, 142
Blood vessels, 69, 222–227
    tumors, 74
Blount disease, 41, 55
Blount displacement osteotomy, 194
Blount osteotomy, 194
Blount plate, 200
Blount procedure, 238
Blount staple, 200
Blue foot syndrome, 331
Blue toe syndrome, 70
Blumensaat line, 107
Blundell Jones varus osteotomy, 194
Blunt dissection, 265
BMP, 99
Board, spinal, 167
Body casts, 157
Body jacket, 185
Boeck sarcoid, 55

Böhler angle, 103
Böhler nail, 200
Böhler splint, 160
Bohlman pin, 200
Bohlman fusion, 286
Bollard, 200
Bone
    age, 110
    anatomy of, 189–193
    block, 199
    cell tumors, 47
    cyst, unicameral, 55
    death, 50
    densitometry, 99
    formation tests, 146
    fracture healing devices, 199–204
    general surgery of, 193–194
    healing and metabolism, 360–361
    infarct, 51
    island, 51
    matrix, 190
    morphogenic protein, 360
    resorption tests, 146
    salts, 360–361
    scan, 97, 114
    scintigraphy, 114
    specific alkaline phosphatase, 146
    spur, 51, 310
    suture fixation, 193
    turnover markers, 145
Bone diseases, 40–49
    eponymic, 55–57
    infectious, 44–45
    miscellaneous, 49–55
    osteo- root, 40–44
    tumors, 45–49
        staging, 45
"Bone Gla protein," 146
Bone grafts, 196–199
    classification, 198–199
        by shape, 199
        by species source, 197
    eponymic terms for, 199
    general terminology of, 197
    preserving, 197–198
    revascularization of, 198–199
Bone marrow, 189–190
    biopsy, 142, 193
    pressure, 99
    transplant, 193
Bonola technique, 317
Bony ankylosis, 69

Boot-top fracture, 11
Borden, Spender, and Herndon os-
    teotomy, 195
Borden and Gearen osteotomy, 195
Bose procedure, 339
Bossing, 89
Boston bivalve, 159
Boston brace, 185
Bosworth arthrodesis, 215
Bosworth fracture, 11
Bosworth procedure, 231, 238, 257,
    339
Bouchard node, 55, 312
Bouldering, 35
Boutonnière deformity, 301–302, 311
    posttraumatic, 308
Boutonnière reconstruction, 320
Bouvier maneuver, 127
Bowers arthroplasty, 315
Bowers fracture, 34
Bowers "hemi" resection, 238
Bowler's thumb, 34
Bowstring sign, 124
Boxer's elbow, 8
Boyd amputation, 339
Boyd and Anderson procedure, 238
Boyd and Griffin fracture
        classification system, 16
Boyd and McLeod procedure, 238
Boyd and Sisk procedure, 231
Boyd side plate, 200
Boyes test, 127
Bozan maneuver, 130
Bracelet test, 127
Brachial artery, 229, 236
Brachial cutaneous nerve, 237
Brachial plexus, 229
Brachial vein, 236
Brachialgia statica paresthetica, 303
Brachialis muscle, 235
Brachioradialis muscle, 235
Brachydactyly, 306
Brackett osteotomy, 195
Bradford frame, 166
Bradford procedure, 288
Brady and Jewett procedure, 238
Bradycardia, 74
Bragard sign, 124
Brahms procedure, 339
Brailsford disease, 41, 55
Brattstrom fusion, 286
Braun procedure, 231

Breaststroker's knee, 34–35
Brendt and Harty fracture classifica-
    tion system, 15
Brett and Campbell, 257
Brett arthrodesis, 215
Brett osteotomy, 195
Brett procedure, 257
Breuerton view, 100–101
Bridle procedure, 339
Brisement, 264
Brisement procedure, 231
Bristow procedure, 231
Bristow-Laterjet procedure, 231
British test, 133
Brittain arthrodesis, 215
Brittain procedure, 231
Brittle bones, 42
Brittle failure, 366
Broaching, 264
Brockman procedure, 339
Brockman-Nissen arthrodesis, 314
Broden view, 101
Brodie abscess, 44, 55
Brooker classification of ectopic
    ossification, 53
Brooker-Willis nail, 200
Brooks and Jenkins fusion, 286
Brooks and Saddon procedure, 231
Broom-stick, 158
Brown procedure, 257
Brown tumor, 51
Brown-Séquard syndrome, 78
Brudzinski sign, 136
Bruit, 74, 89
Bryant sign, 125
Bryant traction, 164
BSAP, 146
BTE, 354
Buchman disease, 50, 55
Bucholtz fracture classification
        system, 16
Buck traction, 164
Bucket-handle fracture, 9
Bucket-handle tear, 84
Buck-Gramko procedure, 321
Budin splint, 188
Buerger disease, 70–71, 309
Buford complex, 82
Bugg-Boyd procedure, 339
Bulb dynamometer, 354
Bumper fracture, 10
BUN, 142

Bunion, 331
Bunionectomy, 339
Bunionette, 331
Bunkbed fracture, 11
Bunnell opponensplasty, 319
Bunnell procedure, 231
Bura view, 101
Burlap bone, 193
Burnham view, 101
Burns, from casts, 160
Burns disease, 41, 55
Burrows procedure, 231
Bursa sac, 213
Bursae, 217
Bursal projection, 330
Bursa-related diseases, 66
Bursectomy, 217
Bursitis, 66, 331
Bursocentesis, 217
Bursography, 99
Bursolith, 66
Bursopathy, 66
Bursotomy, 217
Bursting fracture, 4
Burton sign, 138
Butterfly fracture, 4

C

C bar, 182
Ca, 146
  P, 142
CABG, 225
Cable nerve grafts, 316
Cable twister orthosis, 180
Cachexia, 89
CAD-CAM, 174
Café-au-lait spots, 89, 138
Caffey disease, 55
Caisson disease, 51
Calandruccio device, 200
Calandruccio nail, 200
Calbinden, 361
Calcaneal branch artery/nerve, 330
Calcaneal spur pad, 188
Calcaneal spur syndrome, 331
Calcaneal tendon, 221
Calcaneofibular sprain, 33–34
Calcaneus, 324
  radiographic views, 102
Calcar, 240
Calcidiol (25(OH)D), 146

Calcific bursitis, 66
Calcific tendonitis, 65
Calcification, 89, 189
Calcified cartilage, 216
Calcinosis circumscripta, 73
Calcitonin, 146, 361
Calcitriol 1,25(OH)2D, 146
Calcium, 190
Calcium 47, 114, 146
Calcium binding protein, 361
Calcium pyrophosphate deposition
  disease, 82–83
Caldwell and Durham procedure, 253,
  257
Calf band, 180
Callahan and Scuderi approach, 259
Callahan approach, 260
Callahan fusion, 286
Callaway test, 125
Callosities, 89, 331
  devices for, 188
Callotasis, 193, 264
Callus, 12, 89, 331
Calnan-Nicole prosthesis, 206
Cambium layer, 191, 193
Camelback sign, 133
Camitz procedure, 320
Campanacci lesion, 42
Campbell and Akbarnia procedure,
  238
Campbell arthrodesis, 215
Campbell procedure, 238, 245, 254,
  255, 339
Camptocormia, 276
Camptodactyly, 306
Canale procedure, 245
Canale view, 101
Canale-Kelly fracture classification
  system, 16
Canaliculus, 191
Canal-to-calcar isthmus ratio, 107
Cancellous bone, 191
Cancellous graft, 198
Cancellous screw, 200
Canes, 161
Cannulated nail, 200
Cannulated screw, 200
Cantelli sign, 136
Capacitive coupling, 205, 362
Capacitor, 362
Capillaries, 223–224
Capital epiphysis, 242

Capitellocondylar prosthesis, 206
Capitellum, 233
Capner procedure, 288
Capsotomy, 217
Capsular arthroplasty, 244
Capsular release, 321
Capsule, 213, 217
Capsulectomy, 217, 314, 321
Capsulitis, 69
Capsulo-, 69, 217
Capsulodesis, 217, 321
Capsuloplasty, 217
Capsulorrhaphy, 217
Capsulotomy, 217
Carbon Copy II/III foot, 175
γ-Carboxyglutamic acid, 361
Carboxyterminal propeptide, 146
Carcar femorale, 240
Cardiovascular, 224
Carducci test, 127–128
Caries, 89
Caries sicca, 89
Carotid artery, 272
Carotid endarterectomy, 225
Carotid subclavian bypass, 225
Carotid tubercle, 272
Carpal bone, 291
Carpal bossing, 312
Carpal coalition, 306
Carpal compression test, 128
Carpal height ratio, 107
Carpal instability, 311
Carpal instability dissociative, 310
Carpal instability nondissociative, 310
Carpal pedal spasm, 308
Carpal tunnel, 298
Carpal tunnel release, 321
Carpal tunnel syndrome, 303
Carpal tunnel view, 101
Carpectomy, 321
Carpus, 291
Carroll arthrodesis, 314
Carroll arthroplasty, 314
Carroll procedure, 257
Carrying angle, 103
Carstan reverse wedge osteotomy, 317
Carter-Rowe view, 101
Cartilage, 213, 216–217
  bone, 191
  diseases, 60–63
    chondro- root diseases, 60–61
    epiphyses abnormalities, 62

Cartilage *(cont.)*
 metabolic, 62–63
 miscellaneous, 61–62
 mucopolysaccharidoses, 62–63
 research, 362–363
 space narrowing, 281
 surgical procedures, 217
 tumors, 47–48
 types of, 216–217
Cartilage-hair hypoplasia, 61
Cartwheel fracture, 10
CASH orthosis, 185
Cast boot, 158, 159
Cast brace, 2, 159
Cast cutter, 156
Cast padding, 156
Cast protectors, 159
Cast shoe, 159
Cast sock, 176
Cast syndrome, 160
Castle and Schneider procedure, 245
Casts, 155–156
 abbreviations, 376
 complications of, 160
 devices applied to, 159–160
 immobilization, 157–159
 materials, 156–157
CAT, 114
CAT scan, 97, 114
Cata-, 387
Cathepsins, 362
Catheter, 98
Catheterization, 264
Cathode, 362
Cathode ray tube, 98
Catterall hip score, 110
Cauda equina syndrome, 280
Caudad, 387
Caudal, 387
Causalgia, 75
Cauterization, 265
Cautery, 265
Cave and Rowe procedure, 256
Cave approach, 260
Cavus foot, 335
CAWO, 339
CBC, 141–142
CC, 148
CDH, 32
CE angle, 103
Cedell fracture, 11
Cell components, 358
Cellular cartilage, 217

Cellulitis, 89
Cement line, 361
Cementless total hip replacement, 210
Cement-wedge sign, 109
Center edge angle, 103
Center of gravity, 366
Center of mass, 366
Central cord syndrome, 283
Central dislocation, 32
Central fracture, 9
Central polydactyly, 307
Central slip repair/reconstruction, 319
Central slip tendon, 298
Centri-, 387
Centroid, 366
Cephalic, 387
Cephalic vein, 229, 236
Cerebral palsy, 76
Cerebroside reticulocytosis, 55–56
Cerebrospinal fluid, 148
Cerebrovascular, 224
Cerebrovascular accident, 71
Cervical dislocations, 31
Cervical halter traction, 164
Cervical lordosis, reversal of, 279
Cervical orthoses, 185–186
Cervical plexus, 272
Cervical rib, 277
Cervical spine
 anatomy of, 270, 271–273
 arteries of, 272
 bones of, 271–272
 fusion, 286
 muscles of, 272
 nerves of, 272
 radiographic views, 102
 veins of, 272
Cervical traction, 349
Cervicothoracolumbosacral orthoses, 186
Chaddock reflex, 136
Chaddock sign, 136
Chadwick and Bentley fracture classification system, 16
Chairback orthosis, 184
Chalk-stick fracture, 109
Chamberlain line, 107
Chamfer, 265
Chance fracture, 9
Chandler arthrodesis, 215
Chandler procedure, 245, 257
Chaput fracture, 11
Chaput tubercle, 247

Charcot disease, 75
Charcot joint disease, 78
Charcot restraint orthotic walker, 178
Charcot-Marie-Tooth disease, 78, 304
Charleston bending brace, 185
Charley horse, 35
Charnley and Henderson arthrodesis, 215
Charnley arthrodesis, 215
Charnley hip scale, 139
Charnley screw, 200
Charnley-Müller approach, 260
Chauffeur's fracture, 8
Chaves-Rapp procedure, 231
Check socket, 176
Cheilectomy, 339
Chemistry profiles, 142–143
Chemonucleolysis, 285
Chemosterilized grafts, 198
Chest
 radiographic views, 102
 straps, 172
Chevron arthrodesis, 313
Chevron osteotomy, 339
Chevron procedure, 338
Chiene test, 130
Chilblains, 71
Children, special shoes for, 188
Chip fracture, 4
Chip graft, 199
Chisel fracture, 8
Cho procedure, 254
Cholesterol, 142
Chondralgia, 60
Chondrectomy, 217
Chondritis, 60
Chondro-, 60, 216–217
Chondroblastoma, 47
Chondroblasts, 218
Chondrocalcin, 362
Chondroclasts, 218
Chondrocytes, 218
Chondrodiatasis, 217
Chondrodynia, 60
Chondrodysplasia, 60
Chondrodysplasia punctata, 61
Chondrodystrophia, 61
Chondrodystrophia fetalis, 61
Chondroepiphysitis, 61
Chondrofibroma, 61
Chondroitin sulfate, 363
Chondrolipoangioma, 61

Chondrolipoma, 61
Chondrolysis, 61
Chondroma, 48
  periosteal, 48
Chondromalacia, 61
Chondromatosis, 61
  Henderson-Jones, 41
Chondrometaplasia, 61
Chondromyoma, 61
Chondromyxoid fibroma, 48
Chondromyxoma, 61
Chondromyxosarcoma, 61
Chondronecrosis, 61
Chondroosteodystrophy, 61, 63
Chondropathia tuberosa, 57
Chondropathy, 61
Chondrophyte, 61
Chondroplasty, 217
Chondroporosis, 61
Chondrosarcoma, 48
  clear cell, 48
  dedifferentiated, 48
  mesenchymal, 48
  parosteal, 48
  secondary, 48
Chondrosarcomatosis, 61
Chondrosteoma, 61
Chondrosternoplasty, 217
Chondrotomy, 217
Chop amputation, 264
Chopart amputation, 173, 339
Chopart dislocation, 32
Choppy sea sign, 109
Chordoma, 49
Chorea, 76
Chrisman-Snook procedure, 339
Chromonychia, 311
Chromosomal conditions, 80–82
Chronic, 89
Chronic osteomyclitis, 45
Chronic sclerosing osteomyelitis of
  Garré, 45
Chuinard and Petersen arthrodesis,
  215
Chvostek sign, 138
Chvostek test, 138
Chvostek-Weiss sign, 138
Chylothorax, 90
Cicatrix, 90
CID, 310
Cincinnati incision, 339
Cinefluoroscopy, 114
Cineplastic amputation, 264

Cineradiography, 114
Cineroentgenogram, 114
Circadian, 358
Circular amputation, 264
Circumduction, 383
Circumduction maneuver, 128
Circumference, 387
Circumflex, 387
CK, 144
Clancy procedure, 254
Clark pectoralis major transfer, 319
Claudication, 71
Clavicectomy procedure, 231
Clavicle, 227
  fractures, 14
  orthosis, 184
  radiographic views, 102
Clavicotomy procedure, 231
Clavus, 331–332
Clavus durum, 333
Clawhand deformity, 304
Clawhand sign, 128
Clawtoes, 332
Claw type basic frame, 166
Clay shoveler's fracture, 9
Clayton procedure, 339
Clear cell chondrosarcoma, 48
Cleavage fracture, 4
Cleeman sign, 132
Cleft hand, 306
Cleido-, 227
Cleidocranial dysostosis, 51
Cleland ligament, 298
Clenched fist view, 101
Clinodactyly, 306
Cloacae, 45
Clonus, 90
Closed amputation, 264
Closed biopsy, 264
Closed chain exercise, 350
Closed dislocation, 31
Closed fracture, 3
Closed reduction, 194
Closing abductory wedge osteotomy,
  339
Closing wedge, 159
Closing wedge osteotomy, 195
Closure
  primary, 267
  secondary, 267
Cloth binder, 184
Clothespin graft, 199
Cloverlead nail, 200

Cloward fusion, 286
Clubbing, 311
Clubfoot, 332, 335
Cluneal nerve, 241
Co-, 387
Coach's finger, 35
Coalition, 332
Coaptation splint, 160
Cobb method, 110
Coccyalgia, 277
Coccydynia, 277
Coccygeal spine, anatomy of, 270
Coccygectomy, 288
Coccygodynia, 277
Coccygotomy, 288
Coccyodynia, 277
Coccyx, 273
  anatomy of, 270
  radiographic views, 102
Cocked-half flap, 317
Cock-up splint, 181
Codfish vertebrae, 109
Codivilla procedure, 256
Codman angle, 103
Codman approach, 260
Codman exercises, 350
Codman sign, 126
Codman triangle, 103
Codman tumor, 47
Coefficient of friction, 366
-coele, 90
Coffin-Lowry syndrome, 81
Cofield procedure, 231
Cognitive skills, 356
Cogwheel phenomenon, 138
Cogwheel sign, 138
Cole osteotomy, 195
Cole procedure, 339
Coleman lateral standing block test,
  135
Coleman procedure, 339
Collagen, 218
  research terminology, 364
Collagen vascular disorders, 72–74
Collagenase, 364
Collagenases, 359
Collar and cuff, 159
Collar-button abscess, 312
Collateral circulation, 224
Collateral ligament, 221, 329
Colles fracture, 8
  reverse, 9
Colonna capsular arthroplasty, 244

Colonna fracture classification system, 16–17
Colony count, 148
Colton fracture classification system, 17
Com-, 387
Comatose, 90
Combined arch support, 187
Combined stenosis, 279
Commemorative sign, 138
Comminuted fracture, 4
Commissural myelorrhapy, 288
Common digital arteries, 299
Common digital nerves, 299
Common peroneal nerve, 253
Common tendon, 221
Comolli sign, 126
Compact bone, 191
Compartment syndrome, 71
Compensatory curve, 278
Compere and Thompson fusion arthrodesis, 215
Complete aphalangia, 87
Complete blood count, 141–142
Complete dislocation, 31
Complete fracture, 4
Complete paraxial hemimelia, 87
Complete phocomelia, 87
Compliance, 366
Complicated dislocation, 31
Composite graft, 198
Composite nail bed flap, 317
Compound dislocation, 31
Compression, 366
Compression arthrodesis, 215
Compression dressing, 162
Compression fracture, 4
Compression of nerve root, 280
Compressive neuropathy, 303
Computed axial tomography, 114
Computed axial tomography scanning, 97
Computed tomography, 114
quantitative, 99
Con-, 387
Concave, 387
Concentric contraction, 350
Condensing osteitis of the clavicle, 51
Condylar cuff, 175
Condylar fracture, 4, 8
Condylar-plateau angle, 103
Condyle, 191

Condylectomy, 194, 339
Condylotomy, 194
Cone arthrodesis, 339
Coned-down view, 101
Confidence interval, 358
Configuration of fracture, 6
Confrontational test, 128
Congenital, 90
Congenital bars, 332
Congenital convex pes valgus, 332, 335
Congenital dislocation, 31, 85
Congenital dysplasia of hip, 32
Congenital hypotonia, 59
Congenital limb absences, 87–88
Congenital myotonia, 59
Congenital pancytopenia, 91
Congenital pseudarthrosis, 51
Congenital rocker-bottom flatfoot, 332
Congenital scoliosis, 278–279
Congenital trigger thumb, 305, 306
Congenital ulnar drift, 308
Congenital vertical talus, 332
Congestive heart failure, 74
Congruence angle, 103
Conjoined tendon, 221, 229
Connecting cartilage, 217
Connective tissues, 217–218
Connexus intertendineus, 296
Conrad-Bugg trapping, 11
Consecutive dislocation, 31
Constitutional stenosis, 279
Constrictive edema, from casts, 160
Contagious, 90
Contractions, 90
Contracture, 90
Contralateral, 387
Contralateral sign, 136
Contralateral straight leg raising test, 124
Contrast, 98
Contrast agents, 98
Contrast baths, 349
Contrast radiography, 98
Contrast study, 98
Contrecoup, 90
Control cables, 171
Controlled ankle walker, 188
Contusion, 90
Convalescence, 90
Conversion disorder, 90

Convex, 387
Convulsion, 90
Coonrad prosthesis, 206
Coopernail sign, 124
Coordination extremity test, 136
Copeland and Howard procedure, 231
Coracobrachialis, 227
Coracobrachialis muscle, 235
Coracoclavicular ligament, 229
Coracohumeral ligament, 229
Coracoid, 227
Coracoid impingement syndrome, 35
Cordotomy, 288
Core protein, 363
Corner sign, 110
Coronal, 387
Coronal plane, 381–382
Coronary artery bypass graft, 225
Coronoid process, 235
Corpectomy, 288
Corrective cast, 159
Corset front, 186
Cortical bone, 191
Cortical defect
fibrous, 54
subcortical, 54
Cortical fibrous dysplasia, 51
Cortical fracture, 4
Cortical graft, 198
Corticocancellous graft, 199
Corticotomy, 194
Costectomy, 231
Costo-, 273
Costochondral junction, 273
Costoclavicular maneuver, 123
Costoplasty, 265
Costotransversectomy, 231
Costovertebral angle, 273
Costovertebral joint, 273
Cotrel cast, 157
Cotrel traction, 164
Cotrel-Dubousset instrument, 287
Cotting, 339
Cotton fracture, 11
Cotton osteotomy, 195
Cotton roll, 156
Cotton-loader position cast, 158
Couch, DeRosa, and Throop procedure, 245
Couple, 366
Coupling, 366
Coventry osteotomy, 195

Coxa adducta, 83
Coxa breva, 82
Coxa magna, 82
Coxa plana, 50, 57, 82
Coxa saltans, 82
Coxa senilis, 83
Coxa valga, 83
Coxa vara, 83
Coxa vara luxans, 83
Coxalgia, 83
Coxarthria, 83
Coxarthritis, 83
Coxarthrocace, 83
Coxarthropathy, 83
Coxarthrosis, 83
Coxitis, 83
Coxotomy, 245
CP, 76
CPA, 103
c-PCP, 146
CPK, 144
CPPD, 82–83
Cr, 142
Cracchiolo procedure, 339
Cramp, 90
Craniad, 388
Craniomandibular cervical syndrome, 279
Crankshaft phenomenon, 277
Crawford small parts dexterity test, 354
Crawford-Adams pin, 200
C-reactive protein, 144
Creatine kinase, 144
Creatine phosphokinase, 144
Creatinine, 142, 144
Creep, 366
Creeping substitution, 198
Crego osteotomy, 195
Crego procedure, 244
Crepitus, 90
Crescent sign, 109
Crescentic osteotomy, 339
CREST syndrome, 73
Cricoid ring, 272
Crossed intrinsic transfer, 319
Cross-finger flap, 318
Cross-linking, 364
Cross-over syndrome, 35
Cross-table lateral view, 101
Cross-training, 350
Crossunion, 13

CROW, 178
CRP, 144
Crucial angle if Gissane, 103
Cruciate screw, 201
Cruciform anterior spinal hyperexten-
    sion orthosis, 185
Crush syndrome, 304
Crutches, 161
Crutchfield tongs, 164
Cryoprecipitate, 151
Crystalline arthropathy, 301
C&S, 147
CSF, 148
CT, 114
CT scan, 114
C-telopeptide, 147
CTS, 303
C-tx, 147
Cubbins approach, 259
Cubbins procedure, 231
Cubital tunnel, 238
Cubital tunnel syndrome, 303
Cuboid, 324
Culture and sensitivity, 147
Cuneiform osteotomy, 195
Cuneiforms, 324
Cup arthroplasty, 244
Curettage, 265
Curette, 265
Curly toe, 332
Curvilinear, 388
Cushing disease, 80
Custom-molded shoes, 187, 188
Cutaneous ligaments, 298
Cutaneous nerve
    of arm, 237
    of forearm, 237
Cut-back zone, 191
Cuticle, 299, 330
Cutting cone, 191
CVA, 71
Cyanosis, 74, 90
Cylinder cast, 158
Cylindrical osteotomy, 339
Cyst, 90
    antefemoral, 68
    anteromedial, 68
    ganglion, 64
    mucous, 65
    popliteal, 68, 71
    synovial, 68
    tibiofibular, 68

Cystic arthrosis, 67
Cystic osteomyelitis, 45

D

Dactylitis, 332
DANA total shoulder, 206
Danis-Weber fracture classification
    system, 29
Darrach resection, 314
Darrach-McLaughlin approach, 260
Das Gupta procedure, 231
Dashboard fracture, 9
DAT, 149
d'Aubigne procedure, 253, 257
Davis arthrodesis, 215
Dawbarn sign, 126
DCP, 201
De-, 388
de Andrade and MacNab fusion, 286
de la Caffinière prosthesis, 206
de Quervain disease, 66, 308
de Quervain fracture, 8
de Quervain release, 320
De Rosa and Graziano procedure, 238
Debeyre procedure, 231
Débridement, 90, 265
Decalcification, 90
Decompression, 265
    of spine, 285
Decompressive laminectomy, 285
Decorin, 363
Decubitus ulcer, from casts, 160
Dedifferentiated chondrosarcoma, 48
Deep, 388
Deep compartment, 249
Deep femoral artery, 243, 250
Deep peroneal nerve, 253
Deep space infection, 312
Deep transverse intermetacarpal liga-
    ment, 297
Deep transverse metacarpal ligament, 296
Deep venous thrombosis, 70
Defervescence, 90
Degenerate tear, 85
Degenerative, 90
Degenerative disk disease, 281
Degenerative stenosis, 279
Degrees of freedom, 366
Dehiscence, 90, 265
Dehne cast, 157

Dejerine disease, 78
Dejerine sign, 124
Dejerine-Sottas syndrome, 78
Delayed primary closure, 265
Delayed union, 12
Delayed-onset muscle soreness, 59
Delbert cast, 158
Delbet fracture classification system,
      16–17
DeLorme exercises, 350
Delta, 388
Delta nail, 201
Delta phalanx, 306
Deltoid ligament, 297, 330
Deltoid muscle, 227
Deltoid splitting approach, 259
Deltoid sprain, 33
Demarcation line, 107
Demianoff sign, 124
Demineralized bone graft, 198
Denis Browne bar, 178
Dennison brace, 186
Deossification, 90
Deoxypyridinoline, 147
Dependent drainage, 265
Depressed fracture, 4
Derangement, 90
Derby nail, 201
Dermatomal pain, 39
Dermatome, 280–281
Dermatomycosis pedis, 331
Dermatomyositis, 73
Dermodesis, 321
Derotation osteotomy, 195
Desault sign, 131
Descot fracture, 11
Designed After Natural Anatomy
      total shoulder, 206
Desmalgia, 65
Desmectasis, 65
Desmitis, 65
Desmo-, 65, 221–222
Desmocytoma, 65
Desmodynia, 65
Desmoid, 65
   extraabdominal, 65
   periosteal, 65
Desmoma, 65
Desmopathy, 65
Desmoplasia, 65
Desmoplastic, 65
Desmoplastic fibroma of bone, 49
Desmorrhexis, 65

Desmosis, 65
Desmotomy, 222
Dessault dislocation, 310
Destot sign, 131
Developmental dysplasia, 31
   of hip, 32, 83
Dewar and Barrington procedure, 231
DEXA, 99
Dexter, 388
Dextrorotoscoliosis, 278
Deyerle pin, 201
DHS, 201
Dia-, 388
Diabetes, 81
   foot, devices for, 188
Diabetic cheirarthropathy, 302
Diacondylar fracture, 4
Diagnosis, 90
Dial lock, 180
Dial osteotomy, 195
Diamond inlay, 199
Diaphragm, 273
Diaphysectomy, 194
Diaphysis, 191
Diaplasis, 194, 265
Diarthrodial cartilage, 217
Dias and Giegerich procedure, 339
Dias-Tachdjian fracture classification
      system, 17
Diastasis, 2
   ankle mortise, 10
Diastematomyelia, 284
Diastole, 224
Diastrophic dwarfism, 61
Diathermy, 349
Dickson osteotomy, 195
Dickson-Diveley procedure, 339
Diff, 142
Differential WBC, 142
Diffuse, 90, 388
Diffuse idiopathic sclerosing hyper-
      ostosis, 67
Digital artery/nerves, 330
Digital color Doppler, 97
Digital fossa, 242
Digital prosthesis, 339
Digital retinacula, 297
Digital subtraction angiography, 117
Dillwyn-Evans procedure, 339–340
Dimon and Hughston osteotomy, 195
Dimon and Hughston procedure, 245
Dimon osteotomy, 195
Dimple sign, 135, 138

DIP fusion, 340
Diplegic cerebral palsy, 76
Direct anti-human globulin test, 149
Direct blood, 149
Direct Coombs test, 149
Direct electric stimulation, 205
Direct fracture, 4
Direct injury dislocation, 32
Dis-, 388
Disappearing bone disease, 42
Disarticulation amputation, 264
Discectomy, 285
Discoid meniscus, 85
Diseases
   abbreviations, 371–372
   vs. syndromes, 39
DISH, 67
DISI, 310
Disk space infection, 281
Diskitis, 281
Diskography, 99
Dislocation, 2, 31–32
   terminology of, 2–3
Dismemberment, 265
Displaced fracture, 4
Displacement, 366
Dissection, 265
Dissegmental dysplasia, 81
Distal, 388
Distal bypass, 225
Distal femur fractures, 10
Distal finger amputation revision, 316
Distal muscular dystrophy, 60
Distal pad, 176
Distal phocomelia, 87
Distal pulp, 298
Distal radial ulnar joint, 291
Distal thigh band, 180
Distal tingling on percussion sign, 138
Distraction osteogenesis, 194
Divergent dislocation, 32
Diver's disease, 51
Diverticulum, 90
Dolichostenomelia, 87
Doll's eye sign, 136
Dome fracture, 10, 11
Dome plunger, 201
Dominant, 92
DOMS, 59
Dooley nail, 201
Doppler ultrasound, 117
Dorr ratio, 107
Dorsal, 388

Dorsal digital artery, 299
Dorsal digital nerve, 299
Dorsal expansion, 298
Dorsal extensor compartments, 297
Dorsal intercalated segment instability, 310
Dorsal lumbar corset, 185
Dorsal lumbar orthosis, 185
Dorsal radiocarpal ligament, 297
Dorsal scapular nerve, 230
Dorsal wedge osteotomy, 340
Dorsalis pedis artery, 330
Dorsal-V osteotomy, 340
Dorsiflexed metatarsal, 332
Dorsiflexion, 383
Double camelback sign, 133
Double crush syndrome, 304
Double fracture, 4
Double hip spica, 158
Double-action ankle joint, 180
Dowager's hump, 90
Dowel procedure, 286
Down syndrome, 81
DPA, 99
DPD, 99
DpD, 147
DPG-I, 362
DPG-II, 363
DPYD, 147
Drainage, 265
Drawer sign, 133, 135
Drawer test, 126
Drennan procedure, 340
Dressings, 155–156, 161–163, 355
    abbreviations, 376
    general types of, 162
    specialized, 162–163
Drez procedure, 254
Drop arm test, 126
Drop finger, 9
Dropfoot, 161, 332
    from casts, 160
Dropfoot gait, 139
Drop-lock ring, 180
DRUJ, 291
Drummond interspinous segmental spinal instrument, 288
Dry dressing, 162
DSA, 117
DTP sign, 138
du Toit and Roux procedure, 231
Dual onlay graft, 199
Dual photon absorptiometry, 99

Dual photon densitometry, 99, 115
Dual X-ray absorptiometry, 99
Duchenne disease, 78
Duchenne muscular dystrophy, 59
Duchenne sign, 128
Ductile failure, 366
Ductility, 366
Dugas sign, 126
Dugas test, 126
Dunlop traction, 164
Dunn procedure, 245, 288
Dunn-Brittain procedure, 340
Dunn-Brittain triple arthrodesis, 340
Duplay disease, 65
Duplex Doppler, 117
Duplex ultrasound, 118
Dupuytren contracture, 66, 311, 332
Dupuytren contracture release, 321
Dupuytren fracture, 11
Dupuytren sign, 131, 138
Dural ectasia, 76
Durham procedure, 340
Duverney fracture, 10
DuVries plantar condylectomy, 340
DuVries procedure, 340
Dwarfism
    achondroplastic, 61
    diastrophic, 61
Dwyer instrument, 287
Dwyer osteotomy, 195
Dwyer procedure, 340
Dyc-punch fracture, 8
Dyesthesia, 91
Dynamic hinged elbow fracture brace, 182
Dynamic hip screw, 201
Dynamic load, 366
Dynamic orthosis, 178
Dynamic splint, 160
Dynamic-compression plate, 201
Dynamometer, 352
-dynia, 90
Dys-, 90
Dysautonomia, 76
Dyschondroplasia, 60
Dyscollagenoses, 72
Dyscrasic fracture, 12
Dysfunction, 91
Dysostosis, cleidocranial, 51
Dysplasia, 91
    cortical fibrous, 51
    developmental, 31, 32
    of hip, 83

epiarticular osteochondromatous, 48
    osteofibrous, 42
    progressive diaphyseal, 54
Dysplasia epiphyseal multiplex congenita, 62
Dysplasia epiphysealis capitus femoris, 83
Dysplasia epiphysealis hemimelia, 48, 62
Dysraphism, 277
Dystonia, 91
Dystrophinopathy, 59
Dystrophy, 91
    Fröhlich adiposogenital, 55

E

Eagle-Barrett syndrome, 82
Earle sign, 131
Eaton prosthesis, 206
Eaton volar plate arthroplasty, 314
Ebonation, 194, 265
Eburnation, 91
Ec-, 388
Eccentric contraction, 351
Ecchymosis, 91
ECG, 154
Echogenic, 98
ECIC, 226
Ecker, Lotke, and Glazer procedure, 257
Ectasia, 84
Ectopic, 388
Ectopic ossification
    Brooker classification of, 53
    Hamblen classification of, 53
Ectromelia, 87
ED, 170
Edema, 91
    constrictive, from casts, 160
Eden-Hybbinette procedure, 231
Eden-Lange procedure, 231
Edinburgh method, 110
EDS, 81–82
Edwards instrument, 287
EEG, 154
Effusion, 91
Eggers plate and screw, 201
Eggers procedure, 257
Eggshell procedure, 288
Egyptian foot, 332
Ehlers-Danlos syndrome, 81–82

Elastic behavior, 366
Elastic cartilage, 217
Elastic knee cage, 178
Elastic modulus, 366
Elastic orthosis, 178
Elastic stable intramedullary nailing, 201
Elastic twister orthosis, 180
Elastofibroma, 63
Elbow
    disarticulation, 170
    dislocations, 32
    fractures, 8
    hinges, 171
    orthoses, 182
    prostheses for, 207
    radiographic views, 102
    surgical approaches to, 260
Elbow-wrist-hand orthoses, 182
Electric stimulation of fracture healing, 205
Electrical stimulation, 349
Electrical switch control, 171
Electrical testing, 353
Electrobiology, 361–362
Electrocardiogram, 118, 154
Electrocautery, 265
Electroencephalogram, 154
Electromyography, 353
Eleventh cranial nerve, 272
ELISA, 358
Elliott plate, 201
Ellis Jones procedure, 340
Ellis procedure, 238
Ellison procedure, 254
Elmslie procedure, 340
Elongation, 366
Elson middle slip test, 128
Ely sign, 136
Ely test, 131, 136
Em-, 388
Emaciation, 91
Embolus, 71
Emergency stabilization, 166–167
EMG, 353
Emslie-Cholmely procedure, 340
Emslie-Trillat procedure, 255
En-, 388
Enchondral bone, 191
Enchondroma, 48
Enchondromatosis, 48, 57
Encirclage, 201

Endarterectomy, 225
Ender nail, 201
Endo-, 388
Endocrine fracture, 12
Endolite foot, 175
Endoskeletal prosthesis, 173, 176–177
Endosteum, 191
End-to-end anastomosis, 225
End-to-side anastomosis, 226
Endurance limit, 367
Energy, 366
Energy conservation, 356
Energy storing feet, 174
Engebretsen procedure, 254
Engelmann disease, 55
Enneking procedure, 253
Enthesis, 66
Enthesitis, 66
Enthesopathy, 66
Entrapment syndrome, 76
Enucleate, 265
Enucleation, 91
Enzyme-linked immunosorbent assay, 358
Eosinophilia-myalgia syndrome, 59
Eosinophilic granulomas, 48, 49
Ependymoma, 283
Epi-, 388
Epiarticular osteochondroma, 48
Epiarticular osteochondromatous dysplasia, 48
Epicondylar fracture, 8
Epicondylitis, 66
Epidermoid cyst, 311, 312
Epidural block, 259
Epilepsy, 76
Epineural fibrosis, 281
Epineural repair, 316
Epineurotomy, 316
Epiphyseal cartilage, 191
Epiphyseal dysplasias, 62
Epiphyseal exostosis, 48
Epiphyseal fracture, 4, 25
Epiphyseal hyperplasia, 62
Epiphyseal osteochondroma, 48
Epiphyseal plate, 191
Epiphyseal slip fracture, 4
Epiphyseodesis, 194
Epiphyseolysis, 194
Epiphysiodesis, 62
Epiphysiolysis, 62

Epiphysiopathy, 62
Epiphysis, 41, 191–192
    abnormalities of, 62
    pressure, 41
    slipped, 62
    slipped capital femoral, 54
    stippled, 62
    traction, 41
Epiphysitis, 62
Epithelioid sarcoma, 49
Epitrochlea, 234
Eponychia, 312
Eponychium, 299, 330
Eponymic terms, ICD codes for, 404–409
Equilibrium, 366
Equinovarus outflare shoes, 188
Equinus, 332
Erb disease, 59
Erb palsy, 78
Erb paralysis, 60
Erb-Goldflam disease, 57
Ergotism, 73
Erichsen sign, 124
Ericksson procedure, 254
Erosion, 91
Erythema, 91
Erythrocyte sedimentation rate, 144
Escarotomy, 318
Eschar, 91
ESIN, 201
Esmarch bandage, 162
Eso-, 388
Esophagus, 272
ESR, 144
Essex-Lopresti fracture, 8
Essex-Lopresti fracture classification system, 17
Essex-Lopresti procedure, 340
Esthesia, 91
Etiology, 91
Etymology of orthopaedics, 390–403
Eurotaper, 211
Evacuate, 265
Evans procedure, 340
Evans-Wales fracture classification system, 18
Eversion, 384
Ewing's sarcoma, 48
Ex-, 388
Exacerbation, 91

Exchange nailing, 201
Excise, 265
Excision, 265
Excursion amplifier sleeve, 171
Exercises, physical therapy, 350–352
Exo-, 388
Exoskeletal prosthesis, 173
Exostectomy, 340
Exostosis, 53, 332
    epiphyseal, 48
    hereditary multiple, 53
    hypertrophic, 53
Exploration, 265
Extended counter, 187
Extended steel shank, 180
Extension, 383
Extension aid, 176
Extension body cast, 157
Extension exercises, 351
Extensor carpi radialis brevis, 235
Extensor carpi radialis longus, 235
Extensor digitorum longus, 249
Extensor digitorum longus/brevis, 329
Extensor hallucis longus, 249
Extensor hallucis longus/brevis, 329
Extensor hood, 298
Extensor retinacula, 297
Extensor wad of three, 235
External, 388
External malleolus sign, 136
External rotation, 385
    fracture from, 14
External rotation recurvatum test, 133
External rotators, 242–243
External skeletal fixation devices, 204–205
Externally powered tenodesis orthosis, 181
Extirpation, 265
Extra-, 388
Extraabdominal desmoid, 65
Extraanatomic bypass, 226
Extraarticular arthrodesis, 215
Extracapsular ankylosis, 69
Extracapsular fracture, 4, 10
Extracranial/intracranial bypass, 226
Extraction, 265
Extrinsic muscles, 329
Extrinsic tightness test, 128
Extubation, 265
Exudate, 91

Eyler flexorplasty, 240
Eyler procedure, 231

F

Fabere test, 124
Face climbing, 35
Facet, 192, 388
Facet joint, 271
Facet subluxation, 33
Facet tropism, 277
Facetectomy, 288
Factitious edema, 309
Factitious injury, 91
Factor IX, 150–151
Factor VIII, 150–151
Fadire sign, 124
Fadire test, 124
Fahey and O'Brien procedure, 257
Fahey approach, 260
Failure of segmentation, 284
Fairbanks and Sever procedure, 231
Fairbanks changes, 111
Fajersztajn crossed sciatic sign, 124
False ankylosis, 69
False profile view, 101
Familial dysautonomia, 76
Familial expansile osteolysis, 42
Familial interstitial hypertrophic neuritis, 78
Familial lymphedema, 82
Familial periodic paralysis, 59
Fan sign, 136
Fanconi anemia, 91, 306
Fanconi syndrome, 79
Farmer procedure, 340
Fascia lata, 222
Fasciae, 222
Fasciaplasty, 222
Fascia-related diseases, 66
Fasciectomy, 222, 318
Fasciitis, 66
Fasciodesis, 222
Fasciorrhaphy, 218, 222
Fascioscapulohumeral muscular dystrophy, 60
Fasciotomy, 222, 318
Fasting blood sugar, 144
Fat pad, 330
Fat sat, 115
Fat saturation, 115
Fat suppression, 115

Fatigue failure, 366
Fatigue fracture, 11, 12, 367
Fatigue limit, 367
Fatigue strength, 367
Fatigue wear, 369
FBS, 144
Febrile, 91
Feeding/eating, 355
Feiss line, 330
Feldon wafer resection, 238
Felon, 312
Felt padding, 156
Felty syndrome, 73
Fem-fem bypass, 226
Femoral arteriography, 98, 99
Femoral artery, 243, 250
Femoral condylar shaving, 256
Femoral condyles, 247
Femoral cortical index, 107
Femoral head, 242
    avascular necrosis
        International Classification system, 50
        Ratcliff classification system, 50–51
    prosthesis, 244
Femoral neck, 242
    fracture, 10, 19, 25
Femoral nerve, 241, 243
    stretch test, 136
    traction test, 124
Femoral offset, 108
Femoral popliteal bypass, 226
Femoral shaft fractures, 22, 30
Femoral vein, 250
Femoral-femoral bypass, 226
Femorotibial angle, 103
Femur, 242, 247
    cavitary defect, 84
    deficiencies, 83–84
    intercalary defect, 84
    radiographic view, 105
    radiographic views, 102
    segmental defect, 84
    surgery of, 253–254
    surgical approaches to, 260–261
Femur fractures, 20, 21
    distal, 10
    femoral neck, 10, 19, 25
    femoral shaft, 22
    intertrochanteric, 18, 20, 27
    proximal, 9–10, 16, 27

Femur fractures *(cont.)*
  subtrochanteric, 18, 27
  trochanteric, 21
Fenestrate, 159
Fenestration, 194
Ferguson-Thompson-King-Moore
  osteotomy, 195
Fergusson method, 111
Ferkel-Cheng fracture classification
  system, 18
Ferkel-Sgaglione fracture classifica-
  tion system, 18
Fernandez procedure, 238
FFP, 151
Fiber, 364
Fiberglass cast, 157
Fibril, 364
Fibrillation, 91
Fibro-, 63
Fibroblasts, 218
Fibrocartilage, 217
Fibrocytes, 218
Fibrodysplasia ossificans progressiva,
  53
Fibroma, 63
  chondromyxoid, 48
  desmoplastic, 49
  nonossifying, 49, 54
  ossifying, 42
    of jaw, 54
  periosteal, 64
Fibromatosis, 63
  aggressive, 65
  juvenile hyaline, 64
  pseudosarcomatous, 64
  solitary, of bone, 54
Fibromuscular disease, 71
Fibrosarcoma, 49, 65
Fibrosis, 63
Fibrositis, 63
  periarticular, 64
Fibrositis ossificans progressiva, 53
Fibrous ankylosis, 69
Fibrous cortical defect, 54
Fibrous dysplasia
  monostotic, 64
  polyostotic, 64
Fibrous histiocytoma, 63
  malignant, 63
Fibrous tumors, 49
Fibroxanthoma, 54
Fibroxanthosarcoma, 64

Fibula, 247
  fractures, 10
  radiographic views, 102
Fibular collateral sprain, 33
Fibular facet, 247
Fibular neck, 247
Ficat and Marcus grading system for
  avascular necrosis of femur,
  111–112
Fick angle, 139
Fielding-Magliato fracture classifica-
  tion system, 18
Figure eight dressing, 162
Figure of 4 test, 124
Fillauer bar, 178
Finger, bent, 306
Finger extensors, 294, 320
Finger flaps, 316
Finger flexors, 294, 320
Finger nail, 299 *(see also* Nail)
  disorders of, 311–312
Finger to nose test, 136
Fingers, 298–299
  abbreviations, 374
  arthrodeses of, 313
  radiographic views, 102
  short, 306
Finkelstein sign, 128
First dorsal interosseous assist, 182
Fish osteotomy, 195
Fish procedure, 245
Fisk-Fernandez volar wedge, 316
Fissure fracture, 4
Fissures, 91
Fistula, 71
Five-in-one repair, 254
Fixation, 265
Fixed anatomic prosthesis, 213
Flaccid, 91
Flaccid cerebral palsy, 76
Flail, 91
Flail foot, 332
Flail joint, 67
Flail-elbow hinge, 182
Flaps *(see also* Bone grafts)
  rotational, 258–259
Flat bones, 192
Flatfoot, 332, 335
  devices for, 187
Flatt prosthesis, 206
Flattening of normal lumbar curve,
  279

Flex foot, 175
Flexible hinges, 171
Flexible orthoses, 178
Flexible pes planus, 334
Flexion, 383
Flexion body cast, 157
Flexion contracture, 85
Flexion exercises, 352
Flexion rotation drawer test, 133–
  134
Flexor digitorum longus, 249
Flexor digitorum longus/brevis, 329
Flexor hallucis longus, 249
Flexor hallucis longus/brevis, 329
Flexor origin syndrome, 35, 312
Flexor pronator slide, 319
Flexor retinacula, 297
Flexor tendons, of wrist, 295
Flexor tenolysis, 319
Flexor wad of five, 235, 295
Flexure, 388
Flipper hand, 306
Floating cartilage, 217
Floating knee fracture, 21
Floating ribs, 273
Floating thumb, 306
Floor reaction orthosis, 178
Florid reactive periostitis, 54–55
Flow cytometry, 148
Fluidotherapy, 349
Fluorescent treponemal antibody, 148
Fluoroscopy, 99
Flynn procedure, 238
Focal dystonia, 304
Focal fibrocartilaginous dysplasia, 85
Focal scleroderma, 73
Foot
  abbreviations, 374–375
  anatomy of, 323–331
  arteries/veins/nerves of, 330–331
  bones of, 324–329
  cramps, 332
  diseases/conditions of, 331–335
  dislocations, 32
  fractures, 10–12
  insensitive, devices for, 188
  muscles/tendons/ligaments of,
    329–330
  orthoses for, 178
  prosthetic components, 174–175
  radiographic views, 102
  surgery for, 336–345

surgical approaches, 345
tests, signs, and maneuvers for, 135
Football ankle, 35
Football finger, 35
Footdrop, 332
Foramen, 271
Foraminotomy, 285
Forbes procedure, 257
Force, 367
Forced adduction test, 126
Fore, 388
Forearm
  anatomy of, 233–238
  lift assist, 172
  muscles of, 235
  surgery of, 238–240
  surgical approaches to, 260
Forefoot, 324
Forefoot equinus, 332
Forefoot valgus, 332
Forefoot varus, 332
Foreign body, 91
Foreman fractures, 8–9
Forestier disease, 276
Fork strap, 175
Formication sign, 138
Fossa, 291
Fossae, 291
Foster frame, 166
Four-bar linkage, 175
Fournier test, 136
Four-poster orthosis, 185
  with thoracic extension, 186
  with waist extension, 186
Fovea centralis, 242
Fowler maneuver, 128
Fowler metacarpophalangeal arthro-
    plasty, 315
Fowler procedure, 340
Fowler release, 321
Fowler tenodesis, 319
Fowler test, 126
Fowler-Phillip angle, 103
Fowles procedure, 239
Fox-Blazina procedure, 254
FPB, 226
Fracture, 1–2 (*see also* specific types)
  classification, 1–6
    by anatomic location, 6–12
    general appearance, 4–6
    by grades, types, mechanisms,
      14–30

International Classification
    System, 13–14
  open vs closed, 3
  Orthopaedic Trauma Associa-
    tion, 14
  portion of bone involved, 3–4
  position and alignment of frag-
    ments, 6
  Trauma Registry System, 13–14
  contributing factors, 12
  degree and nature of healing, 12–13
  external skeletal fixation devices,
    204–205
  healing, electric/magnetic stimula-
    tion of, 205
  internal fixation devices, 199–204
  line, 108
  of neccessity, 9
  terminology of, 2–3
Fracture-dislocation, 2
Fragile-X syndrome, 87
Fragilitas ossium congenita, 42
Fragments of fracture, 6
Frames, 166
Frank dislocation, 31
Frankel line, 108
Frankel neurological assessment, 139
Fränkel sign, 136
Free graft, 199
Free pyridinium cross-links, 147
Free-body analysis, 367
Freeman-Sheldon syndrome, 308
Free-motion ankle joint, 180
Free-revascularized autograft, 198
Freeze-dried grafts, 198
Freiberg disease, 41, 50, 55
Freiberg infraction, 334
Freid-Green procedure, 340
Frejka orthosis, 180
French osteotomy, 195
French procedure, 239
Fresh frozen plasma, 151
Fretting, 91
Friable, 92
Friedreich ataxia, 78
Frog splint, 161
Frog-leg lateral view, 101
Fröhlich adiposogenital dystrophy, 55
Froimson and Oh procedure, 239
Froimson arthroplasty, 314
Froment sign, 128
Frontal plane, 381–382

Frost procedure, 340
Frostbite, 71
Frozen shoulder, 65, 67
Frykman fracture classification
    system, 18
FTA, 103, 148
Fulcrum test, 126
Fulford procedure, 340
Fulguration, 265
Full-thickness skin graft, 258
Fully constrained knee replacement,
    212
Functional capacities assessment,
    354
Functional communication, 355
Functional fracture bracing, 356
Functional impairment rating scales,
    139–140
Functional mobility, 355
Functional scoliosis, 279
Fundiplication, 267
Fungal organisms, 148
Funiculectomy, 316
Fusiform, 92
Fusion, 265

G

^{67}Ga, 115
Gadolinium-enhanced MRI, 115
Gadopentetate dimeglumine, 115
Gaenslen sign, 124
Gaenslen spikes, 201
GAG, 363
Gage procedure, 253
Gage sign, 109
Gaille procedure, 239
Gait patterns, 139
Gait training, 351
Galeazzi fracture, 8
Galeazzi procedure, 255
Galeazzi sign, 131
Galleazzi procedure, 257
Gallie fusion, 286
Gallie procedure, 340
Gallium scan, 115
Galveston metacarpal brace, 181
Gamekeeper thumb, 311
Gamekeeper's thumb, 35
Gamma camera, 115
Gamma GT, 142
Gamma nail, 201

Gamma-glutamyltransferase, 142
Gamma-glutamyltranspeptidase, 142
Ganglion, 312, 332
Ganglion cyst, 64
Ganglionectomy, 321
Ganglioneuroma, 76
Gangrene, 92
Gant osteotomy, 195
Ganz osteotomy, 195
Garceau-Brahms procedure, 340
Garden fracture classification system, 19
Garden screws, 201
Gardner syndrome, 55
Gardner-Wells tongs, 164
Gargoylism, 63
Garrod fibromatosis, 64
Garrod pads, 64
Garth view, 101
Gartland fracture classification system, 19
Gas gangrene, 313
Gastrocnemius, 250
Gastrocnemius equinus, 332
Gastrocsoleus muscle, 249
Gaucher disease, 55–56
Gauntlet case, 158
Gauze dressing, 162
Gear-stick sign, 131
Gel cast, 158
Gelatinase, 359
Gelman procedure, 340
Genu, 84
Genu recurvatum, 84
    surgical procedures, 257
Genu valgum, 84
Genu varum, 84
Gerdy tubercle, 247
Germinal matrix, 299
Getty procedure, 288
GGTP, 143
Ghormley arthrodesis, 215
Ghormley osteotomy, 195
Giannestras procedure, 340
Giant cell reparative granuloma, 53
Giant cell tumors, 49
Gibney bandage, 162
Giebel blade plate, 201
Gilbert procedure, 257
Gill arthrodesis, 215
Gill procedure, 231, 239, 257, 340
Gillies flap, 317
Gillies procedure, 321

Gill-Stein arthrodesis, 314
Girdle resection, 232
Girdlestone procedure, 340
Girdlestone resection, 245
Gla protein, 361
Glenoid fossa, 227
Glenoid fractures, 20
Glenoid labrum, 227, 229
Glioma, 76
Glomus tumor, 76, 312
Glucosamine, 363
Gluteal lines, 240
Gluteal lurch, 139
Gluteus maximus gait, 139
Gluteus maximus muscle, 243
Gluteus medius gait, 139
Gluteus medius muscle, 243
Gluteus minimus muscle, 243
Glycocalyx, 92
Glycosaminoglycans, 363
Gobies, 35
Godoy-Moreira stud-bolt, 201
Goldstein procedure, 288
Goldthwait sign, 124
Golfer's elbow, 35
Gordon reflex, 136
Gore AO screw, 201
Gorham disease, 42, 56
Gosselin fracture, 11
Gouffon pin, 201
Gould procedure, 341
Gout, 82, 301, 333
Gouty arthritis, 82
Gouty node, 82
Gower sign, 138
Graber-Duvernay procedure, 245
Gracilis muscle, 242
Grafts (see Bone grafts)
Gram stain, 148
Grand mal epilepsy, 76
Grant, Surrall, and Lehman procedure, 253
Granulation, 92, 265
Granuloma, 265
    subperiosteal giant-cell reparative, 54–55
Grashey view, 101
Grayson ligament, 298
Greater sciatic notch, 240
Greater trochanter, 242
Greater tuberosity, 227
Greek foot, 333
Green procedure, 232

Green transfer, 319
Greenfield filter, 226
Green-Seligson-Henry nail, 201
Greenstick fracture, 4, 5
Greifer prosthesis, 172
Greisinger foot, 175
Grice procedure, 341
Grice-Green procedure, 341
Grimace test, 134
Grip strength test, 128
Grisel syndrome, 277
Gristina and Webb prosthesis, 206
Grommet, 201
Grooming, 355
Gross-Kemph nail, 201
Group fascicular repair, 316
Growth plate, 191
Growth-arrest line, 108
Gruca procedure, 257
Gruen zones, 112
GSH nail, 201
GSU nail, 201
Guillain-Barré syndrome, 78
Guilland sign, 136
Guillotine amputation, 264
Gustilo fracture classification system, 19
Gutter splint, 161
Guyon canal, 298

H

Haas disease, 41, 56
Habitual dislocation, 31
Haboush universal nail, 201
Haddad-Riordan arthrodesis, 314
Hagie pin, 201
Haglund deformity, 333
Haglund process, 330
Haglund syndrome, 333
Hairline fracture, 5
Hairpin splint, 161
Hajdu-Cheney syndrome, 56
Half shell, 161
Half-ring Thomas splint, 163
Halifax fusion, 286
Hall and Pankovich procedure, 239
Hallux, 326
Hallux abductus, 333
Hallux adductus, 333
Hallux dolorosa, 333
Hallux elevatus, 333
Hallux extensus, 333

Hallux flexus, 333
Hallux malleus, 333
Hallux rigidus, 333
Hallux valgus, 333
Hallux valgus angle, 103
Hallux valgus interphalanges, 333
Hallux valgus orthosis, 178
Hallux varus, 333
Halo cast, 157
Halo extension, 186
Halo traction, 186
Halo-femoral traction, 164
Halo-pelvic traction, 164
Hamas prosthesis, 206
Hamblen classification of ectopic
    ossification, 53
Hamilton test, 126
Hammer toes, 333
Hammon procedure, 341
Hamstring tendon, 221
Hamstrung knee, 85
Hand
    abbreviations, 373–374
    anatomy of, 291–301
    arthritic deformities of, 301–302
    bones of, 291–292
    congenital anomalies of, 305–308
    congenital deformity repairs, 317
    diseases of, 301–31–
    dislocations, 310–311
    fractures, 9
    infections of, 312–313
    joints of, 293
    ligaments of, 295–297
    microvascular procedures, 317
    muscle disorders of, 308–309
    muscles of, 293–295
    muscle/tendon surgery of, 318
    neurologic procedures, 316
    neuropathies of, 302–305
    orthoses, 181–182
    prosthetic, 172
    radiographic views, 102
    surgery of, 313–322
    surgical approach to, 322
    tendon disorders of, 308–309
    tendon repair techniques, 319
    tests, signs, and maneuvers for,
        127–130
    trauma procedures for, 316–317
    traumatic disorders of, 309–310
    vascular disorders of, 309
Hand-foot syndrome, 312

Handlebar palsy, 35
Hand-Schüller-Christian disease, 48,
    49
Hanging arm cast, 158
"Hanging hip" procedure, 246
Hangman's fracture, 9
Hansen disease, 312
Hansen pin, 201
Hansen-Street nail, 201
Hard clavus, 333
Hard collar, 186
Hard corn, 333
Hardinge expansion bolt, 201
Hardinge procedure, 245
Hardinger approach, 260
Hare traction, 167
Hark procedure, 341
Harmon approach, 259–260
Harmon procedure, 232
Harrington rod, 201, 287
Harris hip scale, 139
Harris line, 108
Harris nail, 201
Harris view, 101
Harris-Beath footprinting mat, 135
Harris-Beath procedure, 341
Hass osteotomy, 195
Hassman, Brunn, and Neer procedure,
    239
Hatchet head deformity, 31
Hatchet head shoulder, 62
Hauser procedure, 255, 341
Haversian canals, 192
Hawkins fracture classification
    system, 19
Hawkins impingement sign, 126
Hawkins sign, 109
Hb, 141
HB$_s$Ag, 150
Hct, PCV, 141
HD, 174
Head and cold testing, 352
Head-shaft angle, 103
Healed fracture, 12
Heart-hand syndrome, 307
Heberden nodes, 56, 312
Hebosteotomy, 245
Heel cord, 329
Heel pad, 188
Heel spur, 35, 333
Heel tendon, 221
Heel wedge, 187
Heel-cord sign, 135

Heffington frame, 166
Heifetz procedure, 341
Height and weight, 154
Helbing sign, 135
Helical axis of motion, 367
Heloma durum, 333
Hemangioendothelioma, 74
Hemangioma, 74
Hemangiomatosis, 42
Hemangiopericytoma, 74
Hemangiosarcoma, 74
Hemarthrosis, 67
Hematocrit, packed cell volume, 141
Hematocrit and hemoglobin, 141
Hematomyelia, 283
Hematorrhachis, 283
Hemicylindric graft, 199
Hemilaminectomy, 285
Hemimelia, 87, 306–307
Hemimelic progressive osseous
    heteroplasia, 54
Hemipelvectomy, 174
Hemipelvectomy suspension, 176
Hemiphalangectomy, 341
Hemiplegia, 76
Hemi-resection interposition arthro-
    plasty, 315
Hemivertebra, 284
Hemodynamic test, 138
Hemoglobin, 141
Hemoglobin electrophoresis, 144
Hemolymphangiomatosis, 42
Hemophilia, 82
Hemorrhage, 92
Henderson arthrodesis, 215
Henderson fracture, 11
Henderson lag screw, 201
Henderson-Jones chondromatosis, 41,
    61
Henschke-Mauch S'n'S, 175
Herbert and Fisher fracture classifica-
    tion system, 19
Herbert screw, 202
Herbert screw osteosynthesis, 316
Hereditary, 92
Hereditary areflexic dystasia, 79
Hereditary multiple exostosis, 53
Hermodsson fracture, 8
Herndon-Heyman procedure, 341
Herniated intervertebral disk, 281
Herniated nucleus pulposus, 282
Herniation, 92
Herpetic whitlow, 313

Herring lateral pillar classification, 112
Hertz, 358
Hessel/Nystrom pins, 202
Heterograft, 197
Heteroplasia
    hemimelic progressive osseous, 54
    progressive osseous, 54
Heterotopic ossification, 53
Heuter line, 108
Hex screw, 202
Hey-Groves procedure, 254
Heyman procedure, 257, 341
Heyman-Herndon procedure, 245
Hgb, 141
H&H, 141
Hibb and Meary angle, 103
Hibbs arthrodesis, 216
Hibbs procedure, 341
Hibbs spinal fusion, 287
Hibernoma, 92
Hickory-stick fracture, 4
HID, 281
High Dye dressing, 162
High riding patella, 86
Highest genicular artery, 250
High-performance liquid chromatography, 358
High-pressure liquid chromatography, 358
Higley side plate, 202
Hilgenreiner angle, 103
Hilgenreiner line, 109
Hill-Sachs fracture, 8
Hill-Sachs lesion, 31
    reverse, 31
Hindfoot, 326
Hindfoot equinus, 333
Hinge joint, 214
Hinges, prosthetic, 171
Hip
    anatomy of, 242–243
    arteries of, 243
    arthrodeses of, 245
    arthroplasty, 243–244
    aseptic necrosis, Steinberg classification system, 51
    bipolar total replacement, 208
    developmental dysplasia, 244
    disarticulation, 174
    disarticulation suspension, 176
    diseases, 82–83
    dislocations, 25, 28, 32

    dysplasia, 32
    fractures, 9–10, 16
    iliopsoas transfers, 244
    joint, 180
    ligaments of, 243
    muscles of, 242–243
    nerves of, 243
    open reduction, 244
    orthoses, 179–180
    osteotomies of, 245
    pointer, 35
    prostheses for, 207, 211
    radiographic views, 102
    resurfacing procedures, 208
    salvage procedures, 211
    spica, 158
    surgery of, 243–247
    surgical approaches to, 260
    tests, signs, and maneuvers for, 130–132
    total replacement, 207–208
Hip-knee-ankle-foot orthoses, 180
Hirayama procedure, 239
Hiroshima procedure, 341
Hirschberg sign, 136
His-Haas procedure, 232
Histiocytes, 218
Histiocytoma, malignant fibrous, 49, 64
Histiocytosis, Langerhans cell, 49
Histiocytosis X, 48
Histocompatibility, 197
Hitchcock procedure, 232, 239
HIV, viral load, 150
HIV-1 antigen, 150
HLA-B27, 144
HNP, 282
Hobb view, 101
Hockey player's hip, 35
Hodgkin tumor, 48
Hodgson procedure, 288
Hoffa fat, 253
Hoffa fracture, 10
Hoffer procedure, 341
Hoffman-Clayton procedure, 341
Hoffmann sign, 136
Hohmann procedure, 239
Hoke procedure, 341
Hoke-Kite procedure, 341
Holstein-Lewis fracture, 8
Holt nail, 202
Holt-Oram syndrome, 92, 307
Homan's sign, 132

Homograft, 197
Hook nail, 311
Hook of hamate, 292, 298
Hooked acromion, 82
Hook-pin fixation, 202
Hooks, prosthetic, 172–173
Hoop stress fracture, 12
Hoover test, 124
Hop test, 134
Horizontal plane, 382
Horseback rider's knee, 32
Horseshoe abscess, 313
Horwitz and Adams arthrodesis, 216
Hot packs, 350
Housemaid's knee, 85
Houston and Akroyd procedure, 256
Hovanian procedure, 232, 239
Howmedica compression screw, 202
Howship lacuna, 192
HPLC, 358
Hsu and Hsu procedure, 258
Hubbard side plate, 202
Huber transfer, 320
Huckstep nail, 202
Hueter sign, 138
Hueter-Mayo procedure, 341
Hughston and Degenhardt procedure, 254
Hughston and Jacobson procedure, 254
Hughston jerk test, 134
Hughston procedure, 255, 257
Hughston view, 101
Human immunodeficiency virus, viral load test, 150
Human immunodeficiency virus-1 antigen, 150
Humeral head, 227
    fracture, 23
Humerus, 227
    anatomy of, 233
    radiographic views, 102
    surgical approaches to, 260
Humerus fractures
    condylar, 15, 21, 23
    distal intercondylar, 26
    humeral head, 23
    proximal, 6–8
    supracondylar, 19
Hunter rod, 206, 320
Hunter syndrome, 63
Hunter-Scheie syndrome, 63
Huntington chorea, 76
Huntington sign, 136

Hurler syndrome, 63
Hutchinson fracture, 8
Hutchinson sign, 128
Hyaline cartilage, 217
Hyaluronic acid, 363
Hyaluronidase, 363
Hydrarthrosis, 67
Hydrotherapy, 349, 350
Hydroxylisinonorleucine, 364
Hydroxylysine, 364
Hydroxyproline, 147, 364
Hydroxypyridinoline, 364
Hyoid bone, 272
HYP, 147
Hypalgesia, 92
Hyper-, 388
Hyperalgesia, 92
Hypercholesteremia, 74
Hypercholesterinemia, 74
Hypercholesterolemia, 74
Hyperextension, 92
Hyperextension orthosis, 184
Hyperglycemia, 92
Hyperlordosis, 283
Hyperostcoidosis, 40
Hyperostosis, diffuse idiopathic
    sclerosing, 67
Hyperparathyroidism, 40, 79
Hyperphalangism, 307
Hyperplasia, 92
Hyperplasia fascialis ossificans
    progressiva, 53
Hypertension, 74, 92
Hyperthyroidism, 40, 80
Hypertonia, 92
Hypertrophic arthritis, 67
Hypertrophic exostosis, 53
Hypertrophic zone, 191
Hypertrophy, 92
Hypo-, 388
Hypochondrodysplasia, 61
Hypoglycemia, 92
Hyponychium, 299, 330
Hypoparathyroidism, 79
Hypophosphatasia, 80
Hypoplasia, 92
    cartilage-hair, 61
Hypoplastic thumb, 307
Hypotension, 74, 92
Hypothenar eminence, 297
Hypothenar hammer syndrome, 309
Hypothenar muscles, 294
Hypothenar space, 297

Hypothyroidism, 80
Hypotonia, congenital, 59
Hypovolemia, 74
Hypoxia, 74
Hysteresis, 367
Hz, 358

I

IAT, 150
Iatrogenic, 92
Iatrogenic osteomyelitis, 45
ICD codes for eponymic musculo-
    skeletal disease terms, 404–
    409
I&D, 266
Idiopathic, 92
Idiopathic refractory anemia, 91
Idiopathic scoliosis, 279
Ikuta procedure, 239
Ilfeld splint, 179
Iliac crest, 240
Iliac fossa, 240
Iliopectineal line, 240
Iliopsoas muscle, 243, 274
Iliopsoas transfers, 244
Iliotibial band syndrome, 35
Ilium, 240
Imaging techniques, 97–118
    abbreviations, 376
    general radiologic terms, 98–99
    invasive and noninvasive, 114–117
    orthopaedic techniques and proce-
        dures, 99–100
    radiation therapy, 118
    radiographic angles, lines, signs,
        methods, 103–114
    routine radiographic views, 100–
        103
    vascular diagnostic studies, 117–
        118
Imbrication, 266
Immediate postsurgical fitting, 176
Immobilization, cast, 157–159
Immovable joint, 214
Immune serum globulins, 151
Immunosuppression, 197
Impacted fracture, 5
Impedance plethysmography, 118
Impingement, 92
    sign, 126
Impingement syndrome, 35
    coracoid, 35

Implant, 197, 266
Impulse, 367
In-, 388
In situ, 266, 388
In situ bypass, 226
In toto, 266
In vitro, 266, 359
In vivo, 266, 359
Incision and drainage, 266
Inclan-Ober procedure, 232
Inclusion cyst, 312
Incomplete dislocation, 31
Incomplete fracture, 4, 5
Incomplete paraxial hemimelia, 87
Incorporation, 198
Indices, radiographic, 107–109
Indirect anti-human globulin test,
    150
Indirect Coombs test, 150
Indium leukocyte scan, 115
Indium scan, 115
Induration, 92
Inertia, 367
Infantile cortical hyperostosis, 53
Infantile scoliosis, 279
Infants, special shoes for, 188
Infarct, 71, 92
Infection, 92
Inferior, 388
Inferior gluteal artery, 243
Inferior pubic ramus, 240
Infiltration, 266
Inflammation, 92–93
Inflammatory arthritis, 301
Inflammatory fracture, 12
Inflatable splint, 167
Infra, 388
Infraction fracture, 5
Infrapatellar fat pad, 253
Infrapatellar ligament, 250
Infrapatellar straps, 181
Infraspinatus muscle, 227
Infusion, 266
Ingram osteotomy, 195
Ingram procedure, 341
Ingrown nail, 333
Inguinal area, 242
Injection, 266
Inlay graft, 199
Inlet view, 101
Innervation, 222
Innominate bone, 240
Innominate osteotomy, 195

Ino-, 388
INR, 145
Insall and Hood procedure, 254
Insall procedure, 254, 255
Insidious, 93
Install ratio, 108
Instantaneous axis of rotation, 367
Insufficiency fracture, 12
Insulin-like growth factor I, 361
Integrated shape imaging system, 115
Integumentary injury, 13
Inter-, 388
Intercalary, 388
Intercalary graft, 199
Intercarpal arthrodesis, 313
Intercondylar notch, 247
Intercostal muscles, 273
Interferential current, 350
Intermediate bursa, 298
Intermediate ligament, 297
Intermediate phalangectomyl, 341
Intermediate prosthesis, 176
Intermittent compression, 350
Intermittent hydrarthrosis, 73
Internal, 388
Internal derangement of joint, 68
Internal fixation devices for fracture
         healing, 199–204
Internal neurolysis, 316
Internal rotation, 385
Internal rotators, 242–243
International Classification for
         Surgery of Hand in Tetra-
         plegia, 128–129
International Classification of Dis-
         eases codes for eponymic
         disease terms, 404–409
International Classification of femoral
         head deformities from avascu-
         lar necrosis, 50
International normalizing ratio, 145
Interossei muscles, 329
Interosseous cartilage, 217
Interosseous membrane, 238, 253
Interperiosteal fracture, 4
Interphalangeal arthrodesis, 313
Interscapulothoracic forequarter
         amputation, 170
Intersection syndrome, 308
Interspinal disk, 273
Interspinous ligament, 273
Interspinous pseudarthrosis, 277, 284
Interstitial, 388

Intertrochanteric, 242
Intertrochanteric fracture, 10
         of femur, 4
Intertrochanteric fractures, 29
         of femur, 27
Intervertebral disk, 273
Intervertebral disk narrowing, 282
Intima, 224
Intra-, 388
Intraarticular arthrodesis, 215
Intraarticular fracture, 9
Intraarticular osteochondroma, 48
Intracapsular ankylosis, 69
Intracapsular fracture, 4
Intractable, 93
Intractable plantar keratosis, 333
Intramedullary, 271
Intramedullary graft, 199
Intramedullary nail, 202
Intraneural fibrosis, 281
Intraoperative autologous transfusion,
         150
Intraosseous lipoma, 53
Intraosseous pneumatocyst, 53
Intraspongy nuclear herniation, 282
Intravenous block, 259
Intrinsic minus hand, 304
Intrinsic muscles, 294, 329
Intrinsic plus hand, 304
Intrinsic tightness test, 129
Intro-, 388
Intubation, 266
Inversion, 385
Inversion ankle stress view, 101
Inverted radial reflex, 124
Involucrum, 45
Inyo nail, 202
Iodoform dressing, 162
Iowa hip scale, 139
IPSF, 176
Ipsilateral, 388
Irradiation sterilized grafts, 198
Irrigation, 266
Irwin osteotomy, 195
Irwin procedure, 258
Ischemia, 71, 93
Ischemic contracture, 59
Ischial containment sockets, 174
Ischial spine, 240
Ischial tuberosity, 241
Ischial weight-bearing band, 180
Ischial weight-bearing ring, 180
Ischiectomy, 246

Ischiohebotomy, 246
Ischiopubiotomy, 246
Ischium, 241
Iselins disease, 50, 56
Ishihara cervical spine curve index,
         112
ISIS, 115
Iso-, 388
Isoantibodies, 150
Isogeneic, 197
Isograft, 197
Isokinetic exercise, 351
Isola instrument, 287
Isometric exercises, 351
Isotonic exercises, 351
Isotropic, 367
Isovue myelography, 99
Isthmus, 192
IV-type basic frame, 166

J

Jaccoud syndrome, 73
Jacksonian epilepsy, 76
Jacob test, 134
Jacobs locking hook instrument, 287
Jaffe disease, 56
Jahss procedure, 341
Jamar dynamometer, 354
Janecki and Nelson procedure, 232
Jansen disease, 61
Jansen test, 131
Jansey procedure, 341
Japas osteotomy, 195
Japas procedure, 341
Jarcho-Levin syndrome, 284
Javelin thrower's elbow, 34
Jeanne sign, 129
Jebsen-Taylor hand function test, 354
Jefferson fracture, 9
Jendrassik maneuver, 136
Jersey finger, 35
Jewett nail, 202
Jewett orthosis, 184
Jobe and Kvitne procedure, 232
Jobe test, 126
Jockey cap patella, 86
Jogger's heel, 35
Johansson nail, 202
John C. Wilson arthrodesis, 216
Johnson and Barington procedure, 339
Johnson and Spiegl procedure, 341
Joint capsule, 250

Joint diseases, 66–69
Joint manipulation, 351
Joint mice, 68
Joint mobilization, 351
Joint motions, range of, 383–386
Joint play, 351
Joint protection, 356
Joint replacement, 206
Joint stabilizer, 182
Joints
    anatomy of, 213–214
    arthrodesis, 215–216
    general surgery of, 214–215
    internal derangement of, 68
    research, 362–363
    types of, 214
Joints of Luschka, 272
Jones abduction frame, 166
Jones fracture, 11
Jones procedure, 254, 341–342
Jones transfer, 319
Joplin procedure, 342
Joule, 367
Judet quadricepsplasty, 256
Jugular vein, 272
Jumper's knee, 36, 86
Juncturae tendinum, 296
Juvara procedure, 342
Juvenile hyaline fibromatosis, 64
Juvenile rheumatoid arthritis, 73
Juxta-, 388
Juxtaposition, 388

K

Kager triangle, 103
Kanavel sign, 129, 313
Kanavel spaces, 297
Kaneda instrument, 287
Kapandji fixation, 316
Kapandji thumb opposition score, 129
Kapel procedure, 239
Kappis disease, 50, 56
Karakousis and Vezeridis procedure, 246
Karlsson procedure, 342
Kashin-Beck disease, 82
Kashiwagi procedure, 342
Kates-Kessel-Kay procedure, 342
Kaufer procedure, 342
Kawasaki disease, 68
K/B, 174
Keen sign, 135

Kelikian procedure, 257
Keller procedure, 342
Kellgren osteoarthritis grade, 112
Kellogg Speed procedure, 289
Ken nail, 202
Kendrick procedure, 342
Kenny-Howard splint, 162
Keratan sulfate, 363
Keratoma, 331
Kerlix dressing, 162
Kernig sign, 136
Kerr sign, 136
Kessel-Bonnel procedure, 342
Kessler prosthesis, 206
Key arthrodesis, 216
Key pinch, 129, 316
Keyhole procedure, 239
Kickaldy and Willis arthrodesis, 216
Kidner procedure, 342
Kidneys, radiography, 99
Kiehn-Earle-DesPrez procedure, 342
Kienböck disease, 41, 50, 56, 309
Kilfoyle fracture classification system, 21
Kilopond, 367
Kinematics, 364, 367
Kineplastic amputation, 264
Kinesiology, 364
Kinetic apraxia, 75
Kinetic energy, 367
King and Richards procedure, 246
King maneuver, 131
King procedure, 216
Kinking, 71
Kirner deformity, 307
Kirschner wire, 165, 202
Kissing spine, 276
Kleinert technique, 319
Kleinert-Atosoy flaps, 317
Kleinman shear test, 129
Klemm nail, 202
Klenzak orthosis, 180
Klinefelter syndrome, 82
Kling dressing, 162
Klippel-Feil syndrome, 56
Klumpke palsy, 76
KMFTR, 211
Knee
    arthrodeses of, 257
    bearing, 174
    disarticulation, 174
    disarticulation suspension, 175
    dislocation, 32

disorders, 84–86
fractures, 10
instability tests, 132–133
joint, 180
orthoses, 178–179
prostheses for, 211–212
prosthetic components, 175
radiographic views, 102
sprains, 33
surgery of, 254–257
surgical approaches to, 261
tendon transfers, 256–257
tests, signs, and maneuvers for, 132–134
Knee Society clinical rating system, 140
Knee Society total knee arthroplasty roentgenographic evaluation and scoring system, 112
Knee-ankle-foot orthoses, 179
Kneist dysplasia, 62
Knight-Taylor orthosis, 185
Knodt distraction rod, 287
Knowles pin, 202
Knuckle pad, 299
Kocher approach, 259–260
Kocher fracture, 8
Kocher maneuver, 126
Koch-Mason dressing, 162
Köhler disease, 41, 50, 56, 334
Kohler fracture, 11
Kohler line, 108
König disease, 41, 56
Konstram angle, 103–105
Kortzeborn procedure, 320
Kostuick-Harrington instrument, 287
Kotz modular femur and tibia resection system, 211
Krag instrument, 288
Kramer, Craig
    and Noel osteotomy, 195
    and Noel procedure, 246
Kristiansen and Kofoed procedure, 232
KUB, 99
Kümmell disease, 275
Kuntscher modified arthrodesis, 216
Küntscher nail, 202
Küntscher rod, 202
Kurkenberg procedure, 317
Kurosaka screw, 202
K-wire, 165, 202
K-wire fixation, 321

Kyle fracture classification system, 21
Kyphectomy, 288
Kyphoscoliosis, 279
Kyphosis, 279

L

Laboratory evaluations, 141–154
    abbreviations used, 151–153
    annotation of units, 153–154
    bacteriologic, 147–148
    blood and serum tests, 143–145
    blood bank procedures and products, 149–151
    routine, 141–143
    routine physiologic parameters, 154
    serum and urine, for metabolic disease, 145–147
LAC, 158
Laceration, 93
Lachman test, 134
Lactate dehydrogenase, 143
Lacteratus fibrosus, 238
LAD composite graft, 254
Lag screw, 202
Laing H-beam nail, 202
Lambda ratio, 367
Lambrinudi procedure, 342
Lamellar bone, 192
Lamina, 271
Laminectomy, 285
Laminoplasty, 286
Laminotomy, 286
Lance disease, 50, 57
Landouzy-Dejerine disease, 60
Landsmeer ligament, 297
Lane plate, 202
Lange procedure, 244, 342
Langenskiöld osteotomy, 195
Langenskiöld procedure, 258
Langer line, 138
Langerhans cell histiocytosis, 49
Langoria sign, 131
Laparotomy, 226
Lapidus procedure, 342
Laquesna and Deseze angle, 105
Larmon procedure, 342
Larsen syndrome, 88
Lasègue sign, 124, 125
Laser, 266
Laser endarterectomy, 226

Last shoes, 188
Lat-, 388
Lateral, 388
Lateral bands, 299
Lateral collateral ligament, 250, 330
Lateral collateral sprain, 33
Lateral compartment, 249
Lateral cutaneous nerve of forearm, 299
Lateral distal femoral angle, 105
Lateral epicondyles, 234
Lateral facets, 247
Lateral ligament, 221
Lateral malleolus, 247
Lateral mass, 272
Lateral menisci, 253
Lateral monopodal stance view, 101
Lateral patellofemoral angle, 105
Lateral plica, 86
Lateral spring-loaded lock, 180
Lateral view, 101
Latero-, 388
Latissimus dorsi muscle, 227
Latus, 388
Lauenstein procedure, 315
Lauge-Hansen fracture classification system, 21
Laugier sign, 127
Laugler fracture, 8
Laurin angle, 105
Lavage, 266
LC/DCP, 202
LDH, 143
Le Fort fracture, 12
Le prep, 144
Lead line, 108, 138
Lead pipe fracture, 5
Leadbetter maneuver, 131
Lee procedure, 258
Leeds procedure, 288
Leeds-Keio procedure, 254
Legg procedure, 246
Legg-Calvé-Perthes disease, 41, 50, 57
Legg-Perthes disease, 50, 57
Legg-Perthes disease orthosis, 179
Legs (see Lower extremities)
Lehman procedure, 246
Leichtenstern sign, 136
Leinbach screw, 202
Length, annotation of units, 153
L'Episcopo Zachary procedure, 232

Leprosy, 312
Leptomeningitis, 283
Leptomeningopathy, 283
Leri sign, 136
Lesion, 93
Lesser trochanter, 242
Lesser tuberosity, 227
Letournel and Judet fracture classification system, 21–22
Letterer-Siwe disease, 49, 57
Letts-Vincent-Gouw fracture classification system, 21
Leukonychia, 311
LeukoScan, 115
Levator scapula, 228
Levine Drenan angle, 105
Leving-Edwards fracture classification system, 22
Levo, 389
Levoratatory scoliosis, 278
Lewis and Chekofsky procedure, 253
Lewis nail, 202
Lexan jacket, 185
Lhermitte sign, 136
Lichtman classification for Kienböck disease, 309
Lichtman classification of lunate deformities from aseptic necrosis, 50
Lichtman test, 129
LIDO lift and workset, 354
Liebolt arthrodesis, 314
Liebolt procedure, 239, 342
LIFO, 202
Lift-off test, 126
Ligament diseases, 65–66
    eponymic, 65
Ligamentotaxis, 266
Ligamentous advancement, 254
Ligamentous ankylosis, 69
Ligamentous anterior dislocation composite graft, 254
Ligamentous control braces, 179
Ligaments, 221–222
    surgical procedures, 222
    synthetic, 370
Ligaments of Henry and Wrisberg, 250
Ligamentum flavum, 273
Ligamentum mucosa, 250
Ligamentum mucosum, 86
Ligamentum teres, 243

Ligation, 266
Ligatures, 266
Light amplification by stimulated
    emission of radiation, 266
Limb casts, 157–159
Limb girdle muscular dystrophy, 60
Limb salvage, 226
Limbs (*see also* Lower extremities;
        Upper extremities)
    congenital absence of, 87–88
Limbus annulare, 277
Limited scleroderma, 73
Limited-contact dynamic-
        compression plate, 202
Limited-motion ankle joint, 180
Lindeman procedure, 255
Linder sign, 124
Lindholm procedure, 342
Line, 192
Line of demarcation, 93
Linea aspera, 247, 389
Linear, 389
Linear acceleration, 365
Linear fracture, 5
Linebacker's arm, 36
Linen bone, 193
Lines, radiographic, 107–109
Link protein, 363
Lipid, 224
Lipid reticuloendotheliosis, 82
Lipid storage disease, 82
Lipo-, 64
Lipocalcinogranulomatosis, 82
Lipochondrodystrophy, 63, 64
Lipodystrophy, 64
Lipofibroma, 64
Lipoma, 64
Lipoma arborescens, 68
Liposarcoma, 49
Lipping, 93, 110
Lippman screw, 202
Lipscomb procedure, 342
Lisfranc amputation, 173, 342
Lisfranc dislocation, 32
Lisfranc fracture, 11
Lisfranc injury, 36
Lisfranc ligament, 330
List, 125
Lister tubercle, 234, 292, 298
Litter, 167
Little leaguer's elbow, 36
Little leaguer's shoulder, 36

Littler procedure, 321
LLC, 158
Lloyd-Roberts procedure, 342
LLWC, 158
Load and shift test, 126
Load deformation curve, 368
Loading, 367
Lobstein disease, 42
Lobstein syndrome, 42
Lobster foot, 333
Local anesthesia, 259
Localio procedure, 288
Locked intramedullary osteo-
        synthesis, 202
Locked scapula, 31
Locomotor ataxia, 76, 78
Long Beach pedicle screw, 287
Long bone fracture, 4, 13
Long ligament, 297
Long opponens orthosis, 181
Long plantar ligament, 330
Long thoracic nerve, 230
Long tract sign, 137
Long-arm cast, 158
Long-arm splint, 161
Longissimus colli, 272
Longitudiinal, 389
Longitudinal epiphyseal bracket, 53
Longitudinal plane, 382
Long-leg cast, 158
Long-leg splint, 161
Long-leg walking cast, 158
Loose procedure, 255
Lopamidol myelography, 99
Lordoscoliosis, 279
Lordosis, 283
Lorenz osteotomy, 195
Lorenz procedure, 244
Lorenz sign, 125
Lorenzo screw, 202
Lorry driver's fracture, 8
Lottes nail, 202
Lou Gehrig disease, 75
Loughheed and White procedure, 288
Lovett test, 129
Low Dye dressing, 162
Low friction arthroplasty, 244
Lowenstein view, 101
Lower extremities
    amputation levels, 262–264
    anatomy of, 247–253
    arteries of, 250

bones of, 247
casts for, 158–159
compression fracture, 15
ligaments of, 250
muscles of, 247–250
nerves of, 253
orthoses for, 177–181
prostheses for, 173–176
radiographic views, 102
surgery of, 253–258
surgical approaches to, 261
tests, signs, and maneuvers for, 132
veins of, 250
Lower motor neuron disease, 77
Lower obstetrical palsy, 76
Lower scapular nerve, 230
Lowman procedure, 342
Loxoscelism, 93
LRTI-Burton, 315
Lubrication, 367
Lucas and Cottrell osteotomy, 195
Lucas and Murray arthrodesis, 216
Luck nail, 202–203
Luck procedure, 321
Ludloff procedure, 342
Ludloff sign, 131
Lumbago, 277
Lumbar curve, 279
Lumbar kyphosis, 279
Lumbar lordosis, 275
Lumbar plexus, 241
Lumbar spine, 273–274
    anatomy of, 270, 273–274
    bones of, 273
    disk, 273
    muscles of, 274
    radiographic views, 102
    spinal canal, 273
Lumbar stabilization, 351
Lumbar thecoperitoneal shunt syn-
        drome, 76
Lumbarization, 277
Lumbodorsal support, 185
Lumbosacral corset, 184
Lumbosacral curve, 279
Lumbosacral joint angle, 275
Lumbosacral orthoses, 184
Lumbosacral series, 101
Lumbrical plus finger, 310
Lumen, 224
Lunate, aseptic necrosis, Lichtman
        classification system, 50

Lunate dislocation, 310
Lundholm screw, 203
Lunula, 299, 330
Lupus erythematosus, 73
Lupus erythematosus preparation,
    144–145
Luque instrumentation, 287
Luque ISF, 287
Luxatio, 2
Luxatio coxae congenita, 32
Luxatio erecta, 31
Luxatio imperfecta, 2
Luxatio perinealis, 32
Lyden procedure, 246
Lyman-Smith traction, 165
Lyme disease, 68
Lymphangiography, 99
Lymphangiomatosis, 42
Lymphoma, 49
    primary, 49
Lynholm knee-scoring scale, 140
Lynn procedure, 342
Lynne and Katcheria procedure, 246
Lyophilized grafts, 198
Lysinonorleucine, 364
Lysosomal proteases, 359
Lytic, 93

M

MacAusland procedure, 239
MacCarthy procedure, 288
Maceration, 93
Macewen and Shands osteotomy, 195
Macindo procedure, 318
MacIntosh procedure, 255
Macintosh test, 134
Macrodactyly, 307, 333
Macronychia, 311
Maddigan, Wissinger, and Donaldson
    procedure, 256
Madelung deformity, 307
Madura foot, 333
Maffucci syndrome, 61
Mageri fusion, 286
Magnetic field, 362
Magnetic resonance imaging, 97,
    115–116
Magnetic resonance spectroscopy,
    116
Magnetic stimulation, 205
Magnetic stimulation of fracture
    healing, 205

Magnuson procedure, 256
Magnuson-Stack procedure, 232
Ma-Griffith procedure, 342
Maisonneuve fracture, 11
Maisonneuve sign, 129
Majestro-Ruda-Frost procedure, 342
Major histocompatibility complex,
    197
Malacoplakia, 53
Malaise, 93
Malawer procedure, 258
Malgaigne fracture, 8, 10
Malignant, 93
Malignant fibrous histiocytoma, 49,
    63, 64
Malignant fibrous xanthoma, 64
Malignant giant cell tumor of soft
    tissue, 64
Malingering, 93
Malleolar artery, 330
Malleolar osteotomy, 342
Malleolus, 326
Mallet finger, 34, 302
Mallet finger deformity, 9
Mallet finger revision, 321
Mallet fracture, 9
Mallet toes, 333
Mallory fracture classification
    system, 22
Malmo splint, 179
Malum coxae senilis, 83
Malum deformans, 333
Malunion, 13
Malunited fracture, 13
Mancini plate, 203
Maneuvers, orthopaedic, 119–123
Mangled Extremity Severity Score, 22
Manipulation, 266
Manktelow procedure, 239
Mann procedure, 342
Manubrium, 273
Maquet line, 105, 108
Maquet procedure, 256
Marathoner's toe, 37
March fracture, 11, 12
Marcove, Lewis, Horos procedure,
    232
Marcus, Balourdas, Heiple arthro-
    desis, 216
Marfan syndrome, 82
Marginal osteophyte, 276
Marginal osteophytes, 277
Marie-Bamberger disease, 57

Marie-Charcot-Tooth disease, 78
Marie-Foix sign, 135
Marie-Strümpell disease, 73, 280
Maroteaux-Lamy syndrome, 63
Marshall knee-scoring scale, 140
Marshall procedure, 255
Marsupialization, 266
Martin bandage, 162
Martin osteotomy, 195
Martin procedure, 246, 256
Martin screw, 203
Martin Vigorimeter, 354
Martin-Gruber anastomosis, 299
Martin-Gruber connection, 299
Mason fracture classification system,
    22–23
Mass moment of inertia, 367
Masses sign, 129
Massie nail, 203
Massive osteolysis, 42
Massive sliding graft, 199
MAST, 167
Mastocytosis, 45
Mast-Spiegel-Pappas fracture classifi-
    cation system, 23
Matched ulnar resection, 315
Matev lengthening, 317
Matev sign, 109
Matricectomy, 342
Matrix seating system, 186
Matrix unguis, 299
Matrix vesicles, 361
Matta and Saucedo procedure, 246
Matte finish, 266
Mauch S'n'S, 175
Mauck procedure, 255
Mauclair disease, 41, 57
Maximum surgical blood order
    schedule, 150
Mayer procedure, 342
Mayo fracture classification system,
    23
Mayo procedure, 342
Mayo Thomas collar, 186
Mazur ankle rating, 140
McAffee fusion, 286
McBride procedure, 343
McCarty procedure, 246
McCash procedure, 321
McCauley procedure, 343
McConnell taping, 351
McCune-Albright syndrome, 55
McElvenny maneuver, 131

McElvenny procedure, 343
McGregor line, 108
MCH, 142
MCHC, 142
McKay osteotomy, 195
McKeever and Buck procedure, 239
McKeever patellar resurfacing
McKeever procedure, 232, 343
McKenzie exercises, 351
McLaughlin plate, 203
McLaughlin procedure, 232, 256
McLaughlin screw, 203
McMurray circumduction maneuver, 134
McMurray osteotomy, 195
McMurray sign, 134
McRae line, 108
McReynolds procedure, 343
McShane, Leinberry, Fenlin procedure, 232
MCV, 142
McWhorter approach, 259–260
Mean corpuscular hemoglobin, 142
Mean corpuscular hemoglobin concentration, 142
Mean corpuscular volume, 142
Mechanical axis, 105
Medi-, 389
Medial, 389
Medial arteriosclerosis, 73
Medial circumflex artery, 243
Medial collateral ligament, 250
Medial collateral sprain, 33
Medial epicondylectomy, 316
Medial epicondyles, 234
Medial epicondylitis, 35
Medial facets, 247
Medial heel wedge, 187
Medial ligament, 221
Medial malleolus, 247
Medial menisci, 253
Medial proximal tibial angle, 105
Medial shelf/medial plica, 86
Medial swivel dislocation, 32
Medial tibial stress syndrome, 36
Medialization ratio, 108
Median basilic vein, 236
Median cephalic vein, 236
Median nerve, 230, 299
Median plane, 381
Medical antishock trousers, 167
Medical Research Council sensory grade, 137

Mediian neuropathy, 303
Medoff sliding plate, 203
Medullary canal, 192
Medullary rod, 203
Megahorn meniscus, 86
Megalo-, 389
Meisenbach procedure, 343
Meissner's corpuscles, 300
Meleney infection, 313
Meliodosis, 93
Mellesi cable graft, 222
Melorheostosis, 53–54
Membranous bone, 192
Mendel-Bekhterev reflex, 137
Meningioma, 283
Meningism, 283
Meningismus, 283
Meningitis, 283
Meningocele, 283
Meningoencephalomyelitis, 283
Meningomyelitis, 283
Meniscal flounce, 86
Meniscectomy, 255
Meniscus, 85, 213
Meniscus tear, 84
Menkes kinky hair syndrome, 82
Mennell sign, 125
MENS, 349
Menson and Scheck procedure, 246
Mental reflex, 138
Meralgia, 76
Merchant angle, 105
Merchant view, 101
Merle d'Aubigne and Postel hip scale, 140
Mesenchymal chondrosarcoma, 48
Mesenchymoma, 93
Meso-, 389
Met-, 389
Meta-, 389
Metabolic disease, serum and urine tests for, 145–147
Metabolic diseases, 79–82
Metabolic tests, 138–139
Metacarpal lengthening, 317
Metacarpals, 291
Metal alloy, 369
Metal foot plate, 180
Metal orthosis, 178, 179
Metalloproteases, 359
Metalloproteinases, 359
Metallosis, 82
Metaphyseal chondrodysplasia

Jansen type, 61
Schmid type, 62
Metaphyseal head resection with prosthesis, 343
Metaphyseal osteotomy, 343
Metaphyseal-disphyseal angle, 105
Metaphysis, 192
Metastasis, 93
Metastron, 118
Metatarsal bars, 187
Metatarsal cuneiform exostosis, 333
Metatarsal pads, 187
Metatarsal supports, 187–188
Metatarsalgia, 333
Metatarsals, 326
Metatarsophalangeal joint dislocation, 32
Metatarsus abductus, 333
Metatarsus adductocavus, 333
Metatarsus adductus, 334
Metatarsus equinus, 334
Metatarsus latus, 334
Metatarsus primus varus, 334
Metatarsus stavicus, 334
Methylmethacrylate, 206
Meyer dysplasia, 83
Meyer fusion, 286
Meyer line, 330
Meyer-Burgdorff osteotomy, 195
Meyers-McKeever fracture classification system, 23
Meyn and Quigley maneuver, 127
MGHL cord, 65
MI, 74
Michael Reese prosthesis, 206
Microamperage electrical nerve stimulation, 349
Microgeodic disease, 93
Micronychia, 311
Microscopy, replantation, 261–262
Microsphere, 359
Midfoot, 327
Midnight fracture, 11
Midpalmar space, 298
Midsagittal plane, 381
Midtarsal joint, 327
Migration index, 109
Mikulicz angle, 105
Milch fracture classification system, 23
Milch procedure, 239
Milgram test, 125
Military brace maneuver, 123

Milk-alkali disease, 54
Milk-alkali syndrome, 80
Milkmaid's dislocation, 32
Milkmaid's elbow, 32
Milkman syndrome, 57
Miller procedure, 343
Mills test, 127
Milroy disease, 82
Milwaukee cervicothoracolumbo-
    sacral orthoses, 186–187
Milwaukee orthosis, 186
Mimocausalgia, 75
Minerva jacket, 157
Minimization of debilitation, 356
Minnesota rate of manipulation test,
    354
Minor sign, 125
Mirror hand, 307
Mital procedure, 239
Mitchell procedure, 343
Mitochondrial myopathy, 59
Miyakawa procedure, 256
Mizuna, Hirohata, and Kashiwagi
    procedure, 239
Moberg dowel graft, 313
Moberg flap, 318
Moberg procedure, 232, 316, 342
Mobility, functional, 355
Modified French osteotomy, 194
Modified Kessler suture, 319
Modified Ollier approach, 260
Modified Westergren method, 144
Modular prosthesis, 176
Modular prosthetics, 211
Modulus of elasticity, 367
Moe plate, 203
Mold arthroplasty, 244
Molded Thomas collar, 186
Moleskin, 157
Moment, 367
Moment of inertia in an area, 367
Momentum, 367–368
Mönckeberg sclerosis, 73
Monkey paw, 304
Monodactyly, 307
Mononeuritis multiplex, 76
Monostotic fibrous dysplasia, 64
Monteggia dislocation, 32
Monteggia fracture, 8, 15
Monteggia fracture-dislocation, 32
Montercaux fracture, 11
Moore fracture, 8

Moore osteotomy, 195
Moore plate, 203
Moore procedure, 253
B.H. Moore procedure, 232
J.R. Moore procedure, 232
Morbid, 93
Morbidity, 93
Morcellation, 266
Morcellized graft, 199
Morel syndrome, 57
Moro reflex, 137
Morquio sign, 137
Morquio syndrome, 41, 63
Morrisay procedure, 246
Morscher plate, 203
Morse taper, 211
Mortise view, 101
Morton foot, 334
Morton neuroma, 78, 334
Morton test, 135
Mose concentric rings, 112–113
Motor and sensory neuropathy, 78
Motor apraxia, 75
Motor neuron disease, 76–77
Mouchet fracture, 8
MRC sensory grade, 137
MRI, 97, 115–116
MSBOS, 150
Muco-, 63, 64
Mucopolysaccharides, 64, 147, 363
Mucopolysaccharidosis, 65
Mucopurulent, 93
Mucosanguineous, 93
Mucous cyst, 65, 312
Mucus, 64
Mulder sign, 135
Müller arthrodesis, 216
Müller osteotomy, 195
Müller plate, 203
Muller procedure, 255
Multiangular, 389
Multiaxial, 175
Multi-flex foot, 175
Multiple epiphyseal dysplasia, 62
Multiple fracture, 5
Multiple myeloma, 49
Multiple osteochondromatosis, 48
Multiple sclerosis, 77
Mumford-Gurd procedure, 232
Munster cast, 158
Murphy nails, 203
Murphy sign, 135

Muscle, 218
    atrophy, 59
        from casts, 160
    contracture, 59
        ischemic, 59
        organic, 59
        postpoliomyelitic, 59
    cramps, 36, 59
    diseases, 57–60
        miscellaneous, 59–60
        myo- root, 57–59
    energy technique, 351
    fibers, 218
    guarding, 59
    injury, 13–14
    insertion, 218
    ischemia, 59
    origin, 218
    reeducation, 348
    soreness, delayed-onset, 59
    spasm, 59
    surgical procedures, 218
    wasting, 59
Muscular dystrophy, 59–60
    Becker, 59
    Duchenne, 59
Musculocutaneous nerve, 230
Musculoskeletal disease, 39–91
    eponymic terms, ICD codes, 404–
        409
Musculoskeletal research, 357–370
    abbreviations, 378
    bone healing/metabolism, 360–361
    cartilage and joints, 362–363
    electrobiology, 361–362
    measurements, 360
    terminology for, 358–360
Mustard iliopsoas transfer, 244
Myalgia, 58
Myasthenia, 57
Myasthenia gravis, 57
Myatrophy, 57
Myectomy, 218
Myelalgia, 282
Myelanalosis, 282
Myelapoplexy, 282
Myelasthenia, 282
Myelatelia, 283
Myelatrophy, 282
Myelauxe, 282
Myelencephalitis, 282
Myeleterosis, 282

Myelo-, 282
Myeloblastoma, 49
Myelocele, 283, 284
Myelocystocele, 283
Myelocystomeningocele, 283
Myelodiastasis, 284
Myelodysplasia, 284
Myeloencephalitis, 282
Myelofibrosis, 54
Myelogram, 100
Myelography, 99–100
Myeloma, multiple, 49
Myelomalacia, 282
Myelomeningitis, 282
Myelomeningocele, 284
Myeloneuritis, 282
Myeloparalysis, 282
Myelopathy, 282–283
Myelophthisis, 283
Myeloplegia, 283
Myeloradiculitis, 283
Myeloradiculopathy, 283
Myelorrhagia, 283
Myelosclerosis, 283
Myelosyphillis, 283
Myelotomy, 288
Mylctoma, 334
Myo-, 57, 218
Myoblastoma, 58
Myoblasts, 218
Myobock system, 172
Myobradia, 58
Myocardial infarction, 74
Myocele, 58
Myocelialgia, 58
Myocelitis, 58
Myocellulitis, 58
Myocerosis, 58
Myoclasis, 218
Myoclonia, 58
Myoclonus, 58
Myocoele, 58
Myocytes, 218
Myocytoma, 58
Myodegeneration, 58
Myodemia, 58
Myodiastasis, 58
Myodynia, 58
Myodystonia, 58
Myoedema, 58
Myoelectric control, 172
Myofascial release, 351

Myofascitis, 58
Myofibroma, 58
Myofibrosis, 58
Myogelosis, 58
Myoglobinuria, 58
Myohypertrophia, 58
Myoischemia, 58
Myokerosis, 58
Myolipoma, 58
Myolysis, 58
Myoma, 58
Myomalacia, 58
Myomatectomy, 218
Myomatosis, 58
Myomectomy, 218
Myomelanosis, 58
Myoneuralgia, 58
Myoneurasthenia, 58
Myoneurectomy, 218
Myoneuroma, 58
Myoneurosis, 58
Myopachynsis, 58
Myopalmus, 58
Myoparalysis, 58
Myoparesis, 58
Myopathy, 58
  mitochondrial, 59
Myopathy hand, 77
Myophagism, 58
Myoplasty, 218
Myopsychopathy, 58
Myorrhaphy, 218
Myorrhexis, 58
Myosalgia, 58
Myosarcoma, 58
Myosclerosis, 58
Myoseism, 58
Myositis, 58
Myositis fibrosa generalista, 53
Myositis ossificans, 58
Myositis ossificans circumscripta, 58
Myositis ossificans progressiva, 53
Myospasia, 58
Myospasm, 58
Myospasmia, 59
Myostasis, 59
Myosteoma, 59
Myosuture, 218
Myosynizesis, 59
Myotenontoplasty, 218
Myotenositis, 59
Myotenotomy, 218

Myotomy, 218
Myotonia, 59
  congenital, 59
Myotonia intermittens, 59
Myotonic dystrophy, 60
Myxedema, 93
Myxo-, 64
Myxofibroma, 64
Myxoma, 64
Myxosarcoma, 64

N

Naffziger sign, 125
Naffziger syndrome, 78, 282
Nail (*see also* Finger nail; Toe nail)
  ingrown, 333
Nail bed, 299
Nail matrix, 299, 330
Nail plate, 299, 330
Nail-patella syndrome, 57
Nalebuff arthrodesis, 314
Namaqualand hip dysplasia, 83
Natatory ligament, 298
Naughton-Dunn procedure, 343
Navicular, 327
Navicular pads, 187
NCV, 353
Neal-Robertson litter, 167
Neck
  diseases of, 274–277
  tests, signs, and maneuvers for, 123
Neck shaft angle, 105
Neck sign, 136
Necropsy, 264
Necrosis, 74, 93
  aseptic, 50
  avascular, 50
Needle biopsy, 264
Neer fracture classification system,
  23–24
Neer impingement sign, 126
Neer lateral view, 101
Neer procedure, 232
Neer prosthesis, 206
Neer staging system, 35
Neer transscapular view, 101
Neer-Horowitz fracture classification
  system, 24
Negative predictive value, 359
Neibauer prosthesis, 315
Nélaton dislocation, 32

Nélaton line, 108, 131
Neoplasm, 93
Neoplastic fracture, 12
Nerve conduction velocity, 353
Nerve of Bell, 230
Nerves, 222
    surgical procedures, 222
Nested nails, 203
Neufeld nail, 203
Neufeld pin, 203
Neufeld roller traction, 165
Neural tube defect, 77
Neuralgia, 77
Neuralgic amyotrophy, 79
Neurectomy, 222, 316, 343
Neuritis, 77, 280
Neuro-, 222
Neurofibroma, 64, 281
Neurogenic, 77
Neurologic disease, 75–79, 77
Neurologic examination, tests, signs,
        and maneuvers for, 135–138
Neurological assessment, 139
Neurolysis, 77, 222
Neuroma, 77
Neuromuscular scoliosis, 279
Neuropathy, 77
Neuroplasty, 222
Neuropraxia, 77
Neurorrhaphy, 222
Neurosyphillis, 78
Neurotization, 316
Neurotmesis, 77
Neurotomy, 222
Neurotripsy, 222
Neurovascular injury, 14
Neurovascular island transfer, 318
Neutron radiography, 116
Neviaser procedure, 232
Neviaser test, 126
Nevus, 93
New York Orthopedic front-opening
        orthosis, 185
New York University insert, 180
Newington orthosis, 179
Newman fusion, 286
Newton, 368
Newton's law, 366
Nicholas procedure, 254
Nicola procedure, 232
Nicoll procedure, 258
Nidus, 94
Niebauer prosthesis, 206

Niemann-Pick syndrome, 57
Night splint, 161
Nightstick fracture, 8
Nirschl procedure, 239
"No man's land," 309
"No touch" test, 134
Node, 94
Nodular fasciitis, 66
Nodule, 94
Nonarticular fracture, 9
Nonionic contrast agents, 98
Nonossifying fibroma, 49, 54
Nonphyseal fracture, 4
Non-plantar grade foot, 334
Nonsuppurative osteomyelitis, 45
Nonunion, 12
Normal last shoes, 188
Normal strain, 368
Normal stress, 368
Normotensive, 74
Norton-Brown orthosis, 184
Notch view, 101
Noyes test, 133–134
N-PCP, 146
N-telopeptide, 147
NTx, 147
Nuchal ligament, 273
Nuchocephalic reflex, 137
Nuclear medicine studies, 97
Nudge control, 172
Nutritional index, 94
NYU insert, 180

O

OAWO, 343
Ober and Barr procedure, 232
Ober procedure, 343
Ober test, 131
Ober-Barr procedure, 246
Obesity, 94
Objective sign, 138–139
Oblique, 389
Oblique fracture, 5, 9
Oblique ligament, 238
Oblique view, 101
Oblongata, 389
O'Brien procedure, 232
Observation hip, 83
Obstetrical palsy, 76, 78
Obturator artery, 243
Obturator foramen, 241
Obturator gemelli, 242–243

Obturator nerve, 241, 243
Obturator sign, 131
Obturator/brim line, 108
OC, 146
Occipital nerve, 272
Occiput, 272
Occlusion, 74, 94
Occlusive dressing, 162
Occult, 94
Occult fracture, 5
Occupational therapy, 353–356
    abbreviations, 377–378
    assessment, 354
    evaluations/tests/devices for, 354–
        355
    services, 353–354
    treatments, 355–356
Ochronosis, 54
O'Connor finger dexterity test, 354
Ocular muscular dystrophy, 60
Oculoplethysmography, 118
O'Donoghue procedure, 255
Odontoid fractures, 14
Odontoid process, 272
Odontoid view, 101
-odynia, 94
Ogden fracture classification system,
        24–25
Ogden plate, 203
Ogston line, 108
OKC system, 175
Oklahoma cable system, 175
Old dislocation, 31
Olecranon, 235
Olecranon fossa, 234
Olecranon fractures, 17, 23, 25
Olisthy, 277
Olive wire, 203
Ollier disease, 48, 57, 61
ON, 146
Onco-, 94
One-legged hop test, 134
Onlay graft, 199
Onychalgia, 311
Onychauxis, 334
Onychectomy, 318
Onychia, 311
Onychocryptosis, 333, 334
Onychogryphosis, 311
Onycholysis, 311
Onychomadesis, 311
Onychomycosis, 311, 334
Onychophagia, 311

Onychoptosis, 311
Onychorrhexis, 311
Onychotomy, 318, 343
Open amputation, 264
Open biopsy, 264
Open chain exercise, 351
Open dislocation, 31
Open fractures, 3, 19
Open reduction, 194
Opening abductory wedge osteotomy, 343
Opening wedge, 159
Opening wedge osteotomy, 343
Open-wedge osteotomy, 195
Opera-glass hand, 302
OPG, 118
Ophthalmoplegia, progressive dystrophic, 60
Oppenheim disease, 59
Oppenheim sign, 137
Opponens bars, 182
Opponensplasty, 320
Opposition, 385
Orbicular ligament, 238
Organic contracture, 59
-orrhagia, 94
-orrhea, 94
-orrhexis, 94
Orthopaedic abbreviations, 371–380
Orthopaedic procedures, list of, 190
Orthopaedic surgery, 189–268
Orthopaedic tests, signs, and maneuvers, 119–140
  gait patterns, 139
  list of, 120–123
  scales and ratings, 139–140
Orthopaedic Trauma Association classification system, 14
Orthopaedics, etymology of, 390–403
Orthoroentgenogram, 100
Orthoroentgenography, 100
Orthoses, 177–187
  abbreviations for, 177
  lower limb, 177–181
  spinal, 184–187
  upper limb, 181–184
Orthotics, 169, 356
  abbreviations, 376–377
  shoe modifications, 187–188
Orthotist, certified, 169
Ortolani click, 131
Ortolani sign, 131
Os, 327

Os calcis fractures, 17
Os intecuneiforme, 327
Os intermetatarseum, 327
Os peroneum, 327
Os sustentaculum, 327
Os talocalcaneus, 327
Os tibiale externum, 324, 327, 335
Os trigonum, 327
Os vesalianum, 327
Osborne and Cotterill procedure, 239
Osborne fascia, 238
Oscilloscope, 98
Osgood osteotomy, 195
Osgood-Schlatter disease, 50, 57
-osis, 94
Osmone-Clarke procedure, 343
Ossa tarsi, 327
Ossicles, 40
Ossification, 189, 192
Ossifying fibroma of long bones, 42
Ossifying fibroma of the jaw, 54
Ostealgia, 40
Ostectomy, 194
Osteitis, 40
Osteitis condensans, 40
Osteitis deformans, 40
Osteitis fibrosa cystica, 40
Osteitis fragilitans, 42
Osteitis ossificans, 40
Osteitis pubis, 40
Ostemia, 40
Ostempycsis, 40
Osteo, 40
Osteo-, 189
Osteoarthritis, 40, 67
Osteoarthropathy, 40
  pustulotic, 68
Osteoarthrosis, 40
Osteoarthrotomy, 194
Osteoarticular, 40
Osteoarticular graft, 199
Osteoblast, 192
Osteoblastoma, 47
Osteocachexia, 40
Osteocalcin, 146, 361
Osteochondral graft, 199
Osteochondral talus lesions, 18
Osteochondritis, 40, 41
Osteochondritis dissecans, 41
  of talus, 15
Osteochondrodesmoplasia, 41
Osteochondrodystrophy, 41
Osteochondrofibroma, 41

Osteochondrolysis, 41
Osteochondroma, 48
  epiphyseal, 48
Osteochondromatosis, 41
  multiple, 48
  synovial, 41, 68
Osteochondropathy, 41
Osteochondrophyte, 41
Osteochondrosis, 40, 41, 334
Osteochondrosis deformans tibia, 55
Osteochondrosis dissecans, 41
Osteoclasia, 41
Osteoclasis, 194
Osteoclast, 193
Osteoclastoma, 49, 51
Osteocopy, 41
Osteocystoma, 41
Osteocyte, 193
Osteodiastasis, 41
Osteodynia, 42
Osteodystrophy, 42
  pulmonary, 54
Osteofibrochondrosarcoma, 42
Osteofibroma, 42
Osteofibromatosis, 42
Osteofibrous dysplasia, 42
Osteogenesis imperfecta, 42
Osteogenesis imperfecta congenita, 42
Osteogenesis imperfecta tarda, 42
Osteogenic sarcoma, 45
Osteohalisteresis, 42
Osteoid osteoma, 47
Osteolipochondroma, 42
Osteolipoma, 42
Osteolysis, 42–43
Osteoma, 47
  solitary, of long bone, 54
Osteomalacia, 43, 79
Osteomatosis, 48
Osteomesopyknosis, 43
Osteomyelitis, 43, 44
  terms related to, 45
Osteomyelodysplasia, 43
Osteonal bone, 193
Osteonecrosis, 43, 50
Osteoneuralgia, 43
Osteopathia striata, 43
Osteopathy, 43
Osteopenia, 43
  transient, 55
Osteoperiosteal graft, 199
Osteoperiostitis, 43
Osteopetrorickets, 43

Osteopetrosis, 43
Osteophlebitis, 43
Osteophyte, 43, 110
Osteoplastica, 43
Osteoplasty, 194
Osteopoikilosis, 43
Osteoporosis, 43
    regional migratory, 54
Osteopsathyrosis idiopathica, 42
Osteoradionecrosis, 43
Osteosarcoma, 47
Osteosclerosis, 43
Osteosclerosis fragilis, 43
Osteosis, 43
Osteospongioma, 43
Osteosynovitis, 43
Osteosyntheses, 199–204
Osteosynthesis, 2, 194
Osteotabes, 43
Osteothrombophlebitis, 43
Osteothrombosis, 44
Osteotomies, 194–196
Osteotripsy, 343
Otto pelvis, 32
Outerbridge-Kashiwagi procedure, 239
Outlet view, 101
Outrigger, 182
Outside locking hinge, 172
Overhead exercise test, 123
Overhead suspension, 164
Overlapped upright extension, 181
Overlapping toe, 334
Over-the-top procedure, 255
Overton fusion, 286

P

PA, 301
PA view, 101
Pachydysostosis, 54
Pachyonychia, 334
Packing, 162
Pads, 162
Pagddu procedure, 255
Paget disease, 40, 57
Pain
    dermatomal, 39
    phantom, 267
    radicular, 280
    rating scales, 139–140
    referred, 39, 277

rest, 72
    sclerotomal, 39
Painful arc syndrome, 82
Palindromic rheumatism, 73
Palliative, 266
Palm, 297–298
Palmar, 389
Palmar fascia, 298
Palmar fasciectomy, 321
Palmar fasciotomy, 321
Palmar fibromatosis, 311
Palmar flexion, 383
Palmar skin crease, 298
Palmar space infection, 312
Palmar wrist splint, 181
Palmer classification for triangular
        fibrocartilage injury, 309
Palpitation, 74
Pancytopenia, congenital, 91
Panmetatarsal head resection, 343
Panner disease, 41, 50, 57
Pantalar fusion, 343
Pantopaque, 98
Par-, 389
Para-, 389
Paracentesis, 266
Parachute jumper's dislocation, 32
Paraffin bath, 350
Paralysis, 77
    familial periodic, 59
Paralysis agitans, 77
Paraplegia, 77
Parapodium orthosis, 180
Parasympathetic nervous system, 269
Parathyroid hormone, 146, 361
Paratonia, 137
Paratrooper fracture, 11
Paravertebral muscle spasm, 277
Parenteral, 266–267
Paresis, 77
Paresthesia, 77
Parham band, 203
Parkinson disease, 79
Paronychia, 313, 334
Paronychium, 299
Parosteal chondrosarcoma, 48
Parosteal osteosarcoma, 47
Parosteitis, 44
Parosteosis, 44
Parrot pseudoparalysis, 79
Parrot-beak tear, 84
Pars, 389

Pars interarticularis, 271
Pars interarticularis defect, 275
Parsonage-Andrew-Turner syndrome,
        79
Partial adactylia, 87
Partial aphalangia, 87
Partial dislocation, 31
Partial hand amputation, 170
Partial hemimelia, 87
Partial osteotomy, 343
Partial patellectomy, 256
Partial thromboplastin time, 145
Partridge band, 203
Parvin maneuver, 127
Pascal, 368
Passive tendon implant, 321
Patch angioplasty, 226
Patella, 247
    radiographic views, 102
    subluxation of, 255–256
    surgery of, 256
Patella alta, 86
Patella baja, 86
Patella clunk syndrome, 86
Patella dislocation, 32
Patella subluxation, 32
Patella subluxation ratio, 108
Patellar fracture, 10
Patellar implant designs, 212–213
Patellar pad, 181
Patellar retraction test, 134
Patellar tendon, 221
Patellar tendon bearing orthosis, 178
Patellar tendon weight-bearing cast,
        159
Patellectomy, 256
Patellofemoral syndrome, 86
Patency, 224
Patent, 389
Pathologic dislocation, 31
Pathologic fracture, 12
Patrick test, 124
Pauciarticular, 68
Paulos procedure, 255
Pauwels angle, 107
Pauwels fracture classification
        system, 25
Pauwels osteotomy, 195
Pauwels-Y osteotomy, 195
Pavlik harness, 179–180
Pavlov ratio, 108
Payr sign, 132

PCV, 141
PE, 70
Peabody procedure, 343
Pearson attachment, 164
Pectineus, 242
Pectoralis major/minor muscle, 228
Pectus carinatum, 94
Pectus excavatum, 94
Pedicle, 271
Pedicle flap, 318
Pedicle graft, 199
Pedicle grafts, 318
Peg graft, 199
Pellagra, 77
Pellegrini-Stieda disease, 65
Pelvic femoral angle, 107
Pelvic girdle, 241
Pelvic ring, 241
Pelvic rock text, 125
Pelvic sling, 165
Pelvic traction, 165, 350
Pelvis
  anatomy of, 240–242
  blood vessels of, 241
  fractures, 9–10, 16, 20, 28, 30
  ligaments of, 241
  muscles of, 241
  nerves of, 241
  radiographic views, 102
  surgery of, 243–247
  surgical approaches to, 260
Pemberton osteotomy, 195
PEMF, 362
Pennsylvania bimanual worksample, 354
Per primam, 267
Perdriolle torsimeter, 113
Peri-, 389
Periarticular fibrositis, 64
Periarticular fracture, 4
Perichondral autografts, 315
Perilunate dislocation, 310
Perineal loops, 187
Perionychium, 299
Periosteal chondroma, 48
Periosteal desmoid, 65
Periosteal fibroma, 64
Periosteal osteosarcoma, 47
Periosteotomy, 194
Periosteum, 193
Periostitis, 54
  florid reactive, 54–55

Periostitis ossificans, 54–55
Periostomy, 194
Peripheal, 389
Peripheral nerves, 269
Peripheral neuropathy, 77, 304
Peritendinous fibrosis, 309
Peritoneum, 242
Perkin line, 108
Peroneal artery, 250
Peroneal muscles, 329
Peroneal spastic flatfoot, 334
Peroneus brevis, 249
Peroneus longus, 249
Peroneus tertius, 249
Perpendicular, 389
Perry procedure, 257, 343
Persian slipper foot, 334
Perthes disease, 50, 57
Perthes-Bankhart lesion, 31
Pertrochanteric fracture, 10
Pes, 334
Pes anserinus, 249
Pes calcanovarus, 335
Pes cavovalgus, 335
Pes cavovarus, 335
Pes cavus, 334, 335
Pes equinovalgus, 335
Pes equinovarus, 335
Pes planovalgus, 335
Pes planus, 334, 335
PET, 97
Petaling edges, 159
Petechiae, 94
Petit mal epilepsy, 76
Petric spica cast, 158
-pexy, 267
PGP nail, 203
Phalangectomy, 321
Phalanges, 291
Phalanx, 327
Phalen test and maneuver, 129
Phantom bone disease, 42
Phantom limb syndrome, 94
Phantom pain, 267
Phelps procedure, 232
Phemister osteotomy, 195
Phenolization, 343
Philadelphia collar, 186
Phillips screw, 203
Phlebitis, 70
Phlebography, 117, 118
Phlebothrombosis, 70

Phlegmasia cerulea dolens, 74
Phocomelia, 87, 306
Phonophoresis, 350
Phosphoproteins, 361
Photon densitometry, 99
Photoplethysmography, 118
PHPT, 80
Phrenic nerve, 272
-phyma, 94
Physeal angle, 107
Physeal slope, 107
Physical medicine and occupational
  therapy, abbreviations, 377–378
Physical sign, 138–139
Physical therapist, 347
Physical therapy, 347–353
  abbreviations, 377–378
  consultation services, 349
  evaluation, 348
  modalities for, 349–350
  procedures, 350–352
  services, 348–349
  tests and measurements, 352–353
  treatment techniques, 348–349
Physis, 191
Physis fractures, 27
Physis pubis, 241
Piano key sign, 129
PICP, 146
Pidcock pin, 203
Piedmont fracture, 8
Pierrot-Murphy procedure, 343
Piezoelectric potentials, 362
Pigeon toe, 334
Pigmented villonodular synovitis, 69
Pillion fracture, 10
Pillow orthosis, 180
Pilon fracture, 26
Pin tract infection, from casts, 160
Pinch, 354
Pinched nerve, 280
Pinprick test, 352
Piotrowski sign, 137
PIP fusion, 344
Pipkin fracture classification system, 25
Piriform sclerosis ilium, 40
Piriformis, 242–243
Piriformis fossa, 242
Piriformis syndrome, 283
Piston sign, 131

Pitted nail, 311
Pivot, 389
Pivot-shift test, 134
Plafond fracture, 11
Plantar, 389
Plantar aponeurosis, 330
Plantar arch, 331
Plantar arch support, 187
Plantar artery, 330
Plantar axial view of foot, 101
Plantar fascia, 330
Plantar flexed metatarsal, 334
Plantar flexion, 383
Plantar nerve, 331
Plantar wart, 334
Plantaris, 250
Plasmacytoma, 49
Plastazote collar, 186
Plastazote shoes, 188
Plaster rolls, 157
Plastic behavior, 368
Plastic bowing fracture, 5
Plastic collar, 186
Plasticity, 368
Plastics, 370
Platelet concentrate, 151
Platelets, 142
Platou osteotomy, 195
Platysma, 272
Pleomorphic, 94
Plethysmography, 118
Plexiform, 94
Plica, 253
Plica syndrome, 86
Plication, 267
PLIF, 287
Plt, 142
Pneumatic compression boot, 161
Pneumatic compression sleeve, 161
Pneumatocyst, intraosseous, 53
Pneumoarthrogram, 100
Pneumoarthrography, 100
Podagra, 334
Poisson's ratio, 368
Poland fracture classification system,
    25
Poland syndrome, 307
Polar moment of inertia, 368
Polarized light microscopy, 149
Poliomyelitis, 77
Pollicization, 321
Pollock sign, 129
Polyacetyl rod, 267

Polyarteritis nodosa, 73
Polyarthritis, 68
Polydactyly, 307, 335
Polyostotic fibrous dysplasia, 55, 64
Polyps, 94
Polysyndactyly, 307, 335
Polytetrafluoroethylene, 226
Popliteal artery, 250
Popliteal cyst, 68, 71, 86
Popliteal entrapment, 71–72
Popliteal pterygium syndrome, 86
Popliteal vein, 250
Popliteus muscle, 249
Portal, 267
Posada fracture, 8
Positive predictive value, 359
Positive work, 350
Positron emission tomography, 97
Post-, 389
Postaxial deficiency, 308
Posterior, 389
Posterior approach, 259–260
Posterior bow, 6
Posterior cervical spinal fusion, 287
Posterior compartment, 249
Posterior cruciate ligament, 250
Posterior cruciate sprain, 33
Posterior displacement, 32
Posterior drawer test, 134
Posterior element fracture, 9
Posterior fracture-displacement, 32
Posterior hiatal sign, 109
Posterior inferior iliac spine, 241
Posterior interosseous nerve, 238
Posterior intraosseous nerve syn-
    drome, 303
Posterior lip, 242
Posterior lumbar spinal fusion, 287
Posterior malleolus, 247
Posterior neck muscles, 272
Posterior oblique sprain, 33
Posterior shoulder dislocation, 31
Posterior spinal fusion, 287
Posterior spinal muscle segments, 274
Posterior splint, 167
Posterior superior iliac spine, 240
Posterior tibial artery, 250
Posterior tibial artery/nerve/vein, 331
Posterior tibial nerve, 253
Posterior tibial spine, 247
Posterior tibial tendon, 329
Postero-, 389
Posterolateral fusion, 287

Posterolateral interbody fusion, 287
Postphlebitic syndrome, 70
Postpoliomyelitic contracture, 59
Posttraumatic reflex dystrophy, 75
Postural fixation, 125
Potential energy, 368
Potenza arthrodesis, 313
Pott disease, 57, 280
Pott eversion osteotomy, 195
Pott fracture, 11
Potter arthrodesis, 216
Pouce floutant, 306
Poupart inguinal ligament, 241
Power Doppler, 97
PPD, 149
PPG, 118
Prader-Willi syndrome, 88
Prayer view, 101–102
Prehallux, 335
Prehension, 129
Preiser disease, 312
Prenyl jacket, 185
Prepatellar bursa, 253
Prescriptions, abbreviations for, 380
Pressure dressing, 162
Pressure epiphysis, 41, 192
Pressure sore, from casts, 160
Pressure testing, 352
Preston screw, 203
Prevention/minimization of debili-
    tation, 356
Pridie-Koutsogiannis procedure, 344
Primary center of ossification, 192
Primary closure, 267
Primary lymphoma, 49
Primary subacute osteomyelitis, 45
Primitive dislocation, 31
Pro time, 145
Procollagen, 364
Procollagen propeptide, 146
Procurvatum, 94
Profundus, 236
Profundus artery, 243
Prognosis, 94
Progressive diaphyseal dysplasia, 54,
    55
Progressive dystrophic ophthalmo-
    plegia, 60
Progressive osseous heteroplasia, 54
Progressive systemic sclerosis, 73,
    301
Proliferating zone, 191
Pronation, 335, 383

Pronation sign, 137
Pronator quadratus, 235
Pronator syndrome, 303
Prone, 389
Prone external rotation test, 134
Proper volar digital nerve/artery, 300
Prophylaxis, 94
Proprioception, 94
Proprioceptive testing, 352
Prostheses, 170–177, 267
    components, materials, and techniques for, 176
    internal, 206
    lower limb, 173–176
    specialized systems, 176–177
    upper limb, 170–173, 206–207
Prosthetics, 169, 356
    abbreviations, 376–377
    modular, 211
Prosthetist, certified, 169
Protective dressing, 162
Proteoglycan, 363
Proteoglycan aggregate, 363
Proteoglycan subunit, 362
Proteoglycans, 62
Prothrombin time, 145
Proton density, 116
Protract, 389
Protrusio acetabuli, 83
Provisional calcification, 191
Proximal, 389
Proximal femur fractures, 9–10
Proximal focal femoral deficiency, 83
Proximal humerus fractures, 6–8
Proximal phocomelia, 87
Proximal row carpectomy, 315
Proximal thigh band, 181
Proximal tibial fractures, 27
Proximal tibiofibular ligament, 250
Proximal tibiofibular facet, 247
Prune belly syndrome, 82
Pseudarthrosis, congenital, 51
Pseudoarthrosis, 12, 68
Pseudo-Babinski sign, 137
Pseudoclaudication, 277
Pseudogout, 82–83, 301
Pseudohypertrophic muscular dystrophy, 60
Pseudohypoparathyroidism, 80
Pseudomalignant fibroosseous tumors, 54–55
Pseudosarcomatous fibromatosis, 64
Pseudostability test, 129

Psoriatic arthritis, 301
PT, 145
PTA, 225
PTB, 159
PTB orthosis, 178
PTBS, 174
PTB-SC, 174
PTB-SP, 174
PTFE, 226
PTH, 146, 361
PTS, 174
PTT, 145
Pubic bone, 241
Pubic osteolysis, 42
Pubiotomy, 246
Pubis, 241
Pudendal nerve, 241
Pugh nail, 203
Pulley exercises, 351
Pulleys, 295
Pulmonary embolism, 70
Pulmonary osteodystrophy, 54
Pulp pinch, 129
Pulse volume recorder, 118
Pulsed Doppler, 97, 117
Pulsed electromagnetic fields, 362
Pulver-Taft weave, 319
Pump bumps, 335
Punctum ossificationis, 192
Punctum ossificationis primarium, 192
Punctum ossificationis secundarium, 192
Purdue pegboard, 354
Purified protein derivative, 149
Purpura, 94
Purulent, 94
Push-pull ankle stress, 102
Push-pull test, 126
Pustulotic osteoarthropathy, 68
Putti arthrodesis, 216
Putti procedure, 232
Putti screw, 203
Putti-Mayer procedure, 344
Putti-Platt procedure, 232
PVR, 118
PYD, 147
Pyknodysostosis, 54
Pylon, 176
Pyoderma gangrenosum, 94
Pyogenic, 94
Pyogenic arthritis, 301
Pyogenic granuloma, 313

Pyomyositis, 60
Pyramidal tract, 273274
Pyrexia, 94
Pyridinium collagen cross-links, 147
Pyridinoline, 364
Pyridinoline collagen cross-links, 147

Q

Q angle, 107
QCT, 99
Quadratus, 389
Quadratus femoris, 242–243
Quadratus lumborum, 274
Quadratus plantae, 329
Quadregia, 308
Quadriceps active test, 134
Quadriceps muscle, 249
Quadriceps reflex, 138
Quadriceps test, 139
Quadricepsplasty, 256
Quadrilateral brim, 181
Quadrilateral ischial weight-bearing socket, 174
Quadriplegia, 77
Quantitative computed tomography, 99
Quantum foot, 175
Queckenstedt sign, 137
Quengle cast, 158
Quénu and Küss modified fracture classification system, 25–26
Quenu procedure, 344
Quiescence, 94
Quigley traction, 165

R

RA factor, 145
Rachialgia, 276
Rachicentesis, 288
Rachio-, 276
Rachiochysis, 276
Rachiodynia, 276
Rachiokyphosis, 276
Rachiomyelitis, 276
Rachioparalysis, 276
Rachiopathy, 276
Rachioplegia, 276
Rachioscoliosis, 276
Rachiotomy, 288
Rachisagra, 276
Rachischisis, 276

Rachitomy, 288
Racket nail, 311
Rad, 98, 118
Radial artery, 236, 300
Radial bursa, 298
Radial clubbed hand, 307
Radial collateral ligament, 238, 297
Radial deviation, 383
Radial drift, 302
Radial fractures, distal, 18
Radial head
    anatomy of, 234
    fractures, 9, 15, 22–23
Radial nerve, 230, 300
Radial neuropathy, 303
Radial reflex, inverted, 124
Radial sensory nerve entrapment, 303
Radial styloid fracture, 9
Radial styloidectomy, 315
Radial tunnel syndrome, 77, 303
Radial vein, 237
Radialis sign, 137
Radialization/centralization, 317
Radiation therapy, 118
Radicotomy, 222
Radicular pain, 280
Radiculectomy, 222, 288
Radiculitis, 77, 280
Radiculoneuritis, 77
Radiculopathy, 281
Radioactive tracers, 359
Radiocampsis, 276
Radiocarpal arthrodesis, 313, 314
Radiograph, 98
Radiography, 98 (see also Imaging
    techniques)
Radiohumeral synostosis, 308
Radioisotope imaging, 97
Radiologist, 98
Radiology, 98
Radiolucent, 98
Radiopaque, 98
Radioulnar fusion, 314
Radioulnar subluxation, 33
Radius (see also Radial entries)
    anatomy of, 234
    radiographic views, 102
Radley, Liebig
    and Brown approach, 260
    and Brown procedure, 246
Raimiste sign, 137
Range of motion exercises, 351
Rarefaction, 94

Ratchet flexor tenodesis splint, 181
Ratcliff classification of femoral head
    deformities from avascular
    necrosis, 50–51
Ratios, radiographic, 107–109
Ray, 330
Ray amputation, 321
Raynaud disease, 73
Raynaud phenomenon, 73, 139
RBC, 142
Re-, 389
Reagent, 359
Recent dislocation, 31
Recessive, 92
Reciprocal finger prehension, 181
Reciprocating gait orthosis, 179
Recrudescence, 94
Rectus femoris muscle, 243
Rectus femoris syndrome, 71
Recurrent dislocation, 31
Recurvatum, 94, 389
Red blood count, 142
Red cells, 151
Reedy nail, 311
Reefing, 267
Referred pain, 39, 277
Reflect, 267
Reflex sympathetic dystrophy, 75, 302
Refsum syndrome, 79
Regenerated meniscus, 85
Regimen, 267
Regional anesthesia, 259
Regional migratory osteoporosis, 54
Regressive remodeling, 94
Reichenheim-King procedure, 239
Reimers index, 109
Reiter syndrome, 68
Release, 267
Relocation test, 126
Rem, 118
Renal osteodystrophy, 80
Replantation, 321
Replantation microsurgery, 261–262
Research grant, 358
Resection, 267
Residual, 389
Residual nerve root irritabiliity, 280
Resistive exercise table, 352
Rest pain, 72
Resting zone, 191
Reticular cartilage, 217
Reticulocyte count, 145
Retract, 389

Retraction, 267
Retrad, 389
Retro-, 389
Retrocalcaneal exostosis, 333
Retroflex, 389
Retroflexion, 385
Retrograde, 389
Retrolisthesis, 277
Retropatellar fat pad, 253
Retropharyngeal tendonitis, acute
    calcific, 66
Retroversion, 385
Rett syndrome, 77–78
Reverdin-Green procedure, 344
Reversal of cervical lordosis, 279
Reverse Bankhart lesion, 31
Reverse Barton fracture, 9
Reverse Bigelow maneuver, 131–132
Reverse Colles fracture, 9
Reverse Hill-Sachs lesion, 31
Reverse last shoes, 188
Reverse Mauck procedure, 255
Reverse pivot-shift test, 134
Reverse tennis elbow, 35, 312
Reversed vein bypass graft, 226
Revised carpal height ratio, 107
Revision, 267
Revision polydactyly, 322
RGD, 361
RGO, 179
Rhabdomyolysis, 60
Rhabdomyosarcoma, 49
Rheumatoid arthritis, 73–74
Rheumatoid factor, 145
Rheumatoid spondylitis, 73
Rheumatology, 72
Rhizomelic, 86, 88
Rhizotomy, 222, 288
Rhomboid fossa, 227
Rhomboideus major/minor muscle,
    228
Rib belt, 184
Ribs, radiographic views, 102
RICE, 350
Rice bodies, 68
Richard screw, 203
Richardson procedure, 344
Riche-Cannieu connection, 300
Rickets, 54, 80
Ridlon procedure, 244
Rigid dressing, 176
Rigid orthoses, 178
Rigidity, 368

Rigidus, 94
Ring fracture, 10
Ring man shoulder, 36
Ring sign, 109–110
Riordan procedure, 321
Riseborough and Radin fracture
classification system, 26
Risser localizer, 157
Risser procedure, 288
Risser sign, 110
Roaf, Kirkaldy-Willis, and Cattero
procedure, 288
Robert Jones bandage, 162–163
Robert view, 102
Roberts approach, 259
Robinson and Riley fusion, 286
Rocker sole modification, 188
Rocker-bottom foot, 335
Rockwood fracture classification
system, 26
Rockwood procedure, 233
Roentgen, 98, 118
Roentgen absorbed dose, 118
Roentgen ray, 99
Roentgen stereophotogrammetry, 100
Roentgen-equivalent-man, 118
Roentgenography, 98
Roentgenology, 98
Roger fusion, 287
Roger procedure, 233
Rogozinski instrument, 287
Rolando fracture, 9
ROM exercises, 351
Romberg test, 137
Rongeur, 267
Roos test, 123
Root and Siegel procedure, 246
Root procedure, 246
Root sleeve fibrosis, 281
Roper-Day prosthesis, 206
Rose procedure, 344
Rosenberg view, 102
Rotary control, 187
Rotating prosthesis, 213
Rotation, 389
Rotator cuff, 228, 235
Rotator cuff injury, 36
Rotator interval, 229
Rotator unit, 176
Rotter-Erb syndrome, 41
Round cell tumors, 48–49
Roussy-Lévy syndrome, 79
Roux sign, 132

Roux-Goldthwait procedure, 256
Rowe and Lowell fracture classifica-
tion system, 26
Rowe and Zarins procedure, 233
Rowe approach, 259–260
Roy-Camille fusion, 286
Roy-Camille instrument, 288
RSD, 302
Rubor, 72, 94
Rudimentary, 94
Rudimentary ribs, 277
Rüedi and Allgöwer fracture classifi-
cation system, 26
Ruger jersey finger, 35
Rugger jersey spine, 110
Ruiz-Mora procedure, 344
Runner's bump, 36
Runner's knee, 36
Rupture, 94
Ruptured disk, 282
Rush nail/rod/pin, 203
Russe bone graft, 317
Russell procedure, 258
Russell traction, 165
Russell-Taylor fracture classification
system, 27
Russell-Taylor nail, 203
Rust sign, 123
Rydell nails, 203

S

Sabeceous, 95
Saber-cut approach, 259, 260
SAC, 158
SACH foot, 175
Sacral ala, 273
Sacral cyst, 281
Sacral spine, 273
anatomy of, 270
Sacralgia, 277
Sacralization, 277
Sacralized transverse process, 277
Sacrodynia, 277
Sacroiiliac joint, 273
Sacroiliac, 241
Sacroiliac belt, 184
Sacroiliac joints, radiographic views,
102
Sacroiliac line, 108–109
Sacroiliac orthoses, 184
Sacroiliac subluxation, 33
Sacroiliac/symphysis line, 109

Sacroiliitis, 277
Sacrospinous ligament, 241
Sacrotuberous ligament, 241
Sacrovertebral angle, 107
Sacrum, 273
anatomy of, 270
radiographic views, 102
Saddle prosthesis, 211
SAFE foot, 175
Safety, 175
Safety pin orthosis, 181
Sage procedure, 253
Sage rod, 203
Sager traction splint, 167
Sagittal plane, 381
Sagittal stress test, 135
Saha procedure, 233
Sailboarder's injury, 36
Salicylates, 145
Saline dressing, 162
Salter fracture, 4
Salter osteotomy, 195
Salter sling, 179
Salter-Harris fracture, 4
Salter-Harris fracture classification
system, 27
Salter-Thompson classification, 113
Samilson procedure, 344
Samilson-Preito fracture classification
system, 27
Sanfilippo syndrome, 63
Sanguineous, 94
Santana elbow extension splint, 182
Saphenous nerve, 253
Saphenous vein, 250
SAPHO, 45
Saponification, 95
Sarbó sign, 137
Sarcoidosis, 95
Sarcomas, 48
Sargent procedure, 256
Sarmiento nail, 203
Sarmiento osteotomy, 195
Sarmiento procedure, 246
Sarotrius muscle, 243
Saturday night palsy, 304
Saucerization, 267
Sauve-Kapandji procedure, 239
SBO, 284
Scaffold, 267, 370
Scalene block, 259
Scalenus, 272
Scanning electron microscopy, 359

Scanography, 100
Scaphoid, 292, 327
Scaphoid fracture, 19
Scaphoid pads, 187
Scaphoid test, 129–130
Scapholunate advanced collapse, 301
Scapholunate advanced collapse
　　procedure, 314
Scapula, 227
　locked, 31
　radiographic views, 102
Scapula fractures, 6–8, 20
Scapular flaps, 317
Scapular sign of Putti, 126–127
Scapulectomy, 233
Scapulpexy, 267
SCFE, 54
Schanz pins, 203
Schatzker fracture classification
　　system, 27
Scheie syndrome, 63
Scheuermann disease, 50, 57, 280
Schlesinger sign, 132
Schmid disease, 62
Schmorl nodes, 280
Schneider arthrodesis, 216
Schneider nail/rod, 203
Schollner costoplasty, 288
Schreiber maneuver, 137
Schrock procedure, 233
Schultze-Chvostek sign, 138
Schwann tumor, 64
Schwannoma, 79
Sciatic nerve, 241, 243, 253
Sciatic plexus, 241
Sciatica, 277, 280
Scintigraphy, 97, 114
Scleroderma, 74, 311
　limited, 73
Sclerotomal pain, 39
Scoliorachitis, 277
Scoliosis, 278
Scoliosis cast, 157
Scotch terrier sign, 110
Scott procedure, 233, 288
Scottish Rite orthosis, 180
Scotty dog sign, 110
Scout film, 98
Scout radiograph, 98
Screw-home mechanism, 135
SC-SP, 174
Scudari procedure, 256

SD, 170
Seattle foot, 175
Secondary center of ossification, 192
Secondary chondrosarcoma, 48
Secondary closure, 267
Secondary fracture, 5
Secondary osteosarcoma, 47
Secondary union, 13
Secretan edema, 309
Sed. rate, 144
Seddon arthrodesis, 314
Seddon procedure, 289
Sedimentation rate, 144
Segmental fracture, 5
Segmental graft, 199
Segmental instability, 279
Segmental spinal dysgenesis, 284
Segond fracture, 10
Seidel nail, 204
Seinsheimer fracture classification
　　system, 27
Selesian bandage, 175–176
Selesian belt, 175–176
Selig procedure, 246
SEM, 359
Semiconstrained knee replacement,
　212
Semi-Fowler position, 166
Semilunar menisci, 253
Semimembranosus, 249
Semitendinosus, 249
Semm and Weinstein monofilament
　　test, 130
Semmes-Weinstein monofilament,
　355
Senegas approach, 260
Sensitivity, 359
Sensorimotor skills, 355–356
Sensory testing, 352
Sentinel fracture, 9
Sepsis, 95, 267
Septa, 298
Septic, 267
Septicemia, 95
Sequela, 95
Sequestrectomy, 194
Sequestrum, 45
Serendipity view, 102
Serial cast, 159
Serological tests, abbreviations, 152–
　153
Seropurulent, 95

Serosanguineous, 95
Serous, 95
Serratus anterior muscle, 229
Serum alkaline phosphatase, 142
Serum calcium, 146
Serum chemistries, abbreviations,
　　152–153
Serum lead, 145
Serum protein electrophoresis, 145
Serum tests, 143–145
　for metabolic disease, 145–147
Server disease, 50
Sesamoid, 193, 327
Sesamoids, 291–292
Sever disease, 334
Severin hip dysplasia scale, 113
Sex linked, 92
SGOT, 143
SGP, 362
SGPT, 143
Shaffer plate, 187
Shaft fracture, 10
Shands dressing, 163
Sharp angle, 107
Sharp dissection, 265
Sharpey fibers, 221
Sharp-Purser test, 123
Sharrard iliopsoas transfer, 244
Shear modulus, 368
Shear strain, 368
Shear stress, 368
Sheath, 176
Sheet wadding, 157
Sheffield rod, 204
Shelf procedure, 244
Shenton line, 109
Shepherd fracture, 11
Shepherd's crook deformity, 57
Sherk and Probst procedure, 239
Sherman plate, 204
Shin splints, 36
Shirt-stud abscess, 312
Shoe modifications, 187–188
Short fingers, 306
Short ligament, 297
Short opponens orthosis, 181
Short plantar ligament, 330
Short tau inversion recovery, 115
Short-arm cast, 158
Short-arm splint, 161
Short-leg case, 158–159
Short-leg splint, 161

Short-leg walking cast, 159
Shoulder
    anatomy of, 227–230
    apprehension, 36
    arteries, veins, branches around,
        229
    conditions, 82
    disarticulation, 170
    dislocation, 27, 31
        anterior, 31
        posterior, 31
    fractures, 6–8
    frozen, 65, 67
    girdle, 229
    harness, 172
    ligaments around, 229
    muscles around, 227–229
    nerves around, 229–230
    orthoses, 182
    pointer, 36
    radiographic views, 102
    spica, 158
    sprains, 33
    subluxation, 33
    surgery of, 231–233
    surgical approaches, 259–260
    tests, signs, and maneuvers for,
        125–127
Shoulder-elbow-wrist-hand orthoses,
    182
Shwachman syndrome, 83
SI units, 368
Sickle cell anemia, 83
Sideswipe fracture, 8
Siffert-Foster-Nachamie procedure,
    344
Sigmoid notch, 292
Signs
    orthopaedic, 119–123
    radiographic, 109–110
Silfverskiöld procedure, 256
Silicone gel socket insert, 176
Silver procedure, 344
Silverskjold disease, 50, 57
Simmons fusion, 286
Simmons procedure, 289
Simmons test, 132
Simple button prosthesis, 213
Simple dislocation, 31
Simpson catheter, 225
Sinding-Larsen-Johansson disease, 57
Singh index, 113

Single axis, 175
Single hip spica, 158
Single photon emission computerized
        tomography, 116
Sinister, 389
Sinography, 100
Sinus, 45
Sinus tarsi, 330
Site of fracture, 6
Sjögren syndrome, 74
Skeletal amyloidosis, 54
Skeletal traction, 166
Skew foot, 335
Skier's injury, 11
Skillern fracture, 9
Skin, disorders of, 311–312
Skin creases, 299
Skin grafts
    full-thickness, 258
    pedicle, 258
    rotational flaps, 258
    split-thickness, 258
Skiving, 256
SLAC procedure, 314
Slap foot gait, 139
SLAP lesion, 36
SLC, 158–159
SLE, 301
Sleeve, 176
Sleeve fracture, 10
Slide plate, 204
Slider crank mechanism, 298
Sliding arthrodesis, 216
Sliding inlay, 199
Slings, 356
Slipped capital femoral epiphysis, 54
Slipped disk, 282
Slipped epiphysis, 62
Slipped upper femoral epiphysis, 54
Slipper cast, 159
Slocum procedure, 255
Slocum test, 134
Slomann view, 102
Slough, 95
SLR test, 125
SLWC, 159
Sly syndrome, 63
Small-patella syndrome, 86
Sm-C, 361
Smillie nail, 204
Smith and Ross test, 130
Smith dislocation, 32

Smith fracture, 9
Smith maneuver, 132
Smith PCE, 354
Smith Peterson procedure, 289
Smith physical capacities evaluation,
        354
Smith prosthesis, 206
Smith-Albin flap, 318
Smith-Petersen approach, 260
Smith-Petersen arthrodesis, 216, 314
Smith-Petersen nail, 204
Smith-Robinson fusion, 286
Smyth pin, 204
Snapping hip, 82
Snapping knee syndrome, 86
Snapping scapula, 82
Snapping tendon release, 320
Snapping tendons, 312
Snowstorm knee, 86
Socket, 176
Sofield osteotomy, 195
Soft collar, 186
Soft cosmetic cover, 176
Soft socket insert, 176
Soft tissue
    classification, 13
    injury to, 22
Soft tissue diseases, 63–65
Sole inserts, 188
Soleus, 250
Solitary fibromatosis of bone, 54
Solitary osteoma of long bone, 54
Somatic sign, 139
Somatization disorder, 95
Somatomedin C, 361
SOMI orthosis, 186
Sonography, 97, 116
Soto-Hall sign, 125
Southwick angle, 103
Southwick fusion, 287
Southwick osteotomy, 195
Southwick slide procedure, 256
Soutter procedure, 246
Space of Poirer, 297
Space shoes, 187
Spasm, 95
Spastic, 95
Spastic cerebral palsy, 76
SPC, 174
SPE, 145
Spear tackler's spine, 36
Specificity, 359

SPECT 116
Speed and Boyd procedure, 239
Speed osteotomy, 195
Speed procedure, 233, 289
J.S. Speed procedure, 239
Speed test, 127
SPEP, 145
Spetzler fusion, 286
SPGR, 115
Sphincter ani, 241
Spica casts, 157
Spike osteotomy, 195
Spilled teacup sign, 130
Spina bifida, 284
Spina bifida occulta, 284
Spinal accessory nerve, 272
Spinal block, 259
Spinal board, 167
Spinal canal, 273–274
Spinal cord, 273274
    diseases of, 282–283
Spinal instrumentation, 287–288
Spinal region, radiographic views,
    102
Spinal stenosis, 279
Spine, 269–289
    anatomy of, 269–275
    approaches to, 289
    congenital disorders of, 283–284
    deformities of, 277–278
    diseases of, 274–277
    disk diseases of, 281–282
    dislocations, 32
    fractures, 9
    fusions of, 286–287
    nerve root diseases of, 280–281
    orthoses for, 184–187
    procedures for, 288–289
    of scapula, 227
    sign, 125
    spondylo- root diseases, 275
    structural anomalies of, 278
    surgery of, 284–286
Spinoglenoid notch, 227
Spinous process, 271
Spira procedure, 233
Spiral fracture, 6
Spiral groove, 234
Spittler procedure, 240
Splay foot, 335
Splaying, 95
Splintered fracture, 4

Splints, 155–156, 160–161, 167, 356
    abbreviations, 376
    accessories for, 161
Split stirrup, 181
Split-thickness skin graft, 258
Spoiled grass, 115
Spondylalgia, 275
Spondylarthritis, 275
Spondylarthrocace, 275
Spondylexarthrosis, 275
Spondylitis, 275
Spondylizema, 275
Spondylodynia, 275
Spondyloepiphyseal dysplasia, 62,
    275
Spondyloepiphyseal dysplasia of
    Maroteaux, 62
Spondylolisthesis, 32, 275
    classification of, 275
Spondylolysis, 32, 275
    classification of, 275
Spondylomalacia, 275
Spondylopathy, 275
Spondyloptosis, 9
Spondylopyosis, 275
Spondyloschisis, 275
Spondylosis, 276
Spondylosyndesis, 289
Spondylotomy, 289
Sponge test, 125
Spontorno index, 109
Spoon nail, 311
Sports-related injuries, 34–37
Sprain-ligament rupture, 2
Sprains, 33–34
Spray and stretch, 352
Spreader bar, 181
Spring ligament, 330
Spring swivel thumb, 182
Spring wire orthosis, 178
Springlight foot, 175
Spring-loaded crutches, 161
Sprinter's fracture, 10
Spur, 110
Spurious ankylosis, 69
Spurling test, 123
Spurs, 95
Squatters, 335
Squinting patella, 86
St. Vitus dance, 76
Staheli procedure, 246
Stahl index, 113

Stairs sign, 138
Stamm procedure, 216
Standard orthosis, 180
Standing apprehension test, 134
Standing frame orthosis, 180
Stanisavljevic procedure, 256
Staples arthrodesis, 216
Staples-Black-Brostrom procedure,
    344
Stasis, 75, 268
-stasis, 267
Static orthosis, 179, 182
Static tendon transfer, 319
Statics, 368
Station test, 138
Stee procedure, 246
Steel shank, 180
Steffee plate, 288
Steffee thumb arthroplasty, 315
Steinberg classification of hip
    deformities from aseptic
    necrosis, 51
Steinberg staging system for avascu-
    lar necrosis of femur, 113
Steindler arthrodesis, 216
Steindler flexorplasty, 240, 320
Steindler matricectomy, 344
Steindler procedure, 233, 344
Steinmann pin, 166, 204
Stellate fracture, 6
Stener and Gunterberg procedure, 246
Stener lesion, 310
Stenosing tenosynovitis, 312
Stenosis, 75, 95
Stent, 268
Step down osteotomy, 344
Sternal attachment, 187
Sternal occiput mandibular immobi-
    lization orthosis, 186
Sternoclavicular joint, 227
Sternoclavicular joint separation, 31
Sternoclavicular ligament, 229
Sternocleidomastoid, 272
Sternocleidomastoid muscle, 229
Sternum, 273
    radiographic views, 102
Stewart and Harley procedure, 216
Stewart and Milford fracture classifi-
    cation system, 28
Stewart procedure, 233, 240
Stewart-Morel syndrome, 57, 60
Stickler syndrome, 62

Stieda fracture, 10
Stiff man syndrome, 60
Stiff ray, 335
Stiffness, 368
Stiffness coefficient, 368
Stigma, 95
Still disease, 73
Stimson maneuver, 132
Stippled epiphysis, 62
STIR, 115
Stirrup, 181
Stockinette, 157, 176
Stone arthrodesis, 216
Stone procedure, 344
Straddle fracture, 10
Straight last shoes, 188
Straight leg raising test, 125
  contralateral, 124
Strain, 2–3, 368
Strain energy, 368
Strains, 33–34
Strap muscles, 272
Strayer procedure, 344
Streaming potentials, 362
Street medullary pin, 204
Street nail, 204
Strength, 368
Stress, 368
Stress fracture, 12
Stress fractures, 28
Stress injury to bone, 28
Stress reaction to bone, 12
Stress-generated potentials, 362
Stress-strain diagram, 368
Striate, 389
Stroke, 72
Stromelysin, 359, 363
Strontium-89, 118
Strontium-85 resorption rate, 116
Structural curve, 279
Strümpell sign, 132, 137
Strunsky sign, 135
Strut graft, 198
Stryker frame, 166
Stryker notch view, 102
Stulberg method, 113
Stump revision, 264
Stump shrinker, 176
Stump sock, 176
Styloid process, 235
Styloids, 292
Suave Kapanje procedure, 315

Sub-, 389
Subastragalar dislocation, 32
Subcapital fracture, 10
Subchondral bone, 193, 213
Subchondral plate, 213
Subclavian artery, 229
Subclavian carotid bypass, 226
Subclavian vein, 229
Subcoracoid dislocation, 31
Subcortical defect, 54
Subcutaneous, 268
Subcuticular, 268
Subglenoid dislocation, 31
Subliminal, 95
Subluxation, 2
  unilateral facet, 32
Subluxations, 33
Subperiosteal ABC, 54–55
Subperiosteal fracture, 6
Subperiosteal giant-cell reparative
  granuloma, 54
Subscapularis muscle, 229
Substitution bone, 191
Subtalar arthrodesis, 344
Subtalar arthroereisis, 344
Subtalar joint, 327
Subtrochanteric, 242
Subtrochanteric fracture, 10
Subtrochanteric fractures, 30
  of femur, 27
Subungual abscess, 313
Subungual exostosis, 311, 335
Subungual hematoma, 311
Subungual space, 299
Subungual tissue, 299
Succinylcholine test, 139
Suction for below-knee suspension,
  175
Suction socket suspension for below-
  knee prosthesis, 174
Sudeck atrophy, 72, 75
SUFE, 54
Sugar tong cast, 161
Sugar tong splint, 161
Sugiuka osteotomy, 195
Sulcus, 268
Sulcus angle, 107
Sulcus sign, 127
Summit, 389
Sunderland classification, 302
Sunrise view, 102
Sunset view, 102

Super-, 389
Superficial, 389
Superficial palmar arterial arch, 300
Superficial peroneal nerve, 253
Superficial radial nerve, 238
Superficial transverse intermetacarpal
  ligament, 297
Superior, 389
Superior dome, 242
Superior gemellus, 242–243
Superior gluteal artery, 243
Superior mesenteric artery syndrome,
  from casts, 160
Superior pubic ramus, 241
Superior radial head dislocation, 32
Supernumerary, 95
Supernumerary digits, 307
Supero-, 389
Superoxide radical, 359
Supination, 335, 383
Supinator muscle, 235
Supinator syndrome, 77
Supine, 389
Suppan procedure, 344
Suppurative, 95
Suppurative arthritis, 68
Suppurative osteomyelitis, 45
Supra-, 389
Supracondylar cast, 158
Supracondylar cuff, 174, 175
Supracondylar fracture, 8, 10
  of femur, 4
  of humerus, 4
Supracondylar-suprapatellar cuff, 174
Suprapatellar plica, 86
Suprapatellar pouch, 253
Suprapatellar straps, 181
Suprascapular nerve, 230
Supraspinatus muscle, 229
Supraspinatus outlet view, 101
Sural nerve, 253
Surfer's knots, 36
Surgical approaches, 259–261
Surgical blocks, 259
Surgical boot, 187
Surgical corset, 184
Surgical incisions, 261
Surgical neck, 227
Surgical neck fracture, 8
Surgical procedures
  abbreviations, 375
  orthopaedic, 189–268

Surgical shoe, 187
Suspension, 163–164, 268
Suspensionplasty, 315
Sustenaculum tail, 327
Sutherland procedure, 246, 253, 257
Suture, 268
Swafford and Lichtman procedure, 233
Swallow-tail sign, 127
Swan-neck deformity, 302
Swan-neck revision, 321
Swanson arthroplasty, 315
Swanson prosthesis, 206, 315
Swedish knee cage, 178
Swimmer's view, 102
Swiss ball exercises, 352
Sym-, 389
Symbrachidactyly, 307
Syme amputation, 173, 264
Symmetric, 389
Symmetric fusion, 284
Sympathetic nervous system, 269
Symphalangism, 307
Symphysis pubis, 241
Syn-, 389
Synarthrosis, 68
Synchondrosis, 62
Synchondrotomy, 217
Syncope, 78, 95
Syndactylization, 344
Syndactyly, 307, 335
Syndesmectomy, 222
Syndesmopexy, 222
Syndesmoplasty, 222
Syndesmorrhaphy, 222
Syndesmosis, 221
Syndesmotomy, 222
Syndromes
    abbreviations, 371–371
    vs. diseases, 39
Synergy, 218
Synostosis, 13, 194, 307
Synovectomy, 322
Synovial cell sarcoma, 49
Synovial cyst, 68
Synovial fluid evaluation, 149
Synovial joint, 214
Synovial osteochondromatosis, 41, 68
Synovio-, 68
Synoviochondromatosis, 62, 69
Synovioma, 49

Synovitis, 69
    pigmented villonodular, 69
    villous, 69
Synovitis-acne-pustulosis-
    hyperostosis-osteomyelitiis
    syndrome, 45
Synovium, 213
Synthetic ligaments, 370
Syringomyelia, 78, 283
Systemic connectivitis, 72
Systemic lupus erythematosus, 73, 301
Systole, 224

T

T3, 145
T4, 145
T fracture, 8
Tabes dorsalis, 78
Taboparesis, 78
Tachdjian orthosis, 179
Tachdjian procedure, 254, 257
Tachycardia, 75
Tackler's arm, 36
Tailor's bunion, 335
TAL, 344
Talar fractures, 15, 16
Talar neck fracture, 19
Talar tilt test, 135
Talectomy, 344
Talipes, 335
Talipes calcaneocavus, 335
Talipes calcaneus, 335
Talipes calcanovarus, 335
Talipes cavovalgus, 335
Talipes cavovarus, 335
Talipes equinovalgus, 335
Talipes equinovarus, 335
Talipes planovalgus, 335
Talipes planus, 335
Talipomanus, 307
Talocalcaneal bar, 329
Talocrural angle, 107
Talofibular sprain, anterior, 33
Talus, 329
Talus lesions, osteochondral, 18
Tamai procedure, 257
Tamponade, 268
Tangential view, 102
TAR syndrome, 95, 307
Tardy, 95

Tardy ulnar palsy, 304
Tarsal bars, 332
Tarsal dislocation, 32
Tarsal pronator shoes, 188
Tarsometatarsal articulation, frac-
    tures-dislocations, 25–26
Tartrate-resistant acid phosphatase, 146
Taylor, Townsend, and Corlett proce-
    dure, 246
Taylor orthosis, 185
Taylor procedure, 258
T&C, 149
Teardrop, radiographic, 109
Teardrop fracture, 9
Technetium scan, 116
Technetium-99m, 116
Telangiectatic osteosarcoma, 47
Teleroentgenography, 100
Telfa dressing, 162
TEM, 359–360
Temporary prosthesis, 176
Temporomandibular joint syndrome, 279
Tendinoplasty, 221
Tendinosuture, 221
Tendo-, 65
Tendocalcaneus, 221, 329
Tendolysis, 221, 318
Tendon, diseases, 65–66
Tendon Achilles lengthening, 344
Tendon advancement, 318
Tendon injury, 13–14
Tendon reflex examination, 353
Tendon reflexes, 138
Tendon release, 221
Tendon transfer, 319–320
Tendonitis, 65
Tendonitis ossificans traumatica, 65
Tendons, 221
    surgical procedures, 221
Tendoplasty, 221
Tendotomy, 221
Tenectomy, 221
Tennis elbow, 37
    reverse, 35, 312
Tennis leg, 37
Tennis toe, 37
Teno-, 65, 221
Tenodesis, 221, 318
Tenodesis orthosis, 182
Tenodesis test, 130

Tenodynia, 65
Tenolysis, 221
Tenomyoplasty, 221
Tenomyotomy, 221
Tenonectomy, 221
Tenonitis, 65
Tenontagra, 65
Tenontitis, 65
Tenontodynia, 65
Tenontomyoplasty, 221
Tenontomyotomy, 221
Tenontophyma, 65
Tenontoplasty, 221
Tenontothecitis, 65
Tenoperiostitis, 65
Tenophyte, 65
Tenoplasty, 221
Tenorrhaphy, 221, 318
Tenositis, 65
Tenostosis, 65
Tenosuture, 221
Tenosynovectomy, 221, 320
Tenosynovitis, 66, 313
Tenotomy, 221
Tenovaginotomy, 319
TENS, 349
Tensilon test, 138
Tension, 368
Tensor fascia lata, 222
Tensor fascia lata muscle, 243
Tenth cranial nerve, 272
Teres major/minor muscle, 229
Terminal, 389
Terminal devices, 172–173
Terminology, etymology of, 390–403
Terri-Thomas sign, 130
Tests, orthopaedic, 119–123
Tetany, 95
Tethered patellar tendon syndrome, 86
Tetraplegia, 308
Texas Scottish Rite Hospital instrumentation, 288
Thalassemia, 83
Thenar eminence, 298
Thenar flap, 318
Thenar muscles, 294–295
Thenar space, 298
Therapeutic adaptations, 356
Therapeutic exercise, 348
Therapeutic massage, 352
Thermography, 116
Thermoplastic orthosis, 178, 179

Thermoplastic/metal orthosis, 180
Thermoplastics, 356
Thiemann disease, 41, 50, 57
Thigh atrophy, 86
Thomas, Thompson, and Straub procedure, 246
Thomas heel, 187
Thomas procedure, 344
Thomas sign, 132, 138
Thomas splint, 163
Thomas test, 132
Thompson and Epstein fracture classification system, 28
Thompson and Henry approach, 259
Thompson nail, 204
Thompson quadricepsplasty, 256
Thompson telescoping V osteotomy, 195
Thompson test, 132
Thomsen disease, 59
Thoracic curve, 279
Thoracic orthoses, 184
Thoracic outlet syndrome, 279–280, 304
Thoracic region, radiographic views, 102
Thoracic spine
  anatomy of, 270, 273
  radiographic views, 102
Thoracodorsal nerve, 230
Thoracolumbar curve, 279
Thoracolumbosacral orthoses, 184–185
Thorax, 273
Thornton nail, 204
THR, 207–208
Three-finger spica, 157
Three-phase bone scan, 114
Thromboangiitis obliterans, 309
Thrombocytopenia, absent radius syndrome, 307
Thrombolytic therapy, 227
Thrombophlebitis, 70
Thrombosis, 70
Thrower's elbow, 35
Thumb abduction, 320
Thumb abductors, 294
Thumb adduction, 320
Thumb adductors, 294
Thumb extensors, 294
Thumb interphalangeal extension assist, 182

Thumb IP extension assist, 182
Thumb post, 182
Thumb spica, 158
Thumbnail test, 134
Thumb-to-forearm test, 139
Thurston-Holland sign, 110
Thyroid cartilage, 272
Thyroid gland, 273
Thyroid-stimulating hormone, 145
Thyroxine, 145
TIA, 72
Tibia, 247
  fractures, 10, 21, 29
    distal, 16, 23
    intercondylar eminence, 23
    pilon, 26
    plateau, 10, 20, 27
    proximal, 27
    tuberosity, 24–25, 29
  osteotomies, 257
  radiographic view, 105
  radiographic views, 102
  surgery of, 253–254
Tibia vara, 55
Tibial bolt, 204
Tibial dysplasia, 88
Tibial gaiter, 158, 159
Tibial plateau, 247
Tibialis anterior, 249, 329
Tibialis posterior, 249, 329
Tibialis sign, 138
Tibiofibular cyst, 68
Tibiofibular ligament, 250
Tibiofibular sprain, 34
Tic, 78
Tic douloureux, 78
Tieman-Jewett nail, 204
Tietze syndrome, 57
Tikhoff-Linberg procedure, 233
Tile fracture classification system, 28
Tillaux Kleiger fracture, 11
Tine test, 149
Tinea pedis, 331
Tinel sign, 138
Tissue inhibitor of metalloproteinase, 359
TLSO, 184–185
TMJ, 279
Toddler fracture, 10
Toe nail, 330
Toe sign, 136
Toe spica, 159

Toe spread sign, 135
Toes, radiographic views, 102
Toggle, 204
Tohen procedure, 344
Toilet hygiene, 355
-tome, 268
Tomography, 100
Tongue fracture, 11
Tönnis system for hip dysplasia,
    113–114
Tonus, 95
Too many toes sign, 135
Tophus, 302
Torn meniscus, 84
Torode and Zieg fracture classifica-
    tion system, 29
Toronto orthosis, 179
Torque, 368
Torque heels, 188
Torr, 368
Torsion, 369
Torsion fracture, 6
Torsion unit, 176
Torsional rigidity, 369
Torticollis, 95–96
Tortus fracture, 6
Torus fracture, 5
Total bilirubin, 143
Total contact, 176
Total hip arthroplasty, 243–244
    outcome evaluation, 140
Total hip replacement, 207–208
    bipolar, 208
    cementless, 210
Total serum protein, 143
Total wrist arthrodesis, 314
Toughness, 369
Tourniquet, 268
Tourniquet test, 132
Toxic, 96, 268
Trabecula, 193
Trabecular pattern, 193
Trachea, 273
Traction bow, 166
Traction devices, 155–156, 164–166
Traction epiphyses, 41, 192
Traction spur, 280
Trans-, 389
Transacromial approach, 260
Transcondylar fracture, 4
Transcutaneous electrical nerve
    stimulation, 349

Transect, 268
Transfemoral amputation, 174
Transfemoral suspension, 175–176
Transforming growth factor super-
    family, 361
Transfusion, 268
Transient ischemic attack, 72
Transient osteopenia, 55
Transitional vertebra, 280
Translucent, 98
Transluminal angioplasty, 225
Transmetatarsal amputation, 344
Transmission electron microscopy,
    359–360
Transplant, 197
Transposition, 268
Transscaphoid perilunate dislocation,
    310
Transthoracic lateral view, 102
Transtibial amputation, 173–174
Transudate, 96
Transverse, 389
Transverse carpal ligament, 296
Transverse fracture, 6
Transverse humeral ligament, 229
Transverse plane, 382
Transverse process, 271
TRAP, 146
Trapezial hemiarthroplasty, 315
Trapeziometacarpal arthritis, 302
Trapeziometacarpal fusion, 313
Trapezium, 292
Trapezius muscle, 229
Trauma, 96
    emergency stabilization in, 166–
    167
Trauma view, 102
Traumatic dislocation, 31
Traumatic neuroma, 77
Tremor, 78
Trendelenburg sign, 132
Trendelenburg test, 132
Triad knee repair, 255
Triangles, 273
Triangular ligament, 296
Triceps muscles, 235
Triceps reflex, 138
Triceps surae, 249
Triceps surae muscles, 249
Tricompartmental knee replacement,
    212
Trident hand, 307

Trigger finger, 312
    acquired, 308
    release, 320
Trigger points, 60
Triiodothyronine, 145
Trilateral orthosis, 179
Trillat procedure, 233
Triphalangeal thumb, 307
Triplane fracture, 11
Triple arthrodesis, 344
Triplicate thumb, 308
-tripsy, 268
Triradiate cartilage, 242
Triscaphe arthrodesis, 314
Trochanteric fractures, 21
Trochanteric slide, 246
Trochanterplasty, 246
Trochlea, 234, 247
Tronzo fracture classification system,
    29
Tronzo nail, 204
True ankylosis, 69
True lateral view, 102
True-Flex nail, 204
Trumble arthrodesis, 216
T&S, 149
Tscherne fracture classification
    system, 29
TSH, 145
Tsuge technique, 319
Tsuli procedure, 289
Tubercle, 193
Tubercle of Tillaux-Chaput, 247
Tubercles, 292
Tuberosity, 193
Tuck sign, 130
Tuft, 292
Tuft fracture, 4
Tumefaction, 96
Tumor, 96
    treatment of, 262
Tumor capsule, 47
Tumor pseudo-capsule, 47
Tumoral calcinosis, 83
Tunnel view, 102
Tupper arthroplasty, 315
Turco procedure, 344
Turf-toe, 37
Turgid, 96
Turnbuckle, 182
Turnbuckle cast, 157
Turner syndrome, 83

Turret exostosis, 310
Turtle-back nail, 312
Turyn sign, 125
T1–weighted image, 115, 116
T2–weighted image, 115, 116
Twelfth cranial nerve, 272
Two-point discrimination, 130, 353, 354
Two-poster orthosis, 186
  with thoracic extension, 186
  with waist extension, 186
Tyloma, 331
Type and cross-match, 149
Type and screen, 149
Typical bacterial species reports, 147–148

U

UA, 143
UCB orthosis, 178
UHMWPE, 370
Ulcer, 96
Ullman line, 109
Ulna
  anatomy of, 235
  radiographic views, 102
Ulnar artery, 237, 300
Ulnar bursa, 298
Ulnar collateral ligament, 238, 297
Ulnar deficiency, 308
Ulnar deviation, 383
Ulnar dimelia, 307
Ulnar drift, 302
Ulnar fractures, 15
  distal, 18
Ulnar nerve, 230, 300
Ulnar neuropathy, 303
Ulnar tunnel syndrome, 304
Ulnar variance, 308
Ultimate load, 369
Ultra, 389
Ultrahigh molecular-weight poly-
  ethylene, 370
Ultrasonography, 97, 116
Ultrasound, 97, 116, 350
Unciform fracture, 9
Uncommitted metaphyseal lesion, 55
Unconstrained knee replacement, 212
Uncovertebral joints, 272
Underarm orthosis, 185
Unguis, 299

Unguis incarnatus, 312, 333
Unicameral bone cyst, 55
Unicompartmental knee replacement, 212
Unilateral, 389
Unilateral facet subluxation, 32
Union of fractures, 12–13
Univalve cast, 159
Universal gutter splint, 161
Universal hand dressing, 163
Unna boot, 158
Upper extremities
  amputation levels, 262–264
  casts for, 157–158
  congenital anomalies of, 305–308
  fractures, 8
  orthoses for, 181–184
  prostheses for, 170–173, 206–207
  radiographic views, 102
  tests, signs, and maneuvers for, 127
Upper motor neuron disease, 76
Upper obstetrical palsy, 78
Upper subscapular nerve, 230
Uppsala screw, 204
Upright, 181
Uprights, 187
Ureters, radiography, 99
Uric acid, 143
Urinalysis, 143
Urine chemical tests, 147
Urine tests
  abbreviations, 153
  for metabolic disease, 145–147

V

Vagus nerve, 272
Vainio metaphalangeal arthroplasty, 315
Valgus, 386
Valgus corrective ankle straps, 181
Valgus knee control pads, 181
Valpar component work sample series, 355
Valpius-Compere procedure, 344
Valsalva maneuver, 125
Van Gorder approach, 260
Van Neck disease, 57
Van Ness procedure, 258
Vanishing bone disease, 42
Vanzetti sign, 125
Varices, 70

Varicose veins, 70
Varus, 386
Varus corrective ankle straps, 181
Varus knee control pads, 181
Vascular, 224
Vascular diagnostic studies, 117–118
Vascular diseases and conditions, 69–75
Vascular system, 222–227
  surgical procedures, 224–227
Vasoconstriction, 74
Vasodilatation, 74
Vasospastic, 74
Vastus medialis advancement, 255
VATER association, 96
VATER syndrome, 308
Vater-Pacini corpuscle, 301
VCA, 105
VDDR, 80
VDRR, 80
Vector, 369
Vein, 224
Velcro splint, 161
Velcanu, Rosianu, and Ionescu proce-
  dure, 246
Velpeau dressing, 163
Venable screw, 204
Venogram, 117
Venous disorders, 70
Venous insufficiency, 70
Venous reflux, 70
Ventral, 389
Ventral inclination angle, 105
Verdan procedure, 321
Verdan technique, 319
Vermont instrument, 288
Verruca vulgaris, 313, 334
Vertebra plana fracture, 9
Vertebrae, 270
Vertebral artery, 272
Vertebral body, 271
Vertex, 389
Vertical, 389
Vertical side to side planes, 381–382
Vertical talus, 335
Vertigo, 78
Veseley-Street nail, 204
Vestigial, 96
Vest-over-pants closure, 268
Viable, 268
Vibration white finger syndrome, 304–305

Vibrator sense examination, 353
Videofluoroscopy, 114
Villous lipomatous proliferation, 68
Villous synovitis, 69
Vincula longa and breva, 296
Vinculae, 301
Vinke tongs, 166
Virgin screw, 204
Viscoelastic stability, 369
Viscoelasticity, 364, 369
Viscosity, 369
Vital signs, 154
Vitamin D, 361
Vitamin D-dependent rickets, 80
Vitamin D-resistant rickets, 80
Volar, 389
Volar Barton fracture, 9
Volar capsular reefing, 321
Volar carpal ligament, 296
Volar flexes intercalated segment
    instability, 310
Volar ligament, 297
Volar plate, 293
Volar splint, 161
Volkmann canals, 192, 193
Volkmann contracture, 72, 309
Volkmann deformity, 57
Volkmann fracture, 11–12
Volkmann ischemic contracture, 57
Volkmann's triangle, 11–12
Volume, annotation of units, 153
Volumeter set, 355
Volz prosthesis, 207
von Bahr screw, 204
von Recklinghausen disease, 57, 79
von Rosen view, 102
VonFrey hair test, 355
Voorhoeve disease, 43, 57
V-Y plasty, 344

W

Wafer procedure, 322
Wagner disease, 50, 57
Wagner procedure, 254, 258
Wagon wheel fracture, 10
Wagstaffe fracture, 12
Waist belt, 175
Waist belts, 172
Waldenström disease, 57
Waldenström sign, 110
Waldenström staging system in Legg-
    Calvé-Perthes disease, 114

Walker, 160
Walkers, 161
Walking heel, 160
Walther fracture, 10
Ward, Thompson, and Vandergriend
    procedure, 247
Ward triangle, 107
Warner-Farber procedure, 344
Wartenberg sign, 130
Wartenberg syndrome, 303
Watch crystal nail, 312
Watson Jones nail, 204
Watson test, 129–130, 130
Watson-Cheyne procedure, 345
Watson-Jones arthrodesis, 216
Watson-Jones fracture classification
    system, 29
Watson-Jones frame, 166
Watson-Jones procedure, 233, 345
WBC, 142
WD, 170
Wear, 369
Weaver and Dunn procedure, 233
Weaver's bottom, 55
Web ligament, 298
Web space, 299, 330
Webb procedure, 246
Weber, Brunner, and Freuler proce-
    dure, 246
Weber fracture classification system,
    29
Weber osteotomy, 195, 233
Weber procedure, 258, 339
Weber-Vasey procedure, 240
Webril, 156
Wedge, 159
Wedge fracture, 9
Wedging, 280
Weight, 369
    annotation of units, 153
Weight and height, 154
Weight-bearing joint, 214
Weight-lifter's shoulder, 37
Weiland procedure, 258
Weiss sign, 138
Weiss spring, 204
Well-leg cast, 159
Well-leg traction, 166
Wellmerling maneuver, 132
Werdnig-Hoffmann disease, 59
Wertheim Bohlman fusion, 287
WEST, 355
West and Soto-Hall procedure, 256

West Point view, 102
Westin procedure, 345
Wet leather sign, 130
Wet reading, 98–99
Wet-to-dry dressing, 162
Whiplash, 37
Whistling face syndrome, 308
White arthrodesis, 216
White blood count, 142
White procedure, 254
White slide procedure, 345
Whitecloud and Larocca fusion, 287
Whiteman talectomy procedure, 345
Whitman frame, 166
Whitman maneuver, 132
Whitman osteotomy, 195
Whitman plate, 187
Whitman procedure, 233
Whitman-Thompson procedure, 345
Wickstrom arthrodesis, 314
Williams exercises, 352
Williams nail, 204
Williams orthosis, 184
Williams rod, 204
Willow fracture, 4
Wilmington jacket, 185
Wilson and Jacob procedure, 345
Wilson and Jacobs procedure, 258
Wilson and McKeever procedure, 233
Wilson approach, 260
Wilson fracture, 9
Wilson plate, 204
Wilson procedure, 216, 339, 345
Wilson procedure, 240
Wilson test, 134
Wiltse plate, 288
Wiltse procedure, 289
Winberger line, 109
Windblown hand, 308
Window, 159
Windshield wiper sign, 110
Windswept hips, 83
Winged scapula, 82
Wingfield frame, 244
Winograd procedure, 345
Winquist-Hansen fracture classifica-
    tion system, 30
Winter procedure, 289
Wire frame collar, 186
Wirth Jager procedure, 255
Wisconsin interspinous segmental
    spinal instrument, 288
Wolf blade plate, 216

Wolf procedure, 345
Wolff's law, 361
Woodward procedure, 233
Work, 369
Work evaluation systems technology, 355
World Health Organization tumor classification system, 45
Wormian bone, 193
Wounds, 96
Woven bone, 193
Wraparound splint, 161
Wright maneuver, 123
Wrisberg-ligament type discoid meniscus, 85
Wrist
  anatomy of, 291–301
  arthrodeses of, 313–314
  bones of, 291–292
  congenital anomalies of, 305–308
  congenital deformity repairs, 317
  disarticulation, 170
  dislocations, 310
  drop, 303
  extension, 320
  extensors, 293
  flexion unit, 173
  flexors, 293
  fractures, 8–9
  joints of, 293
  ligaments of, 295–297
  microvascular procedures, 317
  muscle disorders of, 308–309
  muscles of, 293–295
  neurologic procedures, 316
  neuropathies of, 302–305
  radiographic views, 102
  subluxation, 33
  surgery of, 313–322
  surgical approach to, 322
  tendon disorders of, 308–309
  trauma procedures for, 316–317
  traumatic disorders of, 309–310
  units, 173
  vascular disorders of, 309
Wrist-driven lateral prehension orthosis, 182
Wrist-hand orthoses, 181–182
Wryneck, 96
Wu procedure, 345
Wu sole opposition test, 135

X

Xanthoma, malignant fibrous, 64
Xenogeneic, 197
Xenograft, 197
Xeroform dressing, 162
Xiphoid, 273
X-ray, 98, 99

Y

Y and T fracture, 10
Y fracture, 8
Y scapular view, 102
Yee approach, 259–260
Yellow cartilage, 217
Yergason test, 127
Yield stress, 369
Y-line, 109
Y-osteotomy, 195
Young fracture classification system, 30
Young procedure, 345
Yount procedure, 255

Z

Zachary sensory grade, 137
Zadik procedure, 345
Zancholli capsuloplasty, 315
Zancholli static-lock procedure, 315
Zancholli-Lasso procedure, 315
Zancolli procedure, 240, 321
Zaricznyj procedure, 255
Zarins and Rowe procedure, 255
Zcir procedure, 233
Zeta potential, 362
Zickle fracture classification system, 30
Zickle nail, 204
Zielke instrumentation, 288
Z-plasty, 345
Zuelzer hook plate, 204
Zygoapophyseal joint, 271